Hilar Cholangiocarcinoma

W.Y. Lau
Editor

Hilar Cholangiocarcinoma

人民卫生出版社
PMPH PEOPLE'S MEDICAL PUBLISHING HOUSE

Springer

Editor
W.Y. Lau, MD(CUHK), DSc(CUHK), FRCS,
FACS, FRACS(Hon)
Faculty of Medicine
The Chinese University of Hong Kong, Shatin
New Territories
Hong Kong

ISBN 978-94-007-6472-9 ISBN 978-94-007-6473-6 (eBook)
DOI 10.1007/978-94-007-6473-6
Springer Dordrecht Heidelberg New York London

Library of Congress Control Number: 2013936396

Jointly published with People's Medical Publishing House
ISBN: 978-7-117-16154-1, People's Medical Publishing House

Printed on acid-free paper

Springer is part of Springer Science+Business Media (www.springer.com)

The enormous effort that I have to put into this book could not have been possible without the unfailing support from my wife Corinna. It is with great admiration, respect and love that I dedicate this book to this wonderful lady—she is truly the "wind beneath my wings".

W.Y. Lau

Preface

Hilar cholangiocarcinoma remains one of the tumours which is difficult to treat. It is situated in a region where the anatomy is complicated. Its proximity to the major vascular structures at the hilus of the liver makes resectional surgery technically challenging. It is relatively resistant to chemotherapy and radiotherapy, thus making resectional surgery the mainstay of curative treatment.

Recent advances in the management of hilar cholangiocarcinoma have progressed rapidly, and the paradigms for its treatment have changed in a major way during the past two to three decades. Not too long ago the treatment only aimed at palliation by establishing drainage of the obstructed biliary system to relieve symptoms and to prolong life. The treatment has since evolved from non-operative to operative treatment, and from conservative to radical resectional surgery. All these changes have been brought about not only by safer liver surgery, but also by changes in management which now encompasses a multidisciplinary approach. What was previously considered unresectable and incurable has become resectable and curable.

This is a multi-author book on hilar cholangiocarcinoma, written by an international team of world-renowned expects covering topics in their respective areas of expertise. There are altogether 71 authors from 14 countries/regions, mainly Argentina, Australia, China (including mainland China and Hong Kong), France, Germany, Italy, Japan, Korea, Malaysia, Thailand, the Netherlands, the United Kingdom and the United States of America. The translation of this book into Chinese for the Chinese edition was carried out by a team of experts coming from the Eastern Hepatobiliary Surgery Hospital led by Prof. Wu Meng-chao and Prof. Shen Feng.

The book aims to provide a fully current, complete reference text that is as succinct as possible, but as comprehensive as necessary. It covers all topics in hilar cholangiocarcinoma. It provides the most updated knowledge in the rapidly advancing field of hilar cholangiocarcinoma. There might be some overlap in some areas but this is unavoidable, as controversial areas are discussed by highly regarded authorities who look at the problem from different perspectives. There is a good list of references at the end of each chapter. The extensive use of diagrams, figures and tables make the text easy to read.

The intended readers of this book are clinicians and researchers who are interested in hilar cholangiocarcinoma, including liver surgeons, hepatologists, interventional and diagnostic radiologists and basic researchers. General physicians, general surgeons, trainees, epidemiologists, hospital administrators, pathologists and instrument manufacturers will also find this book useful as a reference. The English and the Chinese editions of this book will be published at the same time by the same publisher.

Shatin, New Territories, Hong Kong W.Y. Lau

We are sad to report the death of Professor Anthony S.-Y. Leong, who passed away in June 2011. Our heartfelt condolences to his family.

Acknowledgements

I owe my deepest gratitude to many people who helped and supported me during the editing of this book. This book would not have been successful without the contributions of the authors from different parts of the world who have helped to bring together this volume of updated information on this important subject of hilar cholangiocarcinoma. I am honored and thankful that so many of my friends who are renowned experts in their respective fields agreed to take time out of their busy schedules and personal lives to organize their thoughts and to share their experience with us. In fact, the list of contributors reads like a "who's who" in the field of hilar cholangiocarcinoma.

For the production side at the People's Medical Publishing House, I am grateful to President Hu Guo-chen, Du Xian and Ji Fang who believed that a comprehensive book on hilar cholangiocarcinoma was needed. I appreciate the dedication and professionalism of the production team to this project.

I am indebted to Prof. Shen Feng and his team who translated this book into Chinese. The English and the Chinese editions will be published at the same time.

Last but not least I am grateful to my secretary Ms. Helena Lee for her support in compiling this book.

Shatin, New Territories, Hong Kong W.Y. Lau

Contents

1 Anatomy of the Hepatic Hilum ... 1
W.Y. Lau, S.H.Y. Lau, and E.C.H. Lai

2 Epidemiology ... 17
G.L. Tyson, S. Keihanian, and H.B. El-Serag

3 Pathology ... 25
A.S.-Y. Leong and C. Pairojkul

4 Staging Systems ... 43
F.G. Rocha and W.R. Jarnagin

5 Preoperative Imaging ... 53
B.I. Choi and J.M. Lee

6 Role of 3D Reconstructive Imaging ... 65
I. Endo, R. Matsuyama, K. Tanaka, N. Wendt, A. Schenk, and H.O. Peitgen

7 Assessment of Liver Function ... 75
D.V. Mann

8 Diagnosis ... 91
X.Y. Yin

9 Differential Diagnosis ... 99
W. Kassahun, P. Stumpp, A. Hoffmeister, and S. Jonas

10 Molecular Markers of Cholangiocarcinoma ... 111
J.Y.H. Chan, K.K.H. Lee, and Y.L. Chui

11 Laparoscopy and Laparoscopic Ultrasound ... 127
N.J. Peel and O.J. Garden

12 Preoperative Optimization of the Liver for Resection ... 133
J. Belghiti and D. Fuks

13 Preoperative Biliary Drainage ... 139
A.T. Ruys, E.A. Rauws, O.R.C. Busch, J.S. Lameris, D.J. Gouma, and T.M. van Gulik

14 Portal Vein Embolization ... 147
T. Hashimoto and M. Makuuchi

15 Anesthesia for Patients with Hilar Chlolangiocarcinoma ... 155
S.S. Ho and M.T.V. Chan

16 Selection of Patients for Liver Resection and Liver Transplantation ... 167
J.J. Schwartz, J. Sorensen, and R. Kim

17 History of Surgery in Hilar Cholangiocarcinoma 187
S.H.Y. Lau and W.Y. Lau

18 Radical Resection and Its Limits 195
T. Sano and Y. Nimura

19 Central Lobectomy 211
Z.Y. Huang and X.P. Chen

20 Extended Resections 223
D. Seehofer and P. Neuhaus

21 Combined Liver Resection and Portal Vein Resection 237
K. Mekeel and A.W. Hemming

22 The Hepatic Artery Reconstruction First Approach in Hilar Cholangiocarcinoma Type IIIb 247
E. de Santibañes, V. Ardiles, and F.A. Alvarez

23 Local Resection Without Hepatectomy 253
L. Capussotti and L. Viganò

24 Ex Situ Ex Vivo Resection and Autotransplantation 263
A.K.K. Chui

25 Liver Transplantation 275
J.C. Hong and R.W. Busuttil

26 Neoadjuvant/Adjuvant Therapy for Liver Resection and Transplantation 281
B.K.P. Goh and C.B. Rosen

27 Palliative Surgical Treatment 291
E.C.H. Lai, S.H.Y. Lau, and W.Y. Lau

28 Palliation by Endoscopic Approach 297
J. Toouli and S.G. Barreto

29 Percutaneous Palliation of Cholangiocarcinoma 303
P.D. Peng, J.F.H. Geschwind, and M.A. Choti

30 Photodynamic Therapy 309
M.A. Ortner and C. Jost

31 Radiation and Chemotherapy 317
H.A. Pitt and A. Nakeeb

Index 323

Contributors

V. Ardiles, MD General Surgery Service, Hospital Italiano de Buenos Aires, Buenos Aires, Argentina

F.A. Alvarez, MD General Surgery Service, Hospital Italiano de Buenos Aires, Buenos Aires, Argentina

S.G. Barreto, MBBS, MS, PhD Department of Surgery, Flinders University, Adelaide, SA, Australia

J. Belghiti, MD Department of Surgery, Hospital Beaujon, Clichy, France

O.R.C. Busch, MD, PhD Department of Surgery, Academic Medical Center, University of Amsterdam, Amsterdam, the Netherlands

R.W. Busuttil, MD, PhD, FACS Department of Surgery, David Geffen School of Medicine, Dumont-UCLA Transplant and Liver Cancer Centers, University of California, Los Angeles, CA, USA

L. Capussotti, MD Department of HPB and Digestive Surgery, Ospedale Mauriziano "Umberto I", Largo Turati, Torino, Italy

J.Y.H. Chan, PhD Joint JNU-CUHK Key Laboratories of Regenerative Medicine, Ministry of Education, Jinan University, Guangzhou, China

M.T.V. Chan, MBBS, FANZCA, FHKCA, FHKAM Department of Anesthesia & Intensive Care, The Chinese University of Hong Kong, Shatin, New Territories, Hong Kong

X.P. Chen, MD Hepatic Surgery Center, Tongji Hospital, Tongji Medical College, Huazhong University of Science and Technology, Wuhan, China

B.I. Choi, MD Department of Radiology, Seoul National University Hospital, Seoul, South Korea

M.A. Choti, MD, FRCS Departments of Surgery, Johns Hopkins University School of Medicine, John Hopkins Hospital, Baltimore, MD, USA

Y.L. Chui, PhD Department of Chemical Pathology, The Chinese University of Hong Kong, Shatin, New Territories, Hong Kong

A.K.K. Chui, MBBS(NSW), FRCS(Ed), FRACS, FCSHK, FHKAM(Surg), MD(UNSW) Central, Hong Kong

H.B. El-Serag, MD, MPH Gastroenterology and Hepatology Section, Houston AV Medical Center and Baylor College of Medicine, Houston, TX, USA

I. Endo, MD Department of Gastroenterological Surgery, Graduate School of Medicine, Yokohama City University, Yokohama, Japan

D. Fuks, MD Department of Digestive Surgery, Hospital Beaujon, Clichy, France

O.J. Garden, BSc, MBChB, MD, FRCS(Glasg), FRCS(Ed), FRCP(Ed), FRACS(Hon), FRCSC(Hon) Clinical and Surgical Sciences (Surgery), University of Edinburgh, Royal Infirmary of Edinburgh, Edinburgh, UK

J.F.H. Geschwind, MD Department of Radiology, Johns Hopkins University School of Medicine, John Hopkins Hospital, Baltimore, MD, USA

B.K.P. Goh, MBBS, MMed, MSc, FRCS(Ed) Department of Surgery, Singapore General Hospital, Singapore, Singapore

D.J. Gouma, MD, PhD Department of Surgery, Academic Medical Center, University of Amsterdam, Amsterdam, the Netherlands

T. Hashimoto, MD, PhD Department of Hepato-Biliary-Pancreatic Surgery, Japanese Red Cross Medical Center, Tokyo, Japan

A.W. Hemming, MD, FRCS, FACS Division of Transplantation and Hepatobiliary Surgery, University of California San Diego, San Diego, CA, USA

S.S. Ho, MBBS, MRCP, FANZCA, FHKCA, FHKAM Department of Anesthesia & Intensive Care, The Chinese University of Hong Kong, Shatin, New Territories, Hong Kong

A. Hoffmeister, MD Faculty of Medicine, Department of Gastroenterology and Rheumatology, University of Leipzig, Leipzig, Germany

J.C. Hong, MD, FACS Division of Liver and Pancreas Transplantation, Department of Surgery, The Pfleger Liver Institute, Ronald Reagan-UCLA Medical Center, Los Angeles, CA, USA

Department of Surgery, David Geffen School of Medicine, Dumont-UCLA Transplant and Liver Cancer Centers, University of California, Los Angeles, CA, USA

Z.Y. Huang, MD Hepatic Surgery Center, Tongji Hospital, Tongji Medical College, Huazhong University of Science and Technology, Wuhan, China

W.R. Jarnagin, MD Hepatopancreatobiliary Service, Department of Surgery, Memorial Sloan-Kettering Cancer Center, New York, NY, USA

S. Jonas, MD Faculty of Medicine, Department of Abdominal, Transplantation, Thoracic and Vascular Surgery, University of Leipzig, Leipzig, Germany

C. Jost, MD Department of Gastroenterology, University Hospital Bern, Bern, Switzerland

W. Kassahun, MD Faculty of Medicine, Department of Abdominal, Transplantation, Thoracic and Vascular Surgery, University of Leipzig, Leipzig, Germany

S. Keihanian, MD Section of Gastroenterology & Hepatology, Michael E. DeBakey Veterans Affairs Medical Center, Baylor College of Medicine, Houston, TX, USA

R. Kim, MD Department of Surgery, University of Utah, Salt Lake City, UT, USA

E.C.H. Lai, MBChB(CUHK), MRCS(Ed), FRACS, FCSHK, FHKAM(Surgery) Department of Surgery, Pamela Youde Nethersole Eastern Hospital, Chai Wan, Hong Kong

Department of Surgery, The Chinese University of Hong Kong, Shatin, New Territories, Hong Kong

J.S. Lameris, MD, PhD Department of Radiology, Academic Medical Center, University of Amsterdam, Amsterdam, the Netherlands

W.Y. Lau, MD(CUHK), DSc(CUHK), FRCS, FACS, FRACS(Hon) Faculty of Medicine, The Chinese University of Hong Kong, Shatin, New Territories, Hong Kong

S.H.Y. Lau, MBChB(CUHK), MRCS(Ed) Department of Surgery, Queen Elizabeth Hospital, Kowloon, Hong Kong

J.M. Lee, MD Department of Radiology, Seoul National University Hospital, Seoul, South Korea

K.K.H. Lee, PhD Stem Cell and Regeneration Thematic Research Program, School of Biomedical Sciences, The Chinese University of Hong Kong, Shatin, New Territories, Hong Kong

A.S.-Y. Leong, MB, BS, MD, FRCPA, FRC(Path), FCAP, FASCP, FHKAM(Pathol), Honorary FHKC(Path), Honorary FRCPT Pathology Laboratories, Sunway Medical Center, Monash University/Malaysian Campus, Bandar Sunway, Malaysia

M. Makuuchi, MD, PhD Department of Hepato-Biliary-Pancreatic Surgery, Japanese Red Cross Medical Center, Tokyo, Japan

D.V. Mann, MS, FRCS Wanchai, Hong Kong

R. Matsuyama, MD Department of Gastroenterological Surgery, Graduate School of Medicine, Yokohama City University, Yokohama, Japan

K. Mekeel, MD, FACS Division of Transplantation and Hepatobiliary Surgery, University of California San Diego, San Diego, CA, USA

A. Nakeeb, MD Department of Surgery, Indiana University, Indianapolis, IN, USA

P. Neuhaus, MD, PhD Department of General-, Visceral- and Transplantation-Surgery, Charité -Universitätsmedizin Berlin, Berlin, Germany

Y. Nimura, MD Division of Gastroenterological Surgery, Aichi Cancer Center Hospital, Nagoya, Japan

M.A. Ortner, MD Department of Gastroenterology, University Hospital Zuerich, Zuerich, Switzerland

C. Pairojkul, MD, Dip BAP(T) Pathology Department, Faculty of Medicine, KhonKaen University, Khon Kaen, Thailand

N.J. Peel, MBChB, BSc, MRCS(Glas) Clinical Research Fellow, University of Edinburgh, Royal Infirmary of Edinburgh, Edinburgh, UK

H.O. Peitgen, MD Department of Gastroenterological Surgery, Graduate School of Medicine, Yokohama City University, Yokohama, Japan

P.D. Peng, MD Department of Surgery, Johns Hopkins University School of Medicine, John Hopkins Hospital, Baltimore, MD, USA

H.A. Pitt, MD Temple University Health System, Philadelphia, PA

E.A. Rauws, MD, PhD Department of Gastroenterology and Hepatology, Academic Medical Center, University of Amsterdam, Amsterdam, The Netherlands

F.G. Rocha, MD Department of Surgery, Memorial Sloan-Kettering Cancer Center, New York, NY, USA

C.B. Rosen, MD Division of Transplantation Surgery, Mayo Clinic and Mayo Clinic College of Medicine, Rochester, MN, USA

A.T. Ruys, MD Department of Surgery, Academic Medical Center, University of Amsterdam, Amsterdam, The Netherlands

T. Sano, MD Division of Hepato-Biliary and Pancreatic Surgery, Aichi Cancer Center Hospital, Nagoya, Japan

E. de Santibañes, MD, PhD General Surgery Service, Hospital Italiano de Buenos Aires, Buenos Aires, Argentina

A. Schenk, MD Department of Gastroenterological Surgery, Yokohama City University, Yokohama, Japan

J.J. Schwartz, MD Department of Gastroenterological Surgery, Graduate School of Medicine, Yokohama City University, Yokohama, Japan

D. Seehofer, MD, PhD Department of General-, Visceral- and Transplantation-Surgery, Charité -Universitätsmedizin Berlin, Berlin, Germany

J. Sorensen, MD Department of Surgery, University of Utah, Salt Lake City, UT, USA

P. Stumpp, MD Faculty of Medicine, Department of Radiology, University of Leipzig, Leipzig, Germany

K. Tanaka, MD Department of Gastroenterological Surgery, Graduate School of Medicine, Yokohama City University, Yokohama, Japan

J. Toouli, MBBS, PhD, FRACS Department of Surgery, Flinders University, Adelaide, SA, Australia

G.L. Tyson, MD Section of Gastroenterology and Hepatology, Baylor College of Medicine, Houston, TX, USA

T.M. van Gulik, MD, PhD Department of Surgery, Academic Medical Center, University of Amsterdam, Amsterdam, the Netherlands

L. Viganò, MD Department of HPB and Digestive Surgery, Ospedale Mauriziano "Umberto I", Torino, Italy

N. Wendt, MD Department of Gastroenterological Surgery, Graduate School of Medicine, Yokohama City University, Yokohama, Japan

X.Y. Yin, MD, PhD Department of Hepatobiliary Surgery, First Affiliated Hospital, Sun Yat-Sen University, Guangzhou, China

Anatomy of the Hepatic Hilum

1

W.Y. Lau, S.H.Y. Lau, and E.C.H. Lai

1.1 Introduction

A thorough knowledge of anatomy around the hepatic hilus is essential to carry out surgery on hilar cholangiocarcinoma.

The term "hepatic" means "of the liver". It originates from the Greek word "hepar", the liver. The term "hilum" means "a slit-like opening through which ducts, blood vessels lymphatics or nerves enter or leave an organ or a gland". Thus, the term "hepatic hilum" refers to the anatomical region where bile ducts, hepatic arterial branches, portal vein branches, lymphatics and nerves enter or leave the liver. The anatomy around this region is complicated, and is confounded by common occurrence of anomalies of bile ducts and blood vessels.

1.2 Surgical Anatomy of the Hepatic Hilum

A key point in the thorough understanding of the surgical anatomy of the liver and its biliary and vascular supply is to realize that there is a prevailing pattern of anatomy. The prevailing pattern is the most common anatomical pattern, and it may be present almost always or in less than 50 % of patients. Variations from the prevailing pattern in the portal triad (bile duct, hepatic arterial branches and portal vein branches) may affect all its components. Furthermore, variation in one component is independent of variations in either or the other two [1].

Anomalies are variations from the prevailing pattern, and may be common or rare. They may be anomalies of position, number, or size of structures. Aberrancy refers to abnormal position of a structure. An accessory structure is one that is in addition to the "normal" structure in the prevailing pattern and whose function can be deleted without loss of overall function of the organ. The term replaced is used synonymously with aberrant when referring to aberrant arteries in the liver [2].

In this chapter, we shall use the Brisbane 2000 Terminology of Liver Anatomy and Resection as recommended by the International HepatoPancreatoBiliary Association [3].

1.2.1 Prevailing Patterns of the Biliary System (Fig. 1.1)

As the hepatic hilum is the region where structures of the intrahepatic portal triad join the extrahepatic portal triad, a brief overview of the whole biliary system is necessary, especially on the surgical anatomy, for treatment of hilar cholangiocarcinoma.

1.2.1.1 Intrahepatic Biliary Tract

Bile canaliculi are formed by parts of the membrane of adjacent liver parenchymal cells, and they are isolated from the perisinusoidal space by junctions. Bile flows from the canaliculi through ductules (canals of Hering) into the subsegmental and segmental bile ducts which are surrounded by the Glissonian sheath.

1.2.1.2 The Right Hepatic Duct

The right hepatic duct is formed by the union of the anterior and the posterior sectoral branches with each of these two sectoral branches further bifurcating into the superior and inferior segmental branches. Thus, the right anterior sectoral

W.Y. Lau, MD (CUHK), DSc (CUHK), FRCS, FACS, FRACS (Hon) (✉)
Faculty of Medicine, The Chinese University of Hong Kong, Shatin, New Territories, Hong Kong
e-mail: josephlau@cuhk.edu.hk

S.H.Y. Lau, MBChB (CUHK), MRCS (Ed)
Department of Surgery, Queen Elizabeth Hospital, Kowloon, Hong Kong

E.C.H. Lai, MBChB (CUHK), MRCS (Ed), FRACS, FCSHK, FHKAM (Surgery)
Department of Surgery, Pamela Youde Nethersole Eastern Hospital, Chai Wan, Hong Kong

Department of Surgery, The Chinese University of Hong Kong, Shatin, New Territories, Hong Kong

W.Y. Lau (ed.), *Hilar Cholangiocarcinoma*,
DOI 10.1007/978-94-007-6473-6_1, © Springer Science+Business Media Dordrecht and People's Medical Publishing House 2013

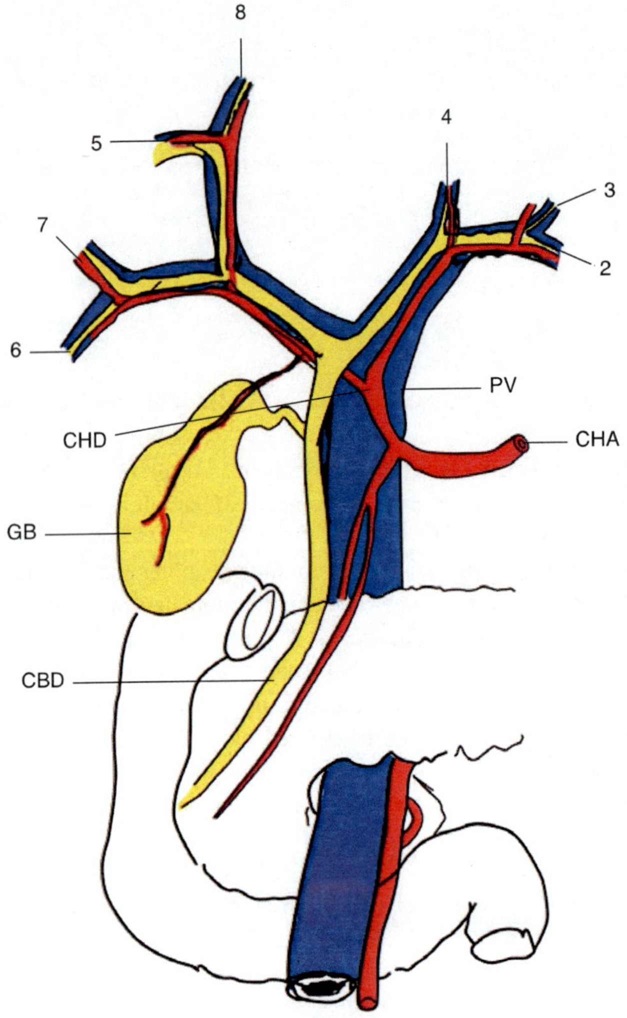

Fig. 1.1 *PV* portal vein, *CHA* common hepatic artery, *CHD* common hepatic duct, *CBD* common bile duct, *GB* gall bladder, *2, 3, 4, 5, 6, 7, 8*, portal triad to segments 2, 3, 4, 5, 6, 7, 8 respectively

branch drains liver segments 8 (right anterior superior segment) and 5 (right anterior inferior segment), while the right posterior sectoral branch drains liver segments 7 (right posterior superior segment) and 6 (right posterior inferior segment). The right hepatic duct, having an average length of 0.9 cm, is formed intrahepatically [4], but it runs a short extrahepatic course to join the left hepatic duct at the bile duct confluence which is totally extrahepatic.

In the prevailing pattern, the right posterior sectoral duct joins the right anterior sectoral duct to form the right hepatic duct, which joins the left hepatic duct to form the confluence of the bile ducts. Instead of the anterior and the posterior sectoral ducts joining together in a Y pattern, the posterior sectoral duct runs superiorly, dorsally, and then inferiorly (Hjortsjo Crook) around the right branch of the portal vein to make a "north-turn" (Fig. 1.2).

Because of this prevailing pattern of the north-turning bile duct branch of the Hjortsjo Crook, resection of the right anterior sector of the liver (segments 5 and 8) can damage the right posterior sectoral duct if the resection is done too close to the bifurcation of the right portal vein into the anterior and posterior sectoral branches. The correct procedure is to stay away from the bifurcation of the right portal vein (Fig. 1.3).

1.2.1.3 The Left Hepatic Duct

The biliary branches of the left medial sectional bile duct (draining liver segment 4) and the left lateral sectional bile duct (draining liver segments 2 and 3) converge to form the left hepatic duct. The medial and the left sectional bile ducts unite at the umbilical fissure (or the left hepatic fissure) in 50 % of cases, to the right in 42 % or to the left in 8 %, according to the study by Healey and Schroy [5]. The left hepatic duct has an average length of 1.7 cm. Again it is formed intrahepatically but it runs extrahepatically to join the right hepatic duct at the bile duct confluence [4]. As the left hepatic duct is longer than the right hepatic duct, palliative bypass is technically easier to the left than the right hepatic duct.

1.2.1.4 Bile Ducts Draining the Caudate Lobe

The caudate lobe can be divided into three parts, each receiving its own vasculo-biliary pedicle: (1) Spiegelian lobe is located to the left of the ligamentum venosum. The prevailing pattern of the vasculo-biliary supply to the Spigelian lobe is by one or two caudate portal triad(s) which originates from the left hepatic pedicle of the portal triad. (2) The paracaval portion lies in front of the retrohepatic portion just to the right of the Spigelian lobe and it is closely attached to the right and middle hepatic veins. It is usually supplied by one or two caudate portal triads which originate from the right posterior sectional pedicle. (3) The caudate process is a small projection between the inferior vena cava and the adjacent portal vein anteriorly. It lies just to the right of the paracaval portion and its vasculo-biliary triad originates from the right hepatic pedicle or from the bifurcation of the main portal triad [6]. As the bile ducts to the caudate lobe arise very near to the confluence of the hepatic ducts, hilar cholangiocarcinoma involves the caudate lobe early. Curative resection of hilar cholangiocarcinoma should be combined with caudate lobectomy.

1.2.1.5 Confluence of Right and Left Hepatic Ducts

The right and left hepatic ducts emerge from the liver and unite at the right margin of the porta hepatis to form the common hepatic duct in a T-shaped manner. The confluence of the right and left hepatic ducts occurs anterior to the portal venous bifurcation and it overlies the origin of the right portal vein. The right hepatic artery usually runs posterior to the common hepatic duct, i.e. posterior and inferior to the confluence of the right and left hepatic ducts. The extrahepatic segment of the right duct is short, but the left duct has a

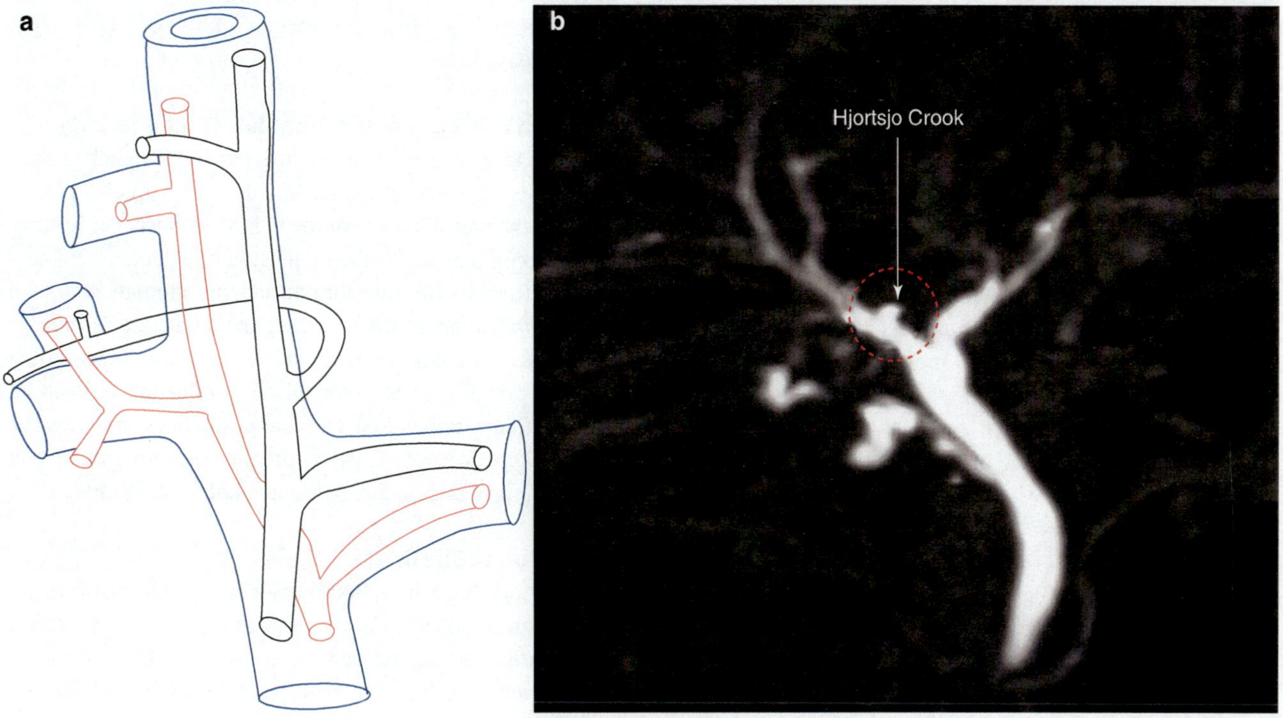

Fig. 1.2 (**a**) Hjortsjo Crook; (**b**) magnetic resonance cholangiopancreatogram showing the Hjortsjo Crook

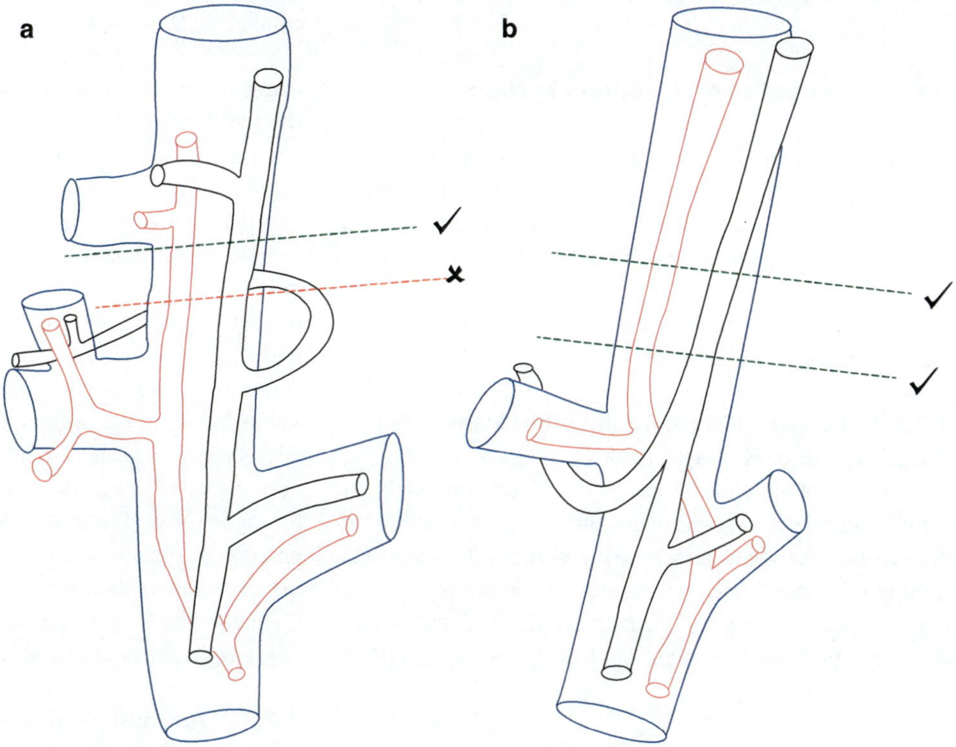

Fig. 1.3 Hjortsjo Crook and its clinical significance. (**a**) The north-turning right posterior sectoral bile duct (majority of people). (**b**) The south-turning right posterior sectoral bile duct (minority of people)

much longer extrahepatic course. The biliary confluence is separated from the posterior aspect of the quadrate lobe of the liver (i.e. segment 4b) by the hilar plate, which is the fusion of connective tissues enclosing the biliary and vascular elements with Glisson's sheath. Because of the absence of any vascular interposition, it is possible to open the connective tissue constituting the hilar plate at the inferior border of the quadrate lobe (segment 4b), and by elevating it to display the biliary convergence and left hepatic duct [7]. This surgical procedure is called lowering of the hepatic hilar plate.

1.2.1.6 Other Components of the Extrahepatic Biliary System

The common hepatic duct is about 4 cm long with a diameter of 4 mm. It lies in the free edge of the lesser omentum in front of the right edge of the main portal vein and with the hepatic artery on its left. The cystic duct usually joins the common hepatic duct on the right, about 1 cm above the first part of the duodenum to form the common bile duct. The common bile duct is about 8 cm long and 8 mm in diameter. It can be divided into the supradudodenal portion which lies in the free edge of the lesser omentum, the retroduodenal portion which runs behind the first part of the duodenum, the paraduodenal portion which runs in the groove between the back of the head of the pancreas and the second part of the duodenum, and the intraduodenal portion which runs obliquely through the wall of the duodenum. The common bile duct joins the pancreatic duct at an angle of about 60° at the ampula of Vater which opens into the posteromedial wall of the second part of the duodenum at the major papilla.

The gallbladder is a reservoir for bile and it is located on the undersurface of the right liver within the gallbladder fossa. It is separated from the liver parenchyma by the cystic plate, which is composed of connective tissue closely applied to the Glisson's capsule and is continuous with the hilar plate.

1.2.2 Anomalies of the Biliary System

It is not the intention of the authors to discuss on all the possible anomalies of the biliary system. Our intention is to discuss on anomalies which are relevant to surgery on hilar cholangiocarcinoma only. As anomalies of the confluence of the right and left hepatic ducts are closely related to either anomalies of the right hepatic duct or the left hepatic duct, these anomalies will be discussed together.

1.2.2.1 Bile Ducts Draining the Right Hemiliver

"South-Turning" Hjortsjo Crook

Instead of making a north-turn as described previously, the right posterior sectoral bile duct courses ventrally and inferiorly around the right branch of the portal vein (the south-turning bile duct branch). This anomaly makes resection of the right anterior sector of the liver (segments 5 and 8) safer than the prevailing pattern, and it is of little clinical significance to recognize.

Absence of Right Hepatic Duct

Absence of the right hepatic duct is an anatomical variation that results during development.

There are three anatomical variations in which the right anterior and posterior sectoral ducts do not come together to form the right hepatic duct, thus resulting in absence of the right hepatic duct (Fig. 1.4) [5, 8–10].

The anomalies which can result in absence of the right hepatic ducts are:

Shifting of the Entry of the Right Bile Duct Inferiorly

This set of anomalies involves the insertion of the right bile duct, or one of its branches, inferiorly into the biliary tree at a lower point than the prevailing site of the biliary confluence (Fig. 1.5).

Low union may affect the main right bile duct, a right sectoral duct (usually the anterior one and this anomaly results in absence of right hepatic duct), a segmental duct, or a subsegmental duct. The duct unites with the common hepatic duct below the prevailing site of the biliary confluence, or in about 2 % of patients, unites first with the cystic duct, and then the common hepatic duct. These anomalies place a greater risk of ductal injury during laparoscopic cholecystectomy.

Trifurcation of Bile Duct

When performing a right hemihepatectomy, a left hemihepatectomy, an anterior right sectionectomy, a right posterior sectionectomy, a right trisectionectomy or a left trisectionectomy, a stricture is likely to develop at the biliary trifurcation site if no normal biliary safety margin is left at the site of the transection. It is always safer to divide the biliary tree with a safety margin of at least 1 cm from the site of the biliary confluence (Fig. 1.6).

Anterior or Posterior Sectoral Branch Joining the Left Hepatic Duct

The right posterior sectoral duct inserts with the left hepatic duct in 20 % of patients and the right anterior sectoral bile duct does so in 6 %. In both cases, there is no right hepatic duct as both join the left hepatic duct, one to the left of the midline and the other in the midplane. A right sectoral bile duct inserting into the left hepatic duct to the left of the midplane is in danger of injury during left hepatectomy, therefore, in left hepatectomy, the left bile duct should be divided close to the umbilical fissure so as to avoid injury to a possible right sectoral duct. If the left duct is divided at the normal site of confluence of the right and left hepatic duct, the right sectoral duct can be injured (Fig. 1.7). It is good practice to obtain an intraoperative cholangiogram through the cystic duct when performing left hepatectomy to detect this anomaly. Please take note that even with these anomalies, a right hepatectomy is safe.

1.2.2.2 Anomalies of Bile Ducts Draining the Left Hemiliver

The prevailing pattern of bile duct draining from the left liver is shown in Fig. 1.8a, and this is present only in 30 % of individuals. Thus, variations are present in the majority of individuals.

The segmental ducts from segments 2 and 3 (B2 and B3 respectively) unite to form the left lateral sectional duct. This

	Presence of a right hepatic duct	Absence of a right hepatic duct		
	Prevailing pattern	Posterior sectoral duct joining to the left hepatic duct	3-branch type	Anterior sectoral duct joining to the left hepatic duct
Variations in the anatomy of the anterior sectoral bile duct	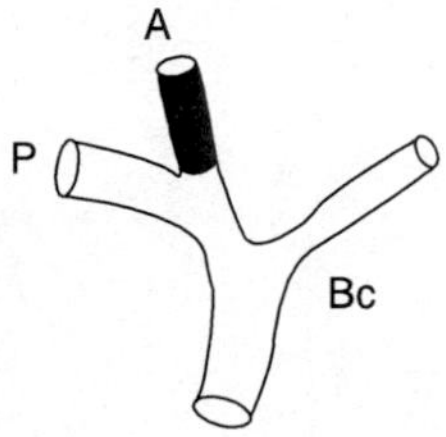	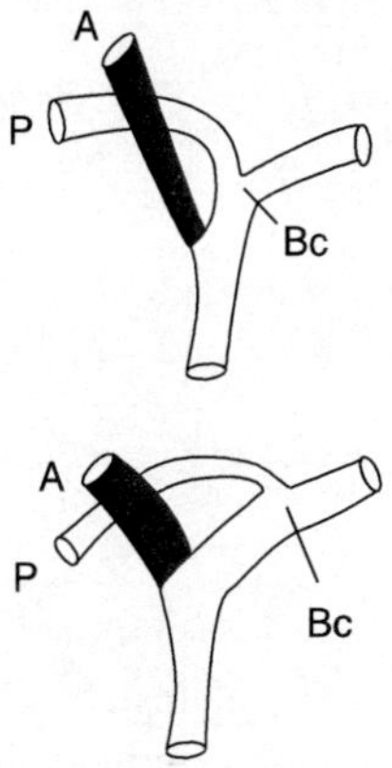	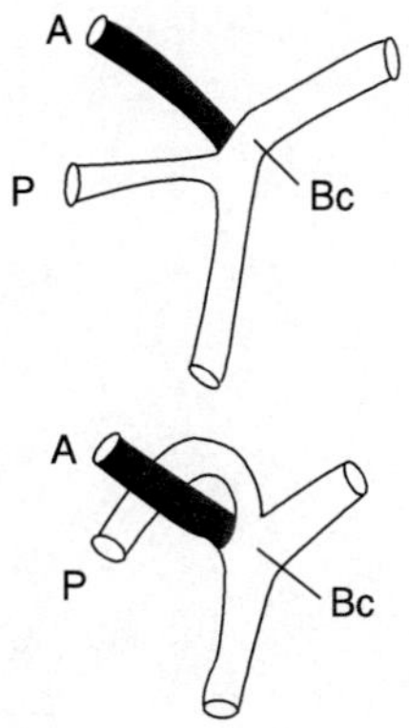	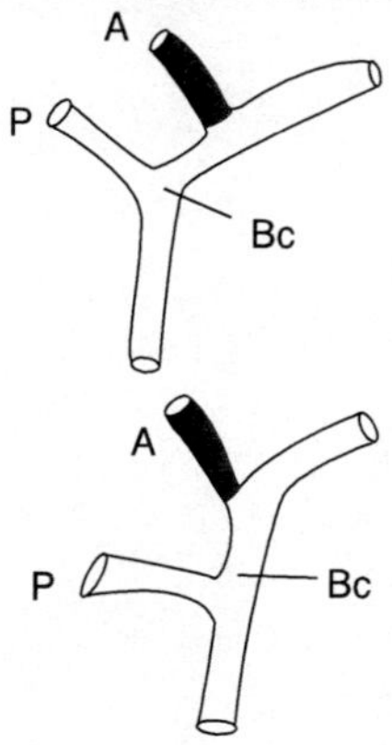
Healey (1953) (n = 96)	72.0 %	22.0 %	—	6.0 %
Couinaud (1981) (n = 102)	53.5 %	24.3 %	14.0 %	8.4 %
Kida (1987) (n = 104)	71.2 %	8.7 %	11.5 %	8.6 %
Ishiyama (1999) (n = 41)	58.4 %	26.9 %	7.3 %	7.3 %

Fig. 1.4 Variations in the anatomy of the right hepatic duct and their incidences, based on analysis of liver casts. *A* anterior sectoral branch, *P* posterior sectoral branch, *Bc* bile duct confluence

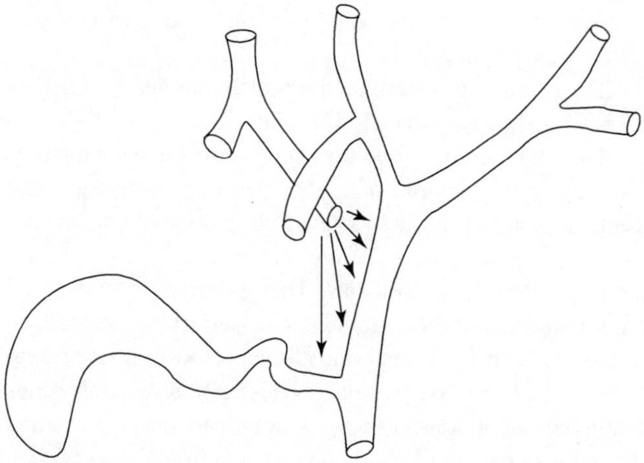

Fig. 1.5 Shifting of entry of right bile duct (or one of its branches) inferiorly

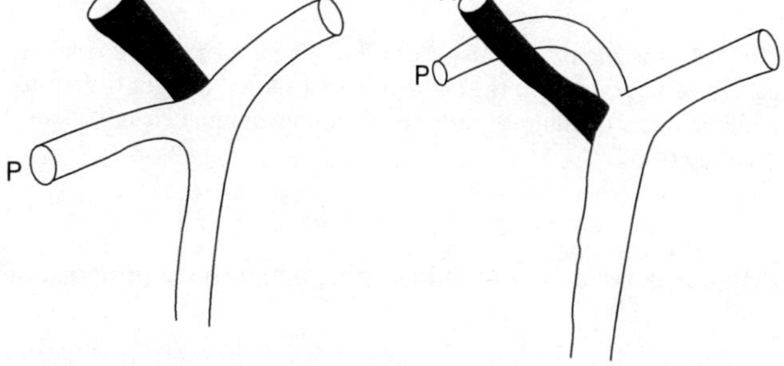

Fig. 1.6 Trifurcation of bile duct. *A* right anterior sectoral branch, *P* right posterior sectoral branch

duct passes behind the umbilical portion of the portal vein and unites with the duct(s) from segment 4 (B4), also called the left medial sectional duct. The union of these ducts to form the left hepatic duct occurs about one third of the

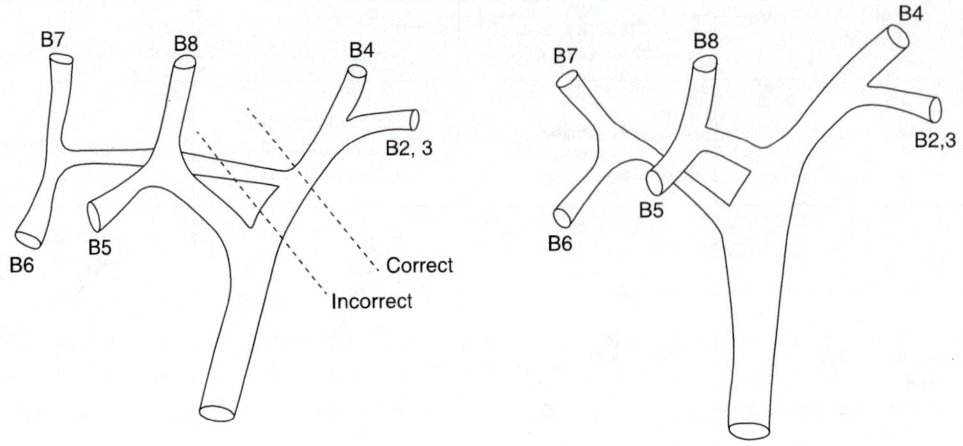

Fig. 1.7 Separate entry of right anterior and right posterior sectoral ducts (no right hepatic duct)

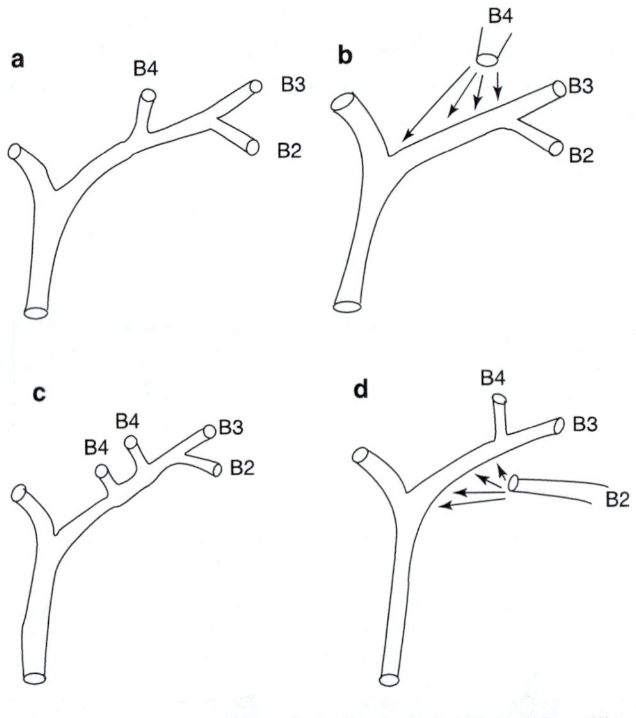

Fig. 1.8 Variations in formation of left hepatic ducts. (**a**) Prevailing pattern of left bile duct; (**b**) insertion of B4 shifted to right or left; (**c**) multiple ducts draining B4; (**d**) B3, B4 form common channel before insertion of B2

distance between the umbilical fissure and the confluence of the left and right ducts.

The surgically important anomalies of the left ductal system involve variations in site of insertion of B4 (Fig. 1.8b), multiple ducts coming from B4 (Fig. 1.8c) and primary union of B3 and B4 with subsequent union of B2 (Fig. 1.8d). B4 may join the left lateral sectional duct to the left or right of its point of union in the prevailing pattern (Fig. 1.8b). In the former case, the insertion may occur at any place to the right of the prevailing location up to the point where the left lateral sectional duct unites with the right bile duct. In the latter instance, which according to Couinaud, is present in 8 % of individuals, there is no left hepatic duct, instead the common hepatic duct is formed by the confluence of three ducts—the right hepatic duct and two left hepatic ducts (B4 and the left lateral sectional duct of B3 and B2).

The commonest variations in the left bile duct are: Type 1 common joining of B2 with B3, B4 then joins near to the left hepatic duct; Type 2 common joining of B4, B3 and B2 near to the same point; Type 3 common joining of B4 with B3 before B2 joins in (Fig. 1.9).

The left hepatic duct runs at a variable angle. In some individuals, it is almost horizontal, but in others it runs sharply upwards. It is much easier to expose a long length of the left hepatic duct in the former type.

1.2.3 Prevailing Pattern of the Portal Venous System

Few variations are found in the major portal vein branches because the portal vein develops during the very earliest part of the gestational period.

The prevailing pattern of the portal vein and its intrahepatic branches are shown in Fig. 1.10.

The main portal vein divides into the right and the left portal vein. The right portal vein subdivides into the right anterior sectoral portal vein which further branches into the segment 8 (superior) and segment 5 (inferior) branches supplying the corresponding liver segments. The posterior sectoral portal vein branches into the segment 7 (superior) and segment 6 (inferior) branches, supplying the corresponding liver segments. The transverse portion of the left portal vein only sends out a few small branches to segment 4 and one or two small branches to segment 1. All large branches from the portal vein to the left liver arise exclusively beyond the attachment of the ligamentum venosum, i.e. from the umbilical portion of the

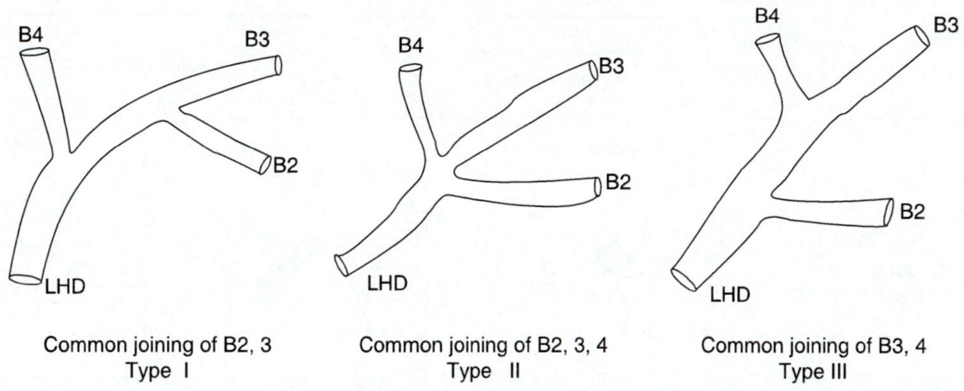

Fig. 1.9 Common variations in the anatomy of the left bile duct

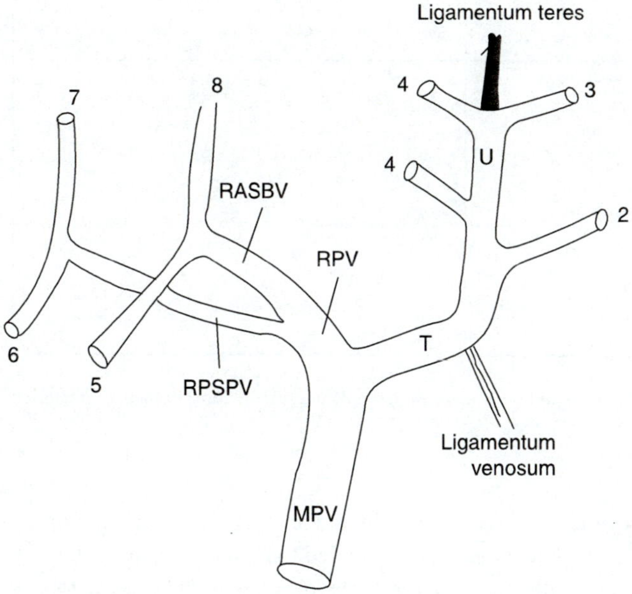

Fig. 1.10 The portal vein and its intrahepatic branches. *MPV* main portal vein, *RPV* right portal vein, *RASPV* right anterior sectoral portal vein, *RPSPV* right posterior sectoral portal vein *U* umbilical portal of left portal vein *T* transverse portion of left portal vein

vein. There are usually more than one branch which supplies segment 4 of the liver coming out from the right side of the umbilical portion of the vein. On the left side, there is usually one branch which goes to segment 2, but one or more branches which go to segment 3. The left portal vein terminates where it joins the ligamentum teres at the free edge of the liver.

1.2.4 Anomalies of the Portal Venous System

Reports by three investigators revealed three principal anomalies of the portal vein in the hilar region (Fig. 1.11) [8, 9, 11].

Kida et al. reported that variations in the anatomy of biliary tract are mostly (81 %), but not invariably, associated with variations in the anatomy of the portal vein.

In operations on patients with trifurcation of the right anterior sectoral vein, right posterior sectoral vein and the left portal vein, it is important to leave a safety margin of at least 1 cm on the portal vein stump to avoid subsequent stricture formation in the portal vein left after liver resection.

In the anomaly where the anterior sectoral vein joins the left portal vein, an unsuspecting surgeon who carries out a right hemihepatectomy may divide the posterior sectoral vein thinking that it is the right portal vein, and will consequently be confused when the anterior sector vein is come upon during hepatic transection. In left hemihepatectomy, the anterior sectoral portal vein is inadvertently damaged, resulting in subsequent ischemia to liver segments 5 and 8.

A very rare but potentially devastating anomaly is the absent extrahepatic left portal vein (Fig. 1.12). In this case, the apparent right portal vein is actually the main portal vein, a structure which enters the liver, gives off the right portal vein, and then loops back within the liver substance to supply the left liver. The vein looks like a right portal vein in position, although it is larger. Transection of this vein results in total portal vein disconnection from the liver. This anomaly should always be searched for in computer tomography, as right hepatectomy is not possible when it is present. Identification of the umbilical portion of the left portal vein in the umbilical fissure on computed tomography can preclude the presence of this problem. A left hepatectomy is possible with this anomaly.

1.2.5 Prevailing Pattern of the Arterial Blood Supply

This occurs in approximately two-third of individuals [1]. The common hepatic artery arises from the coeliac trunk which divides into the common hepatic artery, the left gastric artery and splenic artery. The common hepatic artery divides into the gastroduodenal and the proper hepatic artery (this is referred to in many anatomical textbooks as the common hepatic artery). The proper hepatic artery usually lies lateral and slightly posterior to the common bile duct in the portal pedicle and divides into its terminal branches, usually to the left and below the confluence of the right and left hepatic ducts. The course of the terminal branches is highly variable, they may

	Presence of a right portal vein	Absence of a right portal vein	
	Prevailing pattern	3-branch type	Anterior sectoral vein joining to the left portal vein type
Variations in the anatomy of the anterior sectoral portal vein	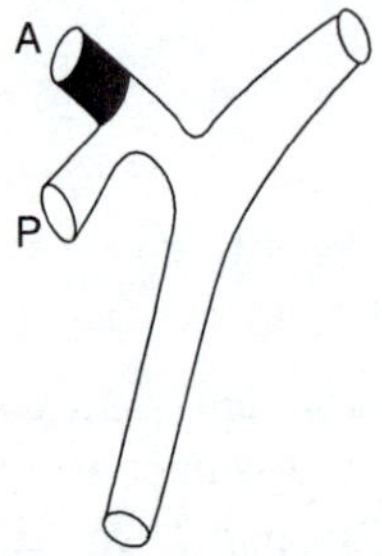	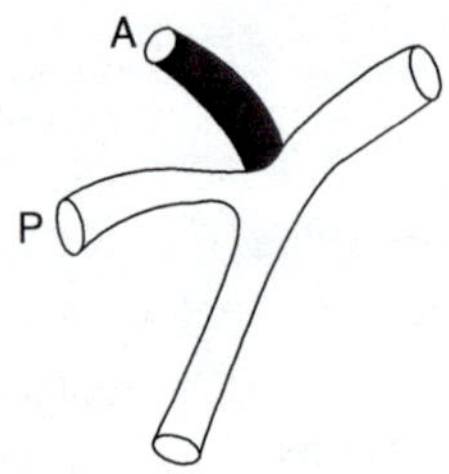	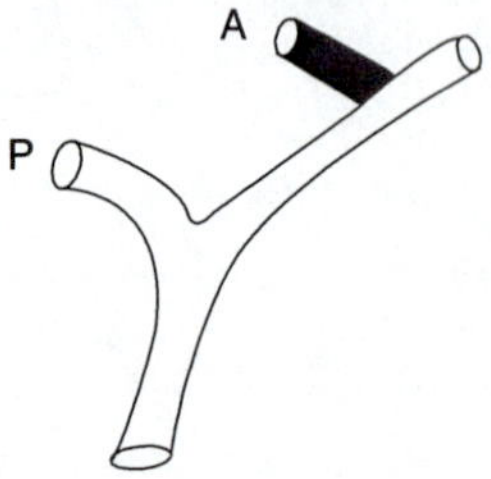
Couinaud (1981) (n = 111)	83.5 %	7.7 %	8.8 %
Kumon (1985) (n = 23)	73.9 %	8.7 %	17.4 %
Kida (1987) (n = 104)	79.8 %	11.5 %	8.7 %

Fig. 1.11 Variations in the anatomy of the right portal vein and their incidences (analysis of liver cyst). *A* anterior sectoral branch, *P* posterior sectoral branch

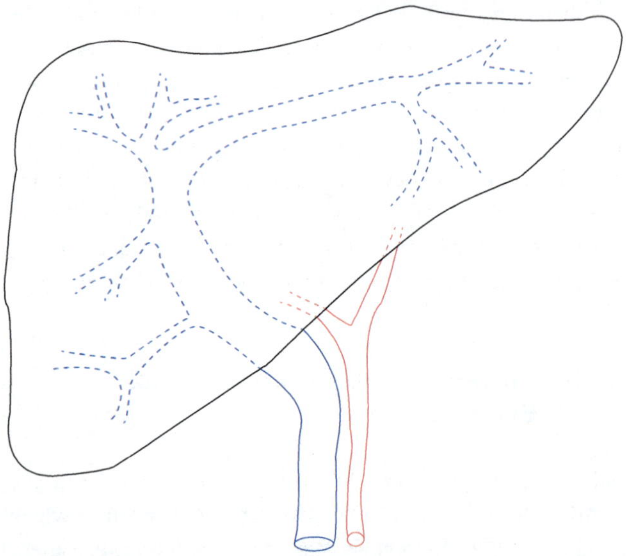

Fig. 1.12 Absent exhraheptic left portal vein

pass posterior (more commonly) or anterior to the bile ducts. The right hepatic artery may lie anterior and to the right of the main bile duct, thereby coming in close contact with the gallbladder where it can be damaged during cholecystectomy. The right hepatic artery generally supplies the right liver and the left hepatic artery the left liver. In 92 % of cases, segment 4 of the liver is supplied by a branch of either the right or the left hepatic artery. This is called the middle hepatic artery by some authors. The arterial blood supply to the caudate lobe is usually from both the right and left hepatic arteries.

1.2.5.1 Variations in Hepatic Arterial Blood Supply

Embryologically, the hepatic artery develops late in the gestational period, and thus variations are common (33–45 %). More than ten variations in the anatomy of the hepatic artery, including an accessory or replaced artery, have been identified [12]. Fortunately some of these variations are rare. Figure 1.13 shows the important variations [13, 14].

Analysis of the anatomy showed the hepatic artery courses dorsal to the hepatic duct in 76 % of the population, and ventrally to it in 24 % of the population. In 9 % of the population, the right hepatic artery runs dorsal to the portal vein, making it necessary to pay special attention to the anatomy of the vessels and ducts of the hilar area during surgical dissection of this area.

1.2.5.2 Blood Supply of the Gallbladder

In 85 % of the population, the cystic artery arises from the right hepatic artery. It divides into an anterior and a posterior branch close to the wall of the gallbladder. The posterior branch of the cystic artery may be anastomosed to the

	Prevailing pattern	Right hepatic a. from the SMA	Left hepatic a. from the LGA	Common hepatic a. from the SMA
	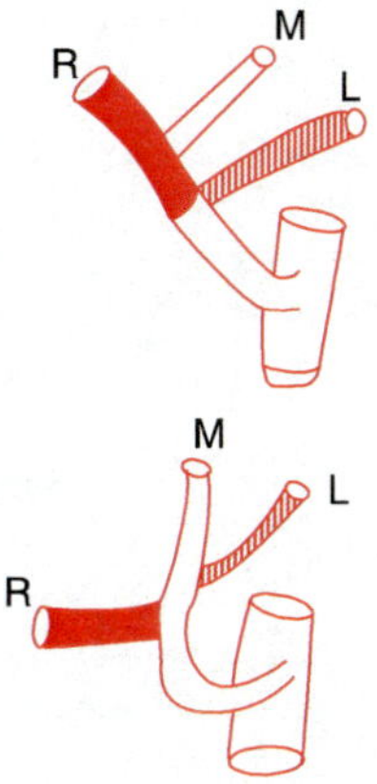	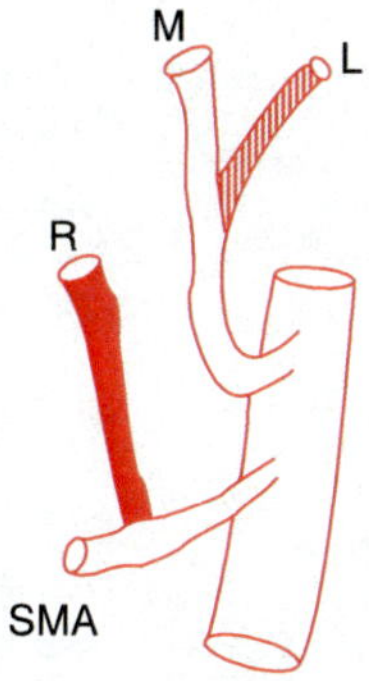	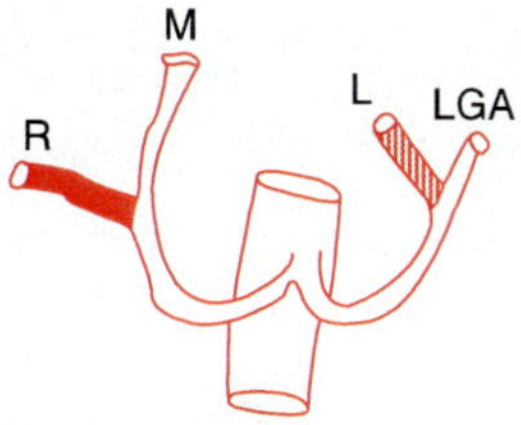	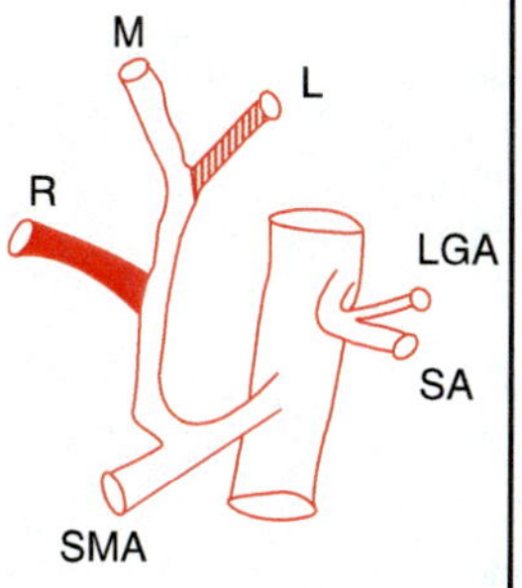
Michels (1966) (n = 200)	71.0 %	13.0 %	11.0 %	5.0 %
Suzuki (1982) (n = 100)	72.0 %	14.0 %	12.0 %	2.0 %

Fig. 1.13 Variations in the anatomy of the main hepatic arteries exclusive of accessory hepatic arterials. *R* right hepatic artery, *M* middle hepatic artery, *L* left hepatic artery, *SMA* superior mesenteric artery, *LGA* left gastric artery, *SA* splenic artery

arterial branches supplying the hepatic parenchyma around the gallbladder fossa.

The origins of the cystic artery may be highly variable, arising from any part of the hepatic artery, coeliac axis, the superior mesenteric artery or any of its branches. If the cystic artery has a low origin, it may participate extensively in the vascularization of the main bile duct [1].

1.2.5.3 Arterial Blood Supply to the Supraduodenal and Retroduodenal Portions of the Extrahepatic Bile Ducts

The arterial blood supply to the supraduodenal and retroduodenal portions of the extrahepatic bile ducts originates from the coeliac and the superior mesenteric arterial branches (Fig. 1.14).

According to the study by Chen et al. [15], the right and left hepatic ducts, the common hepatic duct, and the supraduodenal and retroduodenal portions of the common bile duct are supplied by at least seven arteries which supply different amounts of blood to the different portions of this extrahepatic ductal system. These arterial branches can be divided into the upper and the lower groups according to their distributions as related to the ducts. The upper group includes the cystic artery, right hepatic artery, and left hepatic artery which are located in the region near to the common hepatic duct (Fig. 1.15). The lower group consists of the posterior superior pancreaticoduodenal artery, the gastroduodenal artery, the anterior superior pancreaticoduodenal artery and the retroportal artery, all of which are located near the retroduodenal portion of the bile duct (Table 1.1) (Fig. 1.16).

1.2.5.4 Arterial Blood Supply to the Paraduodenal and Intraduodenal Portions of the Extrahepatic Bile Ducts

The paraduodenal (or pancreatic) and intraduodenal portions of the common bile duct is supplied by arterial branches coming from the posterior superior pancreaticoduodenal artery (coming from the coeliac artery) and the posterior inferior pancreaticoduodenal artery (coming from the superior mesenteric artery) (Fig. 1.16).

There has been some confusion of nomenclature. The term posterior superior pancreaticoduodenal artery whose description by Shapiro [16] in 1948, was the most exact, but it is called the retroduodenal artery in some publications, or less frequently, the right superior pancreaticoduodenal artery. The term posterior superior pancreaticoduodenal artery should be used, whereas the term retroduodenal artery indicates another and quite different artery in some anatomic textbooks [17].

The retroportal artery (R) is worth a more detailed discussion (Fig. 1.15). It was first described by Northover and Terblanche [18] in 1978 and is present in more than 90 % of individuals [15, 18]. It arises from the mesenteric artery in

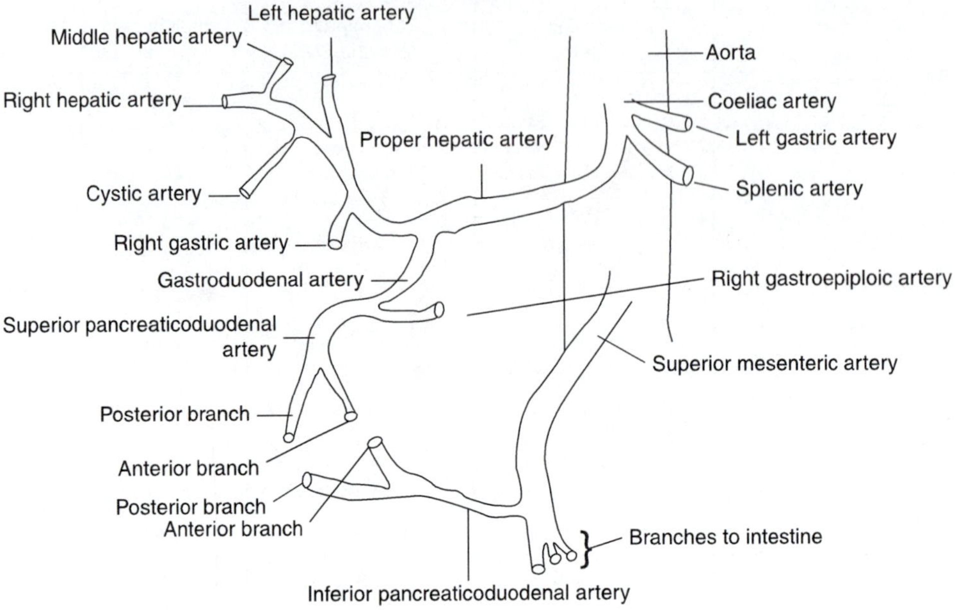

Fig. 1.14 Arterial blood supply to the extrahepatic bile ducts

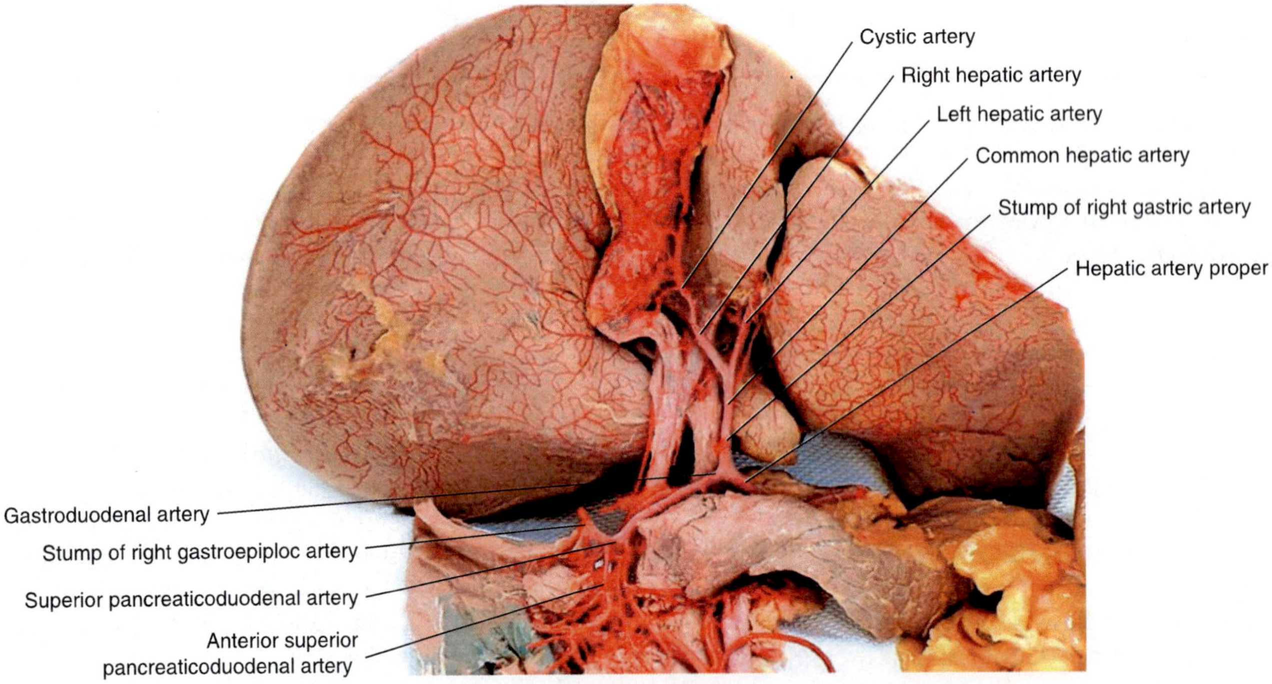

Fig. 1.15 Arterial blood supply to the supraduodenal and retroduodenal portions of the extrahepatic bile duct (anterior view) (Photograph provided by Academician Zhong Shizhen whose injection cast carried out 20 years ago clearly shows the arterial blood supply that we now understand)

58.3 % of individuals, and from the coeliac trunk in 41.7 % according to the study by Chen et al. [15]. After arising from close to the origins of one of these major arteries from the aorta, it passes to the right, posterior to the portal vein and the posterosuperior margin of the pancreatic head to reach the posterior part of the retroduodenal portion of the common bile duct. It then terminates either by joining the posterior superior pancreaticoduodenal artery to form an arterial circle (Type I by Chen et al. [15]), or passing upward along the posterior surface of the supraduodenal part of the bile duct to anastomose with the descending branches of the cystic and the right hepatic artery via two pathways: either joining the right hepatic artery after passing up the posterior surface of the bile duct, or joining the branches of the posterior superior pancreaticoduodenal artery close to the lower end of the common bile duct, from where branches travel superiorly to join the descending branches [1] (Type II by Chen et al. [15]) These two components, anterior as described by Parke et al. [19] in 1963 and posterior as described by Northover and Terblanche [18] in 1978 are freely anastomosed to each other [1]. In about a quarter of patients, the retroportal artery runs inferior to the pancreas [15].

1.2.5.5 Arterial Network of the Extrahepatic Biliary System

Previous investigations on the arterial blood supply to the extrahepatic biliary system are scarce, and most were confined to the common bile duct and/or hepatic ducts [15]. The results were conflicting, and in some cases contradictory [17]. These differences are partly due to the different techniques employed and partly due to the different ages of the subjects studied (adult or fetus). Shapiro and Robillard [16] and Pforriager [20] reported that the bile duct were supplied by end arteries, while studies by Douglas and Cutter [21], Northover and Terblanche [18, 22], Rath et al. [17] and Chen et al. [15] proposed the presence of a rich arterial network around the duct. It is now accepted that arterial anastomoses are found on the surfaces of the extrahepatic biliary system [17]. To understand the arterial blood supply better, it is necessary to divide the extrahepatic biliary system into four portions as each portion has its own special characteristics [15].

First Portion: Cystic Duct and Gallbladder

The cystic artery has two branches, an anterior and a posterior branch which pass closely along the right and left margins respectively (superificial and deep surfaces) of the gallbladder. Arterial branches arborize and anastomose with each other to form a rich arterial network on the wall of the gallbladder (Fig. 1.15). As mentioned previously, the posterior branch of the cystic artery may be anastomosed to the arterial branches supplying the hepatic parenchyma around the gallbladder fossa.

Second Portion: Right and Left Hepatic Ducts

These ducts have a comparatively sparse arterial network. The arteries here run closely along each duct. According to Chen et al. [15], one branch travels on the lateral side of the left hepatic duct. The right hepatic artery and its branches travel on the latero-inferior side of the right hepatic duct (Fig. 1.17).

Third Portion: Common Hepatic duct, and Supra- and Retro-duodenal Portions of the bile duct (Fig. 1.17)

In this portion, a special and sparse longitudinal arterial anastomotic chain is found. This chain passes close to the lateral sides of the duct, where it is named the right or left marginal arteries, respectively (or the 9 O'clock or 3 O'clock marginal arteries, respectively). According to Chen et al. [15], the left margin artery is present in 95 % of individuals, and it arises from the posterior superior pancreaticoduodenal artery in 86 %, or gastroduodenal artery in 13.2 %. It runs distally to join the right hepatic artery (63.2 %) or the cystic artery (26.3 %) or others (5.3 %). The right margin artery is present in 82.5 % of individuals. It arises from the posterior superior pancrea-

Table 1.1 Arterial blood supply to the supraduodenal and retroduodenal portions of the extrahepatic bile ducts

Artery	Percent of contribution of blood flow (%)
Superior group	
Cystic	56.4
Right hepatic	11.9
Left hepatic	0.8
Inferior group	
Posterior superior pancreaticoduodenal	22.8
Retroportal	3.4
Gastroduodenal	1.5
Anterior superior pancreaticoduodenal	1.4
Others	1.8
	100.0

According to Chen et al. [15]

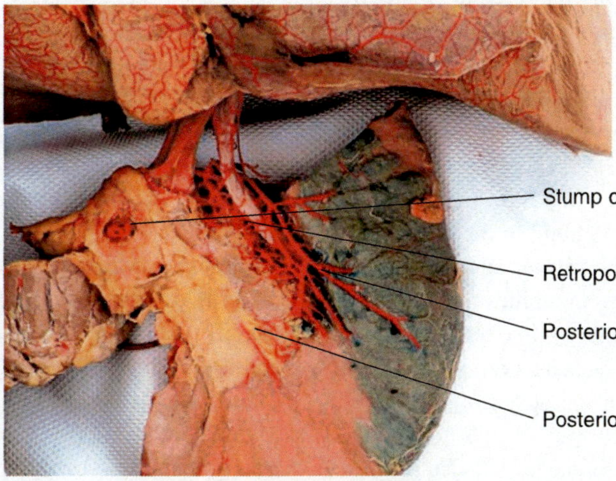

Fig. 1.16 Arterial blood supply to the paraduodenal and intraduodenal portions of the extrahepatic bile ducts (posterior view) (Photograph provided by Academician Zhong Shizhen whose injection cast carried out 20 years ago clearly shows the arterial blood supply that we now understand)

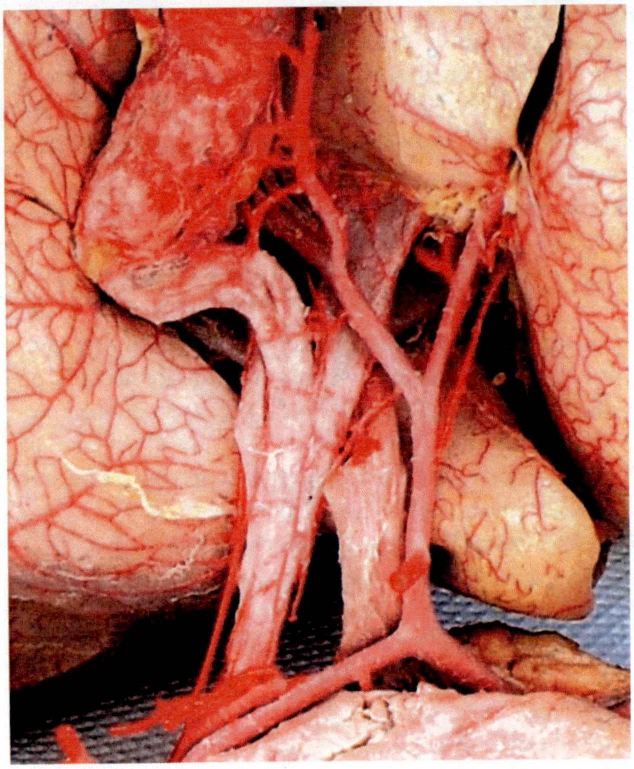

Fig. 1.17 Anterior network on extrahepatic biliary system. Please note the right and left marginal arteries on the right and left borders of the common hepatic and common bile ducts. This specimen represents an axial distribution with two arches in the classification by Rath et al. [17] (Photograph provided by Academician Zhong Shizhen whose injection cast carried out 20 years ago clearly shows the arterial blood supply that we now understand)

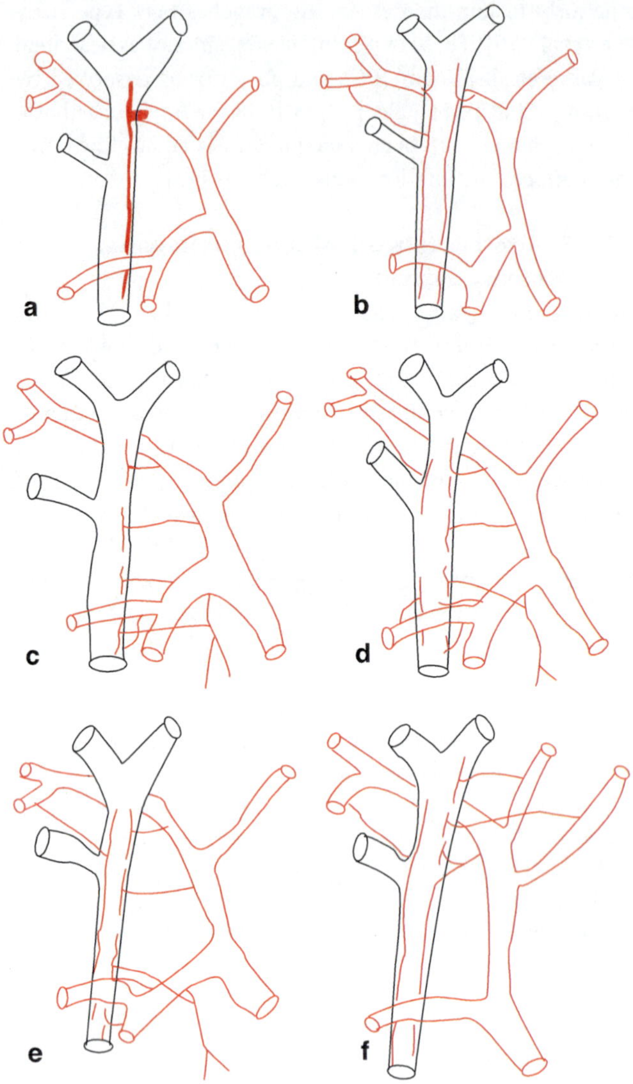

Fig. 1.18 The different types of vascularity of the common hepatic and common bile ducts according to Rath et al. [17] (**a**) axial type with left arch; (**b**) axial type with right and left arches; (**c**) single ladder at left border; (**d**) double ladder, right and up; (**e**) mixed left: left ladder and right arch; (**f**) mixed type, left ladder, left arch and right arch

ticoduodenal artery (87.9 %), or gastroduodenal artery (12.1 %) and runs upward to join the cystic artery (66.7 %) or the right hepatic artery (33.3 %).

Rath et al. [17] identified three types of vascular distribution to this portion of the extrahepatic biliary system (Fig. 1.18):

1. An axial distribution (76.7 %)
   This is represented by a single vascular arch in 18.3 % of individuals in the study by Rath et al. [17], and by two (right and left) arches in 58.3 % of individuals. When only one arch is present, it usually skirts the anterior left aspect of the bile duct. Only very occasionally is an arch formed by a right marginal artery. When two arches are present, they more or less follow the right and left borders of the biliary tract, corresponding to the arterials at 3 and 9 O'clock described by Northover and Terblanche [18]. Anastomosis between the two arches are observed on the arterial aspects of the common bile duct and common hepatic duct. Occasionally there are one or more posterior anastomotic arches in the posterior aspects of these ducts.

The study by Northover and Terblanche [18] also showed that the axial distribution is the most common.

2. Ladder distribution
   This was found to be present in 8.3 % of individuals in the study by Rath et al. [17]. In the majority of patients with a ladder distribution of arterial blood supply to the common ducts, the blood supply comes from both the right and the left sides. The arterial branches divide at the right and the left borders of the biliary tract into ascending and descending branches which anastomose among themselves. In the minority of individuals, the arteries arise exclusively from the left side of the bile ducts, dividing into the ascending and descending branches at the left border of the biliary tree, and anastomosing among themselves.
3. Mixed type
   This type of arterial supply was present in 15 % of individuals in the study by Rath et al. [17]. It can be a combination

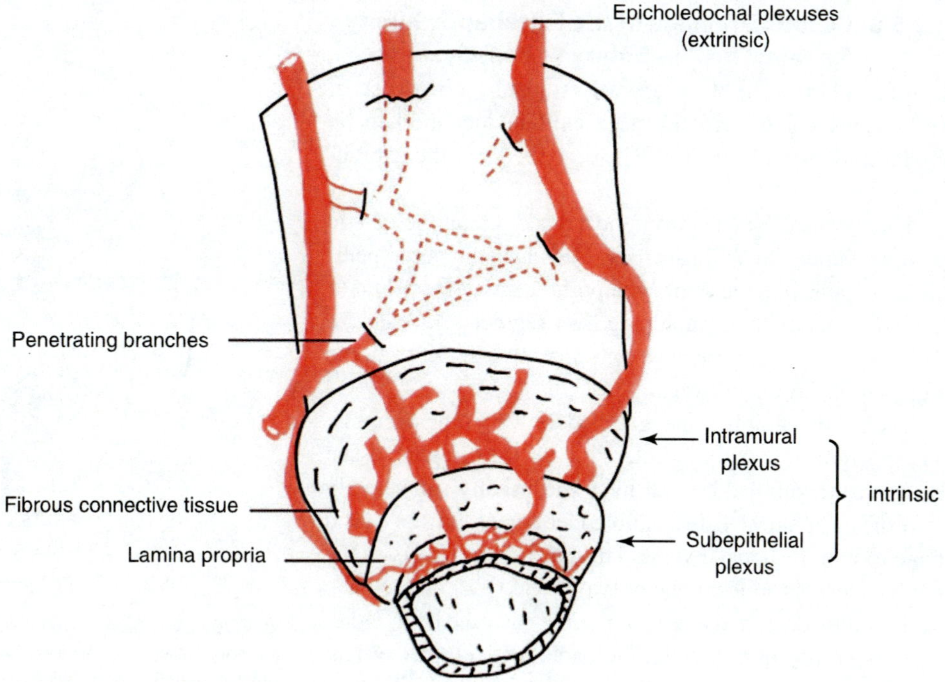

Fig. 1.19 The Anastomosing arterial plexuses of the main bile duct (According to Parkes et al. [19])

of a right marginal arch with a left ladder arrangement, or a right marginal arch with a left ladder arrangement for the common hepatic duct and a left arch for the common bile duct (Fig. 1.18a–f). Other mixed types are possible but are uncommon.

Fourth Portion: Pancreatic and Intraduodenal

The arterial network to this portion of the extrahepatic biliary system is comparatively abundant. It originates mainly from an arterial circle formed by the anastomoses of the retroportal artery, the posterior superior pancreaticoduodenal artery, and the posterior inferior pancreticoduodenal artery located on the posterior surface of the pancreatic portion of the bile duct and the head of the pancreas in the retroportal type I as described by Chen et al. [15] (Fig. 1.16), or from the branches of these arteries in the retroportal type II by Chen et al. [15].

1.2.5.6 Arterial Plexuses of the Main Bile Duct Wall

Parkes et al. [19] in 1963 showed that in addition to the epicholedochal plexus, collateral arterial circulation of the duct is enhanced by two intramural plexuses: an intramural plexus between the connective tissue sheath and the mucosa, and a subepithelial plexuse. The intramural, epicholedochal and subepithelial plexuses anastomose through penetrating branches (Fig. 1.19), thus adding to the anastomotic pathways in the event of compromise to the epicholedochal plexus.

1.2.5.7 Surgical Significance of Arrangement of Arterial Supply to the Major Bile Ducts

The arrangement of the arterial blood supply to the extrahepatic biliary system, especially to the common hepatic and common bile ducts, has considerable surgical significance.

Appleby [23] in 1959 made the following importance recommendations with respect to exposure of the main bile duct and choledochotomy:

1. For exposure of the main bile duct it should never be stripped;
2. It should be opened longitudinally through an area devoid of visible vessels, with its fascial envelop left intact;
3. When resutured, all vessels should be avoided; and
4. Ligate the cystic artery close to the gallbladder.

One point which is still unsettled is that of the advisable level for transection section of the main bile duct with a view to perform bilio-alimentary anastomosis after a Whipple's procedure or a liver transplantation. Both Northover and Terblanche [18] and Parke et al. [19] have recommended transecting the main bile duct closer to the hilum than the duodenum, because the predominant source of blood supply to the main duct is from below (mainly from the gastroduodenal or posterior superior pancreaticoduodenal arteries), while the vessels from above (mainly from the cystic artery and right heptic artery) are more delicate and smaller in diameter and are thus less likely to be able to sustain a long length of the remnant bile duct. This view now seems to be adopted by most hepatobiliary surgeons. However Rath et al. [17] basing on their study on the vascularization of the extraheptic bile duct recommended transection of the main bile duct around the junction of the inferior border of the cystic duct with the common duct in liver transplantation for both donor and recipient. They argued that this would allow simple resection of the two ends should the blood-supply prove unsatisfactory. In this way, end-to-end bilio-biliary anastomosis could be made without tension.

1.2.5.8 Venous Drainage of the Extrahaptic Biliary System: The Parabiliary Venous System

Couinaud [24] in 1989 extensively studied the network of small veins which surrounds the main bile duct and hepatic artery in the portal pedicle and he described it as the parabiliary venous system.

The plexus originates from the veins draining the gastric pylorus, duodenum and pancreas, ascends in the portal pedicle and drains into the segmental portal veins at the hilum of the liver (mainly those supplying liver segments 1, 4 and 5). This plexus is, therefore, a venous anastomosis between the right and the left hemilivers.

The veins draining the gallbladder vary considerably. Those from its upper surface lie in the areolar tissue between the gallbladder and liver and usually run directly into the liver through the gallbladder fossa and the cystic plate to join the hepatic veins. Those from other parts of the gallbladder join to form one or two cystic veins on the neck of the gallbladder, and these commonly enter the liver, either directly or after joining with the parabiliary venous system draining the hepatic ducts and the upper part of the bile duct. Only rarely does a single or double cystic vein drain directly into the right branch of the portal vein.

In patients with portal hypertension, the veins in the parabiliary system may become particularly large, giving rise to troublesome bleeding when the portal pedicle is being dissected. In the event of portal vein thrombosis, the large collaterals venous channel in the portal pedicle are hypertrophied veins of the parabiliary venous system.

1.2.5.9 Lymphatic Drainage of the Extrahepatic Biliary System

The lymphatic drainage of the extrahepatic biliary system was extensively studied and reported by Caplan [25] in 1982 (Fig. 1.20).

1.2.5.10 Lymphatic Drainage of the Supraduodenal and Retroduodenal Portions of the Extrahepatic Bile Ducts

The lymphatic drainage follows two pathways both of which ultimately drain into the thoracic duct:

1. Superior Pathway (or the left pathway by Nimura)
   A superior pathway follows the lymphatics and lymph nodes along the cystic duct (inconstant), the hepatic artery, the anterior and medial aspects of the portal vein and the coeliac axis.

   Using the lymph node station numbers used by the Japanese Gastric Cancer Association [26] published in 1998, the pathway of spread along the nodes is #12a → 8 → 9 → 16.

   The pathway is a more important pathway of spread of malignancy from the extrahepatic bile ducts than the inferior pathway.

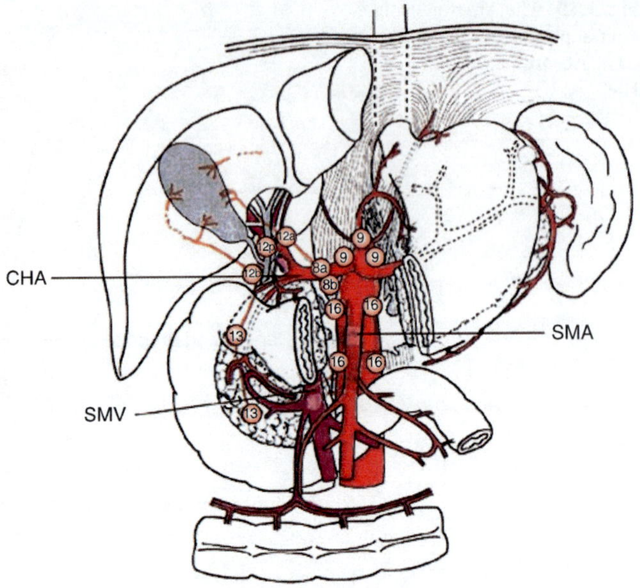

Fig. 1.20 Lymphatic drainage of the extrahepatic biliary system. *SMA* Superior mesenteric artery, *SMV* Superior mesenteric vein, *CHA* Common hepatic artery. *Numbers*: lymph node station numbers used by the Japanese Gastric Cancer Association [26]

2. An inferior pathway (or the right pathway by Nimura)
   The pathway of spread of lymphatics is from the lymph nodes along the cystic duct, the anterior and lateral aspects of the portal vein, the posterior aspect of the pancreas, between the aorta and the inferior vena cava, and the left aspect of the aorta under the left renal vein.

   In the Japanese system, the spread is #12b → 13a → 16.

1.2.5.11 Lymphatic Drainage from the Paraduodenal and Intraduodenal Portions of the Extrahepatic Bile Ducts

The lymphatic drainage from this portion of the bile duct is to the adjacent lymph nodes in the portal pedicle, and then via either the superior (left) or the inferior (right) pathway.

1.2.5.12 Lymphatic Drainage from the Gallbaldder

According to the study by Caplan [25], the lymphatic drainage is more complicated and there are four possible routes of lymphatic drainage from the gallbladder to reach the two pathways as described above:

1. Superior and external pedicle
   Present in 6 % of individuals, draining the fundus of the gallbladder through the hepatic parenchyma of liver segment 5, to join the inferior (or right pathway).
2. Superior and medial pedicle
   Present in 10 % of individuals. Draining the medial aspect of the gallbladder to the hilum after transversing the hepatic parenchyma of liver segment 4 to join the left pathway.

3. Inferior and external pedicle
   Present in 82 % of individuals. Draining the body of the gallbladder to the portal pedicle, finally joining the right pathway.
4. Inferior and medial aspect of pedicle
   This is constant. Drainage from the body of the gallbladder to the lymphatics along the anterior and medial aspects of the portal vein and the left pathway (Fig. 1.20).

1.2.5.13 Clinical Significance of Pattern of Lymphatic Drainage of the Extraheptic Biliary System

The significance is:

1. Lymphatic spread of tumours of the gallbladder and bile duct can be extensive, and it follows two main pathways, thereby making cure by radical surgery even with lymphatic clearance difficult;
2. Carcinoma of gallbladder can spread to the parenchyma of the liver by lymphatic spread making concomitant liver resection necessary for radical surgery.

1.2.5.14 Innervation of the Biliary Tract

A detailed discussion of the innervation of the biliary tract is beyond the scope of this chapter. Only a brief summary of the extrinsic innervation is presented.

The extrinsic nerve supply to the biliary tract is both autonomic (parasympathetic and sympathetic) and sensory. The anterior and posterior vagus nerves carry both parasympathetic motor fibres and sensory fibres. The sympathetic nerve supply is from both the coeliac ganglion and the superior mesenteric ganglion. The pain fibres to the target tissues are post-ganglionic fibres, explaining why sympathetectomy may be effective in the relief of pain.

The intrinsic nerve supply consists of ganglionatic plexuses within the wall of the gallbladder, bile ducts and sphincter of Oddi. Nerve fibres from the ganglia innervate the mucosa, blood vessels and muscle of the biliary tract. The nerve fibres from the extrinsic sources may innervate the target tissues directly, or they may provide neural inputs to the intrinsic ganglia. The arrangement is very complex and this complex neural supply is important in controlling motility of the gallbladder and sphincter of Oddi, blood flow either to the whole biliary tract or to any part thereof, or may even facilitate changes in mucosal transport of water and electrolyte (e.g., in the gallbladder) [1].

1.2.5.15 Hepatic Hilar Plate System

The fusion of Glisson's capsule with the connective tissue sheaths surrounding the biliary and vascular elements at the inferior aspect of the liver constitute to the hepatic hilar plate system. This plate system contains a larger number of lymphatics, nerves and a small vascular network. Although most workers consider the portal triad to be within the plate system,

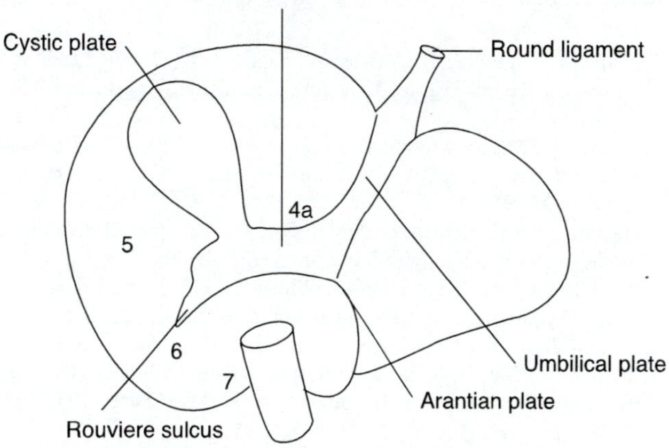

Fig. 1.21 Visceral surface of liver showing the hepatic hilar plate system. Please note that Rouviere sulcus separates the right anterior section (segments 5, 8) and posterior section (segments 6, 7)

Couinaud states that the bile duct and hepatic artery are located within the plate system, but the portal vein is covered with a separate sheath of loose connective tissues. This is the reason why the plate containing the extrahepatic bile duct and hepatic artery can be separated easily from the portal vein [8, 24].

The hepatic hilar plate system includes the hilar plate above the biliary confluence, the cystic plate at the gallbladder fossa, the umbilical plate situated above the umbilical portion of the left portal vein, and the Arantian plate covering the ligamentum venosum [27] (Fig. 1.21).

1.2.5.16 Clinical Significance of the Hepatic Hilar Plate System

The clinical significance is:

1. Hepp and Couinaud in 1956 described a technique where, by lifting the liver segment 4 upwards and incising the Glisson's capsule at its base, good exposure of the hepatic hilar structures can be obtained [28]. This technique is now referred to as lowering of the hilar plate. It can be carried out with safety since there is only exceptionally (in 1 % of cases) any vascular interposition between the hilar plate and the inferior aspect of the liver. The manoeuvre is of particular value in exposing the extrahepatic segment of the left hepatic duct since it has a long courses beneath segment 4. This technique is important for the identification of the left hepatic duct during bile duct repair following injury, or for a palliative side-to-side left duct to jejunum bypass in patients with unresectable hilar or right ductal carcinoma.
2. In treatment of hilar cholangiocarcinoma, it is important to resect the hilar duct confluence en bloc with the hilar plate (and in most cases, combined with liver resection including segment 1 of the liver) because tumour cells can easily invade into the adjacent plate tissues (and along the bile duct branches into segment 1 of the liver).

References

1. Padbury P, Azoulay D. Anatomy. Chapter 1. In: Toouli J, editor. Surgery of the biliary tract. New York: Churchill Livingstone; 1993. p. 3–19.
2. Strasberg SM. Liver terminology and anatomy. Chapter 2. In: Lau WY, editor. Hepatocellular carcinoma. New Jersey: World Scientific; 2008. p. 25–50.
3. Terminology Committee of the IHPBA. The Brisbane 2000 terminology of liver anatomy and resection. HPB. 2000;2:333–9.
4. Skandalakis JE, Shandalakis LE, Shandalakis PW, et al. Hepatic surgical anatomy. Surg Clin North Am. 2004;84:413–35.
5. Healey Jr JE, Schroy IC. Anatomy of the biliary ducts within the human liver: analysis of the prevailing pattern of branchings and the major variations of the biliary ducts. Arch Surg. 1953;66: 599–616.
6. Lau WY. Caudate lobe. Chapter 3. In: Lau WY, editor. Applied anatomy in liver resection and liver transplantation. Beijing: People's Medical Publishing House; 2010. p. 22–30.
7. Blumgart LH, Hann LE. Surgical and radiologic anatomy of the liver, biliary tract and pancreas. Chapter 1. In: Blumgart LH, editor. Surgery of the liver, biliary tract, and pancreas. Philadelphia: Saunders Elsevier; 2007. p. 3–29.
8. Couinaud C. Controlled hepatectomies and exposure of the intrahepatic bile ducts. Anatomical and technical study. Paris: C. Couinaud; 1981.
9. Kida H, Uchimura M, Okamoto K. Intrahepatic architecture of bile and portal vein (in Japanese). Tan To Sui (J Biliary Tract and Pancreas). 1987;8:1–7.
10. Ischiyama S, Yamada Y, Narishima Y, et al. Surgical anatomy of the hilar bile duct carcinoma (in Japanese). Tan To Sui (J Biliary Tract and Pancreas). 1999;20:811–29.
11. Kumon M. Portal vein and bile duct branches of the caudate lobe: analysis of liver casts and clinical cases (in Japanese). Kanzou (Acta Hepatol Jpn). 1985;55:1193–9.
12. Lau WY. Intrahepatic Glissonian triad. Chapter 6. In: Lau WY, editor. Applied anatomy in liver resection and liver transplantation. Beijing: People's Medical Publishing House; 2010. p. 45–59.
13. Michels NA. Newer anatomy of the liver and its variation in blood supply and collateral circulation. Am J Surg. 1966;112:337–46.
14. Syzuki H. Correlation and anomalies of the vascular structure in Glisson's area around the hepatic hilum, from the standpoint of hepatobilairy surgery (in Japanese). Nihon Geka Hokan. 1982;51:713–31.
15. Chen WJ, Ying DJ, Liu ZJ, et al. Analysis of the arterial supply of the extrahepatic bile ducts and its clinical significance. Clin Anat. 1999;12:245–9.
16. Shapiro AL, Robillard GL. The arterial blood supply of the common and hepatic bile ducts with reference to the problems of common duct injury and repair. Surgery. 1948;23:1–11.
17. Rath AM, Zhang J, Bourdelat D, et al. Arterial vascularization of the extrahepatic tract. Surg Radiol Anat. 1993;15:105–11.
18. Northover JM, Terblanche J. Bile duct blood supply. Its importance in human liver transplantation. Transplantation. 1978;26:67–9.
19. Parke WW, Michels NA, Ghosh GM. Blood supply of the common bile duct. Surg Gynecol Obstet. 1963;117:47–55.
20. Pforringer L. Die gerfarbe des ducts choledochus. Acta Anat. 1971;79:389–408.
21. Douglass TC, Cutter WW. Arterial blood supply of the common bile duct. Arch Surg. 1948;57:599–612.
22. Northover JMA, Terblanche J. A new look at the arterial supply of the bile duct in man and its surgical implications. Br J Surg. 1979;66:379–84.
23. Appleby CH. Indwelling common duct tubes. J Int Coll Surg. 1959; 31:631–43.
24. Couinaud C. Surgical anatomy of the liver revisited. Paris: C. Couinaud; 1989.
25. Caplan I. Drainage lymphatique intra at extra-hepatique de la vesicule biliarie. Bulletin Mein. Acad Med Belg. 1982;137:324–34.
26. Japanese Gastric Cancer Association. Japanese classification of gastric cancer—2nd English edition. Gastric Cancer. 1998;1: 10–24.
27. Lau WY. Hepatic Hilar plate system. Chapter 4. In: Lau WY, editor. Applied anatomy in liver resection and liver transplantation. Beijing: People's Medical Publishing House; 2010. p. 31–40.
28. Hepp J, Couinaud C. Approach to and use of the left hepatic duct in reparation of the common bile duct. Presse Med. 1959;64:947–8.

Epidemiology

2

G.L. Tyson, S. Keihanian, and H.B. El-Serag

Cholangiocarcinoma is the second most common primary hepatic malignancy after hepatocellular cancer. It accounts for approximately 10–25 % of all hepatobiliary malignancies. Hilar cholangiocarcinoma is identified based on anatomic location, but the epidemiology is typically aggregated with all cholangiocarcinomas. There are considerable geographic and demographic variations in the incidence of cholangiocarcinoma. These variations are related to risk factors, some of which are established (parasitic infections, primary sclerosing cholangitis, biliary-duct cysts, hepatolithiasis, toxins) and others that are less-established or potential risk factors (inflammatory bowel disease, hepatitis C virus, hepatitis B virus, cirrhosis, diabetes, obesity, alcohol, smoking, host genetic polymorphisms).

2.1 Introduction

Cholangiocarcinoma (CC) accounts for approximately 3 % of gastrointestinal tumors [1–3]. It is the second most common primary hepatic malignancy, representing 10–25 % of primary hepatic malignancies worldwide [1, 4, 5]. Hilar cholangiocarcinoma known as Klatskin tumors, are typically considered extrahepatic (ECC). They are frequently reported to comprise 40–60 % of all CC, but this estimate is derived from a limited number of hospital-based studies, with other hospital and population-based data suggesting a lower proportion of hilar cholangiocarcinomas (5–40 %) [2, 6–8].

There are no population-based studies examining the epidemiology of hilar CC specifically. The epidemiology of hilar CC in terms of incidence and risk factors is aggregated with the epidemiology of CC overall, intrahepatic (ICC) or extrahepatic [9–20].

CC rarely occurs before the age of 40; the typical age at presentation is in the seventh decade of life [3, 4]. There is a higher incidence of CC in men than women, with men to women ratios of 1: (1.2–1.5) [3, 4, 21–25]. The incidence of CC varies greatly by geographic region secondary to variations in risk factors among different regions [3, 5]. The prognosis of CC is poor and, therefore, the mortality and incidence rates are similar.

Population-based CC incidence data are sparse. Most cancer registries tend to combine cases of CC with other liver and biliary malignancies, such as hepatocellular carcinoma and gallbladder cancer [22, 24]. Worldwide the incidence of CC varies greatly (Fig. 2.1) [3, 24]. Thailand has the highest incidence of CC with 113 per 100,000 in men and 50 per 100,000 in women; while in western countries such as Australia the incidence is low at 0.2 per 100,000 in men and 0.1 per 100,000 in women [3, 5]. Differing exposure to risk factors is thought to account for the varying geographic incidences, with parasitic infections and hepatolithiasis being more prevalent in Asia [3, 5]. Studies of temporal trends reported increased incidence of ICC and decreased incidence of ECC [22, 24]. The role of misclassification and reclassification may be substantial as recent data from the United States (US) shows that the incidence of ICC has declined from 0.85 per 100,000 persons in 1995–1999 to 0.58 per 100,000 in 2000–2005, and that of ECC has increased from 0.82 per 100,000 persons in 1998 to 0.88 per 100,000 in 2000–2005 [21].

Differences among studies, registries, and classification of ICC and ECC may account for some of the temporal variations observed in CC (ICC and ECC). For example, hilar cholangiocarcinoma was not given a unique code in Version

G.L. Tyson, MD
Section of Gastroenterology and Hepatology,
Baylor College of Medicine,
Houston, TX, USA

S. Keihanian, MD
Section of Gastroenterology and Hepatology,
Michael E. DeBakey Veterans Affairs Medical Center,
Baylor College of Medicine,
Houston, TX, USA

H.B. El-Serag, MD, MPH (✉)
Gastroenterology and Hepatology Section,
Houston AV Medical Center and Baylor College of Medicine,
Houston, TX, USA
e-mail: hasheme@bcm.edu

W.Y. Lau (ed.), *Hilar Cholangiocarcinoma*,
DOI 10.1007/978-94-007-6473-6_2, © Springer Science+Business Media Dordrecht and People's Medical Publishing House 2013

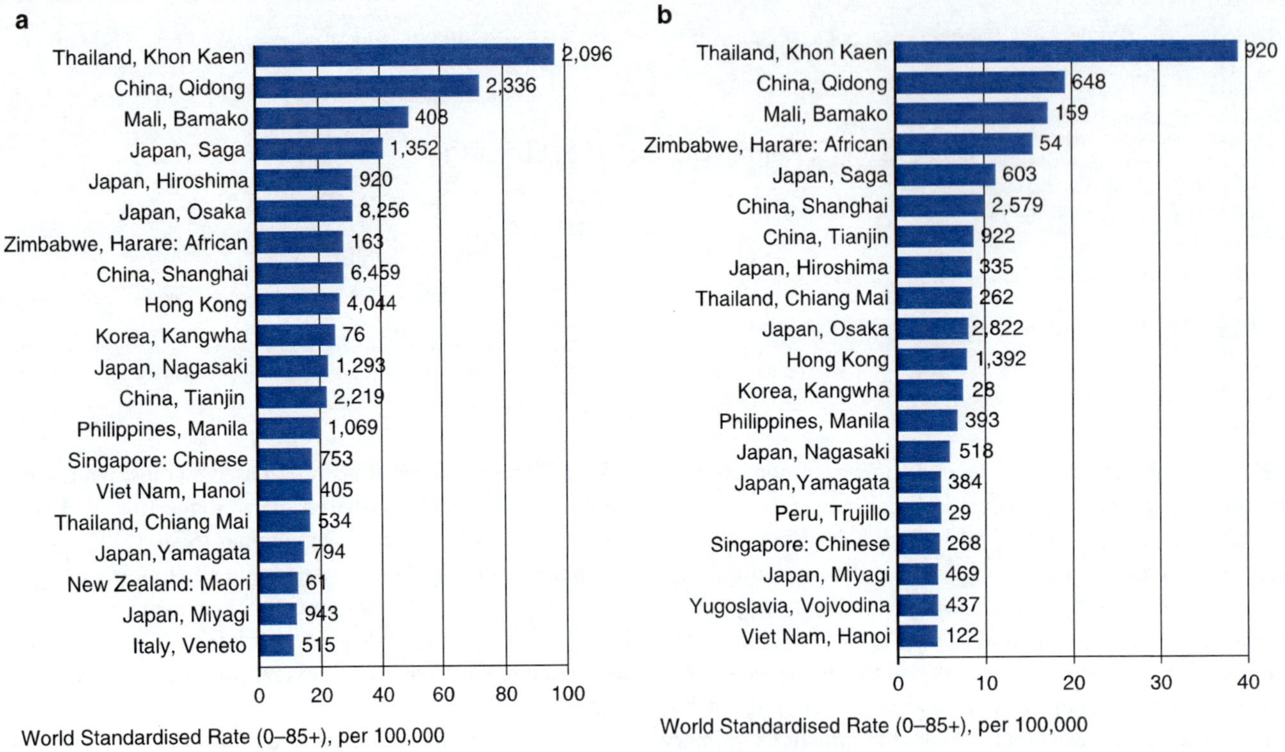

Fig. 2.1 (**a**) The age-adjusted incidence rates of cholangiocarcinoma (CC) in men in 20 different geographic regions. CC has been calculated as primary liver cancer that is not HCC. The frequency of cases is shown to the right of each bar. (**b**) The age-adjusted incidence rates of CC in women in 20 different geographic regions. CC has been calculated as primary liver cancer that is not HCC. The frequency of cases is shown to the right of each bar (Figures obtained from the 1997 publication of the International Agency for Cancer Research)

1 of the ICD-O (International Classification of Diseases for Oncology) (1973–1991); therefore, it could have been characterized topographically as ICC or ECC. In Version 2 of the ICD-O (1992–2000), hilar CC was given a unique histology code that could be linked to ICC rather than ECC. In Version 3 of the ICD-O (2001–present), the histological code for hilar CC could be linked to either ICC or ECC [26].

2.2 Risk Factors for Cholangiocarcinoma

The established risk factors include parasitic infections, biliary-duct cysts, primary sclerosing cholangitis, hepatolithiasis, and toxins. However, most patients do not have identifiable specific risk factors [1, 4]. Other less-established, potential risk factors include inflammatory bowel disease (IBD), hepatitis C virus (HCV), hepatitis B virus (HBV), cirrhosis, diabetes, obesity, alcohol, smoking, and host genetic polymorphisms (Table 2.1). In studies where the distinction between ICC and ECC was used, some potential risk factors seem to have differential effect on CC depending on site. It is unclear how hilar CC factors into these considerations. It is therefore possible that the consistent use of a more refined classification would allow better understanding of risk factors for cholangiocarcinoma.

Table 2.1 Risk factors for cholangiocarcinoma

Established	Less established	Potential[a]
Parasitic infections	Inflammatory bowel disease-likely via PSC	Obesity
Bile-duct cysts	Cirrhosis	Tobacco smoking
Primary sclerosing cholangitis (PSC)	Hepatitis C virus	Genetic polymorphisms
Hepatolithiasis	Hepatitis B virus	
Thorotrast contrast agent	Diabetes	
	Heavy alcohol use	

[a]Inconclusive data

2.2.1 Established Risk Factors for Cholangiocarcinoma

2.2.1.1 Parasitic Infections

The hepatobiliary flukes *Opisthorchis viverrini (O. viverrini)* and *Clonorchis sinensis (C. sinensis)* are associated with the development of CC irrespective of site, particularly in Southeast Asia. They are trematodes that inhabit the bile ducts and, occasionally, the gallbladder and pancreatic duct of mammals. Eggs laid by the adult worms are passed in feces, which may be ingested by snails, where they hatch and then mature into cercariae and subsequently penetrate the flesh of freshwater fish, where they develop into metacercariae. Infestation in humans occurs via ingestion of raw, pickled or undercooked fish [27, 28].

Both parasites increase the susceptibility of cholangiocytes to endogenous and exogenous carcinogens via chronic irritation and increased cellular turnover. Immunopathologic mechanisms, including inflammation and periductal fibrosis combined with proliferative responses, including epithelial hyperplasia, goblet-cell metaplasia, and adenomatous hyperplasia, may enhance susceptibility to carcinogens [27, 28].

One of the early epidemiological studies (1987–1988) to show a relationship between *O. viverrini* and CC was a hospital-based, case-control study conducted in Thailand in which 103 patients with CC were compared with an equal number of age- and sex-matched controls. A strong association was found between elevated *O. viverrini* antibody titers and increased risk of CC (OR 5.0; 95 % CI 2.3–11.0) [29]. A more recent (1999–2001) population-based, case-control study from Thailand compared 129 cases of CC with an equal number of age- and sex-matched controls. Elevated *O. viverrini* antibody levels were again strongly associated with CC (OR 27.09; CI 6.30–116.57) [30]. Based on this study, the population attributable risk due to *O. viverrini* was as high as 88 %.

A case-control study from Korea compared 41 patients with CC with 406 controls and reported a strong association between the presence of *C. sinensis* in the stool and CC (RR 2.7; 95 % CI 1.1–6.3) [31]. A subsequent meta-analysis pooled 912 cases and 4,909 controls and confirmed the strong association between *C. sinensis* and CC (OR 4.7; CI 2.2–9.8). In endemic areas, the population attributable risk based on this study was as high as 27.9 % for men and 16.2 % for women [18].

2.2.1.2 Biliary-Tract Disorders

Bile-Duct Cysts

Bile (choledochal)-duct cysts are rare congenital disorders characterized by cystic dilatation of the extrahepatic and/or intrahepatic bile ducts. There are several types of bile-duct cysts, which include the more commonly known choledochocele (extrahepatic biliary cyst) and Caroli's disease (intrahepatic biliary cysts) [32].

Bile-duct cysts are an established risk factor for CC. It has been postulated that the reflux of pancreatic enzymes, bile stasis, and increased concentration of intraductal bile acids contribute to the formation of malignant cells in patients with bile-duct cysts [32]. The lifetime incidence of CC in these patients ranges from 6 to 30 % [4, 32]. The prevalence of bile-duct cysts is higher in Asian than Western countries [14, 32–35]. The incidence of CC is also higher in Asians with bile-duct cysts, at approximately 18 %, with the US incidence closer to 6 % [19, 33–36]. Patients with bile-duct cysts are reported to have at least 10- to 50-fold increased risk of developing CC compared with the general population [20, 32, 37]. There is an increase in incidence of CC in patients with bile-duct cysts from 0.7 % in the first decade of life to >14 % after the age of 20 [38]. The average age at malignancy detection has been reported to be 32 years, which is younger than the age at presentation of CC in the general population [32, 36]. The risk of malignancy decreases in patients undergoing complete choledochal cyst excision; however, these patients are still at a significantly increased risk of developing CC compared with the general population [14, 19, 32–34].

Primary Sclerosing Cholangitis

Primary sclerosing cholangitis (PSC), an autoimmune disease that results in stricturing of extrahepatic and/or intrahepatic bile ducts, is an established risk factor for CC. Chronic inflammation, proliferation of biliary epithelium, production of endogenous bile mutagens, and bile stasis are postulated mechanisms of carcinogenesis [2]. The lifetime incidence of CC among PSC patients ranges from 6 to 36 % [39, 40]. Although PSC is known to be a strong risk factor for CC, no more than 10 % of CC is attributed to PSC [40].

A hospital-based, retrospective cohort study from the Mayo Clinic followed 161 patients with PSC for a median of 11.5 years; 11 patients (6.8 %) developed CC with an incidence rate of 0.6 % per year. The median time from diagnosis of PSC to diagnosis of CC was 4.1 years (range 0.8–15.0 years), and no association was found between the duration of PSC and the risk of CC [41]. Another hospital-based, retrospective cohort from the Netherlands followed 211 patients with PSC for a median of 9 years; 15 patients (7 %) developed CC with a 10 and 20 year incidence of 7 %. Again there was no association between duration of PSC and the risk of CC; nearly all the cases of CC presented within 3 years of PSC diagnosis [39]. It is unclear whether duration of PSC or underlying IBD correlates with the risk of developing CC, in fact most cases present relatively soon after PSC diagnosis. Cohort studies suggest that CC develops within the first 1–2 years of PSC diagnosis. A European cohort study found that 48 of 394 (12.2 %) PSC patients developed CC, with 24 (50 %) of them being diagnosed within 1 year of the diagnosis of PSC [42]. In a Swedish cohort study 14 of 125 (11.2 %) PSC patients developed CC. Eleven of the 14 (~78 %) were diagnosed with CC within 2 years of the diagnosis of PSC [43].

Two large population-based US studies showed a strong positive association of CC with choledocholithiasis and cholangitis [16, 20]. However, these studies could not definitively exclude PSC-associated cholangitis; therefore, it is unclear if choledocholithiasis and/or cholangitis are independent risk factors for ICC or ECC.

Hepatolithiasis

Hepatolithiasis are calculi or concretions located proximal to the confluence of the right and left hepatic ducts and/or their tributaries. Hepatolithiasis are found mainly in Southeast

Asia (e.g., up to 20 % in Taiwan) and are rare in the West (1–2 %). It has been postulated that prolonged irritation and inflammation of the biliary epithelium by the calculi, bile stasis, and bacterial infections predispose to malignancy [44, 45]. Additionally, infestation with parasites such as *Clonorchis sinensis* and *Ascaris lumbricoides* has been shown in up to 30 % of patients with hepatolithiasis [46].

Hepatolithiasis is an established risk factor for ICC in Asian countries, with 2–10 % of patients with hepatolithiasis developing ICC [4, 44, 45]. A Korean, hospital-based, case-control study found a strong association between hepatolithiasis and ICC, with an OR of 50.0 (95 % CI 21.2–117.3) [37]. A Chinese, hospital-based, case-control study also showed a significant association, with the OR at 5.8 (95 % CI 1.97–16.9) [47]. There is less data on the relationship between hepatolithiasis and ICC in Western countries; but an Italian, hospital-based case-control study also showed a significant association between hepatolithiasis and ICC, with an OR of 6.7 (95 % CI 1.3–33.4) [48].

2.2.1.3 Toxins

The currently banned carcinogenic agent Thorotrast, a radiographic contrast agent used primarily from 1930 to 1960, has been strongly associated with an increased risk of developing CC. Several large studies from Japan, Germany and Denmark have also shown a significantly increased risk of CC among patients exposed to Thorotrast [49–52]. The estimated latency period between exposure and malignancy diagnosis ranges between 16 and 45 years; this is because the biological half-life of Thorotrast is 400 years [51].

2.2.2 Possible Risk Factors for Cholangiocarcinoma

2.2.2.1 Chronic Viral Hepatitis and Cirrhosis

Hepatitis C virus (HCV), hepatitis B virus (HBV) and liver cirrhosis, regardless of etiology, have been postulated as risk factors for CC.

Asian Studies

Hospital based studies including one cohort study and several case-control studies examined viral hepatitis in relation to CC. A prospective cohort study from Japan followed 600 patients with HCV-related cirrhosis for a median of 7.2 years. Fourteen patients (2.3 %) developed CC during the observation period, resulting in incidence rates at 5 and 10 years of 1.6 and 3.5 %, respectively. These rates were 1,000 times higher than in the general Japanese population [13]. A Korean case-control study compared 41 cases of CC with 406 noncancer controls did not find a significant association between HBV or HCV seropositivity and CC. However, having a history of hepatitis was associated with CC, with an RR of 22.4 (95 % CI 3.4–146.2) [31]. In another Korean case-control study that compared 622 cases of ICC with 2,488 controls, there was a significant association between ICC and HBV (OR 2.3; 95 % CI 1.6–3.3) as well as cirrhosis of any etiology (OR 13.6; 95 % CI 6.5–28.5). There was no significant association between HCV seropositivity and ICC [37]. A case-control study from China compared 312 ICC cases with 438 controls and reported a strong association between ICC and HBV seropositivity, with an OR of 8.9 (95 % CI 5.97–13.2) but no significant association with HCV seropositivity [47]. Lastly, a case-control study from Japan reported that HCV was a significant risk factor for ICC, with an OR of 6.02 (95 % CI 1.51–24.1). The presence of cirrhosis merely trended towards significance, whereas HBV infection was not a significant risk factor for ICC [53].

European Studies

Few Western European studies reported an association between CC and both HCV and cirrhosis. A large, population-based cohort study from Denmark examined cancer risk in 11,605 patients with cirrhosis over a mean follow-up period of 6 years, and reported a tenfold increased risk of CC among patients with cirrhosis compared with the expected cancer cases in the general population (standardized incidence ratio of 21 versus 2) [54]. A hospital-based, case-control study in Italy compared 26 ICC cases with 824 controls. Both HCV and HBV seropositivity was analyzed, but only HCV was significantly associated with ICC; OR 9.7 (95 % CI 1.6–58.9) [48].

US Studies

Several US studies have shown an association between the presence of HCV and/or cirrhosis and increased risk of ICC. A hospital-based, case-control study compared 83 patients with ICC and 163 with ECC to 236 controls. HCV was a significant risk factor for ICC with an OR of 7.9 (95 % CI 1.3–84.5). Cirrhosis was not analyzed as a separate variable, but 80 % of HCV-positive patients had cirrhosis. For ECC, neither HCV nor HBV status was a significant risk factor [17]. A large, population-based, case-control study compared 625 cases of ICC with 90,834 controls. In multivariate analysis, HCV was significantly associated with ICC, with an OR of 5.2 (95 % CI 2.1–12.8). It was unclear if patients with HCV also had a recorded diagnostic code for cirrhosis. However, nonspecific cirrhosis was strongly associated with ICC, with an OR of 27.2 (95 % CI 19.9–37.1). In the same study, the prevalence of HBV infection was similar in cases and controls (0.2 %) [16]. A similar population-based, case-control study examined risk factors for both ICC and ECC. There were 549 cases of ECC and 535 cases of ICC compared with 102,782 controls. Similar to the findings of the previous population-based study, significant risk factors for ICC included HCV and nonspecific cirrhosis. Regarding ECC, nonspecific cirrhosis was also a risk factor, but HCV

Table 2.2 Diabetes as a potential risk factor for cholangiocarcinoma. All studies shown in the table were case-control in design

First author (Country)	Study dates	CC type	Cases (% with risk factor)	Controls (% with risk factor)	Risk estimate (95 % CI)
Welzel [56] (Denmark)	1978–1991	ICC	764 (1.96 %)	3,056 (1.41 %)	1.43 (0.8–2.6)
Grainge [57] (United Kingdom)	1987–2002	NS	372 (9.4 %)	5,760 (5.9 %)	1.48 (1.0–2.2)
Yamamoto [53] (Japan)	1991–2002	ICC	50 (22 %)	205 (12 %)	1.95 (0.6–5.8)
Shaib [17] (US)	1992–2002	ICC	83 (14.5 %)	236 (8.5 %)	Not calculated
		ECC	163 (11.7 %)	236 (8.5 %)	Not calculated
Shaib [16] (US)	1993–1999	ICC	625 (26.4 %)	90,834 (15.6 %)	2.0 (1.6–2.4)
Welzel [20] (US)	1993–1999	ICC	535 (33.1 %)	102,782 (22.1 %)	1.8 (1.5–2.1)
		ECC	549 (30.1 %)	102,782 (22.1 %)	1.5 (1.3–1.8)
Lee [37] (Korea)	2000–2004	ICC	622 (15.4 %)	2,488 (5.6 %)	3.2 (2.3–4.3)
Zhou [47] (China)	2004–2006	ICC	312 (4.2 %)	438 (2.5 %)	1.5 (0.6–3.8)

infection was not significant [20]. A large cohort study of US veterans examined the association between HCV and both ICC and ECC in a cohort of 146,394 HCV-infected veterans and 572,293 uninfected controls. The risk for ICC in the HCV-infected cohort, though low at 4 per 100,000 person-years, was more than double that in the controls (HR 2.55; 95 % CI 1.31–4.95). The risk of ECC did not differ between the HCV-infected and uninfected veterans (4.3 vs. 4.2 per 100,000 person-years) [10].

The association of these risk factors with CC is not entirely clear, as studies have differing conclusions; and there is a paucity of population-based or prospective cohort studies. In countries such as Korea and Thailand where both HBV and CC are endemic, data show HBV but not HCV as a risk factor for ICC. On the other hand, countries such as Japan and Western nations, including the United States, where HCV is more prevalent, were more likely to show an association between HCV and ICC [37, 55].

2.2.2.2 Diabetes and Obesity

Population-based case-control studies from the United States and United Kingdom report a significant, but modest association between diabetes and CC (Table 2.2). For example, two large US studies showed a significant positive association between diabetes and CC. The first study looked specifically at ICC and reported an OR of 2.0 (95 % CI 1.6–2.4) with diabetes [16]. The second study found diabetes to be a significant risk factor for both ICC and ECC, with ORs of 1.8 (95 % CI 1.5–2.1) and 1.5 (95 % CI 1.3–1.8), respectively [20]. Another large, population-based, case-control study from the United Kingdom also found a significant association between diabetes and CC, with an OR of 1.48 (95 % CI 1.0–2.2) [57]. Conversely, a population-based study from Denmark did not find a significant association between diabetes and ICC [56]. Additionally, at least three hospital-based, case-control studies failed to show a significant association between diabetes and CC (Table 2.2) [17, 47, 53]. These associations could be confounded by the presence of underlying liver disease which predisposes to diabetes. Case-control studies are typically non informative to this crucial temporal sequence. Given the absence of data from longitudinal cohort studies, the association between diabetes and CC can only be regarded as preliminary.

Obesity was reported as a significant, but weak, risk factor for CC in two population-based, case-control studies. In the UK a BMI $\geq$30 was significantly associated with CC, type not specified, with an OR of 1.52 (95 % CI 1.0–2.2) [57]. The US study reported a significant association between obesity and ICC, with an OR of 1.7 (95 % CI 1.1–2.6), but not between obesity and ECC [20]. However, in the Danish, population-based study there was no significant association between obesity and ICC [56]. The data available on obesity are too limited to make any conclusions.

2.2.2.3 Alcohol Drinking

Several cohort studies and case-control studies have reported a strong association between heavy alcohol use, typically >80 g/day, and CC (Table 2.3). The cohort study from Denmark that examined 11,605 patients with cirrhosis found a significantly increased CC risk, with an RR of 15.3 (95 % CI 8.9–24.5) in individuals with alcoholic cirrhosis [54]. The two US population-based case-control studies also found alcoholic liver disease to be significantly associated with CC. In the first study of ICC, the OR was 7.4 (95 % CI 4.3–12.8) [16]. In the second study of both ICC and ECC, there was an OR of 3.1 (95 % CI 1.3–7.5) and an OR of 4.5 (95 % CI 2.2–9.1), respectively [20]. However, the UK population-based, case-control study did not find alcohol use to be a risk factor for CC [57]. Few hospital-based, case-control studies have shown a significant association between alcohol intake and CC [17, 31, 37]; while others have not (Table 2.3) [47, 48, 53]. Based on the strong magnitude of association (risk estimate range from 2 to 15) and studies with different designs, heavy alcohol use is likely to be a risk factor for CC.

Table 2.3 Alcohol drinking and tobacco smoking as potential risk factors for cholangiocarcinoma. All studies were case–control in design except for Sorensen et al. which was a retrospective cohort

First author (Country)	Study dates	Risk factor	CC type	Cases (% with risk factor)	Controls (% with risk factor)	Risk estimate (95 % CI)
Sorensen [54] (Denmark)	1977–1993	Alcoholic cirrhosis	NS	17	11,605	15.3 (8.9–24.5)
Grainge [57] (United Kingdom)	1987–2002	Smoking (current exposure)	NS	372 (27.5 %)	5,760 (20.9 %)	1.38 (1.0–1.9)
		^Alcohol (problem drinker)	NS	372 (0.3 %)	5,760 (0.7 %)	Not calculated
Shin [31] (Korea)	1990–1993	Heavy smoking (>1 pack/day, >10 years)	NS	41 (36.6 %)	406 (46.8 %)	0.8 (0.2–2.5)
		Heavy alcohol (>80 g/day, >10 years)	NS	41 (22 %)	406 (11.1 %)	4.6 (1.4–15.2)
Yamamoto [53] (Japan)	1991–2002	Smoking (any previous exposure)	ICC	50 (34 %)	205 (44 %)	Not calculated
		Heavy alcohol (>5 go sake/day, >10 years)	ICC	50 (2 %)	205 (5 %)	0.97 (0.5–1.9)
Shaib [17] (US)	1992–2002	Smoking (>25 pack years)	ICC	83 (24.1 %)	236 (15.7 %)	Not calculated
		Smoking (>25 pack years)	ECC	163 (20.9 %)	236 (15.7 %)	Not calculated
		Heavy alcohol (>80 g/day)	ICC	83 (21.7 %)	236 (3.8 %)	5.9 (2.1–17.4)
		Heavy alcohol (>80 g/day)	ECC	163 (17.8 %)	236 (3.8 %)	3.6 (1.5–9.4)
		Mild/moderate alcohol (80 g/day)	ICC	83 (33.7 %)	236 (48.3 %)	Not calculated
		Mild/moderate alcohol (80 g/day)	ECC	163 (26.9 %)	236 (48.3 %)	0.5 (0.3–0.8)
Shaib [16] (US)	1993–1999	^Smoking	ICC	625 (3.8 %)	90,834 (2.1 %)	1.8 (1.2–2.70)
		^Alcoholic liver disease	ICC	625 (2.2 %)	90,834 (0.3 %)	7.4 (4.3–12.8)
Welzel [20] (US)	1993–1999	^Smoking	ICC	535 (2.2 %)	102,782 (1.2 %)	1.8 (1.0–3.2)
		^Smoking	ECC	549 (2.2 %)	102,782 (1.2 %)	1.7 (1.0–3.0)
		^Alcoholic liver disease	ICC	535(0.9 %)	102,782 (0.3 %)	3.1 (1.3–7.5)
		^Alcoholic liver disease	ECC	549 (1.5 %)	102,782 (0.3 %)	4.5 (2.2–9.1)
Donato [48] (Italy)	1995–2000	Heavy alcohol (>80 g/day)	ICC	26 (23.1 %)	824 (33 %)	0.4 (0.2–1.6)
Lee [37] (Korea)	2000–2004	Smoking (any prior exposure)	ICC	622 (47.1 %)	2,488 (45.6 %)	Not calculated
		Heavy alcohol (>80 g/day)	ICC	622 (18 %)	2,488 (3.1 %)	6.6 (4.8–9.2)
Zhou [47] (China)	2004–2006	Smoking (≥4 day/week, ≥6 months)	ICC	312 (13.8 %)	438 (15.3 %)	1.23 (0.7–2.2)
		Alcohol (≥1 drink/week, ≥ 6 months)	ICC	312 (12.5 %)	438 (9.4 %)	0.80 (0.5–1.3)

^Problem drinkers were defined as those with a GPRD code indicating alcohol misuse at any time prior to diagnosis
GPRD General practice research database

2.2.2.4 Tobacco Smoking

The data on a possible association between tobacco smoking and CC are not consistent (Table 2.3). Three large, population-based case-control studies found reported history of tobacco smoking to be weakly associated with CC, with risk estimates from 1.38 to 1.80 [16, 20, 57]; the frequency and duration of smoking was not quantified in these studies. Several other hospital-based case-control studies reported no significant association between smoking and CC [17, 31, 37, 47, 53]. Smoking may be a weak risk factor for CC; but given the conflicting data, a firm conclusion cannot be made.

2.2.2.5 Genetic Factors

Several hospital-based, case-control studies reported that polymorphisms in genes coding for enzymes responsible for metabolism of carcinogens, DNA repair, and inflammation were associated with increased as well as decreased risk of developing CC [12, 58–63]. However, given the varying study populations and lack of study replication in independent cohorts, it is difficult to draw firm conclusions regarding the relevance of genetic polymorphisms.

2.3 Summary

There is limited information of the epidemiology of hilar CC specifically; instead incidence and risk factors data are reported on CC overall or based on ICC and ECC. CC is a rare malignancy in Western countries, but more common in some parts of Asia. This difference is mostly attributed to the higher prevalence of established risk factors like parasitic infestations, bile-duct cysts and hepatolithiasis. However, most cases of CC especially in Western countries are not associated with established risk factors for CC which include parasitic infestations, biliary-duct cysts, primary sclerosing cholangitis, hepatolithiasis and toxins. Less-established risk factors include IBD, HCV, HBV, cirrhosis, obesity, diabetes, alcohol, smoking and genetic polymorphisms. There are not enough consistent data to support that obesity, smoking, or specific genetic polymorphisms confer an increased risk for CC. The available data suggest that diabetes and heavy alcohol drinking may confer an increased risk for CC. The data also suggest that in Western countries HCV is consistently associated with ICC and not ECC. In Asian countries it appears that HBV may be associated with ICC. Cirrhosis is the most consistently illustrated risk factor for ICC, but not ECC. In studies where the distinction between ICC and ECC was used, some potential risk factors seem to have differential effect on CC depending on site.

References

1. Gatto M, Bragazzi MC, Semeraro R, et al. Cholangiocarcinoma: update and future perspectives. Dig Liver Dis. 2010;42(4):253–60.
2. Patel T. Cholangiocarcinoma. Nat Clin Pract Gastroenterol Hepatol. 2006;3(1):33–42.
3. Shaib Y, El-Serag HB. The epidemiology of cholangiocarcinoma. Semin Liver Dis. 2004;24(2):115–25.
4. Blechacz BR, Gores GJ. Cholangiocarcinoma. Clin Liver Dis. 2008;12(1):131–50.
5. Sripa B, Pairojkul C. Cholangiocarcinoma: lessons from Thailand. Curr Opin Gastroenterol. 2008;24(3):349–56.
6. Chamberlain RS, Blumgart LH. Hilar cholangiocarcinoma: a review and commentary. Ann Surg Oncol. 2000;7(1):55–66.
7. Ebata T, Kamiya J, Nishio H, et al. The concept of perihilar cholangiocarcinoma is valid. Br J Surg. 2009;96(8):926–34.
8. Nakeeb A, Pitt HA, Sohn TA, et al. Cholangiocarcinoma. A spectrum of intrahepatic, perihilar, and distal tumors. Ann Surg. 1996;224(4):463–73.
9. Alvaro D, Crocetti E, Ferretti S, et al. Descriptive epidemiology of cholangiocarcinoma in Italy. Dig Liver Dis. 2010;42(7):490–5.
10. El-Serag HB, Engels EA, Landgren O, et al. Risk of hepatobiliary and pancreatic cancers after hepatitis C virus infection: a population-based study of U.S. veterans. Hepatology. 2009;49(1):116–23.
11. Erichsen R, Jepsen P, Vilstrup H, et al. Incidence and prognosis of cholangiocarcinoma in Danish patients with and without inflammatory bowel disease: a national cohort study, 1978–2003. Eur J Epidemiol. 2009;24(9):513–20.
12. Hoblinger A, Grunhage F, Sauerbruch T, et al. Association of the c.3972C>T variant of the multidrug resistance-associated protein 2 Gene (MRP2/ABCC2) with susceptibility to bile duct cancer. Digestion. 2009;80(1):36–9.
13. Kobayashi M, Ikeda K, Saitoh S, et al. Incidence of primary cholangiocellular carcinoma of the liver in Japanese patients with hepatitis C virus-related cirrhosis. Cancer. 2000;88(11):2471–7.
14. Kobayashi S, Asano T, Yamasaki M, et al. Risk of bile duct carcinogenesis after excision of extrahepatic bile ducts in pancreaticobiliary maljunction. Surgery. 1999;126(5):939–44.
15. Rosen CB, Nagorney DM, Wiesner RH, et al. Cholangiocarcinoma complicating primary sclerosing cholangitis. Ann Surg. 1991; 213(1):21–5.
16. Shaib YH, El-Serag HB, Davila JA, et al. Risk factors of intrahepatic cholangiocarcinoma in the United States: a case-control study. Gastroenterology. 2005;128(3):620–6.
17. Shaib YH, El-Serag HB, Nooka AK, et al. Risk factors for intrahepatic and extrahepatic cholangiocarcinoma: a hospital-based case-control study. Am J Gastroenterol. 2007;102(5):1016–21.
18. Shin HR, Oh JK, Lim MK, et al. Descriptive epidemiology of cholangiocarcinoma and clonorchiasis in Korea. J Korean Med Sci. 2010;25(7):1011–6.
19. Watanabe Y, Toki A, Todani T. Bile duct cancer developed after cyst excision for choledochal cyst. J Hepatobiliary Pancreat Surg. 1999;6(3):207–12.
20. Welzel TM, Graubard BI, El-Serag HB, et al. Risk factors for intrahepatic and extrahepatic cholangiocarcinoma in the United States: a population-based case-control study. Clin Gastroenterol Hepatol. 2007;5(10):1221–8.
21. Surveillance, Epidemiology, and End Results (SEER) Program. Research Data (1973–2007), National Cancer Institute, DCCPS, Surveillance Research Program, Cancer Statistics Branch. 2011. www.seer.cancer.gov. Released April 2010, based on the November 2009 submission.
22. Khan SA, Toledano MB, Taylor-Robinson SD. Epidemiology, risk factors, and pathogenesis of cholangiocarcinoma. HPB (Oxford). 2008;10(2):77–82.
23. Patel T. Increasing incidence and mortality of primary intrahepatic cholangiocarcinoma in the United States. Hepatology. 2001; 33(6):1353–7.
24. Patel T. Worldwide trends in mortality from biliary tract malignancies. BMC Cancer. 2002;2:10.
25. Taylor-Robinson SD, Toledano MB, Arora S, et al. Increase in mortality rates from intrahepatic cholangiocarcinoma in England and Wales 1968–1998. Gut. 2001;48(6):816–20.
26. Welzel TM, McGlynn KA, Hsing AW, et al. Impact of classification of hilar cholangiocarcinomas (Klatskin tumors) on the incidence of intra- and extrahepatic cholangiocarcinoma in the United States. J Natl Cancer Inst. 2006;98(12):873–5.
27. Kaewpitoon N, Kaewpitoon SJ, Pengsaa P, et al. Opisthorchis viverrini: the carcinogenic human liver fluke. World J Gastroenterol. 2008;14(5):666–74.
28. Upatham ES, Viyanant V. Opisthorchis viverrini and opisthorchiasis: a historical review and future perspective. Acta Trop. 2003; 88(3):171–6.
29. Parkin DM, Srivatanakul P, Khlat M, et al. Liver cancer in Thailand I. A case-control study of cholangiocarcinoma. Int J Cancer. 1991;48(3):323–8.
30. Honjo S, Srivatanakul P, Sriplung H, et al. Genetic and environmental determinants of risk for cholangiocarcinoma via Opisthorchis viverrini in a densely infested area in Nakhon Phanom, northeast Thailand. Int J Cancer. 2005;117(5):854–60.
31. Shin HR, Lee CU, Park HJ, et al. Hepatitis B and C virus, Clonorchis sinensis for the risk of liver cancer: a case-control study in Pusan, Korea. Int J Epidemiol. 1996;25(5):933–40.
32. Soreide K, Korner H, Havnen J, et al. Bile duct cysts in adults. Br J Surg. 2004;91(12):1538–48.
33. Edil BH, Cameron JL, Reddy S, et al. Choledochal cyst disease in children and adults: a 30-year single-institution experience. J Am Coll Surg. 2008;206(5):1000–5.
34. Mabrut JY, Bozio G, Hubert C, et al. Management of congenital bile duct cysts. Dig Surg. 2010;27(1):12–8.
35. Yamaguchi M. Congenital choledochal cyst. Analysis of 1433 patients in the Japanese literature. Am J Surg. 1980;140(5): 653–7.
36. Todani T, Watanabe Y, Toki A, et al. Carcinoma related to choledochal cysts with internal drainage operations. Surg Gynecol Obstet. 1987;164(1):61–4.
37. Lee TY, Lee SS, Jung SW, et al. Hepatitis B virus infection and intrahepatic cholangiocarcinoma in Korea: a case-control study. Am J Gastroenterol. 2008;103(7):1716–20.
38. Voyles CR, Smadja C, Shands WC, et al. Carcinoma in choledochal cysts. Age-related incidence. Arch Surg. 1983;118(8):986–8.
39. Claessen MM, Vleggaar FP, Tytgat KM, et al. High lifetime risk of cancer in primary sclerosing cholangitis. J Hepatol. 2009;50(1): 158–64.
40. LaRusso NF, Shneider BL, Black D, et al. Primary sclerosing cholangitis: summary of a workshop. Hepatology. 2006;44(3):746–64.

41. Burak K, Angulo P, Pasha TM, et al. Incidence and risk factors for cholangiocarcinoma in primary sclerosing cholangitis. Am J Gastroenterol. 2004;99(3):523–6.
42. Boberg KM, Bergquist A, Mitchell S, et al. Cholangiocarcinoma in primary sclerosing cholangitis: risk factors and clinical presentation. Scand J Gastroenterol. 2002;37(10):1205–11.
43. Kornfeld D, Ekbom A, Ihre T. Survival and risk of cholangiocarcinoma in patients with primary sclerosing cholangitis. A population-based study. Scand J Gastroenterol. 1997;32(10):1042–5.
44. Kubo S, Kinoshita H, Hirohashi K, et al. Hepatolithiasis associated with cholangiocarcinoma. World J Surg. 1995;19(4):637–41.
45. Lesurtel M, Regimbeau JM, Farges O, et al. Intrahepatic cholangiocarcinoma and hepatolithiasis: an unusual association in Western countries. Eur J Gastroenterol Hepatol. 2002;14(9): 1025–7.
46. Huang MH, Chen CH, Yen CM, et al. Relation of hepatolithiasis to helminthic infestation. J Gastroenterol Hepatol. 2005;20(1): 141–6.
47. Zhou YM, Yin ZF, Yang JM, et al. Risk factors for intrahepatic cholangiocarcinoma: a case-control study in China. World J Gastroenterol. 2008;14(4):632–5.
48. Donato F, Gelatti U, Tagger A, et al. Intrahepatic cholangiocarcinoma and hepatitis C and B virus infection, alcohol intake, and hepatolithiasis: a case-control study in Italy. Cancer Causes Control. 2001;12(10):959–64.
49. Andersson M, Vyberg M, Visfeldt J, et al. Primary liver tumors among Danish patients exposed to Thorotrast. Radiat Res. 1994; 137(2):262–73.
50. Kato I, Kido C. Increased risk of death in thorotrast-exposed patients during the late follow-up period. Jpn J Cancer Res. 1987;78(11):1187–92.
51. Lipshutz GS, Brennan TV, Warren RS. Thorotrast-induced liver neoplasia: a collective review. J Am Coll Surg. 2002;195(5): 713–8.
52. van Kaick G, Wesch H, Luhrs H, et al. Neoplastic diseases induced by chronic alpha-irradiation – epidemiological, biophysical and clinical results of the German Thorotrast Study. J Radiat Res (Tokyo). 1991;32 Suppl 2Suppl 2:20–33.
53. Yamamoto S, Kubo S, Hai S, et al. Hepatitis C virus infection as a likely etiology of intrahepatic cholangiocarcinoma. Cancer Sci. 2004;95(7):592–5.
54. Sorensen HT, Friis S, Olsen JH, et al. Risk of liver and other types of cancer in patients with cirrhosis: a nationwide cohort study in Denmark. Hepatology. 1998;28(4):921–5.
55. Songsivilai S, Dharakul T, Kanistanon D. Hepatitis C virus genotypes in patients with hepatocellular carcinoma and cholangiocarcinoma in Thailand. Trans R Soc Trop Med Hyg. 1996;90(5):505–7.
56. Welzel TM, Mellemkjaer L, Gloria G, et al. Risk factors for intrahepatic cholangiocarcinoma in a low-risk population: a nationwide case-control study. Int J Cancer. 2007;120(3):638–41.
57. Grainge MJ, West J, Solaymani-Dodaran M, et al. The antecedents of biliary cancer: a primary care case-control study in the United Kingdom. Br J Cancer. 2009;100(1):178–80.
58. Huang WY, Gao YT, Rashid A, et al. Selected base excision repair gene polymorphisms and susceptibility to biliary tract cancer and biliary stones: a population-based case-control study in China. Carcinogenesis. 2008;29(1):100–5.
59. Ko KH, Kim NK, Yim DJ, et al. Polymorphisms of 5,10-methylenetetrahydrofolate reductase (MTHFR C677T) and thymidylate synthase enhancer region (TSER) as a risk factor of cholangiocarcinoma in a Korean population. Anticancer Res. 2006; 26(6B):4229–33.
60. Marahatta SB, Punyarit P, Bhudisawasdi V, et al. Polymorphism of glutathione S-transferase omega gene and risk of cancer. Cancer Lett. 2006;236(2):276–81.
61. Melum E, Karlsen TH, Schrumpf E, et al. Cholangiocarcinoma in primary sclerosing cholangitis is associated with NKG2D polymorphisms. Hepatology. 2008;47(1):90–6.
62. Prawan A, Kukongviriyapan V, Tassaneeyakul W, et al. Association between genetic polymorphisms of CYP1A2, arylamine N-acetyltransferase 1 and 2 and susceptibility to cholangiocarcinoma. Eur J Cancer Prev. 2005;14(3):245–50.
63. Sakoda LC, Gao YT, Chen BE, et al. Prostaglandin-endoperoxide synthase 2 (PTGS2) gene polymorphisms and risk of biliary tract cancer and gallstones: a population-based study in Shanghai, China. Carcinogenesis. 2006;27(6):1251–6.

3 Pathology

A.S.-Y. Leong and C. Pairojkul

3.1 Introduction

In 1965, Gerald Klatskin, a pathologist at Yale University, drew attention to an adenocarcinoma in the porta hepatis that had distinctive clinical and pathological features. He concluded that the tumor was frequently overlooked because of failure to clinically probe and explore the biliary confluence and tributaries. In the 13 patients studied, death occurred from obstruction causing hepatocellular failure and hepatobiliary infection, rather than massive infiltration of the liver or extrahepatic metastasis [1]. Adenocarcinoma of the bile duct epithelium or cholangiocarcinoma (CC) at the confluence of the right and left hepatic ducts has come to be known as "Klatskin tumor".

Cholangiocarcinoma (CC) is conventionally divided into three groups, intrahepatic or peripheral CC arising in the liver, hilar CC that arise at the confluence of the right and left hepatic ducts (in this chapter, CC arising in the right and left hepatic bile ducts and the common hepatic bile duct are considered as hilar CC), and distal CC that arise between the hepatic hilum and the ampulla of Vater. While this anatomical division is useful and convenient from a clinical standpoint because of differences in epidemiology, presentation, management and prognosis, the histological appearances are very similar among tumors arising at any of these anatomical sites and bear a strong resemblance to adenocarcinoma of the pancreatic ducts. By convention, adenocarcinomas of the gallbladder are grouped separately but they are also closely related to epithelial tumors of the extrahepatic bile ducts, although those in the gallbladder show prominent geographic, gender, and racial differences not observed with extrahepatic bile duct carcinomas.

CC accounts for about 3 % of all gastrointestinal cancers worldwide and intrahepatic CC comprises 10–20 % of all primary liver cancers [2]. It is interesting that the incidence of intrahepatic CC is said to be rising in several parts of the world including Europe, Australia and Japan, whereas, extrahepatic CC has declined slightly [3–5]. The same has been observed in North America where a three-fold increase for intrahepatic CC has been reported between 1975 and 1999 [3, 5]. There are suggestions however, that this apparent increase has been the result of a change in classification. CC are topographically categorized as intrahepatic or extrahepatic by the International Classification of Diseases for Oncology (ICD-O). Hilar CC (Klatskin tumors) are extrahepatic CC but the second edition of the ICD-O assigned them a histology code 8162/3 which cross-referenced to intrahepatic CC. In the United States, studies that included this code (8162/3, Klatskin) grouped what is an extrahepatic or hilar CC with intrahepatic CC, perhaps accounting for an overestimation of intrahepatic CC incidence by 13 % and a corresponding decrease in incidence of extrahepatic CC by 15 %. Similar results have been published from Europe [6] where the same ICD-O codes are employed [7]. However, in one study which examined the incorrect coding of Klatskin tumors as intrahepatic CC, the age-adjusted annual intrahepatic CC incidence remained increased by about 4 % [8]. It has been advocated that terms such as "Klatskin tumor", or "perihilar" CC not be used as they lead to confusion, furthermore, biliary tract cancers should not be "lumped" together in clinical trials, but rather examined and treated as individual, distinct subsets of biliary tract cancers such as intrahepatic and ductal CC [9].

The epidemiology and risk factors for hilar CC are discussed in detail in Chap. 2 and it is suffice to state briefly

A.S.-Y. Leong, MB, BS, MD, FRCPA, FRC (Path), FCAP, FASCP, FHKAM (Pathol), Honorary FHKC (Path), Honorary FRCPT (✉)
Pathology Laboratories, Sunway Medical Center,
Monash University/Malaysian Campus,
Bandar Sunway, Malaysia
e-mail: aleong45@gmail.com

C. Pairojkul, MD, Dip BAP (T)
Faculty of Medicine, Pathology Department,
KhonKaen University,
KhonKaen, Thailand

W.Y. Lau (ed.), *Hilar Cholangiocarcinoma*,
DOI 10.1007/978-94-007-6473-6_3, © Springer Science+Business Media Dordrecht and People's Medical Publishing House 2013

that carcinomas of the extrahepatic ducts are associated with sclerosing cholangitis, ulcerative colitis, abnormal choledochopancreatic junction, choledochal cysts [10, 11] and infestations with the liver flukes *Clonorchis sinensis* and *Opisthorchis viverri* [4, 5]. *C. sinensis* may have been a frequent association of cancer of the bile ducts in China and Korea with an accompanying high prevalence in the local population, but this association is much lower in recent times. Infection with *O. viverrini* in Northeast Thailand, in contrast, remains high and evidence supporting its role in the induction of CC is compelling. Chronic infection and other variables including the host's immune response and the ingestion of dietary carcinogens such as nitrosamines may have a further contributory role [12, 13].

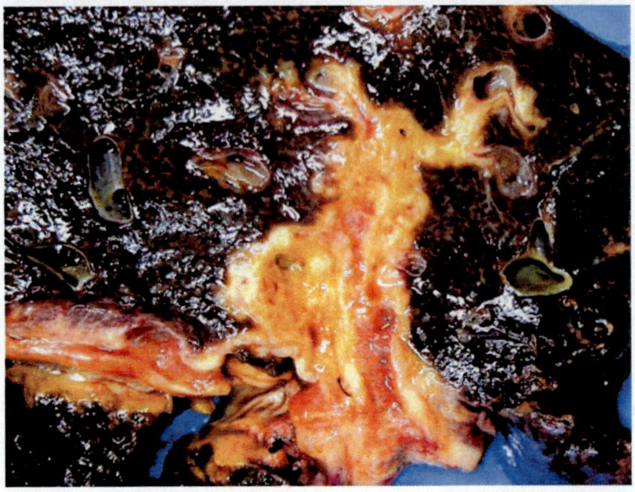

Fig. 3.1 Nodular-sclerosing carcinoma arising in the common bile duct and right hepatic duct with linear extension along the two main intrahepatic tributaries draining the anterior and posterior segments. The periductal tissue is thickened by tumor infiltration and a desmoplastic response, and the proximal intrahepatic bile ducts are dilated. The liver shows marked cholestasis. The gall bladder was collapsed (not shown)

3.2 Clinical Presentation

Hilar CC usually present relatively early with obstructive jaundice that progresses rapidly or fluctuates. Because of their location within the duct confluence, obstruction and accompanying jaundice occurs when the tumor is relatively small and before widespread dissemination or spread into the intrahepatic tributaries occurs. Malaise, weight loss, anorexia, nausea, vomiting, pruritus and right upper quadrant pain are other symptoms. In patients with hilar CC, the intrahepatic bile ducts are dilated, the gallbladder is not palpable and the common duct is often collapsed. In contrast, those patients with carcinoma in the common bile duct or cystic duct have a distended gallbladder and marked dilatation of the proximal bile duct system.

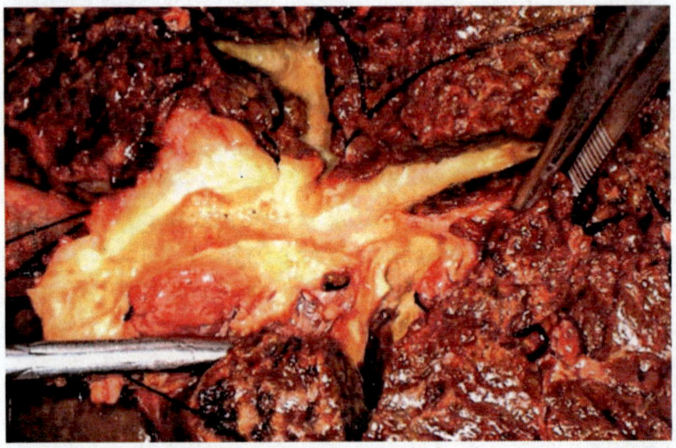

Fig. 3.2 Nodular-sclerosing carcinoma in the common bile duct and right hepatic duct. There is infiltration of the periductal tissues to produce an annular thickening. The segmental bile ducts are dilated and the liver shows marked cholestasis

3.2.1 Gross Appearance

Macroscopically, carcinomas of the extrahepatic bile ducts can be grouped into three types, viz, sclerosing/scirrhous, nodular, or papillary. Sclerosing/scirrhous tumors, the most common, are very firm and cause an annular thickening of the bile duct, often with diffuse infiltration and fibrosis of the periductal tissues. Nodular tumors are characterized by firm, irregular nodules that project into the lumen of the duct. Features of both types are often combined, hence the frequently used descriptor "nodular-sclerosing". The nodular-sclerosing variant is often firm or hard because of the desmoplastic response and varies from white to tan (Figs. 3.1 and 3.2), with a propensity to show radial infiltration into surrounding tissues and is difficult to resect (Fig. 3.3). They may also show diffuse spread linearly along the ducts distally and proximally into intrahepatic tributaries (Figs. 3.1 and 3.2). Necrosis is very uncommon. The papillary variant accounts for approximately 10 % of all CC, and while occasionally seen at the hilus, is more common in the distal bile duct. These tumors are soft and friable, and may show only early transmural invasion. While convenient and useful to guide the operative procedure, extent of resection, and prognosis, macroscopic separation of the variants is often not possible because of overlapping gross features, the exception being the papillary carcinoma which, being largely exophytic is more readily identifiable (Fig. 3.4).

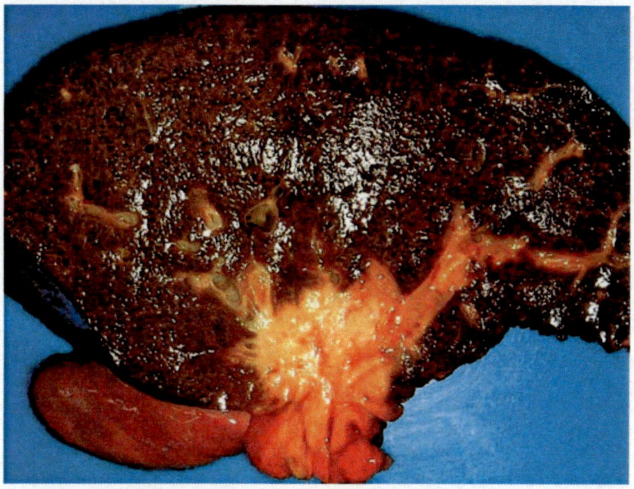

Fig. 3.3 Hilar cholangiocarcinoma arising in the right hepatic duct and showing radial infiltration into the immediate surrounding tissues. While the intrahepatic ducts are edematous, there is no macroscopic involvement. Cholestasis is less pronounced than in the previously illustrated examples of nodular sclerosing cholangiocarcinoma

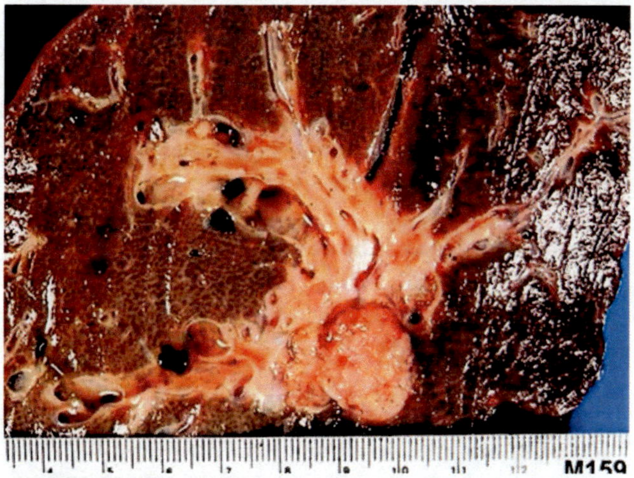

Fig. 3.4 Papillary cholangiocarcinoma at the hilum arising in the left hepatic duct. The polypoid tumor shows no apparent infiltration and appears limited to the wall of the duct. There is dilation of the intrahepatic bile ducts, some of which contain small pigmented calculi

3.2.2 Staging

Several systems have been described for staging of extrahepatic CC. They include the Bismuth-Corlette system [14] employed at Memorial Sloan–Kettering Cancer Center (MSKCC) [15], American Joint Committee on Cancer (AJCC) [16], and Japanese Society of Biliary Surgery (JSBS) [17]. The College of American Pathologists staging system, based on the AJCC/UICC TNM staging (7th edition) is as follows [18]:

Primary tumor (pT)	
pTX	Cannot be assessed
pT0	No evidence of primary tumor
pTis	Carcinoma in situ
pT1	Tumor confined to bile duct, with extension up to muscle layer or fibrous tissue
pT2a	Tumor invades beyond the wall of the bile duct to surrounding adipose tissue
pT2b	Tumor invades adjacent hepatic parenchyma
pT3	Tumor invades unilateral branches of the portal vein or hepatic artery
pT4	Tumor invades main portal vein or its branches bilaterally; or unilateral second-order biliary radicals with contralateral portal vein or hepatic artery involvement
Regional lymph nodes (pN)	
pNX	Cannot be assessed
pN0	No regional lymph node metastasis
pN1	Regional lymph node metastasis (including nodes along the cystic duct, common bile duct, hepatic artery, and portal vein)
pN2	Metastasis to periaortic, pericaval, superior mesentery artery, and/or celiac artery lymph nodes
Specify	Number examined…………..
	Number involved…………….
Distant metastasis (pM)	
pM0	Cannot be assessed
pM1	Distant metastasis, specify site(s), if known……………

It has been argued that existing staging systems are largely applicable only after surgical tumor resection as with the AJCC system [19], or provide little prognostic indication or help in the selection of patients for surgical treatment as in the case of the Bismuth-Corlette system [19–23]. On the other hand, the modified system proposed by Burke et al. [24] not only provided anatomical localization of the tumor but also defined the local extent, allowing better stratification of patients for surgical exploration [22] and can be employed preoperatively with imaging studies [23]. Essentially, the modified staging system classifies hilar CC according the local extent of tumor based on the location and extent of bile duct involvement, the presence or absence of portal venous invasion, and presence or absence of hepatic lobar atrophy [23].

The T staging system for hilar CC [20, 21] is as follows:

T1 Tumor involving biliary confluence ± unilateral extension to secondary biliary radicles. No liver atrophy or portal vein involvement.

T2 Tumor involving biliary confluence ± unilateral extension to secondary biliary radicles with ipsilateral portal vein involvement ± ipsilateral lobar atrophy. No main portal vein involvement.

T3 Tumor involving biliary confluence + bilateral extension to secondary biliary radicles; OR unilateral extension to secondary biliary radicles with contralateral portal vein involvement; OR unilateral extension to secondary biliary radicles with contralateral hepatic lobar atrophy; contralateral hepatic lobar atrophy; OR main or bilateral portal venous involvement.

3.2.3 Microscopic Appearances

A number of histological subtypes is recognized in the World Health Organization [25] and Armed Forces Institute of Pathology [26] classifications. Histological subtypes are most commonly described in the gallbladder with less frequent descriptions of the tumors in the extrahepatic bile ducts. Many of the histological subtypes described below in the gallbladder can be seen in the extrahepatic bile ducts but the spectrum of histological types in the latter is much less.

3.2.3.1 Adenocarcinoma

Adenocarcinomas are the most common, accounting for about 90 % malignant epithelial tumors of the extrahepatic bile ducts. They superficially resemble bile duct epithelium with mucin expression frequently present in the cells and glands and may show three primary forms of differentiation, namely, pancreaticobiliary (Fig. 3.5a, b), intestinal (Fig. 3.6), and gastric (Fig. 3.7). A clear distinction of these forms of adenocarcinoma is often difficult to make as the features overlap. Furthermore, about one third of all such tumors show focal intestinal differentiation with goblet and neuroendocrine cells, the latter may show expression of peptide hormones and serotonin but their presence does not warrant a diagnosis of neuroendocrine carcinoma. An extremely well-differentiated variant may simulate adenoma and Paneth cells may rarely be present. Other histological variants of intestinal type adenocarcinoma can occur, viz, a papillary adenocarcinoma composed predominantly of papillary fronds lined by cuboidal or columnar cells with varying amounts of mucin and intestinal metaplasia with collections of Paneth cells (Fig. 3.8) and occasional neuroendocrine and goblet cells [25, 26]. Such papillary carcinomas may fill the duct lumen before invading the wall (Fig. 3.4) and in a small percentage of cases may show skip lesions. Mucinous adenocarcinoma, another variant, shows abundant mucin secretion and is similar in appearance to those occurring at other sites (Fig. 3.9). Perineural and neural invasion is common, especially with radial spread of these tumors (Fig. 3.10).

Other variants of adenocarcinoma described in the gallbladder such as clear cell and signet ring adenocarcinomas (Fig. 3.6) are very uncommon in the extrahepatic bile ducts. These are generally aggressive tumors.

3.2.3.2 Adenosquamous Carcinoma

Such tumors are composed of two components; a glandular and a squamous component, each varying in quantity and extent of differentiation. Mucin secretion is often evident in the former and intercellular bridges in the latter (Fig. 3.11). Keratin pearls are less common.

3.2.3.3 Squamous Cell Carcinoma

This variant is uncommon and comprises sheets of squamous cells that vary considerably in extent of differentiation (Fig. 3.12). Keratinizing and non-keratinizing types exist and spindle cells may predominate. In the latter, immunohistological stains for cytokeratin are useful to identify their nature.

3.2.3.4 Small Cell Carcinoma

These are endocrine tumors and show varying degrees of differentiation. As such, immunohistological stains for synaptophysin and chromogranin are often necessary to confirm their endocrine nature and serotonin and peptide hormones may be expressed. The tumor is composed of small cells with round or fusiform nuclei with finely stippled chromatin and is arranged in cords, ribbons, trabeculae, nests and sheets with very occasional rosette-like structures (Fig. 3.13). Mixed endocrine-exocrine tumors also exist. These are composite tumors with areas of endocrine carcinoma and adenocarcinoma. Such tumors behave as adenocarcinomas and are clinically more aggressive tumors.

3.2.3.5 Rare Variants of Carcinoma

Other rare variants of carcinoma described in the bile ducts include clear cell carcinoma, hepatoid carcinoma (Fig. 3.14), and signet ring carcinoma.

3.2.3.6 Carcinosarcoma

This tumor needs to be distinguished from squamous cell carcinoma with spindled areas. A true carcinosarcoma, besides displaying the presence of malignant epithelial elements commonly in the form of glands with squamous cell areas, also contains sarcomatous elements in the form of heterologous mesenchymal tissue such as chondrosarcoma, osteosarcoma, and rhabdosarcoma. The mesenchymal component should be devoid of cytokeratin.

3.2.4 Grading

Adenocarcinoma is conventionally divided into three grades. Well differentiated adenocarcinoma requires the presence of glands in 95 % of the tumor, in moderately differentiated adenocarcinoma 40–95 % of the tumor should contain glands and in poorly differentiated adenocarcinoma 5–39 % of the tumor should contain glands [25].

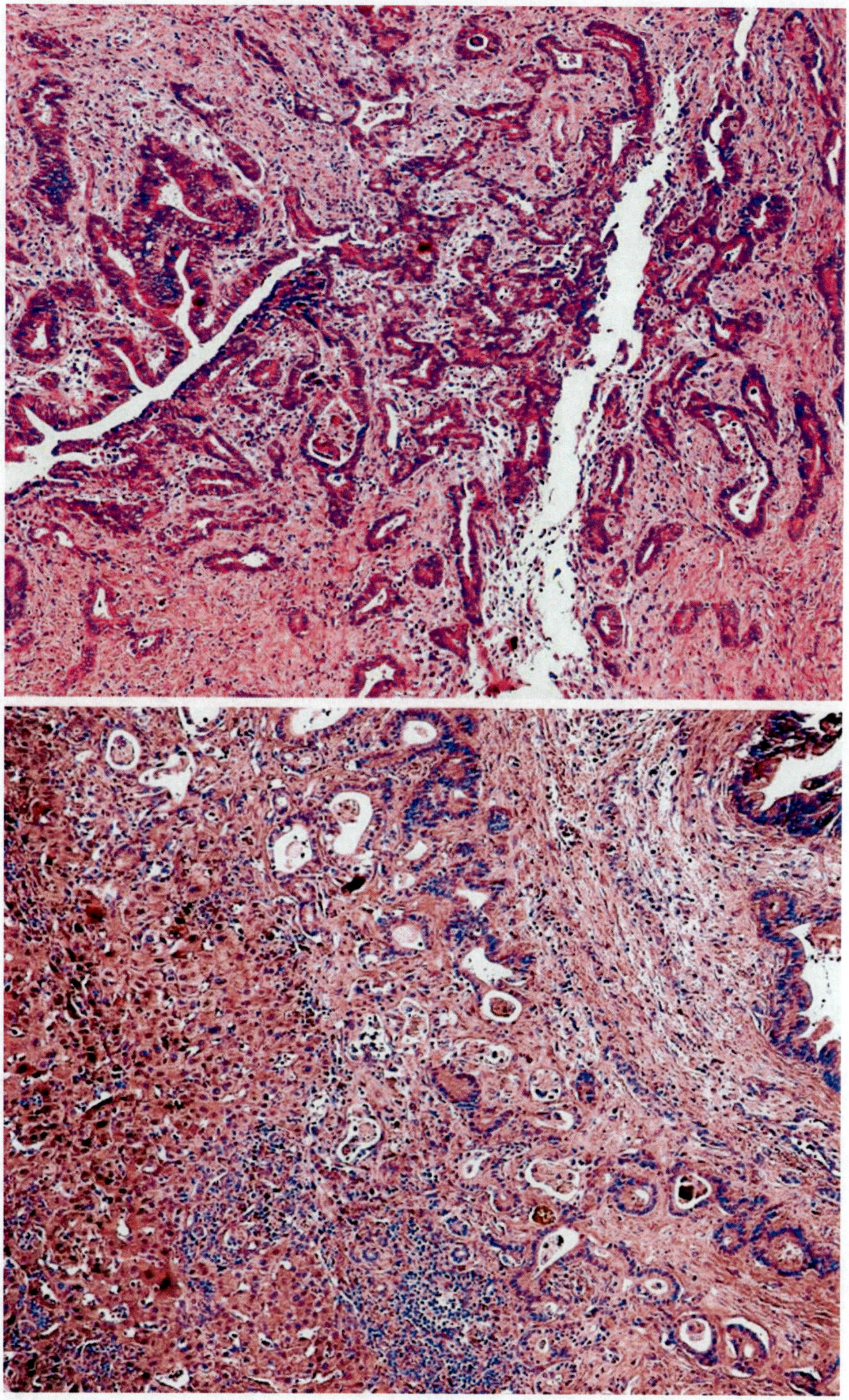

Fig 3.5 (**a**) Cholangiocarcinoma with pancreaticobiliary type differentiation. Atypical glands infiltrate the periductal tissue associated with a densely desmoplastic stroma. (**b**) There is tumor extension along the intrahepatic ducts with infiltration into surrounding hepatic parenchyma by similar-appearing atypical glands which evoke a fibrous response

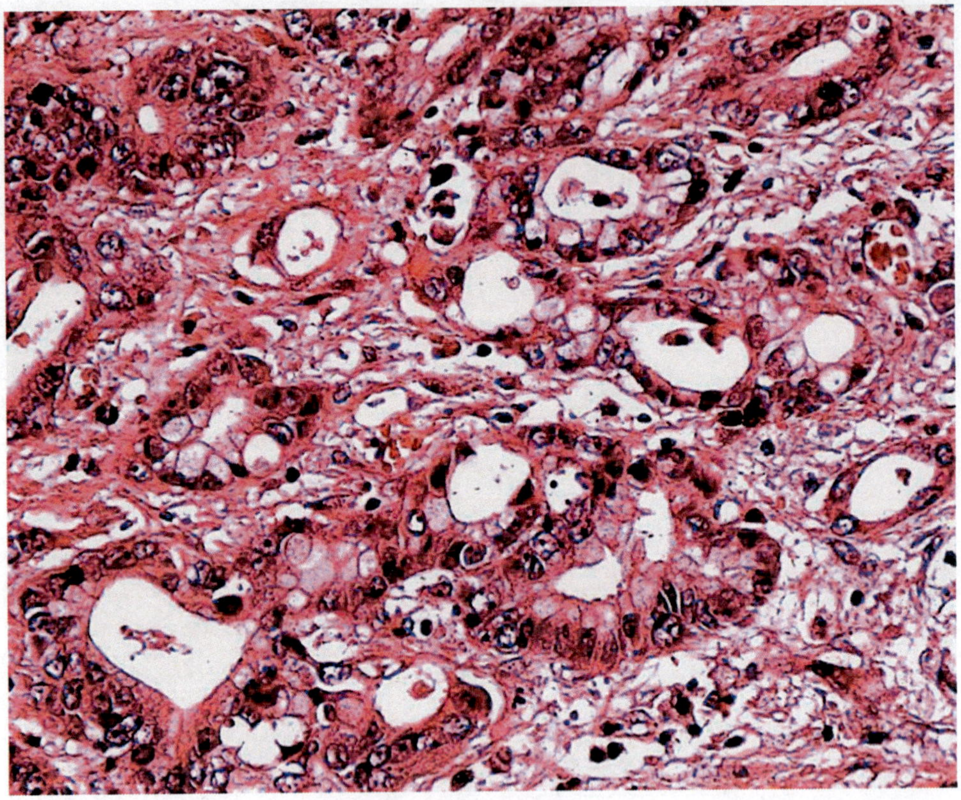

Fig. 3.6 Hilar cholangiocarcinoma with intestinal type differentiation. The atypical infiltrating glands contain cytoplasmic vacuoles of mucin which was also present in the glandular lumen. Scattered cells lining the glands have prominent cytoplasmic vacuoles that displace the crescentic nuclei peripherally to produce a signet cell appearance. When such cells predominate and infiltrate the stroma as single cells, the tumor is designated signet cell carcinoma

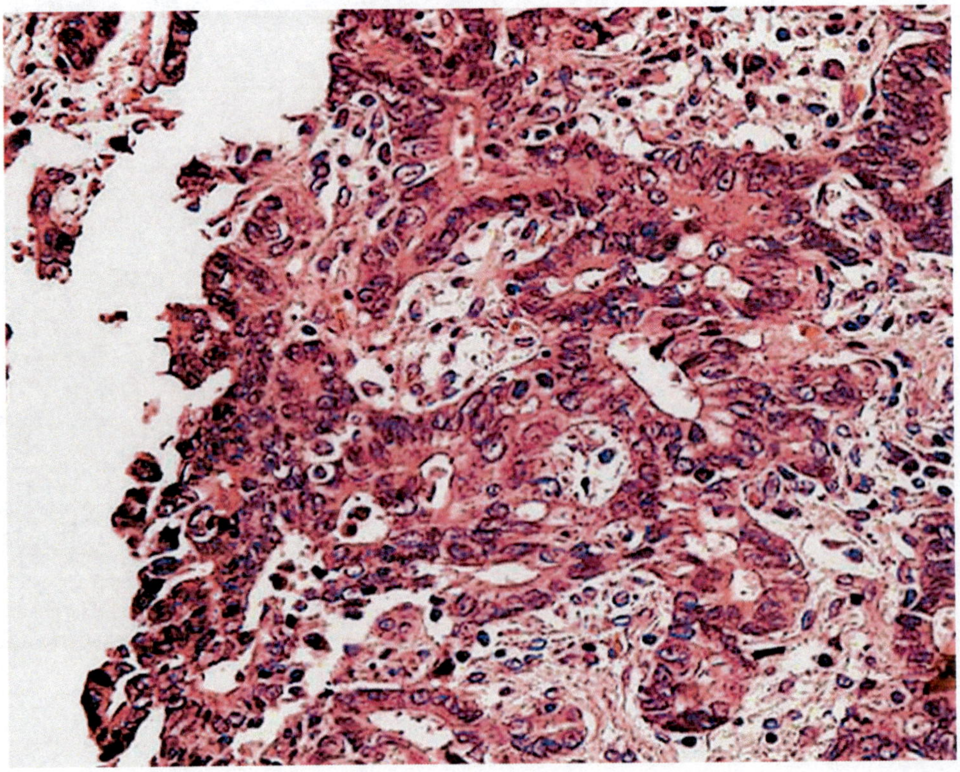

Fig. 3.7 The distinction of intestinal from gastric type differentiation is often difficult as in this example where the tumor is composed of infiltrating atypical glands that also secrete variable amounts of mucin. Unless areas of differentiation into distinct gastric type mucosa such as oxyntic cells are found, the separation cannot be made. The histological distinction has not been shown to be of prognostic relevance

Fig. 3.8 Foci of Paneth cell metaplasia are present in this well-differentiated variant of papillary adenocarcinoma. Occasional neuroendocrine and goblet cells may also be found

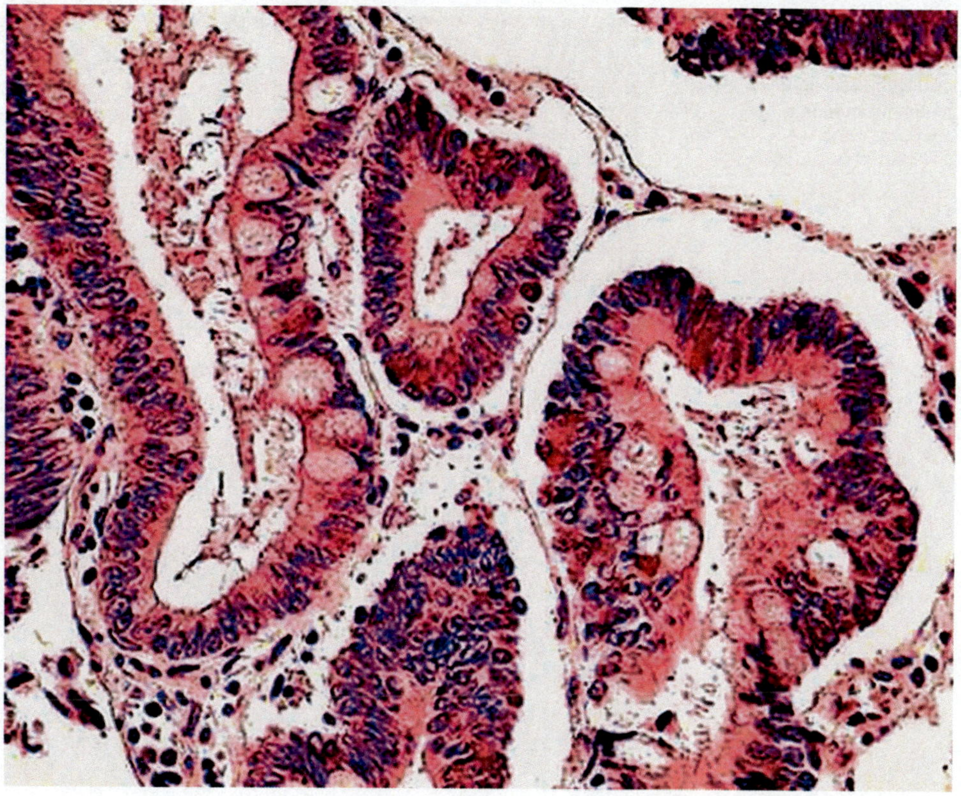

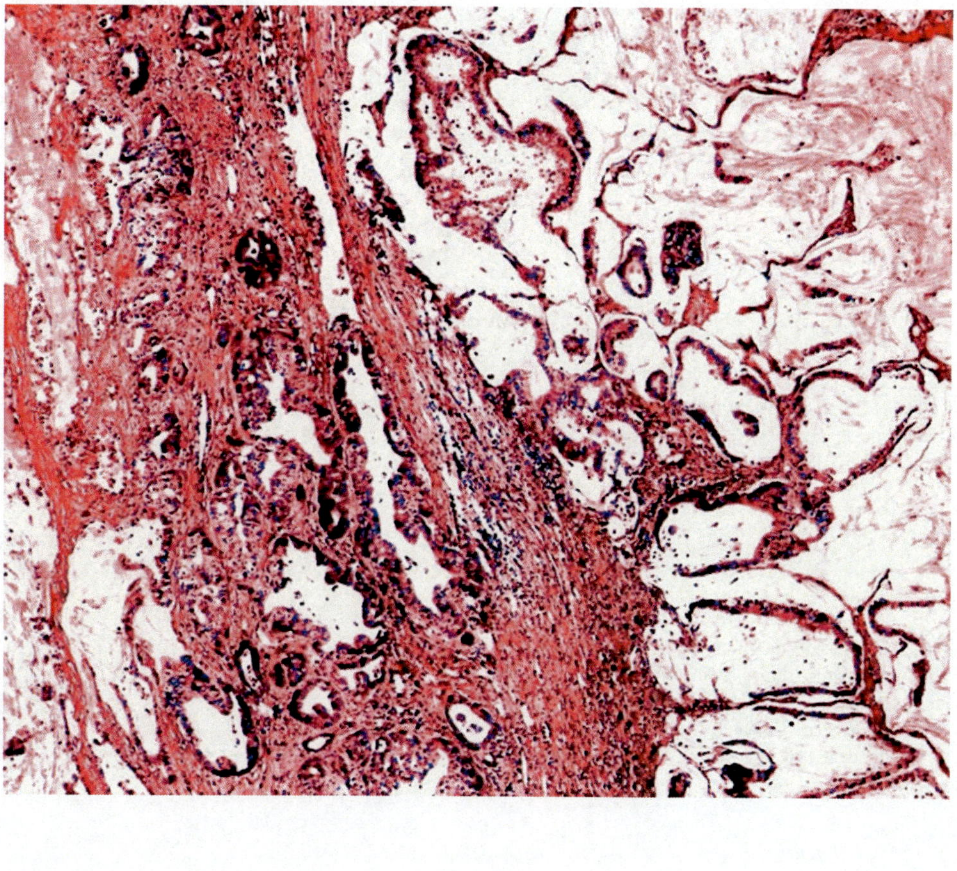

Fig. 3.9 Mucinous adenocarcinoma is not an uncommon form of cholangiocarcinoma. Abundant mucin distends the glands and a mild to moderate inflammatory response is present

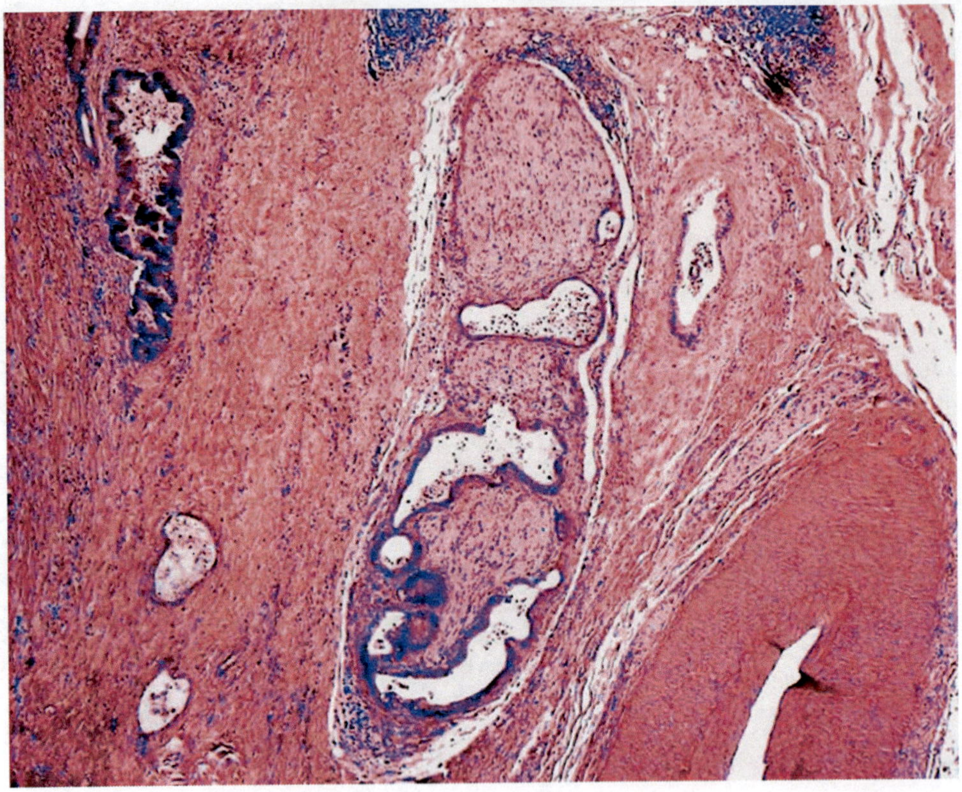

Fig. 3.10 There is prominent neural infiltration in the periductal tissue in this hilar cholangiocarcinoma

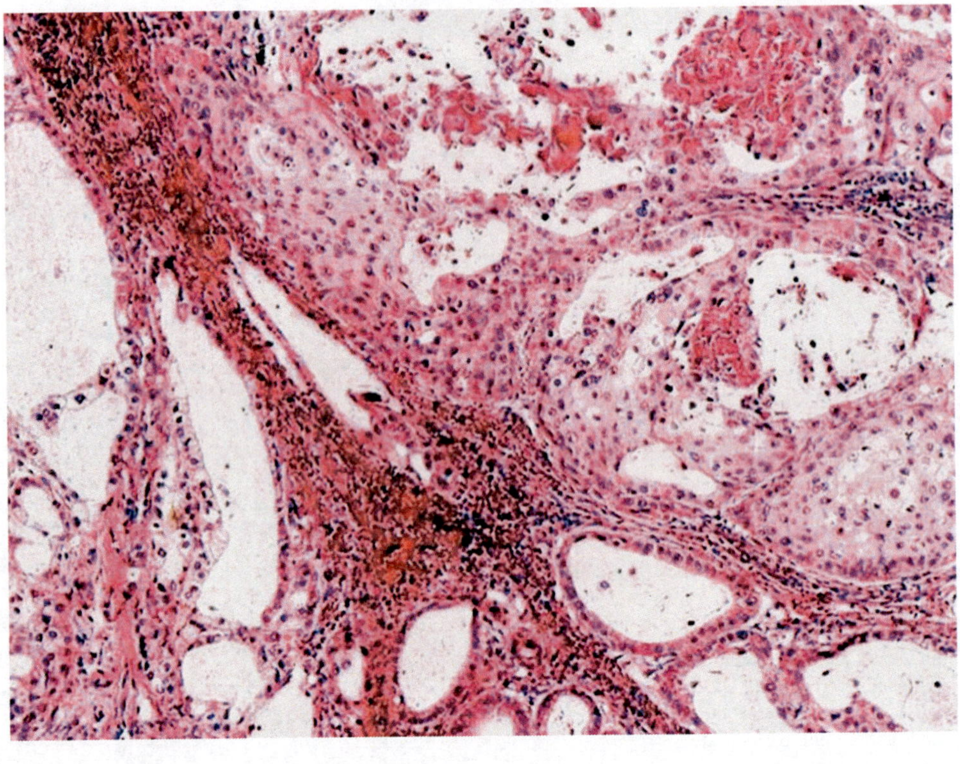

Fig. 3.11 Adenosquamous carcinoma composed of sheets of squamous cells with intercellular bridges. There are distinct glands in the adjacent stroma

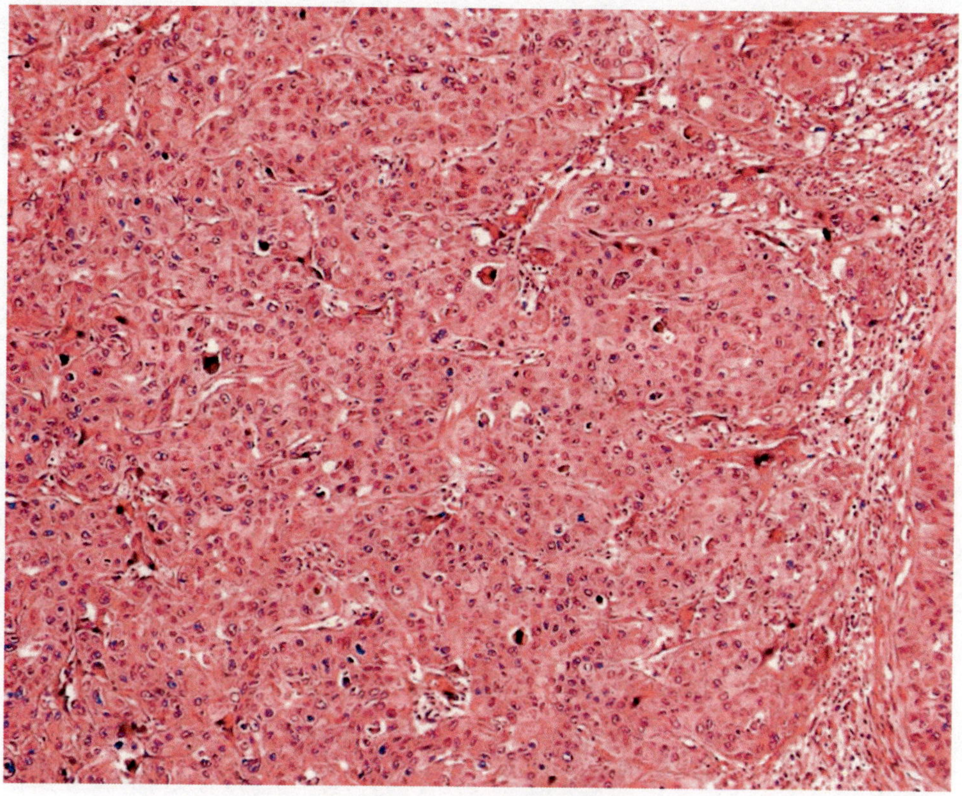

Fig. 3.12 Squamous cells carcinoma composed of sheets of well differentiated squamous cells with distinct intercellular bridges and eosinophilic keratinized cytoplasm. Keratin pearls are not present

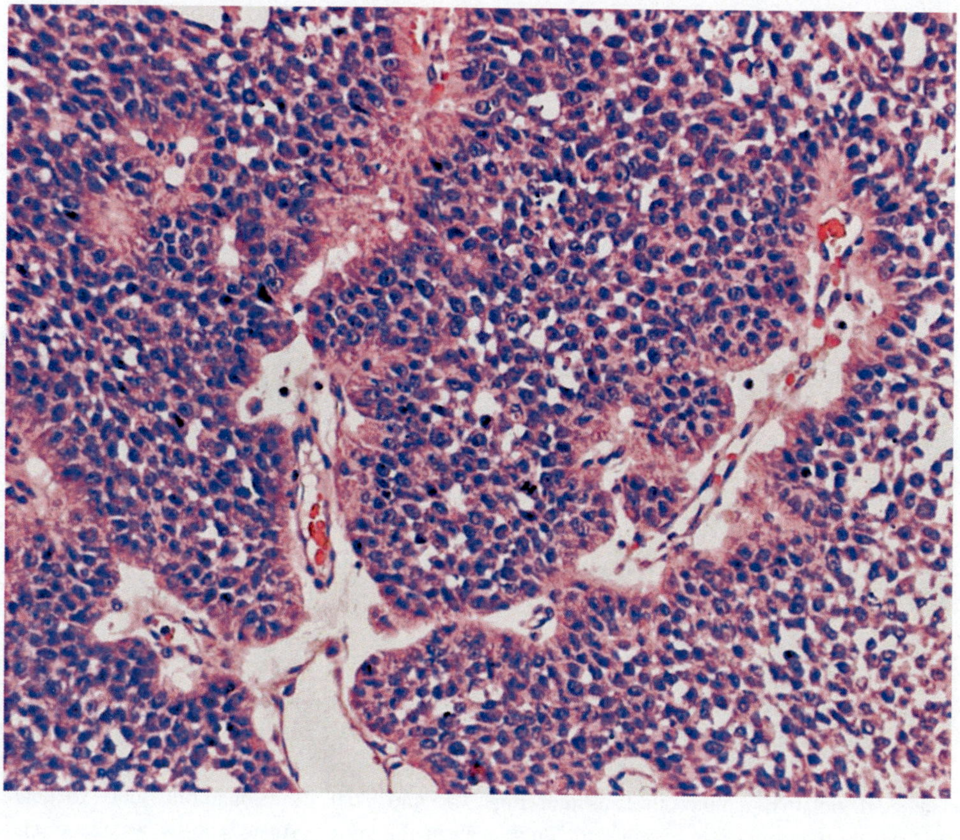

Fig. 3.13 Small cell carcinoma showing small cells with high nuclear cytoplasmic ratio and hyperchromatic nuclei arranged in sheets and nests

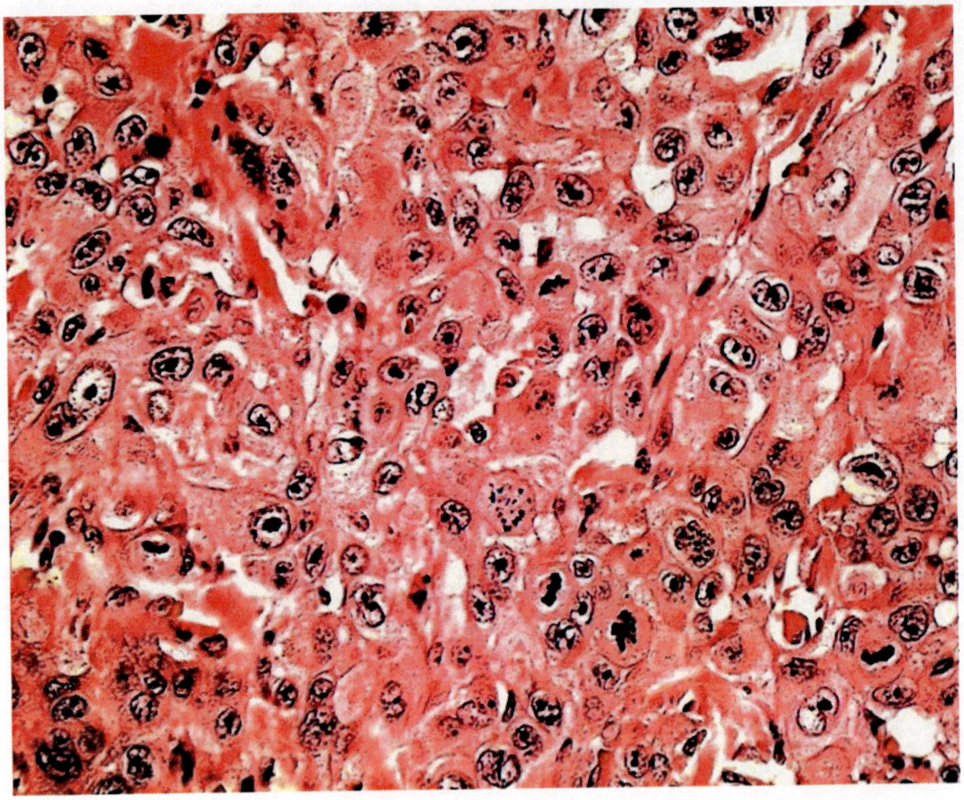

Fig. 3.14 Cholangiocarcinoma with hepatoid features. The large cells with vesicular nuclei and central nucleoli have abundant granular eosinophilic cytoplasm and resemble hepatocytes. This variant is very uncommon

3.2.5 Precursor Lesions

A number of precursor lesions arise in the extrahepatic bile ducts and include adenomas, biliary cystadenoma, papillomatosis (adenomatosis) and various grades of intraepithelial neoplasia (dysplasia) up to carcinoma in situ.

3.2.5.1 Adenoma

Adenomas are benign neoplasms of the biliary epithelium. They are commonly polypoid, single and well-demarcated and are more common in the gallbladder than extrahepatic bile ducts being seen in less than 0.5 % of gallbladders removed for cholelithiasis and chronic cholecystitis. A small proportion is known to progress to carcinoma. Biliary adenomas may be tubular, papillary or tubulopapillary as in the colon, and can show gastric pyloric, intestinal, or biliary type mucosa, the gastric pyloric type adenoma being more common in the gallbladder.

3.2.5.2 Biliary Cystadenoma

These are benign cystic tumors lined by columnar epithelium that resembles bile duct or foveolar gastric epithelium and occur almost exclusively in females. Often they are multiloculated and contain mucinous or serous fluid (Figs. 3.15 and 3.16) and are more common in extrahepatic ducts than in the gallbladder [27, 28]. Occasional endocrine cells may be present and the subepithelial stroma is of varying cellularity and resembles ovarian stroma. This stroma shows immunoreactivity for estrogen and progesterone receptors [29, 30]. Malignant transformation can occur with cystadenocarcinomas occurring equally in both females and males. In these tumors a large papillary mass may be present with areas of grey-white tumor in a thickened bile duct. Adequate sampling is necessary to distinguish benign cystadenomas from cystadenocarcinomas and prognosis is good if curative removal is possible [27, 28].

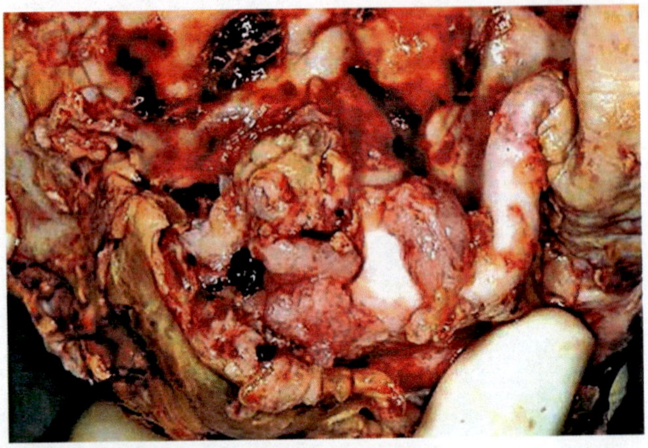

Fig. 3.15 Biliary cystadenoma. The mutilocular cyst contains soft polypoid excrescences and mucinous fluid

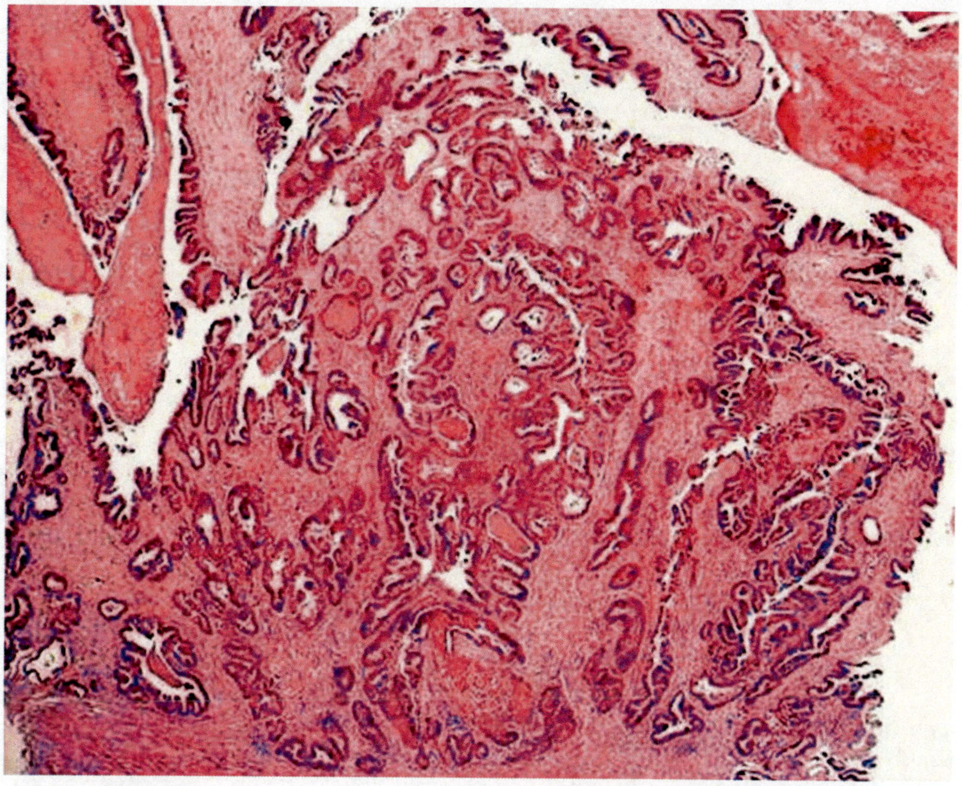

Fig. 3.16 The polypoid masses in biliary cystadenomas are composed of fibrovascular fronds lined by a single layer of cuboidal to columnar cells. Variable nuclear atypia may be seen and focal areas of pseudostrafication may be present. Adequate sampling ensures exclusion of a low-grade carcinoma

3.2.5.3 Papillomatosis

Multiple recurring papillary adenomas may involve large areas of the extrahepatic bile ducts (Figs. 3.17, 3.18 and 3.19) and extend into the gallbladder and intrahepatic bile ducts. Because of their multicentricity complete excision is difficult. The presence of severe dysplastic change in the epithelium lining the papillary adenomas makes distinction from carcinoma difficult hence this lesion is sometimes regarded as a form of low grade carcinoma and is considered a precursor lesion of adenocarcinoma. The potential for malignant transformation is greater compared to solitary adenomas [25, 26].

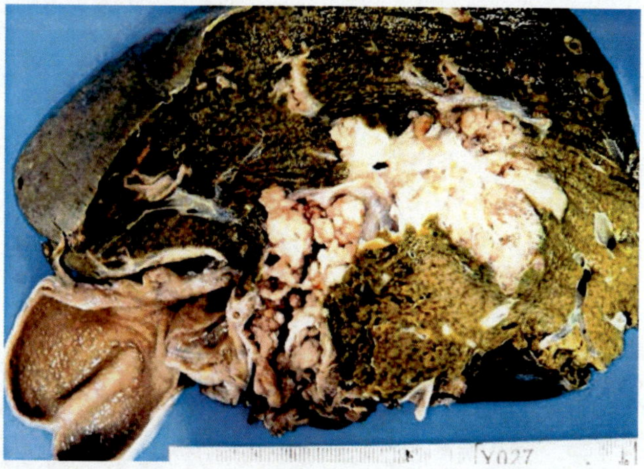

Fig. 3.17 Multiple papillary tumors are seen extending along the hilum into the intrahepatic bile ducts. Focal skip lesions are present

3.2.5.4 Intraepithelial Neoplasia (Dysplasia)

Intraepithelial neoplasia or dysplastic changes are not recognizable grossly as they are often associated with chronic inflammation and are difficult to distinguish from such changes which include fibrosis, thickening and induration of the mucosa. Careful examination may reveal small cauliflower-like excrescences in the mucosa or granularity and trabeculation.

Intraepithelial neoplasia can be papillary or more commonly flat. Papillary intraepithelial neoplasia is characterized by short stumpy fibrovascular fronds covered by dysplastic epithelium which may be columnar, cuboidal, or elongated with varying degrees of nuclear atypia, loss of polarity and occasional mitosis. Pseudostratification may occur in later stages and papillae may form. The cytoplasm is usually eosinophilic and contains non-sulphated acid and neutral mucin. Goblet cells may be seen and an abrupt transition of dysplastic from normal-appearing epithelium is often seen. Distinction of intraepithelial neoplasia from the epithelial atypia of repair is based on the homogeneous population seen in the former which is also often widespread in the mucosa [25, 26]. In addition, the heterogeneous cell population in repair which comprises columnar mucus-secreting

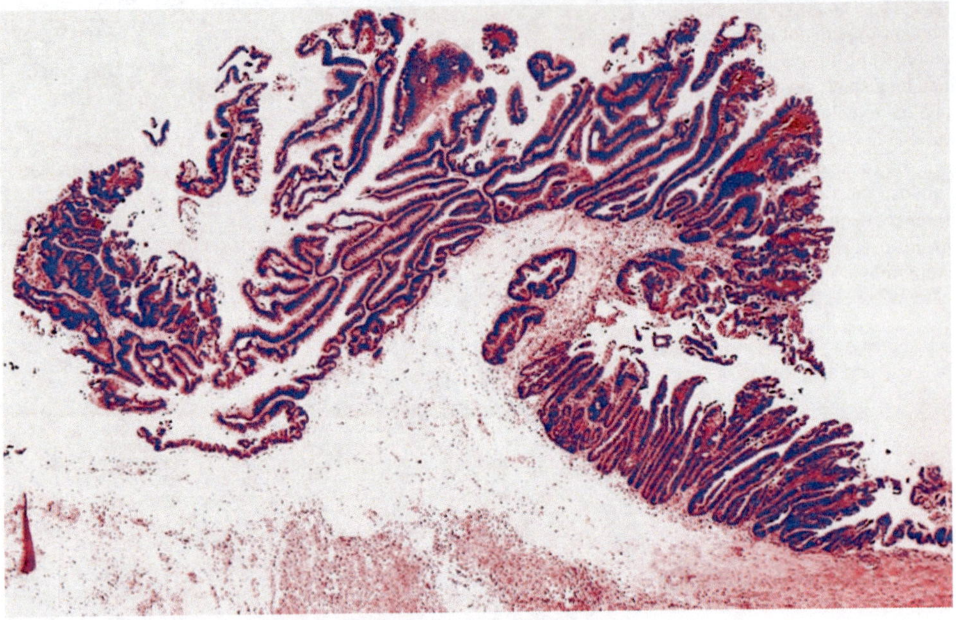

Fig. 3.18 Low power view of a papillary adenoma

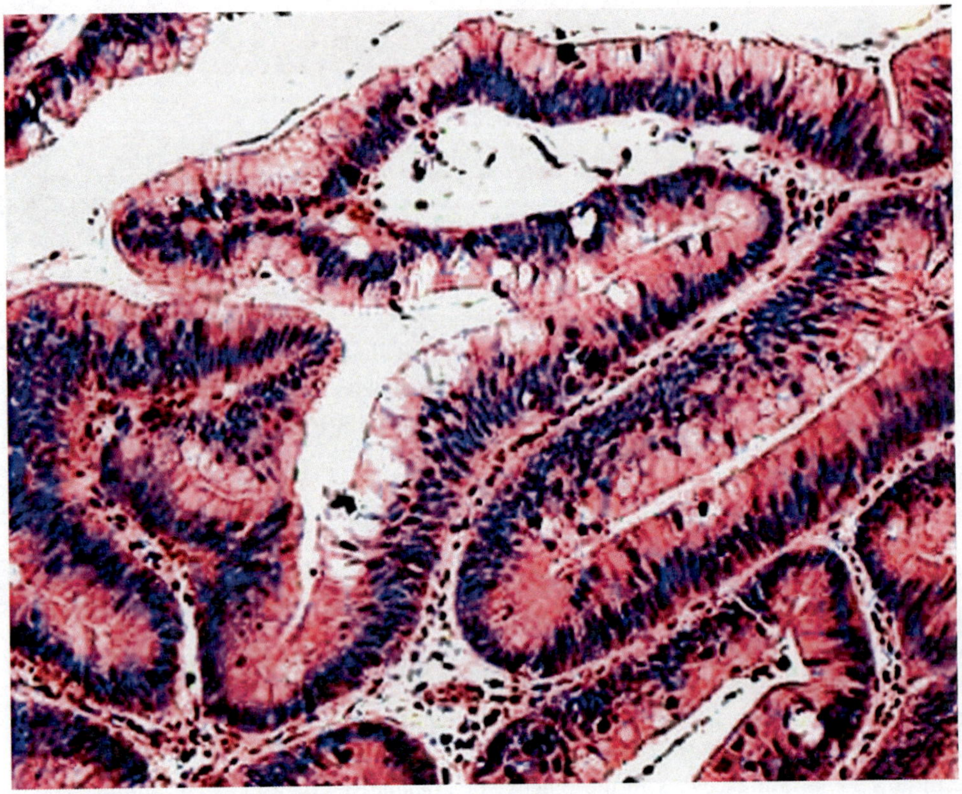

Fig. 3.19 High magnification of papillary adenoma shows papillary fronds lined by a single layer of tall columnar mucin-secreting cells. Nuclear atypia is mild to moderate and pseudostratification is not seen

cells, low cuboidal cells, atropic-appearing epithelium, and pencil-like cells display a gradual transition of the cellular abnormalities unlike the abrupt transition seen in intraepithelial neoplasia (Fig. 3.20). Immunoreactivity for p53 also helps in the identification of true dysplastic changes.

The two morphological forms of intraepithelial neoplasia in the bile ducts have been named biliary intraepithelial neoplasia (BilIN) for the non-papillary type and biliary intraductal papillary neoplasia (biliary IPN) for the papillary type. BilINs are a group of flat, pseudopapillary, or micropapillary

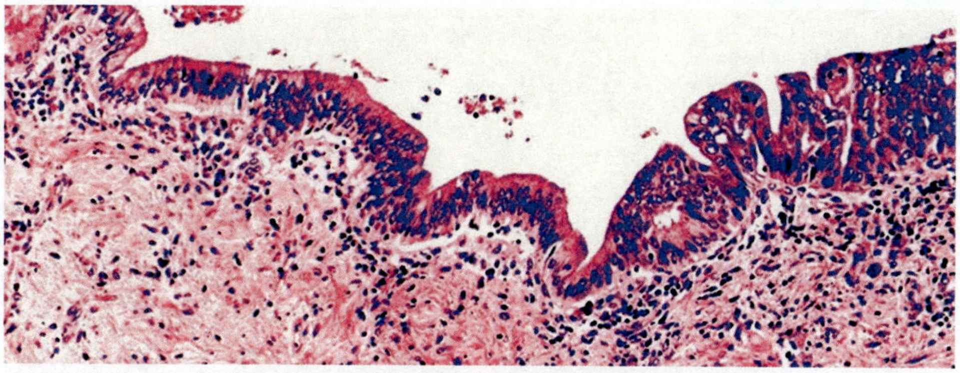

Fig. 3.20 Biliary dysplasia. A sharp transition is seen from the normal biliary epithelium on the left and dysplastic epithelium on the right. This transition can be enhanced by staining for p53 expressed in the dysplastic cells

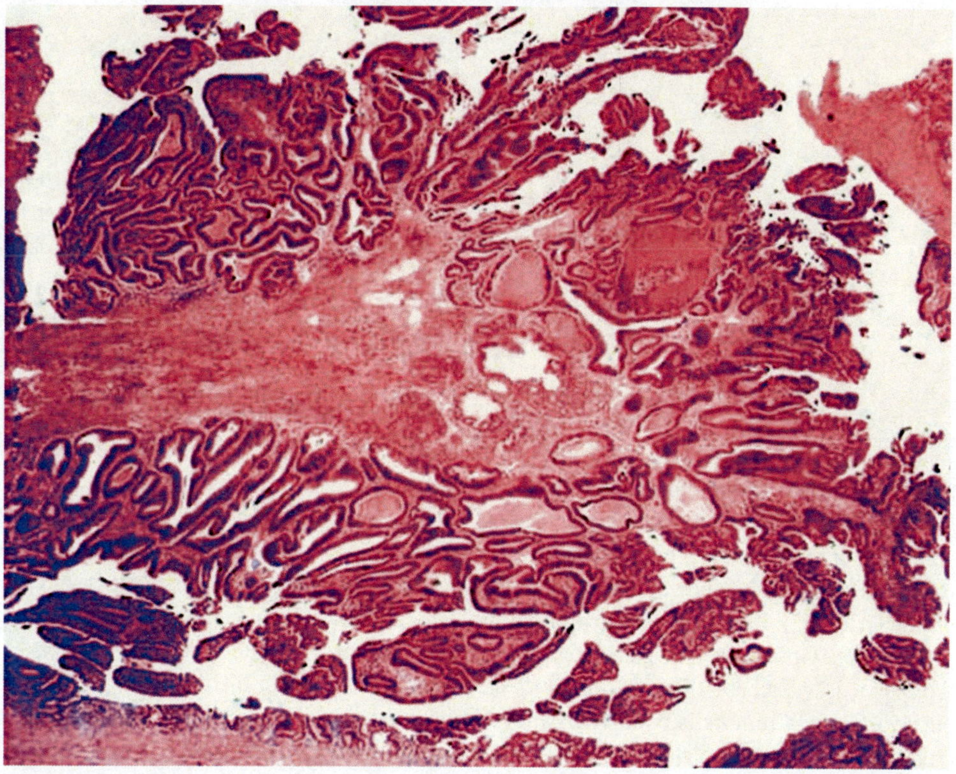

Fig. 3.21 Biliary adenoma. Fibrovascular fronds are lined by columnar cells with minimal atypia. There is no invasion of the fibrous stalk

lesions classified by a recent international consensus into three categories (grades) based on the degree of atypia: BilIN-1, BilIN-2, and BilIN-3, the last-mentioned also include carcinoma in situ (Figs. 3.20, 3.21 and 3.22) [31, 32]. Since BilINs share morphology and expression patterns of mucin core proteins (MUC1 and MUC2) with pancreatic intraepithelial neoplasia (PanIN) [32], it has been suggested that they represent the counterpart of PanIN [33, 34]. Biliary IPNs are grossly visible, non-invasive, intraductal papillary proliferations and resemble pancreatic intraductal papillary mucinous neoplasms (IPMN) [34]. Biliary IPNs, including biliary papillomatosis, show macroscopic mucinous hypersecretion in about 30 % of cases and may display three different forms of differentiation, namely, pancreaticobiliary, intestinal, and gastric. It is currently recognized that these two forms of intraepithelial neoplasia represent at least two pathways of carcinogenesis in bile duct adenocarcinoma, viz, a dysplasia-carcinoma sequence via BilIN and an adenoma-carcinoma sequence via biliary IPN [31].

3.3 Immunohistochemistry

Immunohistology is not particularly helpful in the identification of biliary carcinoma. In the case of distinguishing reactive atypia from intraepithelial neoplasia, as mentioned above, p53 immunoexpression may be useful in identifying the latter.

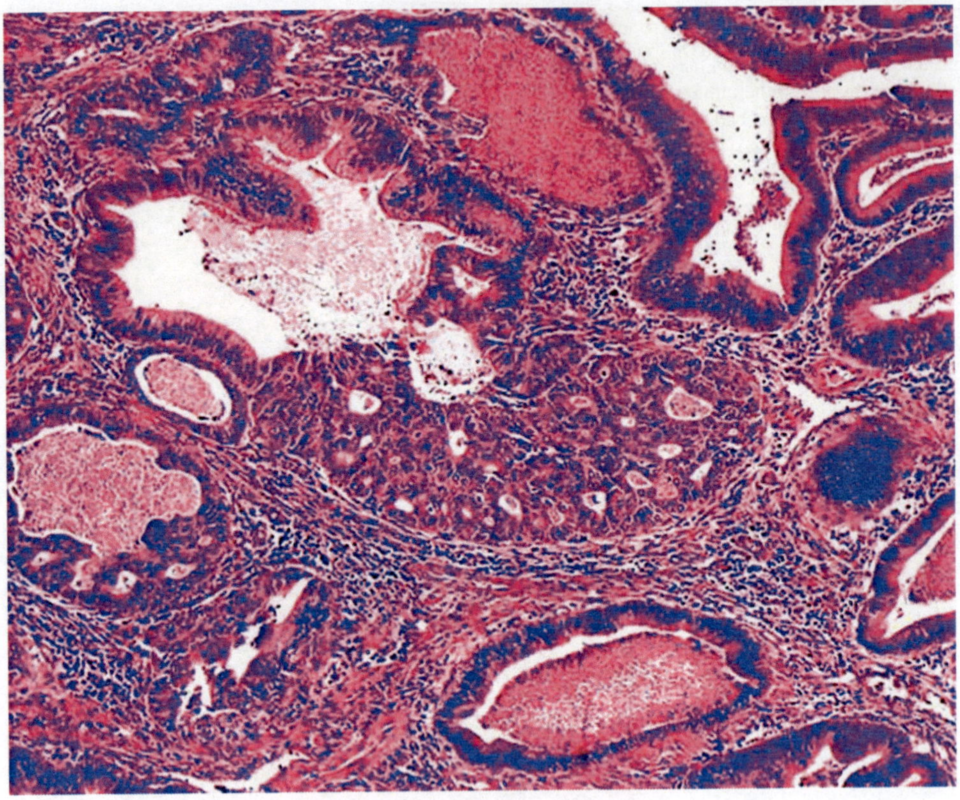

Fig. 3.22 High magnification of another adenoma which shows focal microinvasion of the inflamed fibrovascular stroma by small atypical glands that form a cribriform pattern in the center of the field

Immunohistological studies of hilar CC are uncommon although several studies of intrahepatic CC are available. CC express CK7, CK19, BerEP4 and show cytoplasmic staining for CEA, unlike hepatocellular carcinoma which express HepPar1 and show membranous staining for polyclonal CEA [35]. However, the role of immunohistochemistry to identify possible surrogate prognostic markers suffer from the drawback that correlation is weak as long-term survival in such tumors is poor. HER2/neu overexpression has been shown to correlate with nodal metastasis and with nuclear translocation of β-catenin, both markers showing significant correlation with high histological grade and high Ki-67 proliferation index, as well as with reduced immunoexpression of E-cadherin and FAT, the latter a newly described member of the cadherin superfamily [36]. K-*ras* and *p53* correlate with the microscopic types of CC, with k-*ras* mutations being more common in the periductal infiltrating than in mass-forming CC, whereas *p53* mutations had the reverse association. CDX2 and MUC2 have been employed to identify tumors of the intraductal papillary type of CC and over-expression of c-Met is said to be a feature of longer survival. Other markers studied include B-cell lymphoma-2 (Bcl-2), transforming growth factor β, telomerase, MUC4, p27, cyclin D1 but none has proven reliable [37, 38].

3.4 Molecular Genetics

Much of the published molecular genetics of CC relates to intrahepatic CC and carcinoma of the gallbladder and has been previously described [15, 39]. Mutations of the *RAS* and *TP53* genes are the most common abnormalities identified in both these conditions [39]. The molecular events associated with the development of CC have been investigated but are incompletely understood. Likewise, the changes that distinguish papillary from nodular-sclerosing lesions that are prognostically different (see below) are unclear [15, 40–42]. Abraham et al. [42], in an analysis of 14 cases of papillary bile duct carcinomas, failed to identify any unifying molecular derangements, although the study population was heterogeneous and there was no direct comparison to nodular-sclerosing tumors. Despite gaps in our understanding of these tumors, it is reasonable to postulate differences in the genetic changes between invasive papillary tumors and purely nodular-sclerosing lesions. The finding of highly invasive tumors with some residual papillary carcinoma components would suggest the possibility of overlap between two distinct pathogenetic mechanisms. Alternatively, this finding may represent the slow evolution of noninvasive papillary carcinomas to more invasive and aggressive tumors, an explanation that is possible but would require a long symptom-free period [43, 44].

3.5 Prognostic and Predictive Factors

The extent of the tumor largely determines prognosis with histological type influencing prognosis to a lesser extent. Polypoid tumors are most often papillary carcinomas and have the best prognosis, and non-invasive papillary carcinomas have a better prognosis than other types of invasive carcinomas [44, 45]. In one study of 13 patients with extrahepatic bile duct papillary carcinomas and 174 invasive papillary carcinomas complied by the Surveillance, Epidemiology, and End Results (SEER) program of the National Cancer Institute from 1981 to 1990, papillary carcinomas confined to the ductal wall had better 10-year relative survival rates than adenocarcinoma limited to the wall (21 % versus 12 %). Furthermore, when there was lymph node metastasis, papillary carcinoma had better prognosis than adenocarcinoma (10-year survival rate of 12 % versus 5 %) [45]. When invasive, papillary carcinomas may show a tubular or mucinous pattern and the former is said to show a worse prognosis [39]. The difference in outcome between papillary and nodular-sclerosing CC appears to be related, at least in part, to differences in disease biology. However, the data show that the favorable impact of papillary histology on survival is most pronounced in patients with less invasive cancers, suggesting that once a certain critical degree of invasiveness is reached, the clinical behavior of papillary CC approaches that of nodular-sclerosing tumors [15, 36]. This contrasts somewhat with a recent report from that summarized results from the SEER database that showed a survival advantage of papillary CC even in patients with more invasive tumors and tumors associated with regional lymph node metastases [40]. Whether more invasive CC of papillary origin are distinct from nodular-sclerosing cancers is thus less clear and may be clarified through a better understanding of the pathogenesis of CC.

Perineural and lymphatic permeation are significant prognostic factors. Perineural spread has been reported in 75 % of hilar CC, lymph node metastasis in 50 % and venous invasion in 38 % [46]. In one study of 564 cases of CC, locoregional lymph node metastasis occurred more frequently in distal CC (60 %) compared to hilar CC (28 %) and intrahepatic CC (29 %) [47].

Clearance of the surgical margin is an important prognostic indicator for all forms of CC [48, 49]. The lowest rate of negative margins was found in hilar CC. However, there is no clear-cut definition of margin clearance. Japanese authors require a 5 mm clearance [50, 51] whereas this is not the case in Western countries [18]. Furthermore, the examination of surgical margins with frozen sections will reduce the accuracy of detection of involvement especially of dysplasia and carcinoma-in-situ.

3.6 Differential Diagnoses

A variety of structures and tissues occur at the porta hepatis and both benign and malignant tumors arising in any of these tissues can produce compression of the common bile duct resulting in a clinical presentation similar to that of bile duct epithelial proliferation [52]. The list of such tumors that have been considered in the clinical differential diagnoses include granular cell tumor [53], inflammatory myofibroblastic tumor [54], embryonal carcinoma [55], neurilemmoma [56], malignant lymphoma [57], and heterotopic pancreatic tissue [58] as well as reactive conditions like tuberculosis [59], sclerosing mesenteritis [60], sarcoidosis [61], and IgG4 sclerosing disease [62]. Metastatic tumors can produce similar symptoms and presentation.

References

1. Klatskin G. Adenocarcinoma of the hepatic duct at its bifurcation within the porta hepatis: an unusual tumor with distinctive clinical and pathological features. Am J Med. 1965;38:241–56.
2. Shahip Y, El-Sharag HB. The epidemiology of cholangiocarcinoma. Semin Liver Dis. 2004;24:115–24.
3. Patel T. Increasing incidence and mortality of primary intrahepatic cholangiocarcinoma in the United States. Hepatology. 2001; 33:1353–7.
4. Khan SA, Taylor-Robinson SD, Toledano MD, et al. Changing international trends in mortality rates for liver, biliary and pancreatic tumors. J Hepatol. 2002;37:806–13.
5. West J, Wood H, Logan RFA, et al. Trends in the incidence of primary liver and biliary tracts cancers in England and Wales 1971–2001. Br J Cancer. 2006;94:1751–8.
6. Khan SA, Thomas HC, Davidson BR, et al. Cholangiocarcinoma. Lancet. 2005;366:1303–14.
7. Shaib YB, Davila JA, McGlynn K, et al. Rising incidence of intrahepatic cholangiocarcinoma in the United States: a true increase? J Hepatol. 2004;40:472–7.
8. Welzel TM, McGlynn KA, Hsing AW, et al. Impact of classification of hilar cholangiocarcinomas (Klatskin tumor) on the incidence of intra- and extrahepatic cholangiocarcinoma in the United States. J Natl Cancer Inst. 2006;98:873–5.
9. Blechacz BRA, Sanchez W, Gores GJ. A conceptual proposal for staging ductal cholangiocarcinoma. Curr Opin Gastroenterol. 2009;25:238–9.
10. Kagawa Y, Kashihara S, Kuramoto S, et al. Carcinoma arising in a congenitally dilated biliary tree. Report of a case and review of the literature. Gastroenterology. 1978;74:1286–94.
11. Boberg KM, Bergquist A, Mitchell S, et al. Cholangiocarcinoma in primary sclerosing cholangitis: risk factors and clinical presentation. Scand J Gastroenterol. 2002;37:1205–11.
12. Vatanasapt V, Sripa B, Sithithaworn P, et al. Liver flukes and liver cancer. Cancer Surv. 1999;33:313–43.
13. Migasena P, Reaunsuwan W, Changbumrung S. Nitrates and nitrites in local Thai preserved protein foods. J Med Assoc Thai. 1980; 63:500–55.
14. Bismuth H, Corlette MB. Intrahepatic cholangioenteric anastomosis in carcinoma of the hilus of the liver. Surg Gynecol Obstet. 1975;140:170–8.

15. Jarnagin WR, Fong Y, DeMatteo RP, et al. Staging, resectability, and outcome in 225 patients with hilar cholangiocarcinoma. Ann Surg. 2001;234:507–17.
16. American Joint Committee on Cancer. Extrahepatic bile ducts. In: Greene FL, Page DL, Fleming ID, editors. AJCC cancer staging manual. 6th ed. New York: Springer; 2002. p. 145–50.
17. Japanese Society of Biliary Surgery. Extrahepatic bile ducts. In: Nagakawa T, Kayahara M, Tashiro S, editors. Classification of biliary tract carcinoma. 2nd ed. Tokyo: Kanchara; 2004. p. 11–32.
18. Washington K, Berlin J, Brannton P, et al. Protocol for the examination of specimens from patients with carcinoma of the perihilar bile ducts. 2009. http://www.cap.org/apps/docs/committees/cancer/cancer_protocols/2009/PerihilarBileDucts_09protocol.pdf. Accessed on 30 Nov 2010.
19. Kim HJ. TNM staging of hilar cholangiocarcinoma. Korean J Gastroenterol. 2005;46:20–7.
20. Zervos EE, Osborne D, Goldin SB, et al. Stage does not predict survival after resection of hilar cholangiocarcinomas promoting an aggressive operative approach. Am J Surg. 2005;190:810–5.
21. Weber A, Landrock S, Schneider J, et al. Long-term outcome and prognostic factors of patients with hilar cholangiocarcinoma. World J Gastroenterol. 2007;13:1422–6.
22. Chen R-F, Li Z-H, Zhou J-J, et al. Preoperative evaluation with T-staging system for hilar cholangiocarcinoma. World J Gastroenterol. 2007;21:5754–9.
23. Jarnagin W, Winston C. Hilar cholangiocarcinoma: diagnosis and staging. HPB. 2005;7:244–51.
24. Burke EC, Jarnagin W, Hochwald SN, et al. Cholangiocarcinoma: patterns of spread, the importance of hepatic resection for curative operation, and a presurgical clinical staging system. Ann Surg. 1998;228:385–94.
25. Albores-Saavedra J, Scoazec JC, Wittekind C, et al. Carcinoma of the gallbladder and extrahepatic bile ducts. In: Hamilton SR, Aaltonen LA, editors. World Health Organization classification of tumours. Tumors of the digestive system. Lyon: International Agency for Research on Cancer Press; 2000. p. 206–14.
26. Albores-Saavedra J, Henson DE, Klimstra D. Tumors of the gallbladder and extrahepatic ducts, Atlas of tumor pathology, vol. 3. Washington D.C.: Armed Forces Institute of Pathology; 1999.
27. Devaney K, Goodman ZD, Ishak KG. Hepatobiliary cystadenoma and cystadenocarcinoma. A light microscopic and immunohistochemical study of 70 patients. Am J Surg Pathol. 1994;18:1078–91.
28. Ishak KG, Willis GW, Cummins SD, et al. Biliary cystadenoma and cystadenocarcinoma: report of 14 cases and review of the literature. Cancer. 1977;39:322–38.
29. Abdul-Al HM, Makhlouf HR, Goodman ZD. Expression of estrogen and progesterone receptors and inhibin-alpha in hepatobiliary cystadenoma: an immunohistochemical study. Virchows Arch. 2007;450:691–7.
30. Wheeler DA, Edmondson HA. Cystadenoma with mesenchymal stroma (CMS) in the liver and bile ducts. A clinicopathologic study of 17 cases, 4 with malignant change. Cancer. 1985;56:1434–45.
31. Zen Y, Adsay NV, Bardadin K, et al. Biliary intraepithelial neoplasia: an international interobserver agreement study and proposal for diagnostic criteria. Mod Pathol. 2007;20:701–9.
32. Zen Y, Sasaki M, Fujii T, et al. Different expression patterns of mucin core proteins and cytokeratins during intrahepatic cholangiocarcinogenesis from biliary intraepithelial neoplasia and intraductal papillary neoplasm of the bile duct—an immunohistochemical study of 110 cases of hepatolithiasis. J Hepatol. 2006;44:350–8.
33. Kloppel G, Kosmahl M. Is the intraductal papillary mucinous neoplasia of the biliary tract a counterpart of pancreatic papillary mucinous neoplasm? J Hepatol. 2006;44:249–50.
34. Zen Y, Fujii T, Itatsu K, et al. Biliary papillary tumors share pathological features with intraductal papillary mucinous neoplasm of the pancreas. Hepatology. 2006;44:1333–43.
35. Leong AS-Y, Sormunen RT, Tsui WM-S, et al. Immunostaining for liver cancers. With special reference to Hep Par 1 antibody. Histopathology. 1998;33:318–24.
36. Settakorn J, Kaewpila N, Burns G, et al. Fat, E-cadherin, β-catenin, HER 2/neu, Ki67 immunoexpression and histologic grade in intrahepatic cholangiocarcinoma. J Clin Pathol. 2005;58:1249–54.
37. Leong TY-M, Leong AS-Y. Prognostication in intrahepatic cholangiocarcinoma. Adv Anat Pathol. 2006;13:99–100.
38. Leong TY-M, Wannakrairot P, Lee ES, et al. Review: pathology of cholangiocarcinoma. Curr Diagn Pathol. 2007;13:54–64.
39. Nakanuma Y, Sripa B, Vatanasapt V, et al. Intrahepatic cholangiocarcinoma. In: Hamilton SR, Aaltonen LA, editors. World Health Organization classification of tumors. Tumors of the digestive system. Lyon: International Agency for Research on Cancer Press; 2000. p. 173.
40. Rashid A. Cellular and molecular biology of biliary tract cancers. Surg Oncol Clin N Am. 2002;11:995–1009.
41. Albores-Saavedra J, Murakata L, Krueger JE, et al. Non-invasive and minimally invasive papillary carcinomas of the extrahepatic bile ducts. Cancer. 2000;89:508–15.
42. Abraham SC, Lee JH, Hruban RH, et al. Molecular and immunohistochemical analysis of intraductal papillary neoplasms of the biliary tract. Hum Pathol. 2003;34:902–10.
43. Albores-Saavedra J, Henson DE, Klimstra D. Dysplasia, carcinoma in situ, and invasive carcinoma of the extrahepatic bile duct. In: Rosai J, Sobin LH, editors. Tumors of the gallbladder, extrahepatic bile ducts and ampulla of Vater. Washington D.C.: AFIP; 2000. p. 191–215.
44. Jarnagin WR, Bowne W, Klimstra DS, et al. Papillary phenotype confers improved survival after resection of hilar cholangiocarcinoma. Ann Surg. 2005;241:703–14.
45. Hoang MP, Murakata LA, Katabi N, et al. Invasive papillary carcinomas of the extrahepatic bile ducts: a clinicopathologic and immunohistochemical study of 13 cases. Mod Pathol. 2002;15:1251–8.
46. Yamaguchi K, Chijiiwa K, Saiki S, et al. Carcinoma of the extrahepatic bile duct: mode of spread and its prognostic implications. Hepatogastroenterology. 1997;44:1256–61.
47. DeOliveira ML, Cunningham SC, Cameron JL, et al. Cholangiocarcinoma: thirty-one-year experience with 564 patients at a single institution. Ann Surg. 2007;245:755–62.
48. Nakeeb A, Pitt HA, Sohn TA, et al. Cholangiocarcinoma. A spectrum of intrahepatic, perihilar, and distal tumors. Ann Surg. 1996;224:463–73.
49. Sasaki R, Takeda Y, Funato O, et al. Significance of ductal margin status in patients undergoing surgical resection for extrahepatic cholangiocarcinoma. World J Surg. 2007;31:1788–96.
50. Uenishi T, Hirohashi K, Kubo S, et al. Histologic factors affecting prognosis following hepatectomy for intrahepatic cholangiocarcinoma. World J Surg. 2001;25:865–9.
51. Ogura Y, Takahashi K, Tabata M, et al. Clinicopathological study on carcinoma of the extrahepatic bile duct with special focus on cancer invasion on the surgical margins. World J Surg. 1994;18:778–84.
52. Dumitrascu T, Ionescu M, Clurea S, et al. Klatskin-mimicking lesions—a case series and literature review. Hepatogastroenterology. 2010;57:961–7.
53. Bilanovic D, Boricic I, Zdravkovic D, et al. Granular cell tumor of the common hepatic duct presenting as cholangiocarcinoma and acute acalculous cholecystitis. Acta Chir Iugosl. 2008;55:99–101.
54. Gohy S, Hubert C, Deprez P, et al. Benign biliary inflammatory pseudotumor mimicking Klatskin tumor. Hepatogastroenterology. 2007;54:1348–52.

55. Lee JA, Kim TW, Min JH, et al. A case of undifferentiated (embryonal) liver sarcoma mimicking Klatskin tumor in an adult. Korean J Gastroenterol. 2010;55:144–8.
56. Kamani F, Dorudinia A, Goravanchi F, et al. Extrahepatic bile duct neurilemmoma mimicking Klatskin tumor. Arch Iran Med. 2007;10:264–7.
57. Kang HG, Choi JS, Seo JA, et al. A case of primary biliary malignant lymphoma mimicking Klatskin tumor. Korean J Gastroenterol. 2009;54:191–5.
58. Heer C, Pfortner M, Hamberger U, et al. Heterotopic pancreatic tissue in the bifurcation of the bile duct: rare diagnosis mimicking a Klatskin tumor. Chirurg. 2010;81:151–4.
59. Arora R, Sharma A, Bhowate P, et al. Hepatic tuberculosis mimicking Klatskin tumor: a diagnostic dilemma. Indian J Pathol Microbiol. 2008;51:382–5.
60. Medina-Franco H, Listinsky C, Mel Wilcox C, et al. Concomitant sclerosing mesenteritis and bile duct fibrosis simulating Klatskin tumor. J Gastrointest Surg. 2001;5:658–60.
61. Pungpapong S, Steers JL, Wallace MB, et al. Hepatobiliary sarcoidosis mimicking Klatskin's cholangiocarcinoma. Gastrointest Endosc. 2006;64:124–5.
62. Cheung MT, Lo IL. IgG4-related sclerosing lymphoplasmacytic pancreatitis and cholangitis mimicking carcinoma of the pancreas and Klatskin tumour. ANZ J Surg. 2008;78:252–6.

Staging Systems

4

F.G. Rocha and W.R. Jarnagin

4.1 Introduction

Originally described by Altmeier [1] and Klatskin [2], hilar cholangiocarcinoma is an adenocarcinoma of the extrahepatic biliary tree arising from the main left or right hepatic ducts or their confluence. Along with distal bile duct cancer and intrahepatic cholangiocarcinoma, they comprise the spectrum of bile duct cancers that arise from the biliary epithelium. However, unlike those tumors, which can be usually be removed, respectively, with pancreaticoduodenectomy or liver resection alone, the surgical approach to hilar cholangiocarcinoma often combines bile duct resection with concomitant hepatectomy and/or portal vein resection due to the infiltrative nature of the disease. Therefore, a complete, margin-negative resection can be difficult to achieve.

While curative resection remains the only treatment modality associated with prolonged survival, the majority of patients present with disease not amenable to surgical correction. Over the last several decades, improvements in operative techniques and cross-sectional imaging, a better understanding of tumor biology, and the advent of perioperative interventions such as portal vein embolization and biliary decompression of the liver remnant have been adopted in order to maximize resectability and reduce morbidity associated with a major hepatectomy and bile duct resection. Furthermore, caudate resection has been adopted when the left hepatic duct is involved by tumor given it is the origin of the caudate bile ducts. Despite these advances, the 5-year survival rate following curative resection for hilar cholangiocarcinoma remains in the range of 20–40 % [3].

Therefore, accurate staging of this disease to guide therapy and properly select patients who would benefit from surgical extirpation, while sparing potential morbidity in those patients with advanced disease is of utmost importance. Several systems have been developed to distinguish the extent of disease from an anatomic, pathologic and clinical perspective; however, no uniform, universally accepted standard has been embraced. The purpose of this chapter is to examine the historical basis and current applications of the available staging systems and their role in the management of patients with hilar cholangiocarcinoma.

4.2 Anatomic Staging Systems (Bismuth-Corlette)

Given the significant challenges in the surgical removal of hilar cholangiocarcinoma and the lack of a common terminology for the description of these tumors, a preoperative classification system was initially described by Bismuth and Corlette from the Hospital Paul Brousse in Paris [4]. It is a simple system that attempts to stratify the location of the tumor and its longitudinal extent along the biliary ductal system for the purpose of determining extent of resection. Originally described in 1975 and modified in 1992, it is depicted in Fig. 4.1 as a progression of cholangiocarcinoma from the distal extrahepatic portion of the duct up to the hilus and into the secondary biliary radicles. A type I tumor involves the common hepatic and/or bile duct below the confluence and is sometimes referred to as middle CBD cancer or perihilar cholangiocarcinoma depending on its location with regards to the cystic duct of the gallbladder. Some authors argue this type of tumor can be managed with resection of the extrahepatic ductal system and regional lymphadenectomy without the need for hepatic resection provided the surgical margins are negative by frozen section. Bismuth-Corlette type II lesions are sometimes considered the true Klatskin tumors as they involve the confluence of the right and left hepatic ducts without involvement of the intrahepatic ductal system. Depending on the tumor encroachment, resection of the common hepatic duct and regional lymph

F.G. Rocha, MD
Department of Surgery, Memorial Sloan-Kettering Cancer Center, New York, NY 10027, USA

W.R. Jarnagin, MD (✉)
Hepatopancreatobiliary Service, Department of Surgery, Memorial Sloan-Kettering Cancer Center, New York, NY 10027, USA
e-mail: jarnagiw@mskcc.org

W.Y. Lau (ed.), *Hilar Cholangiocarcinoma*,
DOI 10.1007/978-94-007-6473-6_4, © Springer Science+Business Media Dordrecht and People's Medical Publishing House 2013

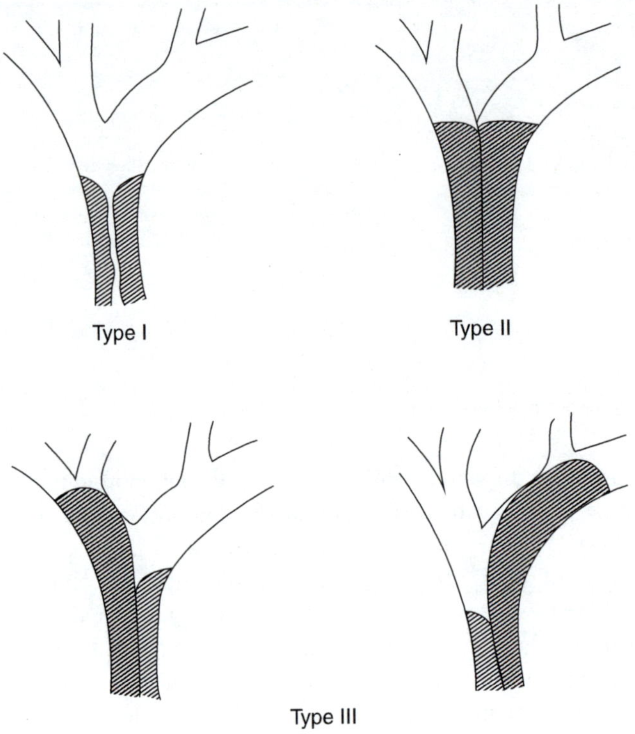

Fig. 4.1 Bismuth-Corlette classification for carcinoma of the hilus. Type I, non-obstructed primary confluence; Type II, obstruction limited to primary confluence; Type III, primary confluence with extension to the right or left secondary confluence (With permission from Bismuth and Corlette [4])

nodes along with a right or left hepatectomy may be warranted. For technical purposes, the longer extrahepatic course and therefore accessibility of the left hepatic duct can be exploited to facilitate bilioenteric reconstruction following resection. In this case, a right hepatectomy should be performed to ensure negative margins. However, if the tumor extends into the left hepatic duct, then a left hepatectomy should be performed, along with caudate lobectomy, for the same reason. This is certainly the case with Bismuth-Corlette type III tumors whereby IIIa tumors involve the confluence along with the right secondary biliary ducts while IIIb tumors involve the left secondary bile ducts. Hepatectomy is universally mandated in these cases in order to achieve complete tumor clearance. Type IV tumors, which by definition extend to involve the bilateral secondary biliary radicles, were traditionally considered unresectable, and patients with this extent of disease are typically referred for palliative treatments or liver transplantation. In addition, patients with multicentric tumors are considered Bismuth-Corlette type IV.

In response to the extension of tumor beyond the traditional Bismuth-Corlette borders, Starzl and others proposed a modification to this classification system, whereby type IIIa+ tumors would include tumors that penetrated both the anterior and posterior sectoral ducts and type IIIb+ in which the tumor extended into the segment 4, 3 and 2 ducts [5]. In addition, he proposed type IVa tumors where the right-sided component extended to the second bifurcation and type IVb which involved the segment 4, 3, 2 ducts. Lastly, type V would comprise the combination of type IVa and IVb.

Pitt and others from Johns Hopkins developed an expanded system that classifies the entire spectrum of cholangiocarcinoma from the intrahepatic ducts down to the ampulla of Vater including the gallbladder using nine stages [6]. Of 196 perihilar tumors comprising the Bismuth types in this series, 106 were resected with a median survival of 19 months and 5-year survival of 11 % [7]. Of note, they did not report a difference in survival for the 15 patients who had a hepatectomy as part of their procedure.

The French group spearheaded by Bismuth, evaluated 136 consecutive patients between 1960 and 1990 with hilar cholangiocarcinoma [8]. With the assistance of preoperative ultrasound, computed tomography, mesenteric angiography, intraoperative ultrasound and cholangiography, 23 of these patients were considered suitable for resection. There were three type I, three type II, 16 type III (9IIa, 7IIIb), and four type IV tumors. In this early series, only nine patients had negative margins with a 50 % 3-year survival. Local excision was performed in eight cases but only those with type I tumors had a margin and recurrence-free resection. In 2 of the 3 type II lesions, where local excision of the bile duct only was performed, both patients developed early recurrence. Conversely, 4 of 7 patients with type III lesions who had a concomitant hepatectomy along with bile duct resection had R0 resections and were disease-free. The authors concluded that some type II tumors may require caudate and/or segment 4 resection if a significant portion of the left hepatic duct is involved. In addition, they also suggested that resection in combination with liver transplantation should be considered for type IV lesions.

A similar study over the same period examined 94 patients with hilar cholangiocarcinoma stratified by Bismuth-Corlette stage [9]. Of the 40 patients that underwent resection, the majority presented with type III disease (62.5 %) followed by type IV (15 %) while type I and type II disease were seen in 12.5 and 10 % of patients respectively. Twenty-five patients had a concomitant hepatectomy along with bile duct resection while 4 of them required liver transplantation (all type IV). The overall resectability rate was 49 % and was dependent on the Bismuth-Corlette type with higher types (III, IV) requiring liver resection. In addition, tumors with bilateral vascular invasion were treated with primary hepatectomy, and reconstruction of contralateral vascular supply. Determining resectability was facilitated by the posterior approach to the hepatic hilus used to separate the remnant inflow structures proximal to the tumor at the biliary confluence in those tumors without hepatic parenchymal invasion and contained in the Glissonian sheath. The mean survival according to tumor location was 31 months for type I, 58 months for type II, 25 months for type III and 22 months for type IV lesions.

Another large report of 95 patients resected for hilar cholangiocarcinoma demonstrated an R0 resection rate of 43 %

for type I/II, 63 % type IIIa, 59 % of type IIIb and 72 % of type IV tumors likely due to the fact that the early stage tumors (I, II) only had hilar bile duct resections [10]. This translated into no 5 year survivors in the type I, II patients, with 48, 40, and 34 % 5 year survivors in type IIIa, IIIb, IV patients.

More recent updates, mainly from Asia, have challenged the traditional paradigm of resectability in advanced hilar tumors. The largest series from Nagoya describes 428 patients diagnosed between 2000 and 2008, of which 298 were resected [11]. They comprised 15 type I tumors (5 %), 21 type II (7 %), 120 type III (40 %), 142 type IV tumors (48 %). The surgical strategy was right hepatectomy for type I, II and IIIA lesions, standard or extended left hepatectomy for type IIIB lesions, and extended right or extended left hepatectomy or central hepatectomy for type IV lesions. With a majority of patients undergoing >50 % of their liver resected due to liberal use of portal vein embolization and aggressive resection of the portal vein (37 %) and hepatic artery (18 %), the authors achieved a 52 % 5 year survival rate for patients with R0, N0, M0 disease. However, there was no mention of whether the Bismuth-Corlette stage correlated with resectability or outcome. Meanwhile, other contemporary reports from Japan have failed to demonstrate a relationship between Bismuth-Corlette classification and survival [12–14].

Although this system simplifies the anatomical location of hilar cholangiocarcinoma, there are several considerations that are not evaluated. For example, the known variability of biliary tree can affect the Bismuth-Corlette classification. Some of the most common variations include a trifurcation at the biliary confluence of the right anterior and posterior sectoral ducts along with the left hepatic duct. Others include the drainage of either the right anterior or right posterior duct directly into the left hepatic duct. These anatomical considerations must be taken into account because they may render type IV tumors resectable. Another potential conflicting factor is the presence of a papillary tumor which may have a long intraductal mucosal component that is underestimated by standard imaging techniques. This is usually not the case with infiltrative tumors whose submucosal extent can be visualized as enhancement of the ductal wall. In summary, while the Bismuth-Corlette classification can be used as a common terminology to determine the likely extent of resection along anatomic borders of the biliary duct system, it has not served as a preoperative stating system in order to determine resectability or survival following resection.

4.3 Pathologic Staging Systems (AJCC, JSBS)

One of the major drawbacks of the Bismuth-Corlette classification however, is that it does not account for the radial extension of tumor away from the biliary ductal system into adjacent hepatic parenchyma, vascular structures and perihilar soft tissues. The American Joint Commission on Cancer (AJCC) developed a pathologic staging system which accounts for both the lateral spread of cancer as well as the presence of lymph node and distant metastases (Fig. 4.2). This tumor, node, metastases model (TNM) has been applied to several disease sites in the hope of stratifying patients to different survival categories based on the invasiveness or biology of the tumor.

Prior to the current 7th edition, the AJCC system separated the primary lesion into 4 T stages of which T1 was tumor confined to the bile duct wall and T2 was tumor

Anatomic stage/Prognostic groups

Stage 0	Tis	N0	M0
Stage I	T1	N0	M0
Stage II	T2a–b	N0	M0
Stage IIIA	T3	N0	M0
Stage IIIB	T1–3	N1	M0
Stage IVA	T4	N0–1	M0
Stage IVB	AnyT	N2	M0
	AnyT	Any N	M1

Primary tumor (T)

TX	Primary tumor cannot be assessed
T0	No evidence of primary tumor
Tis	Carcinoma in situ
T1	Tumor confined to the bile duct, with extension up to the muscle layer or fibrous tissue
T2a	Tumor invades beyond the wall of the bile duct to surrounding adipose tissue
T2b	Tumor invades adjacent hepatic parenchyma
T3	Tumor invades unilateral branches of the portal vein or hepatic artery
T4	Tumor invades main portal vein or its branches bilaterally; or the common hepatic artery; or the second-order biliary radicals bilaterally; or unilateral second-order biliary radicals with contralateral portal vein or hepatic artery involvement

Regional lymph nodes (N)

NX	Regional lymph nodes cannot be assessed
N0	No regional lymph node metastasis
N1	Regional lymph node metastasis (including nodes along the cystic duct, common bile duct, hepatic artery, and portal vein)
N2	Metastasis to periaortic, pericaval, superior mesenteric artery, and/or celiac artery lymph nodes

Distant metastasis (M)

M0	No distant metastasis
M1	Distant metastasis

Fig. 4.2 American Joint Commission on Cancer 7th Edition TNM staging for Perihilar Bile ducts (With permission from AJCC)

beyond the bile duct wall [15]. This is followed by T3 lesions that involve the liver, gallbladder or pancreas or the ipsilateral portal vein or hepatic artery. A T4 lesion was one that extended to the main portal trunk or its left and right branches simultaneously, the common hepatic artery or other adjacent structures such as the colon, stomach, duodenum or abdominal wall. This system created some ambiguity with regard to the definition of "beyond" the bile duct wall. This was further complicated by the 5th edition, which had split T1 lesions into T1a (invading the subepithelial connective tissue) and T1b (invading the fibromuscular tissue) from T2 lesions which were described as those within the perifibromuscular connective tissue of the bile duct [16]. Histologically, the outer muscular layer of the bile duct is variable along its length [17]. While a continuous layer may be found in the distal CBD, intermittent muscle fibers are found along the middle portion of the duct with little or no muscle seen in its proximal portion. Therefore the distinction between a T1 and T2 tumor may be difficult in a densely inflamed bile duct tumor. Furthermore, the correct identification of a T3 lesion is highly dependent on its longitudinal location on the bile duct. For example, a T3 lesion in the middle duct is likely to be more advanced than a T3 lesion in the hilus or distal duct, which is in close proximity to their respective adjacent structures (i.e., the liver and pancreas). However, the separation of T3 lesions into two separate categories of visceral and vascular invasion updated in the 6th edition was noted to improve survival prediction [18].

A better system to separate depth of penetration between T1 and T2 lesions has been proposed by Hong et al. [19]. His group of four experienced pathologists examined 222 bile duct specimens with the operative definition of T1 as tumors confined to the outermost layer of muscle and fibrous tissue and T2 as tumors in the adipose tissue beyond the bile duct while preserving the T3 and T4 nomenclatures. They found that there was a statistically significant difference in survival between patients with T1 and T2 tumors; however, there was no difference in survival between T2 and T3 tumors and therefore no difference between Stages Ib and IIa in the 6th edition. This was likely due to the discrepancy in T staging depending on the location of the tumor whereby proximal and distal tumors were overstaged while middle tumors were understaged. They did note however, that patients with papillary and nodular tumors had an improved outcome than those with infiltrative growth patterns. In an attempt to standardize the T staging of extrahepatic bile duct tumors, the same authors examined the absolute depth of invasion measured in centimeters in the 222 patient cohort and stratified tumors into those with <5 mm of invasion, 5–12 mm of invasion and >12 mm of invasion based on censored local regression and recursive partitioning [20]. Using this technique, they noted a statistically significant decrease in survival as depth of invasion increased between groups. This difference remained significant on multivariate analysis.

Due to these observations, the T staging criteria were amended for the 7th Edition so that T1 are defined to be tumors confined to the bile duct with extension to the muscle layer or fibrous tissue while T2 are separated into T2a which are tumors that invade beyond the bile duct wall into surrounding adipose tissue and T2b which are tumors that invade adjacent hepatic parenchyma. Another important change in the 7th Edition was the separation of perihilar and distal bile duct cancer into separate staging categories. Perihilar carcinomas were defined as extrahepatic bile duct tumors arising anywhere proximal to the cystic duct up to the right and/or left hepatic ducts. Middle bile duct tumors, which are rare, are assigned depending on the type of resection needed for clearance: perihilar group if they required a hilar and hepatic resection or distal group if they required a pancreaticoduodenectomy. This separation allows for the proper staging with regard to invasion of adjacent structures such as the liver and pancreas. The other amendment to the T staging was the adjustment of T3 to unilateral vascular invasion only as this has been demonstrated to have a worse prognosis than hepatic parenchymal involvement which had been included in T3 lesions according to the 6th edition [21]. Lastly, T4 lesions, which are characterized by bilateral vascular invasion, bilateral secondary biliary radical involvement or the combination of unilateral vascular invasion with contralateral secondary biliary radical involvement have been upstaged to Stage IVa disease and differentiated from Stage IVb (distal nodal or metastatic disease) reflecting their low resectability rates while preserving the possibility for neoadjuvant chemotherapy and liver transplantation in that cohort of patients [22].

It is well known that the presence of lymph node metastases is directly correlated with increasing T stage. Overall, positive lymph nodes are found in 30–50 % of cases [23]. Often, the hilar and periductal nodes within the porta hepatis are involved primarily, but extension to periaortic, pericaval, celiac and superior mesenteric nodal basins can occur in advanced cases. In a study of 110 patients with hilar cholangiocarcinoma and 2,652 resected lymph nodes, 47 patients contained lymph node metastases (42.7 %). Out of 382 dissected lymph nodes 14 % contained metastases with the pericholedochal nodes involved most frequently (20.1 %) followed by periportal (15.4 %), common hepatic (15 %), paraaortic (14 %) and posterior pancreaticoduodenal (12.5 %) [24]. The authors found that the presence of nodal metastases was significantly higher in patients with pT3 disease than those with pT2 disease (64.7 % vs. 33.3 %, $P<0.005$) using the AJCC/UICC 5th Edition staging system.

Paraaortic nodal metastases translated to a worse outcome with 3 and 5 year survival rates of 12.3 and 12.3 % compared to patients with no lymph node metastases (55.4 and 30.5 %) or limited to regional nodal involvement (31.8 and 14.7 %). Of note, there were few patients who had isolated paraaortic lymph node involvement alone without positive regional nodes suggesting a progression of disease along existing lymphatic channels. In fact, lymphatic dye staining studies have demonstrated a distinct pathway from pericholedochal nodes to the posterior pancreatic, retroportal, common hepatic and paraaortic nodes [25, 26]. Therefore, in the current 7th Edition the N category has been edited to reflect this finding properly with N1 disease being regional (i.e. periportal) node involvement while presence of tumor in distant mesenteric or aortocaval nodes categorized as N2. Accordingly, N1 has been upstaged from Stage IIb to Stage IIIb while N2 disease is now considered Stage IVb even in the absence of widely metastatic disease reflecting its poor prognosis.

Much like other gastrointestinal tumors, lymph node involvement is also a major prognostic factor for overall and disease-specific survival. However, unlike gastric [27], pancreatic [28] and colon [29] carcinoma where specific guidelines for number of harvested lymph nodes for accurate staging of disease have been established, there are no such recommendations for hilar cholangiocarcinoma. The 6th Edition of the AJCC staging system defined the absence (N0) or presence (N1) of regional nodal disease based on the analysis of three lymph nodes despite minimal support from published studies. In fact, a large epidemiological study using the SEER database have suggested a minimum lymph node harvest of ten nodes for proper stage assignment [30]. From their cohort of 20,068 patients with extrahepatic bile duct cancers including gallbladder and ampullary cancers, those with node-negative tumors who had >10 lymph nodes in their specimen had the highest median survival of 36 months. Although a projection model using linear regression comparing the impact of increasing lymph node count on survival failed to show a statistically significant improvement ($P=0.0742$), the authors concluded that the presence of at least ten negative lymph nodes were predictive of improved survival. Interestingly, this number was consistent among N0 and N1 disease in all anatomic sites except for ampullary cancers.

In response to this observation and the fact that the SEER data was contaminated with gallbladder cancer patients, our group embarked on a study to examine the importance of adequate lymph node assessment in extrahepatic bile duct cancers. Out of a cohort of 247 patients with cholangiocarcinoma, 144 with hilar cholangiocarcinoma were identified and noted to have a median total lymph node count (TLNC) of 3 with a range of 0–16 [31]. Multivariate analysis revealed that lymph node metastasis was an independent prognostic factor for DSS. Additionally, in patients who underwent R0, N0 resection, DSS was higher in those with higher TLNC. Using maximal chi-square analysis, the optimal lymph node harvest for hilar cholangiocarcinoma in our population was determined to be seven. In the 97 patients who had an R0 resection (with concomitant hepatectomy) and found to be node-negative based on a TLNC greater than seven, the 5 year DSS was significantly higher than those whose TLNC was below that number (85 % vs. 48 %). Another study from Japan examined the incidence of lymph node metastases in 209 cases of extrahepatic bile duct cancers excluding intrahepatic and periampullary tumors. The authors found a significant survival cutoff point in patients with at least five lymph nodes examined between those with 1–4 positive nodes and five or greater nodes positive for metastases [32]. They proposed the AJCC nodal classification should be amended to N0 (no regional node metastases), N1 (1–4 regional node metastases) and N2 (five or more regional node metastases). These observations likely reflect more accurate staging of patients with advanced disease as opposed to a therapeutic effect of lymphadenectomy. Although no randomized, controlled trials of lymphadenectomy specifically in cholangiocarcinoma have been performed, data from trials including periampullary tumors do not support the role of extended lymphadenectomy in bile duct tumors [33]. Besides overall number and number of negative lymph nodes, other groups have focused on the ratio of positive lymph nodes to the total number harvested [34]. This lymph node ratio (LNR) has been examined in other pancreatobiliary malignancies and found to have prognostic capabilities. Recently, Oshiro et al. found that a $LNR \geq 0.2$ was an independent predictive factor of survival in multivariate analysis and supported the notion of more aggressive tumor biology [35].

Although the AJCC classification is most commonly used internationally, a separate pathologic staging system has been established by the Japanese Society of Biliary Surgery (JSBS) in 1981 and subsequently revised to its current 5th edition in 2003 (Fig. 4.3). In this system, the T classification is carefully separated into categories of invasion based on histologic landmarks such as mucosa, serosa and subserosa as well as depth of invasion into adjacent structures such as the liver or pancreas which stratified into less than 5 mm, between 5 and 20 mm and greater than 20 mm. Vascular invasion is distinguished between portal and hepatic arterial, with each type having three depths (adventitial, tunica medial, and tunica intimal with stenosis or obstruction) numbered 1–3 respectively. The type of tumor growth is also separated into papillary, nodular, flat types each with their own subcategories of expanding and infiltrating patterns. In addition, nodal metastases are numbered according to

pT classification	
pT	Contents
pT1	m, fm, hinf0, panc0, pv0, a0
pT2	ss, hinf1, panc1, pv0 ,a0
pT3	se, hinf2, panc2 , pv1, a1
pT4	si, hinf3, panc3 , pv2, pv3, a2, a3

Lymph node grouping			
Lymph node (site number)	Group		
	Hilar and proximal	Middle	Distal
Infrapyloric LN (6)	pN3	pN3	pN3
LN around the common hepatic artery (8)	pN2	pN2	pN2
LN at the splenic hilum (10)	pN3	pN3	pN3
LN along the splenic artery (11)	pN3	pN3	pN3
LN at the hepatic hilum (12h)	pN1	pN2	pN2
LN along the hepatic artery (12a)	pN1	pN2	pN2
Periportal LN (12p)	pN1	pN2	pN2
Pericholedochal LN (12b)	pN1	pN1	pN1
LN around the cystic duct (12c)	pN1	pN1	pN1
Posterior superior pancreatoduodental LN (13a)	pN2	pN2	pN2
Posterior inferior pancreatoduodental LN (13b)	pN3	pN3	pN3
LN along the superior mesenteric artery (14)	pN3	pN3	pN2
Para-aortic LN (16)	pN3	pN3	pN3
Anterior superior pancreatoduodenal LN (17a)	pN3	pN3	pN3
Anterior inferior pancreatoduodenal LN (17b)	pN3	pN3	pN3

Stage grouping	H(–) and P(–) and M(–)				H(+) and/or P(+) and/or
	pN0	pN1	pN2	pN3	M(+) and any N
pT1	I	II	III	IVa	IVb
pT2	II	III	III	IVa	IVb
pT3	III	III	IVa	IVb	IVb
pT4	IVa	IVa	IVb	IVb	IVb

m invasion limited to the mucosa, *fm* invasion limited to the fibromuscular layer, *ss* invasion limited to the subserosa, *se* invasion of serosal surface, *si* invasion beyond the serosa and invasion of other organs or structures, *hinf0* no direct invasion of the liver, or direct invasion limited to the fibromuscular layer of intrahepatic bile ducts, *hinf1* direct invasion of fibromuscular layer of intrahepatic ducts and/or liver parenchyma which invasion is not more than 5 mm in depth, *hinf2* direct invasion of liver parenchyma, which invasion is 5 mm or more but not more than 20 mm in depth, *hinf3* direct invasion of liver parenchyma, which invasion is 20 mm or more in depth, *panc0* no invasion of the fibromuscular layer of the inferior bile duct, *panc1* invasion of the fibromuscular layer of the inferior bile duct and/or pancreatic parenchyma of which invasion is not more than 5 mm in depth, *panc2* invasion of the pancreatic parenchyma of which invasion is 5 mm or more but not more than 20 mm in depth, *panc3* invasion of the pancreatic parenchyma of which invasion is 20 mm or more in depth, *pv0* no invasion of portal vein, *pv1* invasion of the adventita, *pv2* invasion of the media, *pv3* invasion of the intima, *a0* no invasion of hepatic arteries, *a1* invasion of the adventita, *a2* invasion of the media, *a3* invasion of the intima, *LN* lymph node, *H(–)* no liver metastasis, *H(+)* liver metastasis, *P(–)* no peritoneal metastasis, *P(+)* peritoneal metastasis, *M(–)* no distant metastasis, *M(+)* distant metastasis

Fig. 4.3 Japanese Society for Biliary Surgery Classification for Cholangiocarcinoma (With permission from Langebecks Archives of Surgery)

location of the node and classified according to location the primary tumor (hilar, middle or distal) in order to more accurately stage the extent of disease. For example, a lymph node at the hepatic hilus (#12 h) is considered N1 for a hilar tumor but N2 for a middle or distal duct tumor. Conversely, a lymph node along the superior mesenteric artery (#14) is considered

N2 for a distal tumor but N3 for a hilar or middle duct tumor. Although the JSBS system permits a very detailed description of tumor extent, there are no studies that report a correlation between JSBS stage assignment and either resectability or outcome. Recently, this system was compared to the AJCC/UICC TNM classification and it was found to provide improved survival stratification of patients according to stage [36]. However outside of Japan, it has not been applied extensively due to its inherent complexity and lack of validation.

Besides depth of invasion, presence and location of nodal and distant metastases, the AJCC recognized that certain stage-independent factors contribute to survival in these patients. Probably, the most well-established is the ability to achieve an R0 resection which is the major contributor to outcome. Additionally, tumor grade and lobar atrophy are features associated with poorer survival. Recently, papillary morphology has been demonstrated to carry a more favorable prognosis than nodular sclerosing tumors [37]. The 7th Edition of the AJCC recommended these factors be incorporated into the reporting of staging information of patients with hilar cholangiocarcinoma.

4.4 Preoperative Clinical Staging Systems (Gazzaniga, Blumgart)

Despite the anatomic and pathologic descriptions of the Bismuth-Corlette and AJCC staging systems, neither classification is associated with ability to determine resectability of the tumor which is the only proven modality for long-term survival. The propensity of hilar cholangiocarcinoma to spread longitudinally along the duct up to 2 cm beyond the location of the primary mass may underestimate the extent of disease on radiographic studies. It is possible that complete tumor clearance may not be appreciated even on palpation during operation highlighting the need for frozen section analysis of the margins. In addition, the presence of vascular invasion suggested on preoperative imaging may be technically difficult to assess intraoperatively given the lateral spread of tumor away from the bile duct to the portal vessels directly beneath it.

Therefore it is important for a clinical staging system to accurately predict resectability, need for hepatectomy and survival following R0 resection. Gazzaniga and colleagues first proposed a system accounting for the extrabiliary growth of tumor into surrounding vasculature in 1985 [38] (Fig. 4.4). The stages were divided into four categories where stage 1 was disease confined to the biliary confluence, stage 2 was disease that extended from the biliary confluence to secondary biliary ducts or vascular structures in the same lobe, stage 3 was disease that extended from the biliary confluence to secondary biliary ducts and/or vascular

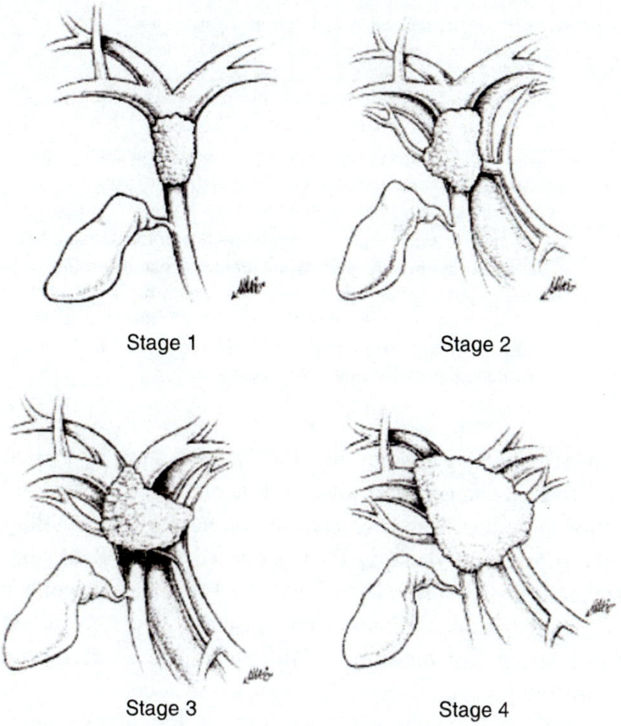

Fig. 4.4 Gazzaniga classification. Stage 1: hilar neoplasm with no extrabiliary involvement. Stage 2: hilar neoplasm with extrabiliary development concerning structures belonging to a single hepatic lobe and/or endobiliary diffusion in second-order branches of a single lobe. Stage 3: hilar neoplasm with endobiliary and/or extrabiliary diffusion to a single lobe, associated with infiltration due to the proximity of the contralateral lobe vascular structures, limited to the first-order branches. Stage 4: hilar neoplasm with large endo- and extrabiliary diffusion

structures in the same lobe and infiltration to the contralateral vascular structures while stage 4 was diffuse disease involving the entire porta hepatis. They proposed a treatment algorithm whereby stages 1–3 could undergo potentially curative resection by bile duct resection and caudate lobectomy for stage 1, a similar operation plus hemihepatectomy for stage 2, and the operation in stage 2 in addition to a vascular resection and reconstruction for stage 3 while surgical palliation would be reserved for stage 4. Using this system, the authors found a 43.5 % resectability rate for stage 1 tumors, 45.6 % for stage 2 tumors and 10.9 % for stage 3 tumors; however, the authors did not report the survival of patients according to stage [39].

At Memorial Sloan-Kettering, we have developed a preoperative clinical staging system for hilar cholangiocarcinoma using factors characterizing local tumor extent regardless of nodal or metastatic disease. In order to evaluate a patient for curative resection, tumor longitudinal growth along the biliary tree must be taken into account in conjunction with its radial growth into adjacent vascular structures as the combination will influence resectability. This is because ipsilateral involvement of vessels and bile ducts can be amenable to resection, whereas contralateral involvement

Table 4.1 Blumgart preoperative T staging system

Stage	Criteria
T1	Tumor involving biliary confluence ± unilateral extension to second-order biliary radicles
T2	Tumor involving biliary confluence ± unilateral extension to second-order biliary radicles **and** *ipsilateral* portal vein involvement ± *ipsilateral* hepatic atrophy
T3	Tumor involving biliary confluence + bilateral extension to second-order biliary radicles; **or** unilateral extension to second-order biliary radicles with *contralateral* portal vein involvement; **or** unilateral extension to second-order biliary radicles with *contralateral* hepatic lobar atrophy; **or** main or bilateral portal venous involvement

cannot be managed surgically. Lastly, lobar atrophy caused by long-standing biliary obstruction or by lack of portal blood flow has been a crucial determinant of resectability and subsequent therapy. First proposed in 1998 as four separate T stages, it was amended in 2001 to the current 3 T stages that include biliary extent, vascular involvement and lobar atrophy of the tumor (Table 4.1). These criteria are evaluated preoperatively using non-invasive, cross-sectional or ultrasound imaging with rare need for direct cholangiography through endoscopic or percutaneous approaches or angiography/portography for staging.

Using the original classification system, 90 patients with hilar cholangiocarcinoma were evaluated between 1991 and 1997 and 48 % of patients deemed T1 were resectable compared to 0 of T4 patients [40]. In addition, 58 % of T1 patients required concomitant hepatectomy for gross tumor clearance compared to 100 % of T2 and T3 tumors. Although the T-staging system does not account for N or M status, 39 % of T1 had evidence of metastatic disease compared to 53 % of those with T3 tumors. This translated into improved median survival of T1 patients compared to T3 tumors and although there was no difference between T3 and T4 tumors, there were no 5 year survivors in the T4 group.

In an updated series of patients, this Blumgart classification system was used to stratify 225 patients with hilar cholangiocarcinoma into 3 T categories including the previous 90 patients that had been staged [41]. Of the 219 that had complete staging information available, 87 were T1, 95 were T2, and 37 were T3 tumors. On logistic regression, increasing T stage significantly reduced the resectability rate and likelihood of R0 resection. While 33 (65 %) T1 patients required hepatectomy with two (4 %) portal vein resections, all T2 patients underwent liver resection with seven (24 %) requiring portal vein resection. Furthermore, distal and N2 nodal metastatic disease was significantly associated with increasing T-stage. Using Cox regression with T stage as a categorical covariate and T1 as a reference, median survival was reduced significantly as T stage increased (20 months for T1, 13 months for T2, 8 months for T3). In order to compare outcome data, 187 patients were staged using the AJCC system. Unlike the Blumgart T staging system, AJCC tumor stage did not correlate with resectability, likelihood of R0 resection and did not predict survival. In fact, 46 out of 80 patients who underwent resection and seven out of nine 5 year survivors were classified as AJCC Stage IV tumors.

The most contemporary series of 118 patients from Memorial Sloan-Kettering with hilar cholangiocarcinoma from 2001 to 2008 were staged by the updated preoperative classification [42]. Forty eight patients had primary tumor involvement of the biliary confluence but without unilateral extension into second-order biliary radicles, portal vein involvement or lobar atrophy and therefore T1 tumors. Forty one patients had T2 tumors due to ipsilateral lobar atrophy or portal vein involvement (n=31 for both). There were 29 patients with T3 tumors, 10 due to main portal vein involvement, 7 due to extension to unilateral second-order biliary radicles and contralateral lobar atrophy, 9 due to extension to unilateral second-order biliary radicles and contralateral portal vein involvement, 2 due to extension to bilateral second-order biliary radicles, and 1 due to tumor encasing the contralateral hepatic artery. Using this system, resectability and feasibility of R0 resection decreased progressively with increasing stage (T1 to T3). Furthermore, the presence of metastatic disease precluding resection correlated with increasing T stage (T1 to T3).

The Blumgart system has also been evaluated by other groups. Hemming et al. evaluated 87 consecutive patients with resected hilar cholangiocarcinoma and retrospectively staged them simultaneously with the Bismuth-Corlette and Blumgart classifications [43]. There was no correlation between resectability and Bismuth-Corlette stage while 84 % of Blumgart T1 lesions were resectable followed by 55 % of Blumgart T2 lesions and 0 of Blumgart T3 lesions. The authors also highlighted the importance of the lobar atrophy/hypertrophy complex in determining survival following resection. However, on their univariate analysis, no staging system was predictive of survival due to a statistical lack of sufficient numbers for analysis. This phenomenon was suggested in another single institution report of 69 patients from the University of Wisconsin where the correlation between Blumgart T stage and resectability had a p-value of 0.06 [44]. Another underpowered study of 42 patients failed to demonstrate prognostic capability of any staging system [45].

Recently, a novel staging system has been proposed by Blechacz et al. [46]. Recognizing the fact that an optimal staging system is required in order to properly evaluate patients in clinical trials, they maintain that such a system would take into the account not only the stage of the tumor but also the physiological consequences of biliary and vascular obstruction as well as the performance status of the patient and effectiveness of available therapies. In their system, tumor stage would include size of the lesion, vascular encasement, lobar atrophy and extent of extrahepatic disease. The authors suggest that the primary tumors should be separated into those that can be visualized on imaging and those that are radiographically occult. In addition, lesions should be stratified according to size greater or less than 3 cm. They also propose the presence of vascular encasement and subsequent lobar atrophy represent long-standing events that have a high likelihood of harboring regional micrometastases. Lastly, given recent evidence that the timing of the resolution of jaundice following biliary stenting leading to recovery of liver functional status, this variable is included in this proposed staging system [47]. This system is currently being validated.

Conclusion

In summary, there are currently several staging systems available in the management of hilar cholangiocarcinoma. Unlike other disease sites, most patients with perihilar malignancies have locoregional and/or distant spread which may be radiographically occult and prevent surgical intervention. Therefore, while pathologic staging of the specimen can provide definitive confirmation of extent of disease, decisions on therapy are often based on clinical judgment and/or intraoperative evaluation in unresectable cases. The Bismuth-Corlette system provides a good introduction to the level of biliary involvement by tumor and allows surgeons to standardize an operative plan. However, the growth pattern of hilar cholangiocarcinoma is such that local vascular (portal and arterial) as well as parenchymal atrophy from longstanding obstruction can adversely affect the potential for surgical resection. Given that long-term survival is dependent not only on tumor characteristics but also the ability to achieve a margin-negative curative resection, better preoperative staging is needed. The Blumgart system provides a more comprehensive framework to base preoperative decisions by predicting not only resectability, but also the likelihood of R0 resection and subsequent survival. However, the ideal system would incorporate this information along with status of regional or distant disease so that all patients could be stratified for clinical trials to test novel therapies for this aggressive malignancy.

References

1. Altemeier WA, Gall EA, Zinninger MM, et al. Sclerosing carcinoma of the major intrahepatic bile ducts. AMA Arch Surg. 1957;75(3):450–60; discussion 460–1.
2. Klatskin G. Adenocarcinoma of the hepatic duct at its bifurcation within the porta hepatis. An unusual tumor with distinctive clinical and pathological features. Am J Med. 1965;38:241–56.
3. Ito F, Cho CS, Rikkers LF, et al. Hilar cholangiocarcinoma: current management. Ann Surg. 2009;250(2):210–8.
4. Bismuth H, Corlette MB. Intrahepatic cholangioenteric anastomosis in carcinoma of the hilus of the liver. Surg Gynecol Obstet. 1975;140(2):170–8.
5. Madariaga JR, Iwatsuki S, Todo S, et al. Liver resection for hilar and peripheral cholangiocarcinomas: a study of 62 cases. Ann Surg. 1998;227(1):70–9.
6. Pitt HA, Dooley WC, Yeo CJ, et al. Malignancies of the biliary tree. Curr Probl Surg. 1995;32(1):1–90.
7. Nakeeb A, Pitt HA, Sohn TA, et al. Cholangiocarcinoma. A spectrum of intrahepatic, perihilar, and distal tumors. Ann Surg. 1996;224(4):463–73; discussion 473–5.
8. Bismuth H, Nakache R, Diamond T. Management strategies in resection for hilar cholangiocarcinoma. Ann Surg. 1992;215(1):31–8.
9. Launois B, Terblanche J, Lakehal M, et al. Proximal bile duct cancer: high resectability rate and 5-year survival. Ann Surg. 1999; 230(2):266–75.
10. Neuhaus P, Jonas S, Bechstein WO, et al. Extended resections for hilar cholangiocarcinoma. Ann Surg. 1999;230(6):808–18; discussion 819.
11. Igami T, Nishio H, Ebata T, et al. Surgical treatment of hilar cholangiocarcinoma in the "new era": the Nagoya University experience. J Hepatobiliary Pancreat Sci. 2010;17(4):449–54.
12. Hirano S, Kondo S, Tanaka E, et al. Outcome of surgical treatment of hilar cholangiocarcinoma: a special reference to postoperative morbidity and mortality. J Hepatobiliary Pancreat Sci. 2010;17(4): 455–62.
13. Miyazaki M, Kimura F, Shimizu H, et al. One hundred seven consecutive surgical resections for hilar cholangiocarcinoma of bismuth types II, III, IV between 2001 and 2008. J Hepatobiliary Pancreat Sci. 2010;17(4):470–5.
14. Unno M, Katayose Y, Rikiyama T, et al. Major hepatectomy for perihilar cholangiocarcinoma. J Hepatobiliary Pancreat Sci. 2010; 17(4):463–9.
15. Greene FL, American Joint Committee on Cancer, American Cancer Society. AJCC cancer staging handbook: from the AJCC cancer staging manual. 6th ed. New York: Springer; 2002.
16. Fleming ID, American Joint Committee on Cancer, American Cancer Society, et al. AJCC cancer staging manual. 5th ed. Philadelphia: Lippincott-Raven; 1997.
17. Hong SM, Kang GH, Lee HY, et al. Smooth muscle distribution in the extrahepatic bile duct: histologic and immunohistochemical studies of 122 cases. Am J Surg Pathol. 2000;24(5):660–7.
18. Nishio H, Nagino M, Oda K, et al. TNM classification for perihilar cholangiocarcinoma: comparison between 5th and 6th editions of the AJCC/UICC staging system. Langenbecks Arch Surg. 2005; 390(4):319–27.
19. Hong SM, Kim MJ, Pi DY, et al. Analysis of extrahepatic bile duct carcinomas according to the new American Joint Committee on cancer staging system focused on tumor classification problems in 222 patients. Cancer. 2005;104(4):802–10.
20. Hong SM, Cho H, Moskaluk CA, et al. Measurement of the invasion depth of extrahepatic bile duct carcinoma: an alternative method overcoming the current T classification problems of the AJCC staging system. Am J Surg Pathol. 2007;31(2):199–206.
21. Ebata T, Nagino M, Kamiya J, et al. Hepatectomy with portal vein resection for hilar cholangiocarcinoma: audit of 52 consecutive cases. Ann Surg. 2003;238(5):720–7.
22. Rea DJ, Heimbach JK, Rosen CB, et al. Liver transplantation with neoadjuvant chemoradiation is more effective than resection for hilar cholangiocarcinoma. Ann Surg. 2005;242(3):451–8; discussion 458–61.
23. Klempnauer J, Ridder GJ, von Wasielewski R, et al. Resectional surgery of hilar cholangiocarcinoma: a multivariate analysis of prognostic factors. J Clin Oncol. 1997;15(3):947–54.
24. Kitagawa Y, Nagino M, Kamiya J, et al. Lymph node metastasis from hilar cholangiocarcinoma: audit of 110 patients who underwent regional and paraaortic node dissection. Ann Surg. 2001;233(3): 385–92.
25. Deki H, Sato T. An anatomic study of the peripancreatic lymphatics. Surg Radiol Anat. 1988;10(2):121–35.

26. Shirai Y, Yoshida K, Tsukada K, et al. Identification of the regional lymphatic system of the gallbladder by vital staining. Br J Surg. 1992;79(7):659–62.
27. Bonenkamp JJ, Hermans J, Sasako M, et al. Extended lymph-node dissection for gastric cancer. N Engl J Med. 1999;340(12):908–14.
28. House MG, Gonen M, Jarnagin WR, et al. Prognostic significance of pathologic nodal status in patients with resected pancreatic cancer. J Gastrointest Surg. 2007;11(11):1549–55.
29. Tepper JE, O'Connell MJ, Niedzwiecki D, et al. Impact of number of nodes retrieved on outcome in patients with rectal cancer. J Clin Oncol. 2001;19(1):157–63.
30. Schwarz RE, Smith DD. Lymph node dissection impact on staging and survival of extrahepatic cholangiocarcinomas, based on U.S. Population data. J Gastrointest Surg. 2007;11(2):158–65.
31. Ito K, Ito H, Allen PJ, et al. Adequate lymph node assessment for extrahepatic bile duct adenocarcinoma. Ann Surg. 2010;251(4):675–81.
32. Hong SM, Cho H, Lee OJ, et al. The number of metastatic lymph nodes in extrahepatic bile duct carcinoma as a prognostic factor. Am J Surg Pathol. 2005;29(9):1177–83.
33. Yeo CJ, Cameron JL, Lillemoe KD, et al. Pancreaticoduodenectomy with or without distal gastrectomy and extended retroperitoneal lymphadenectomy for periampullary adenocarcinoma, part 2: randomized controlled trial evaluating survival, morbidity, and mortality. Ann Surg. 2002;236(3):355–66; discussion 366–8.
34. Kawai M, Tani M, Kobayashi Y, et al. The ratio between metastatic and examined lymph nodes is an independent prognostic factor for patients with resectable middle and distal bile duct carcinoma. Am J Surg. 2010;199(4):447–52.
35. Oshiro Y, Sasaki R, Kobayashi A, et al. Prognostic relevance of the lymph node ratio in surgical patients with extrahepatic cholangiocarcinoma. Eur J Surg Oncol. 2011;37(1):60–4.
36. Sasaki R, Murata S, Oda T, et al. Evaluation of UICC-TNM and JSBS staging systems for surgical patients with extrahepatic cholangiocarcinoma. Langenbecks Arch Surg. 2010;395(6):615–23.
37. Jarnagin WR, Bowne W, Klimstra DS, et al. Papillary phenotype confers improved survival after resection of hilar cholangiocarcinoma. Ann Surg. 2005;241(5):703–12; discussion 712–4.
38. Gazzaniga GM, Faggioni A, Filauro M. Surgical treatment of proximal bile duct tumors. Int Surg. 1985;70(1):45–8.
39. Gazzaniga GM, Filauro M, Bagarolo C, et al. Surgery for hilar cholangiocarcinoma: an Italian experience. J Hepatobiliary Pancreat Surg. 2000;7(2):122–7.
40. Burke EC, Jarnagin WR, Hochwald SN, et al. Hilar cholangiocarcinoma: patterns of spread, the importance of hepatic resection for curative operation, and a presurgical clinical staging system. Ann Surg. 1998;228(3):385–94.
41. Jarnagin WR, Fong Y, DeMatteo RP, et al. Staging, resectability, and outcome in 225 patients with hilar cholangiocarcinoma. Ann Surg. 2001;234(4):507–17; discussion 517–9.
42. Rocha FG, Matsuo K, Blumgart LH, et al. Hilar cholangiocarcinoma: the memorial sloan-kettering cancer center experience. J Hepatobiliary Pancreat Sci. 2010;17(4):490–6.
43. Hemming AW, Reed AI, Fujita S, et al. Surgical management of hilar cholangiocarcinoma. Ann Surg. 2005;241(5):693–9; discussion 699–702.
44. Ito F, Agni R, Rettammel RJ, et al. Resection of hilar cholangiocarcinoma: concomitant liver resection decreases hepatic recurrence. Ann Surg. 2008;248(2):273–9.
45. Zervos EE, Osborne D, Goldin SB, et al. Stage does not predict survival after resection of hilar cholangiocarcinomas promoting an aggressive operative approach. Am J Surg. 2005;190(5):810–5.
46. Blechacz BR, Sanchez W, Gores GJ. A conceptual proposal for staging ductal cholangiocarcinoma. Curr Opin Gastroenterol. 2009;25(3):238–9.
47. Weston BR, Ross WA, Wolff RA, et al. Rate of bilirubin regression after stenting in malignant biliary obstruction for the initiation of chemotherapy: how soon should we repeat endoscopic retrograde cholangiopancreatography? Cancer. 2008;112(11):2417–23.

Preoperative Imaging

5

B.I. Choi and J.M. Lee

5.1 Introduction

Cholangiocarcinomas (CC) are relatively rare tumors, although their incidence is increasing worldwide [1]. CC is classified anatomically as intrahepatic (5–10 % of cases), perihilar (60–70 %), or distal (20–30 %) [2, 3]. Hilar cholangiocarcinoma (HCCA) originally described by Klatskin, is defined as adenocarcinoma of the extrahepatic biliary tree, arising from the biliary confluence and/or the main left or right hepatic ducts, whereas intrahepatic CC arises from the bile ducts peripheral to the secondary bifurcation of the left or right hepatic duct [4, 5]. Cancers arising in the perihilar region have been further classified according to the pattern of involvement of the hepatic ducts (the Bismuth-Corlette classification) (Fig. 5.1) [6]. Despite a great increase in knowledge and major improvements in diagnostic methods as well as surgical techniques, these tumors still are a problematic issue [7]. Preoperative histological confirmation of an HCCA can be difficult to obtain. Percutaneous needle biopsies and endoscopic brush biopsies are reliable only if they identify a malignancy (sensitivity, 50 %), and excessive reliance on negative results may miss the opportunity to resect an early lesion [8, 9]. Whereas the vast majority of hilar strictures are the result of an HCCA, histological diagnosis is not mandatory before exploration. Accurate detection and differentiation from other bile duct pathologies on imaging, such as inflammatory lesions or stone disease, are highly important [7].

Surgical resection remains the only potentially curative treatment modality [10–12]. However, HCCA is a disease characterized by frequent locoregional invasion into porta hepatis structures, and although not necessarily indicative of unresectability, they are associated with both locally advanced tumors and metastatic disease [12]. Therefore, the majority of patients, nearly two-thirds in some series, present with disease that is beyond surgical correction [13]. In general, operation for HCCA requires a supraduodenal bile duct excision, portal lymphadenectomy, cholecystectomy, bilioenteric reconstruction, and, in most cases, a partial hepatectomy, which carry significant risk of morbidity [14–16]. Therefore, accurate disease staging is clearly critical for identifying patients who would benefit from an operation and for avoiding a non-therapeutic laparotomy [12].

Recently, cross-sectional imaging modalities such as multi-row detector computed tomography (MDCT) and magnetic resonance imaging (MRI) with magnetic resonance cholangiopancreatography(MRCP) have made considerable advances, and have contributed to robust biliary imaging with higher temporal and spatial resolution. Therefore, currently, those noninvasive cross sectional imaging modalities are more frequently used for diagnosis and tumor staging, whereas invasive examinations, including diagnostic endoscopic retrograde cholangiography (ERC) or percutaneous cholangiography or endoscopic ultrasound (EUS), have become less important [2, 7]. If HCCAs is diagnosed on preoperative imaging study, the next step is to exclude the established criteria for unresectable tumors, and then to define the tumor spread, and to identify any other combined findings [17]. The diagnosis and staging of CC require a multimodality approach involving laboratory, radiologic, endoscopic, and pathologic analysis [18]. Despite the variety of techniques used, determining the extent of disease still poses a challenge and is often underestimated [19]. Given that these tumors are usually very small, although these imaging tests can suggest the diagnosis, the major issue of imaging with this tumor is to determine whether the tumor is resectable [4]. In the absence of clear evidence of unresectability, all suspected HCCA should be considered for resection [13].

B.I. Choi, MD (✉) • J.M. Lee, MD
Department of Radiology, Seoul National University Hospital, Seoul, South Korea
e-mail: bichoi@snu.ac.kr

W.Y. Lau (ed.), *Hilar Cholangiocarcinoma*,
DOI 10.1007/978-94-007-6473-6_5, © Springer Science+Business Media Dordrecht and People's Medical Publishing House 2013

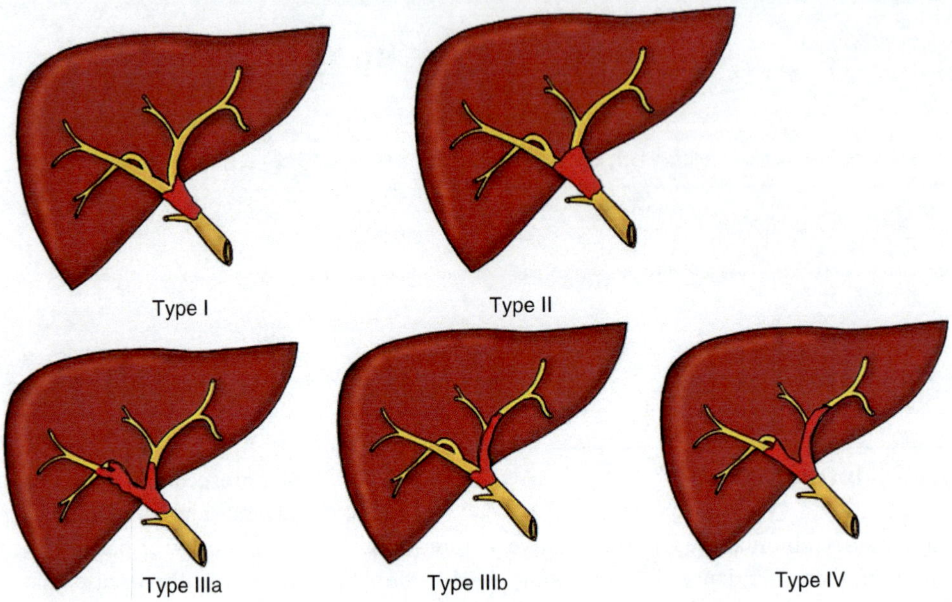

Fig. 5.1 Classification of biliary extent of hilar cholangiocarcinoma according to Bismuth-Corlette

5.2 Imaging Techniques

Imaging studies are essential in establishing the cause of jaundice, whether bile duct strictures are benign or malignant, and planning management in patients with suspected CC. The appropriate selection of radiological tests necessary to evaluate a patient with a suspected HCCA has undergone significant evolution in recent years. The diagnostic procedures include the traditional procedures of diagnosing bile duct pathologies such as transabdominal and endoscopic ultrasonography and ERC or percutaneous cholangiography as well as the modern cross-sectional imaging modalities such as MDCT, MRI with MR angiography (MRA) or MRCP, and positron emission tomography (PET) [7]. Until recently, invasive techniques such as transhepatic percutaneous cholangiography, ERC, and visceral angiography, combined with CT scanning were required to establish the diagnosis and determine resectability. However, besides being invasive in nature, recent studies have found that preoperative biliary instrumentation, particularly when combined with biliary stenting, increases perioperative infectious complications [20, 21]. Advances in imaging technology such as CT or MRI, combined with a philosophical approach aimed at limiting biliary instrumentation, have led us to more frequent use of MDCT with CT angiography, and/or MRI with MRCP with good determination of the disease extent and the potential respectability [22–25].

5.2.1 Ultrasonography

Ultrasound (US) is one of the first-line imaging modalities chosen for the evaluation of biliary disease [19]. At many centers, most jaundiced patients undergo initial transabdominal US to confirm biliary ductal dilatation, localize the site of the obstruction, and exclude gallstones [26]. Although US can effectively demonstrate dilatation of the bile duct, it has only limited value in demonstrating the obstructing lesion in this type of tumor [4]. Most common findings of HCCA on US include nonspecific indirect signs such as intrahepatic bile duct dilatation with an abrupt change in bile duct caliber and nonunion of the right and left ducts. Although perihilar cancers may not be detected, especially if small, indirect signs (ductal dilatation throughout the obstructed liver segments) may point toward the diagnosis of HCCA. With state-of-the-art equipment, an excellent view even of the central hepatic parts with high spatial resolution is possible [27]. With regard to detection of intrahepatic bile duct dilatation, ultrasound reveals up to 100 % sensitivity for experienced examiners [28]. Color Doppler and spectral Doppler are helpful tools for detecting compression and tumor encasement of the portal vein or hepatic artery. However, for direct tumor assessment and differentiation between benign or malignant biliary lesions in the course of the common bile duct, it often has only limited value because of the image degradation from bowel gas and difficult anatomy [28]. In addition, US has poor sensitivity for detecting metastases in the lymph nodes (LN) (37 %), liver (66 %), and peritoneum (33 %) [29]. Overall, the sensitivity and specificity of ultrasound is poor in the diagnosis of HCCA, and staging generally relies on other imaging modalities [26, 30]. On the other hand, EUS is able to provide detailed information about pathologies in the hepatic porta, although it is invasive and its quality also depends on the experience of the examiner [28, 31, 32]. In addition, EUS seems to be more accurate at determination of regional LN and vascular involvement, and has the ability to perform direct-guided, fine-needle aspiration (FNA) on primary tumors as well as local LNs with sensitivity, specificity, and accuracy of 86–89, 100, and 88–91 %, respectively [31, 33, 34]. More recently, intraductal US has been developed and it uses small-diameter probes that can be inserted over a 9-mm guide wire at the time of direct cholangiography, providing US views that are 89 % accurate at determining the benign or malignant nature of biliary strictures and 82 % accurate at determining respectability [31, 35]. As with any US procedure, the accuracy of IDUS is again operator dependent [36].

5.2.2 Direct Cholangiography

Cholangiography through a retrograde endoscopic or percutaneous transhepatic approach may provide the most accurate anatomic information pertaining to which segmental branches are involved [4, 37]. Preoperative cholangiography may be indicated either diagnostically or therapeutically for patients with biliary obstruction.

The choice between ERCP and percutaneous cholangiography (PTC) is dictated by institutional experience and anatomic characteristics of the tumor: hilar and intrahepatic lesions typically can be viewed better with PTC [36]. However, ERCP is preferred in patients with primary sclerosing cholangitis (PSC) since the marked stricturing of the intrahepatic biliary tree makes a percutaneous approach difficult. Both modalities carry an overall sensitivity of 75–85 %, a specificity of 70–75 %, and an accuracy of 95 % in identifying the presence and extent of CC [2, 28, 36]. However, the invasiveness of both procedures is a notable limiting factor, favoring routine use of MRCP with or without EUS during the diagnostic stage of most cases unless the development of cholangitis demands early interventional therapy [38, 39]. Furthermore, direct cholangiography provides information only on the ductal system as a filling defect in the lumen, whereas any data on extraductal extension or the cause of the biliary obstruction cannot be obtained (Fig. 5.2) [7]. Other diseases that can cause hilar obstruction indistinguishable from HCCAs are metastases to periportal lymph nodes, gallbladder cancer invading the hepatoduodenal ligament, lymphadenopathy due to other inflammation, and idiopathic benign focal stricture of the bile duct [4]. However, direct cholangiography affords the opportunity of obtaining brush cytology and/or biopsy specimens, which can assist with making a definitive diagnosis [36]. Although these sampling methods carry sensitivities ranging from 10 to 80 % in the diagnosis of CC, the experience of most authorities has been at the lower end of this range, reflective of the substantial associated desmoplastic reaction and low cellularity seen in many CCs [32, 40]. This limitation has frequently led to the need to make definitive treatment decisions without the advantage of tissue diagnosis [36].

Nevertheless, in some centers, particularly in Japan, direct cholangiography of segmental ducts and cholangioscopy are still used in the evaluation of respectability [41–45]. This approach generally involves placement of multiple percutaneous biliary drainage catheters to allow complete access to the biliary tree. This is frequently combined with preoperative portal vein embolization in an effort to lower the risk of postoperative hepatic failure. Such an aggressive diagnostic evaluation may increase resectability but requires a prolonged hospital stay, and its ultimate value is unclear [46].

5.2.3 MDCT

Because of its widespread availability, CT is commonly obtained in patients with suspected biliary malignancy. It is useful for detecting biliary tumors, the level of biliary obstruction, and the presence of liver atrophy. In addition, MDCT has greatly enhanced the capabilities of CT in the assessment of HCCA. With state-of-the art scanners, the entire upper abdomen can be covered with a sub-millimeter collimation in one breath hold (<5 s). With these data, high-quality multiplanar reconstructions (MPR) in sagittal, coronal, oblique coronal or curved planes can be acquired, which are helpful for assessing the complex anatomy of the biliary system (Fig. 5.2) [47–49]. Moreover, the arterial and portovenous enhancement phases are clearly separated. The detail representation of the hepatic artery or portal vein as well as possible tumor invasion of these vessels at the porta hepatis can be demonstrated adequately [7]. CT can image the primary site of HCCA in 70–90 % of cases as lesions that are hypo- or hyper-attenuating relative to normal hepatic parenchyma during arterial and portal venous phases before showing gradual enhancement during delayed phase images [4, 47]. Although HCCA sometimes is not well demonstrated on CT, ductal dilatation in both hepatic lobes with a contracted gallbladder or nonunion of the right and left hepatic ducts suggest a Klatskin tumor.

Although previous reports have shown only a limited value of CT in diagnosing tumors of the biliary system with tumor detection rates of only 69 % and correct assessment of resectability in only 54 % [50], when performed with modern technology, the detection rate of biliary tumors is much better, with accuracies up to 100 % in hepatic arterial dominant phase scans and 86 % in portovenous phase scans [51]. The overall accuracy of CT for assessing resectability ranges between 60 and 86 % with sensitivities between 56 and 76 % [7, 47, 51–58].

5.2.4 MRI

For many years, biliary MRI was limited by poor spatial resolution as well as motion artifacts related with breathing. However, recently introduced technical improvements including parallel imaging and rapid sequences such as gradient echo, and half Fourier acquired single-shot turbo spin echo (HASTE), and respiratory independent sequences navigator triggering, have contributed to increasing use of MRI, including MRCP for evaluation of biliary tumors [7, 59]. Each of these techniques or in combination, have substantially increased the spatial and temporal resolution as a critical parameter in biliary imaging with reduced blurring. It is important to use sequences with thin-slice thickness (3–4 mm) that provide sufficient signal to obtain good quality images and are sufficiently thin to detect subtle abnormalities. For MRCP, the latest developments are 3D-triggered T2-weighted fast spin echo sequences with a voxel size of approximately 1.5 mm, by which high quality MPR images and maximum intensity projections (MIP) can be obtained

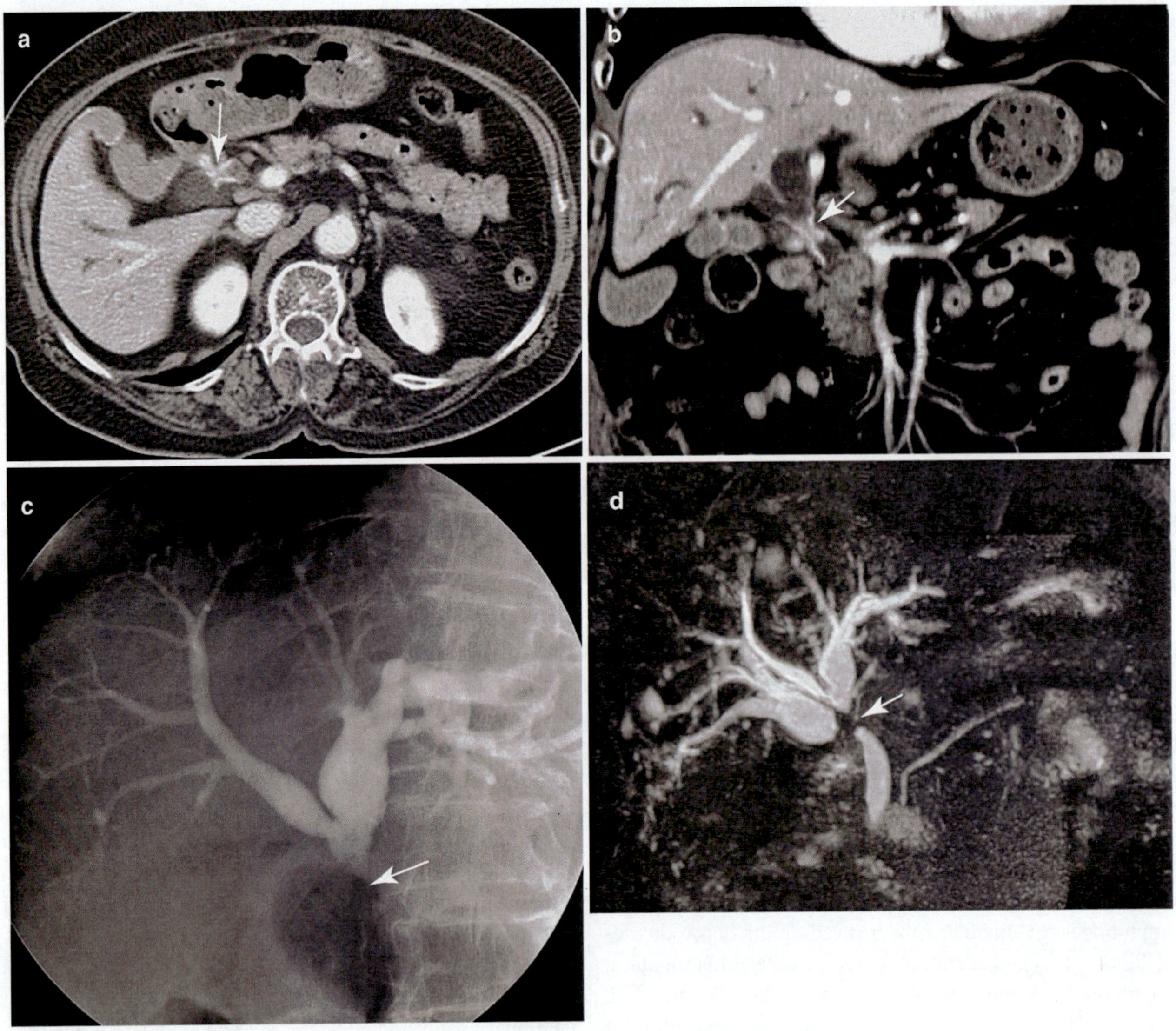

Fig. 5.2 Surgically proven periductal infiltrating type, hilar cholangiocarcinoma (Bismuth-Corlette type II). (**a**) Contrast-enhanced axial CT scan shows a hilar cholangiocarcinoma, which is depicted as a thickened and strongly enhancing wall of the hilar duct (*arrow*), and dilatation of the intrahepatic bile duct. (**b**) Coronal multiplanar reformatted image better demonstrates a longitudinal extent of the hilar cholangiocarcinoma than axial CT (**a**). Note that a hilar cholangiocarcinoma presents as a thickened bile duct wall with enhancement (*arrow*) during the portal venous phase. (**c**) On direct cholangiogram obtained by contrast injection through the percutaneous transhepatic biliary drainage, the proximal common bile duct is obliterated by the tumor. However, bilateral secondary confluences are intact. (**d**) MR cholangiography also demonstrates a stricture (*arrow*) involving hilar duct and proximal common bile duct, with dilatation of upstream intrahepatic bile duct. (**e** and **f**) Axial T2-weighted image (**e**) and T1-weighted image (**f**) show a focally thickened ductal wall (*arrow*) obliterating the lumen. On both T1- and T2-weighted images, the tumor appears slightly hypointense to the liver. (**g**) On contrast-enhanced axial T1-weighted image, the tumor is appreciated as a thickened and strongly enhancing wall of the hilar duct (*arrow*), anterior to the right portal vein branch. (**h**) On coronal T1-weighted image, the tumor involves the hilar portion as well as the proximal common bile duct (*arrow*). (**i**) The macroscopic picture of the resected specimen shows an irregular mucosal lesion (*arrows*) involving the primary biliary confluence as well as right and left intrahepatic bile duct

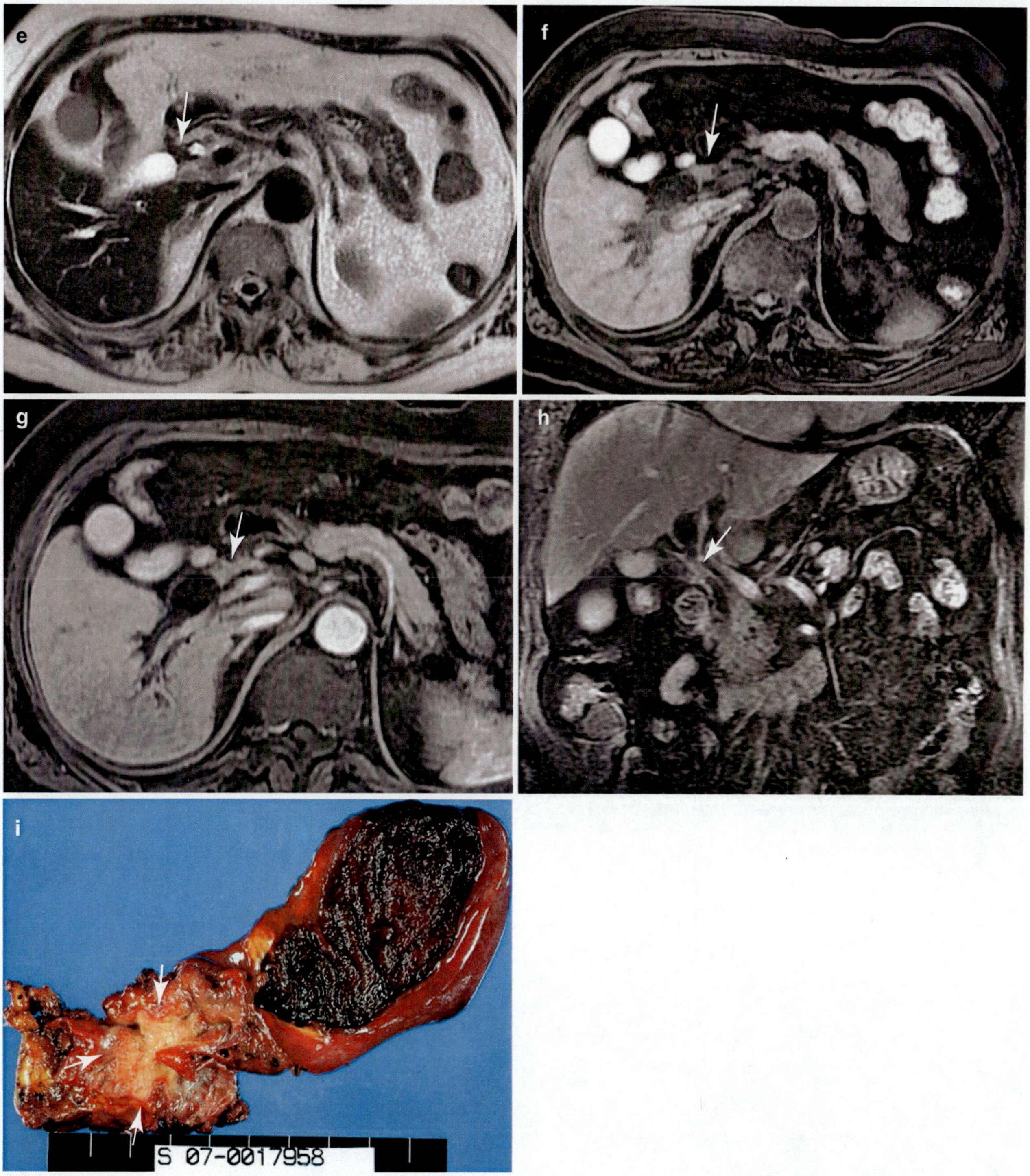

Fig. 5.2 (continued)

(Figs. 5.2 and 5.3). In addition, the axial thick-slab TSE T2-weighted cholangiographic views obtained at the hilum are the most informative about the number of strictures and the involvement of the different liver segments, including the caudate lobe (Fig. 5.4) [59]. MRCP can be very useful in visualization of the exact biliary tree map regarding extent of HCCA, in a non-invasive manner.

The principle sequences used for imaging the biliary system are T2-weighted imaging, MRCP, and pre- and postgadolinium-enhanced volumetric fat-suppressed gradient echo T1-weighted imaging [59]. MRI, in conjunction with MRCP, has proved helpful in diagnosing HCCA and in determining respectability [7, 60, 61]. This is due to MR imaging and MRCP being able to investigate all different

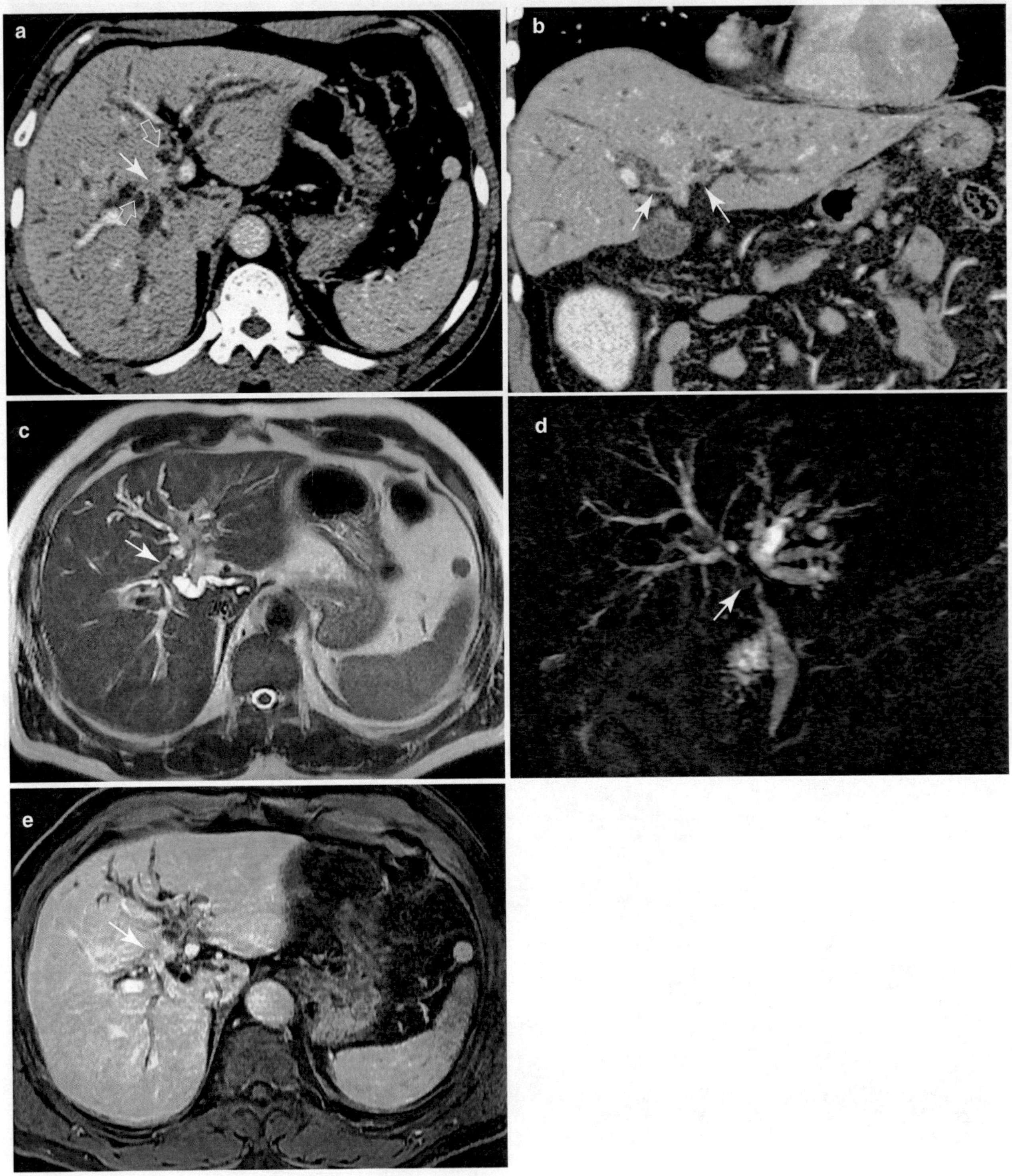

Fig. 5.3 Surgically proven periductal infiltrating type, hilar cholangiocarcinoma (Bismuth-Corlette type IV). (**a**) Contrast enhanced axial CT scan shows a slightly hyperattenuated mass (*arrow*) with heterogeneous enhancement, involving both secondary biliary confluences (*open arrows*). Note that there is a dilatation of the bile duct branches of the caudate lobe. Thus, CT diagnosis was Bismuth-Corlette type IV. (**b**) Coronal multiplanar reformatted image also demonstrates an irregular thickening of the hilar duct with hyperenhacement (*arrows*). (**c** and **d**) Axial T2-weighted image (**c**) and MR cholangiography (**d**) show an obliteration of the hilar duct (*arrow*) by the tumor with a hypointensity compared with adjacent liver parenchyma. (**e**) Contrast-enhanced axial T1-weighted image demonstrates an irregular shaped tumor (*arrow*) with hyperenhancement and upstream ductal dilatation, near the lobar branches of the portal vein

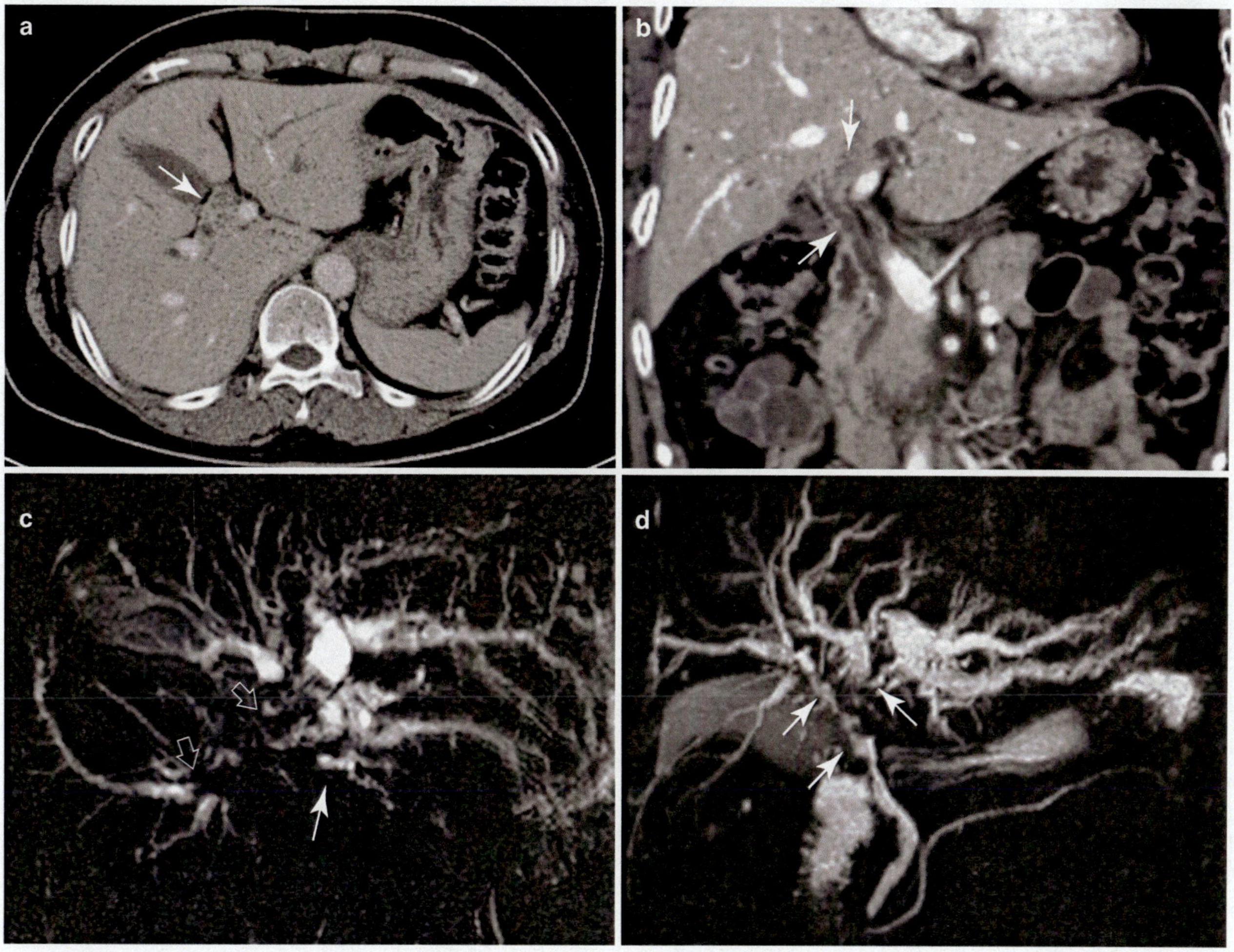

Fig. 5.4 Histolgically proven intraductal polypoid hilar cholangiocarcinoma (Bismuth-Corlette type IV). (**a**) Portal venous phase CT scan shows an intraductal mass (*arrow*) with slight hypoattenuation as compared with the adjacent hepatic parenchyma. (**b**) Coronal multiplanar reformatted image demonstrates multiple intraluminal filling defects (*arrows*) in the left and right intrahepatic ducts, hilar duct, and the common bile duct. (**c**) Axial slab MRCP also demonstrates a long stricture involving hilar duct and bilateral secondary biliary confluences (*open arrows*), and dilatation of intrahepatic bile duct in caudate lobe (*arrow*). Note that axial slab MR cholangiography con provide the most informative about the number of strictures and the involvement of the different liver segments, including caudate lobe. (**d**) Coronal multiplanar reformatted image of 3D-T2-weighted MRC shows irregular narrowing of both intrahepatic bile ducts and hilar duct, caused by multiple polypoid intraductal lesions (*arrows*)

components: bile ducts, vessels, and invasion of adjacent liver parenchyma [17]. The morphology of bile duct stricture detectable on MRCP closely reflects the gross morphologic changes occurring along the biliary ductal walls [4, 62, 63]. In addition, combined use of MRCP and dynamic MRI can display the overall extent of biliary tree involvement and the correct diagnosis of biliary malignancies (Fig. 5.3) [4, 17, 61, 64]. This capability of obtaining both cross sectional MRI and MRCP results in nearly 100 % sensitivity in diagnosing biliary obstruction, 98 % accuracy in identifying the level of obstruction, and an 88–95 % accurate assessment of the cause of obstruction; performance equivalent to that of direct cholangiography [28, 36, 60, 61, 65]. Given this cholangiographic performance, the ability to concurrently evaluate for intra-abdominal local or distant metastasis and its noninvasive nature, MRCP has become the imaging modality of choice in evaluation of biliary strictures and CC [15, 36, 60, 61]. Until now, the place of MRCP in the preoperative evaluation of suspected CC is evolving and somewhat center-dependent [66]. Some consider that the combination of MRCP and spiral CT have largely supplanted invasive cholangiography in patients with obstructive jaundice thought to be due to a proximal lesion. However, one of the disadvantages of MRCP is that current technology does not allow any intervention to be performed, such as stent insertion, or biopsy [28]. An accurate assessment of resectability of CC is rendered by MRI with MRCP in 70–80 % of cases, a rate equivalent to that provided by the combination of CT and direct cholangiography in prospective comparison [67].

From a strategic standpoint, it is important to recognize that stenting and percutaneous drainage procedures cause mild bile duct wall inflammation that is indistinguishable on MRI from CC spread [17]. Consequently, MRCP should be performed before interventional procedures whenever possible [17, 36]. For preoperative assessment of resectability of HCCA, however, several types of invasive imaging such as cholangiography and angiography are sometimes required, when the tumor size is too small to demonstrate its extent clearly on MRI with MRCP [4].

5.2.5 FDG-PET

Evaluation of metastatic disease from several neoplasms has recently been aided with the development of positron emission tomography (PET) scanning, particularly when fused with CT [36]. FDG-PET scan permits visualization of CCs because of the high glucose uptake of bile duct epithelium [68]. PET scans can detect nodular CCs as small as 1 cm but is less helpful for infiltrating tumors [68, 69]. However, the role of FDG-PET in the management of HCCA is yet less clear [70]. Most studies addressing the use of FDG-PET have included few patients and have combined CC with other biliary cancers, making interpretation of these studies difficult. Nonetheless, these studies suggest a potential benefit of FDG-PET; it can be helpful when there is a question of possible metastatic disease [32, 36, 71, 72]. In a study of 62 patients with CC who underwent preoperative PET staging at the Memorial Sloan-Kettering Cancer Center, 78 % of the tumors were PET-avid, and PET identified occult metastatic disease that altered management in 24 % of patients [71]. However, pending further data, PET does not currently have a routine role in preoperative evaluation of HCCA.

5.3 Imaging Findings

HCCAs can be classified as exophytic, infiltrative, polypoid, or a combination of these based on their typical growth pattern [73–75]. At the hilar portion, CCs are most commonly of the infiltrative type (>70 %) and less frequently they manifest as exophytic or polypoid lesions [59, 74]. Radiologic studies can show different imaging features of HCCAs based on their growth pattern [63, 76, 77]. Those of unusual histologic type (e.g., mucin-hypersecreting CC, squamous adenocarcinoma, biliary cystadenocarcinoma, and mucinous carcinoma) show a different growth pattern compared with that of the typical ones (i.e., ductal), and also may show different imaging features [78]. For example, mucin-producing intraductal papillary neoplasm (adenocarcinoma/adenoma) in the bile duct bears a striking similarity to intraductal papillary mucinous neoplasms of the pancreas with regard to its histopathologic features and is becoming recognized as a specific type of neoplasm [79]. CCs frequently develop in patients with any of a variety of preexisting bile duct diseases, some of which are considered precursors of CC (e.g., biliary lithiasis, clonorchiasis, recurrent pyogenic cholangitis, and primary sclerosing cholangitis) [75]. Although imaging tests can suggest the diagnosis of a HCCA, in some patients with those precursors, early diagnosis of a HCCA can be difficult [74]. In patients with primary sclerosing cholangitis, early diagnosis of a CC can be challenging, because CCs or significant intrahepatic biliary dilatation are infrequently identified on imaging. Similarly, in patients with recurrent pyogenic cholangitis in whom severe periductal fibrosis and hepatolithiasis have developed, diagnosis of a CC can be very difficult, due to the presence of severe biliary stricture and ductal wall thickening [80]. Therefore, a high index of suspicion and multidisciplinary investigative procedures are needed in those patients.

5.3.1 Periductal-Infiltrating Hilar Cholangiocarcinoma

Periductal infiltrating CA is the most common type of HCCA (70 % of cases). At pathologic analysis, infiltrating HCCA manifests as a sclerotic lesion with abundant fibrous tissue [74, 80]. US shows dilatation of the intrahepatic bile duct and normal-size extrahepatic bile ducts, as well as nonunion of the right and left ducts. This association suggests the diagnosis of HCCA. Although the tumor can appear as a mural thickening or an encircling mass along the bile duct wall, a definite mass is rarely seen on sonograms [81]. On CT and MRI, the key diagnostic features of periductal infiltrating hype HCCA include a long segment stricture with an irregular margin, asymmetric narrowing and peripheral ductal dilatation, ductal enhancement, and periductal soft tissue lesion (Figs. 5.2 and 5.3) [59]. Benign stenoses usually appear as regular, symmetric, and smooth-shaped narrowing of the lumen [82]. Although it is not a sensitive feature, thickening of the ductal wall more than 5 mm is suggestive of CCs [61]. Nonunion of the right and left hepatic ducts with or without a visibly thickened wall is a typical finding of infiltrating HCCA [83]. On contrast-enhanced CT, infiltrating tumors are seen as an asymetrically thickened ductal wall obliterating the lumen, and approximately 80 % of these tumors are hyperattenuating relative to the liver on arterial or portal phase or both (Fig. 5.2) [77, 84]. On either direct cholangiography or MRCP, HCCA frequently shows a long segment stricture with an irregular margin, asymmetric narrowing and peripheral ductal dilatation (Fig. 5.3). The involved bile duct lumen may be completely obstructed or markedly narrowed. On cross-sectional MR images, the lesion appears hypointense to the liver on T1-weighted images and slightly or moderately hyperintense on T2-weighted images.

5.3.2 Mass-Forming Exophytic Hilar Cholangiocarcinoma

Mass-forming exophytic HCCA manifests as hilar ductal stricture and a parenchymal mass with connection to the hilar duct. The parenchymal mass frequently present as a low-attenuation mass with peripheral rim enhancement during the arterial dominant phase, and homogeneous hypoattenuation in the portal dominant phase, findings that are similar to those for peripheral intrahepatic CC [47, 63, 75, 83]. It can be difficult or even impossible to ascertain whether the carcinoma arises at the main hepatic juncture or represents a peripheral CC that secondarily obliterates the hilar area [4, 86].

5.3.3 Intraductal Polypoid Hilar Cholangiocarcinoma

On pathology, intraductal papillary CCs can present as an polypoid mass or cast-like intraductal growth, superficial spreading growth or cyst-forming bile duct dilatation [73, 76, 78]. Variable degrees of bile duct dilatations may be observed. On CT or MRI with MRCP, intraductal HCCAs manifest as single or multiple intraductal soft tissue masses that are hypoattenuating or hypointense relative to the hepatic parenchyma or cast-like filling defects in bile duct on either CT or dynamic MRI (Fig. 5.4) [63, 77, 86]. On cross-sectional MR images, the lesion appears hypointense to the liver on T1-weighted images and moderately hyperintense with a high signal on T2-weighted images [59, 63]. The tumors are frequently multiple or disseminated within the biliary system and involve the intrahepatic and extrahepatic bile ducts [67, 84, 87]. A subtype of intraductal papillary CCs is intraductal papillary mucin producing neoplasm of the bile duct, which can secrete mucin. This tumor often demonstrates dilatation of the upstream bile duct as well as the downstream bile duct, or entire biliary tree because of excessive mucin discharge or compression by the primary tumor [79]. When bile duct dilatation is prominent and associated aneurismal dilatation occurs, mucin production and consequent bile flow obstruction should be suspected [59]. At MR imaging, mucin may have the same signal intensity as bile or manifest as multiple cordlike filling defects that are better diagnosed at ERCP.

5.4 Preoperative Evaluation and Staging

The surgical management of HCCA and the indications for operative exploration are complex. Precise preoperative staging is necessary to determine whether the patient's disease is potentially resectable and warrants operative exploration and to guide the surgeon in planning the operation [46]. Comprehensive preoperative imaging of biliary tumors should: (1) show the size and location of a primary lesion and assess the longitudinal and radial extent of bile duct involvement; (2) show involvement of the hepatic artery (main and lobar branches) and portal vein (main and lobar branches) with the tumor, for the purpose of surgical planning; (3) Depict the presence and extent of liver invasion and lobar atrophy or hypertrophy; and (4) enable the detection of regional lymph nodes and metastases [59, 62]. Despite that several staging systems for CC have been proposed based on pathologic evaluation of the surgical specimen, for surgical planning, preoperative staging based on the information that is garnered from imaging of patients with HCCA is necessary. The two most commonly used are the tumor, node, metastasis staging system, devised by the American Joint Committee on Cancer (AJCC), and the modified Bismuth-Corlette classification for HCCA (Fig. 5.1) [88–91]. Both systems are based mainly on the extent of primary tumor involvement within the hepatic ductal system. In an attempt to improve the preoperative clinical and prognostic usefulness of the AJCC tumor, node, metastasis system, modified T-stage criteria for HCCA have been proposed by Memorial Sloan-Kettering Cancer Center [14, 92]. This modified T staging that takes into consideration of both vascular involvement by local tumor extension and the presence or absence of liver atrophy. This proposed T staging system is predictive of resectability, the likelihood of nodal or distant metastases, and overall survival [92].

The major determinants of resectability are the extent of tumor within the biliary tree, the amount of hepatic parenchyma involved, vascular invasion, hepatic lobar atrophy, and metastatic disease. The infiltrative growth pattern and the close proximity to the portal vein and the hepatic artery of HCCA result in a low resectability rate, ranging between 20 and 40 % [18, 40, 93]. Although there is some disagreement about the criteria for resectability among surgeons, unsectability of HCCA is suggested by (a) cholangiographic evidence of severe bilateral involvement of the secondary confluence, (b) involvement of the main trunk of the portal vein, (c) involvement of both branches of the portal vein or bilateral involvement of the hepatic artery and portal vein, or (d) vascular involvement on one side of the liver and extensive bile duct involvement on the other side [4, 13, 62].

Understaging of CCs on preoperative imaging may frequently occur due to a lack of recognition of submucosal spread in involved bile ducts on imaging or limitation of imaging for detection of metastases [32, 94–96]. Even multiphasic CT is limited in its ability to establish the extent of intraductal tumor spread and resectability. In one report of 29 patients with histologically-proven HCCA, all of whom underwent multiphasic CT (arterial and portal venous phase), resectability was correctly predicted in only 60 % [51]. In the study by Park and colleagues, overall accuracy rates for predicting involvement of the bilateral secondary biliary confluences were 90.7 and 85.1 %, respectively, for MR imaging with MRCP and MDCT compared with direct cholangiography [67]. However, in general, the relationship of the tumor to the vessels and surrounding organs is regarded as being more easily evaluated on CT as opposed to MRI [97]. However, precise preoperative evaluation of tumor extent often requires several imaging or combined use of imaging with endoscopy such as cholangioscopy or laparoscopy [2, 46, 98]. Despite the enhanced diagnostic capability of newer radiologic studies such as MRI with MRCP and dynamic CT, unless there is clear evidence of metastatic disease, true resectability can be determined only by operative evaluation [96, 99].

References

1. Shaib YH, Davila JA, McGlynn K, El-Serag HB, et al. Rising incidence of intrahepatic cholangiocarcinoma in the United States: a true increase? J Hepatol. 2004;40(3):472–7.
2. Aljiffry M, Walsh MJ, Molinari M. Advances in diagnosis, treatment and palliation of cholangiocarcinoma: 1990–2009. World J Gastroenterol. 2009;15(34):4240–62.
3. Nakeeb A, Pitt HA, Sohn TA, et al. Cholangiocarcinoma—a spectrum of intrahepatic, perihilar, and distal tumors. Ann Surg. 1996;224(4):463–73.
4. Choi BI, Lee JM, Han JK. Imaging of intrahepatic and hilar cholangiocarcinoma. Abdom Imaging. 2004;29(5):548–57.
5. Klatskin G. Adenocarcinoma of hepatic duct at its bifuration within porta hepatis—an unusual tumor with distinctive clinical and pathological features. Am J Med. 1965;38(2):241–56.
6. Bismuth H, Castaing D, Traynor O. Resection or palliation: priority of surgery in the treatment of hilar cancer. World J Surg. 1988; 12(1):39–47.
7. Zech CJ, Schoenberg SO, Reiser M, et al. Cross-sectional imaging of biliary tumors: current clinical status and future developments. Eur Radiol. 2004;14(7):1174–87.
8. Wetter LA, Ring EJ, Pellegrini CA, et al. Differential diagnosis of sclerosing cholangiocarcinomas of the common hepatic duct (klatskin tumors). Am J Surg. 1991;161(1):57–62; discussion 62–53.
9. Ryan ME. Cytologic brushings of ductal lesions during ERCP. Gastrointest Endosc. 1991;37(2):139–42.
10. Nagorney DM, Kendrick ML. Hepatic resection in the treatment of hilar cholangiocarcinoma. Adv Surg. 2006;40:159–71.
11. Nakeeb A, Tran KQ, Black MJ, et al. Improved survival in resected biliary malignancies. Surgery. 2002;132(4):555–63.
12. Rocha FG, Matsuo K, Blumgart LH, et al. Hilar cholangiocarcinoma: the memorial Sloan-Kettering Cancer Center experience. J Hepatobiliary Pancreat Sci. 2010;17(4):490–6.
13. Chamberlain RS, Blumgart LH. Hilar cholangiocarcinoma: a review and commentary. Ann Surg Oncol. 2000;7(1):55–66.
14. Jarnagin WR, Fong Y, DeMatteo RP, et al. Staging, resectability, and outcome in 225 patients with hilar cholangiocarcinoma. Ann Surg. 2001;234(4):507–17.
15. Khan SA, Thomas HC, Davidson BR, et al. Cholangiocarcinoma. Lancet. 2006;366:1303. Lancet. 2006;367(9523):1656.
16. Jonas S, Benckert C, Thelen A, et al. Radical surgery for hilar cholangiocarcinoma. Eur J Surg Oncol. 2008;34(3):263–71.
17. Masselli G, Manfredi R, Vecchioli A, et al. MR imaging and MR cholangiopancreatography in the preoperative evaluation of hilar cholangiocarcinoma: correlation with surgical and pathologic findings. Eur Radiol. 2008;18(10):2213–21.
18. Blechacz B, Gores GJ. Cholangiocarcinoma: advances in pathogenesis, diagnosis, and treatment. Hepatology. 2008;48(1):308–21.
19. Blechacz BR, Gores GJ. Cholangiocarcinoma. Clin Liver Dis. 2008;12(1):131–50, ix.
20. Heslin MJ, Brooks AD, Hochwald SN, et al. A preoperative biliary stent is associated with increased complications after pancreatoduodenectomy. Arch Surg. 1998;133(2):149–54.
21. Hochwald SN, Burke EC, Jarnagin WR, et al. Association of preoperative biliary stenting with increased postoperative infectious complications in proximal cholangiocarcinoma. Arch Surg. 1999;134(3):261–6.
22. Hochwald SN, Dobryansky MB, Rofsky NM, et al. Magnetic resonance cholangiopancreatography accurately predicts the presence or absence of choledocholithiasis. J Gastrointest Surg. 1998;2(6): 573–9.
23. Hochwald SN, Rofsky NM, Dobryansky M, et al. Magnetic resonance imaging with magnetic resonance cholangiopancreatography accurately predicts resectability of pancreatic carcinoma. J Gastrointest Surg. 1999;3(5):506–11.
24. Kim HJ, Lee DH, Lim JW, et al. Multidetector computed tomography in the preoperative workup of hilar cholangiocarcinoma. Acta Radiol. 2009;50(8):845–53.
25. Uchida M, Ishibashi M, Tomita N, et al. Hilar and suprapancreatic cholangiocarcinoma: value of 3D angiography and multiphase fusion images using MDCT. Am J Roentgenol. 2005;184(5):1572–7.
26. Foley WD, Quiroz FA. The role of sonography in imaging of the biliary tract. Ultrasound Q. 2007;23(2):123–35.
27. Bloom CM, Langer B, Wilson SR. Role of US in the detection, characterization, and staging of cholangiocarcinoma. Radiographics. 1999;19(5):1199–218.
28. Rosch T, Meining A, Fruhmorgen S, et al. A prospective comparison of the diagnostic accuracy of ERCP, MRCP, CT, and EUS in biliary strictures. Gastrointest Endosc. 2002;55(7):870–6.
29. Neumaier CE, Bertolotto M, Perrone R, et al. Staging of hilar cholangiocarcinoma with ultrasound. J Clin Ultrasound. 1995; 23(3):173–8.
30. Slattery JM, Sahani DV. What is the current state-of-the-art imaging for detection and staging of cholangiocarcinoma? Oncologist. 2006;11(8):913–22.
31. Varadarajulu S, Eloubeidi MA. The role of endoscopic ultrasonography in the evaluation of pancreatico-biliary cancer. Surg Clin North Am. 2010;90(2):251–63.
32. Weber A, Schmid RM, Prinz C. Diagnostic approaches for cholangiocarcinoma. World J Gastroenterol. 2008;14(26):4131–6.
33. Eloubeidi MA, Chen VK, Jhala NC, et al. Endoscopic ultrasound-guided fine needle aspiration biopsy of suspected cholangiocarcinoma. Clin Gastroenterol Hepatol. 2004;2(3):209–13.
34. Fritscher-Ravens A, Broering DC, Sriram PV, et al. EUS-guided fine-needle aspiration cytodiagnosis of hilar cholangiocarcinoma: a case series. Gastrointest Endosc. 2000;52(4):534–40.
35. Menzel J, Poremba C, Dietl KH, et al. Preoperative diagnosis of bile duct strictures – comparison of intraductal ultrasonography with conventional endosonography. Scand J Gastroenterol. 2000; 35(1):77–82.
36. Reitz S, Slam K, Chambers LW. Biliary, pancreatic, and hepatic imaging for the general surgeon. Surg Clin North Am. 2011; 91(1):59–92.
37. Yu SA, Zhang C, Zhang JM, et al. Preoperative assessment of hilar cholangiocarcinoma: combination of cholangiography and CT angiography. Hepatobiliary Pancreat Dis Int. 2010;9(2):186–91.
38. Andriulli A, Loperfido S, Napolitano G, et al. Incidence rates of post-ERCP complications: a systematic survey of prospective studies. Am J Gastroenterol. 2007;102(8):1781–8.
39. Loperfido S, Angelini G, Benedetti G, et al. Major early complications from diagnostic and therapeutic ERCP: a prospective multicenter study. Gastrointest Endosc. 1998;48(1):1–10.
40. Lazaridis KN, Gores GJ. Cholangiocarcinoma. Gastroenterology. 2005;128(6):1655–67.

41. Nimura Y. Preoperative biliary drainage before resection for cholangiocarcinoma (Pro). HPB (Oxford). 2008;10(2):130–3.
42. Nimura Y. Staging cholangiocarcinoma by cholangioscopy. HPB (Oxford). 2008;10(2):113–5.
43. Nimura Y. Radical surgery: vascular and pancreatic resection for cholangiocarcinoma. HPB (Oxford). 2008;10(3):183–5.
44. Nimura Y. Extended surgery in bilio-pancreatic cancer: the Japanese experience. Semin Oncol. 2002;29(6 Suppl 20):17–22.
45. Nimura Y, Kamiya J, Kondo S, et al. Aggressive preoperative management and extended surgery for hilar cholangiocarcinoma: Nagoya experience. J Hepatobiliary Pancreat Surg. 2000;7(2):155–62.
46. Miller G, Schwartz LH, D'Angelica M. The use of imaging in the diagnosis and staging of Hepatobiliary malignancies. Surg Oncol Clin N Am. 2007;16(2):343–68.
47. Choi JY, Kim MJ, Lee JM, et al. Hilar cholangiocarcinoma: role of preoperative imaging with sonography, MDCT, MRI, and direct cholangiography. AJR Am J Roentgenol. 2008;191(5):1448–57.
48. Endo I, Shimada H, Sugita M, et al. Role of three-dimensional imaging in operative planning for hilar cholangiocarcinoma. Surgery. 2007;142(5):666–75.
49. Tamm EP, Balachandran A, Bhosale P, et al. Update on 3D and multiplanar MDCT in the assessment of biliary and pancreatic pathology. Abdom Imaging. 2009;34(1):64–74.
50. Nesbit GM, Johnson CD, James EM, et al. Cholangiocarcinoma: diagnosis and evaluation of resectability by CT and sonography as procedures complementary to cholangiography. AJR Am J Roentgenol. 1988;151(5):933–8.
51. Tillich M, Mischinger HJ, Preisegger KH, et al. Multiphasic helical CT in diagnosis and staging of hilar cholangiocarcinoma. AJR Am J Roentgenol. 1998;171(3):651–8.
52. Akamatsu N, Sugawara Y, Osada H, et al. Diagnostic accuracy of multidetector-row computed tomography for hilar cholangiocarcinoma. J Gastroenterol Hepatol. 2010;25(4):731–7.
53. Cho ES, Park MS, Yu JS, et al. Biliary ductal involvement of hilar cholangiocarcinoma: multidetector computed tomography versus magnetic resonance cholangiography. J Comput Assist Tomogr. 2007;31(1):72–8.
54. Choi JY, Lee JM, Lee JY, et al. Assessment of hilar and extrahepatic bile duct cancer using multidetector CT: value of addingmultiplanar reformations to standard axial images. Eur Radiol. 2007;17(12):3130–8. Epub 8 May 2007.
55. Senda Y, Nishio H, Oda K, et al. Value of multidetector row CT in the assessment of longitudinal extension of cholangiocarcinoma-correlation between MDCT and microscopic findings. World J Surg. 2009;33(7):1459–67.
56. Unno M, Okumoto T, Katayose Y, et al. Preoperative assessment of hilar cholangiocarcinoma by multidetector row computed tomography. J Hepatobiliary Pancreat Surg. 2007;14(5):434–40.
57. Watadani T, Akahane M, Yoshikawa T, et al. Preoperative assessment of hilar cholangiocarcinoma using multidetector-row CT: correlation with histopathological findings. Radiat Med. 2008;26(7):402–7.
58. Cha JH, Han JK, Kim TK, et al. Preoperative evaluation of klatskin tumor: accuracy of spiral CT in determining vascular invasion as a sign of unresectability. Abdom Imaging. 2000;25(5):500–7.
59. Matos C, Serrao E, Bali MA. Magnetic resonance imaging of biliary tumors. Magn Reson Imaging Clin N Am. 2010;18(3):477–96, x.
60. Manfredi R, Masselli G, Maresca G, et al. MR imaging and MRCP of hilar cholangiocarcinoma. Abdom Imaging. 2003;28(3):319–25.
61. Manfredi R, Barbaro B, Masselli G, et al. Magnetic resonance imaging of cholangiocarcinoma. Sem Liver Dis. 2004;24(2):155–64.
62. Lee HY, Kim SH, Lee JM, et al. Preoperative assessment of resectability of hepatic hilar cholangiocarcinoma: combined CT and cholangiography with revised criteria. Radiology. 2006;239(1):113–21.
63. Kim JE, Lee JM, Kim SH, et al. Differentiation of intraductal growing-type cholangiocarcinomas from nodular-type cholangiocarcinomas at biliary MR imaging with MR cholangiography. Radiology. 2010;257(2):364–72.
64. Kim HJ, Lee JM, Kim SH, et al. Evaluation of the longitudinal tumor extent of bile duct cancer: value of adding gadolinium-enhanced dynamic imaging to unenhanced images and magnetic resonance cholangiography. J Comput Assist Tomogr. 2007;31(3):469–74.
65. Varghese JC, Farrell MA, Courtney G, et al. A prospective comparison of magnetic resonance cholangiopancreatography with endoscopic retrograde cholangiopancreatography in the evaluation of patients with suspected biliary tract disease. Clin Radiol. 1999;54(8):513–20.
66. Freeman ML, Sielaff TD. A modern approach to malignant hilar biliary obstruction. Rev Gastroenterol Disord. 2003;3(4):187–201.
67. Park HS, Lee JM, Choi JY, et al. Preoperative evaluation of bile duct cancer: MRI combined with MR cholangiopancreatography versus MDCT with direct cholangiography. AJR Am J Roentgenol. 2008;190(2):396–405.
68. Kim YJ, Yun M, Lee WJ, et al. Usefulness of 18F-FDG PET in intrahepatic cholangiocarcinoma. Eur J Nucl Med Mol Imaging. 2003;30(11):1467–72.
69. Anderson CD, Rice MH, Pinson CW, et al. Fluorodeoxyglucose PET imaging in the evaluation of gallbladder carcinoma and cholangiocarcinoma. J Gastrointest Surg. 2004;8(1):90–7.
70. Poultsides GA, Zhu AX, Choti MA, et al. Intrahepatic cholangiocarcinoma. Surg Clin North Am. 2010;90(4):817–37.
71. Corvera CU, Blumgart LH, Akhurst T, et al. F-18-fluorodeoxyglucose positron emission tomography influences management decisions in patients with biliary cancer. J Am Coll Surg. 2008;206(1):57–65.
72. Wakabayashi H, Akamoto S, Yachida S, et al. Significance of fluorodeoxyglucose PET imaging in the diagnosis of malignancies in patients with biliary stricture. Eur J Surg Oncol. 2005;31(10):1175–9.
73. Lim JH, Kim YI, Park CK. Intraductal mucosal-spreading mucin-producing peripheral cholangiocarcinoma of the liver. Abdom Imaging. 2000;25(1):89–92.
74. Lim JH, Park CK. Pathology of cholangiocarcinoma. Abdom Imaging. 2004;29(5):540–7.
75. Lim JH. Cholangiocarcinoma: morphologic classification according to growth pattern and imaging findings. AJR Am J Roentgenol. 2003;181(3):819–27.
76. Kim H, Lim JH, Jang KT, et al. Morphology of intraductal papillary neoplasm of the bile ducts: radiologic-pathologic correlation. Abdom Imaging. 2010;36(4):438–46.
77. Kim NR, Lee JM, Kim SH, et al. Enhancement characteristics of cholangiocarcinomas on mutiphasic helical CT: emphasis on morphologic subtypes. Clin Imaging. 2008;32(2):114–20.
78. Lee WJ, Lim HK, Jang KM, et al. Radiologic spectrum of cholangiocarcinoma: emphasis on unusual manifestations and differential diagnoses. Radiographics. 2001;21(Spec No):S97–116.
79. Takanami K, Yamada T, Tsuda M, et al. Intraductal papillary mucininous neoplasm of the bile ducts: multimodality assessment with pathologic correlation. Abdom Imaging. 2011;36(4):447–56.
80. Park HS, Lee JM, Kim SH, et al. CT differentiation of cholangiocarcinoma from periductal fibrosis in patients with hepatolithiasis. AJR Am J Roentgenol. 2006;187(2):445–53.
81. Hann LE, Greatrex KV, Bach AM, et al. Cholangiocarcinoma at the hepatic hilus: sonographic findings. AJR Am J Roentgenol. 1997;168(4):985–9.
82. Kim JY, Lee JM, Han JK, et al. Contrast-enhanced MRI combined with MR cholangiopancreatography for the evaluation of patients

with biliary strictures: differentiation of malignant from benign bile duct strictures. J Magn Reson Imaging. 2007;26(2):304–12.
83. Han JK, Choi BI, Kim TK, et al. Hilar cholangiocarcinoma: thin-section spiral CT findings with cholangiographic correlation. Radiographics. 1997;17(6):1475–85.
84. Seo H, Lee JM, Kim IH, et al. Evaluation of the gross type and longitudinal extent of extrahepatic cholangiocarcinomas on contrast-enhanced multidetector row computed tomography. J Comput Assist Tomogr. 2009;33(3):376–82.
85. Han JK, Choi BI, Kim AY, et al. Cholangiocarcinoma: pictorial essay of CT and cholangiographic findings. Radiographics. 2002; 22(1):173–87.
86. Lee JW, Han JK, Kim TK, et al. CT features of intraductal intrahepatic cholangiocarcinoma. AJR Am J Roentgenol. 2000;175(3): 721–5.
87. Jung AY, Lee JM, Choi SH, et al. CT features of an intraductal polypoid mass: differentiation between hepatocellular carcinoma with bile duct tumor invasion and intraductal papillary cholangiocarcinoma. J Comput Assist Tomogr. 2006;30(2):173–81.
88. Nathan H, Pawlik TM. Staging of intrahepatic cholangiocarcinoma. Curr Opin Gastroenterol. 2010;26(3):269–73.
89. Farges O, Fuks D, Le Treut YP, et al. AJCC 7th edition of TNM staging accurately discriminates outcomes of patients with resectable intrahepatic cholangiocarcinoma: by the AFC-IHCC-2009 study group. Cancer. 2010;117(10):2170–7.
90. Edge SB, Compton CC. The American joint committee on cancer: the 7th edition of the AJCC cancer staging manual and the future of TNM. Ann Surg Oncol. 2010;17(6):1471–4.
91. Bismuth H, Corlette MB. Intrahepatic cholangioenteric anastomosis in carcinoma of the hilus of the liver. Surg Gynecol Obstet. 1975;140(2):170–8.
92. Burke EC, Jarnagin WR, Hochwald SN, et al. Hilar cholangiocarcinoma – patterns of spread, the importance of hepatic resection for curative operation, and a presurgical clinical staging system. Ann Surg. 1998;228(3):385–92.
93. Blechacz BR, Sanchez W, Gores GJ. A conceptual proposal for staging ductal cholangiocarcinoma. Curr Opin Gastroenterol. 2009;25(3):238–9.
94. Zidi SH, Prat F, Le Guen O, et al. Performance characteristics of magnetic resonance cholangiography in the staging of malignant hilar strictures. Gut. 2000;46(1):103–6.
95. Weber SM, DeMatteo RP, Fong Y, et al. Staging laparoscopy in patients with extrahepatic biliary carcinoma. Analysis of 100 patients. Ann Surg. 2002;235(3):392–9.
96. Callery MP, Strasberg SM, Doherty GM, et al. Staging laparoscopy with laparoscopic ultrasonography: optimizing resectability in Hepatobiliary and pancreatic malignancy. J Am Coll Surg. 1997;185(1):33–9.
97. Zhang Y, Uchida M, Abe T, et al. Intrahepatic peripheral cholangiocarcinoma: comparison of dynamic CT and dynamic MRI. J Comput Assist Tomogr. 1999;23(5):670–7.
98. Fishman DS, Tarnasky PR, Patel SN, et al. Management of pancreaticobiliary disease using a new intra-ductal endoscope: the Texas experience. World J Gastroenterol. 2009;15(11): 1353–8, 21.
99. Su CH, Tsay SH, Wu CC, et al. Factors influencing postoperative morbidity, mortality, and survival after resection for hilar cholangiocarcinoma. Ann Surg. 1996;223(4):384–94.

Role of 3D Reconstructive Imaging

6

I. Endo, R. Matsuyama, K. Tanaka, N. Wendt, A. Schenk, and H.O. Peitgen

6.1 Introduction

Since its introduction to hepatobiliary surgery, three-dimensional (3D) imaging has assumed a growing importance for the visualization of abdominal diseases. The main clinical applications include preoperative simulation for oncologic liver resection [1, 2], and living-donor liver transplantation [3, 4]. The advantages of 3D imaging are the exact visualization of vessels in areas with complex and variable vascular anatomy, determining possible resection margins, and predicting operative risks. Although hepatectomy is increasingly carried out, it is still one of the most difficult operative procedures because of the anatomical complexity and hepatic vascular variability [5]. Moreover, patients with hilar cholangiocarcinoma often have obstructive jaundice, and the impaired hepatic function restricts the volume of liver resection. In addition, a positive resection margin should be avoided in order to achieve a potential cure of the disease. Thus, exact preoperative information on the detailed topography and precise liver resection volume should be obtained for curative and harmless hepatectomy. Concerning hilar cholangiocarcinoma, a successful management requires the following three steps: accurate preoperative estimation of both the tumor extent and anatomical variations, appropriate planning and simulation of the operative procedures, and implementing the planned procedures securely [6–8].

I. Endo, MD (✉) • R. Matsuyama, MD • K. Tanaka, MD •
N. Wendt, MD • H.O. Peitgen, MD
Department of Gastroenterological Surgery,
Graduate School of Medicine, Yokohama City University,
Yokohama, Japan
e-mail: endoit@med.yokohama-cu.ac.jp

A. Schenk, MD
Department of Gastroenterological Surgery,
Yokohama City University, Yokohama, Japan

6.2 Advances in the Imaging Tools for Assessing Tumor Extent in Hilar Cholangiocarcinoma

Currently, direct cholangiography has been used as the reference standard for the diagnosis of the longitudinal ductal infiltration by the tumor [9–12]. MRCP and 3D cholangiography are relatively new techniques that offer improved accuracy for imaging in hilar cholangiocarcinoma [9, 13–16]. Kim et al. [14] correctly determined the tumor extent in 10 of 11 patients with 3D cholangiography. Considering that the accuracy rate of determining the longitudinal extension by direct cholangiography varies from 53 to 90 % [11, 17, 18], these new imaging modalities are at least as good as conventional cholangiography in determining the extent of ductal invasion. A further advantage of 3D cholangiography is that it allows 360° imaging of the biliary tree. This function facilitates accurate assignment of each bile duct branches. The 90° cranial view is particularly useful to resolve overlapping bile ducts on conventional cholangiograms.

MRI has been established as the standard imaging modality for the evaluation of the extent of cholangiocarcinoma because it has several advantages over conventional cholangiographic techniques. It provides an accurate map of the biliary tree even in the undrained segments, and demonstrates extraductal tumors directly and non-invasively. Furthermore, it has the capability of 3-dimensional visualization. Concerning the diagnostic ability of MRCP, Schwartz et al. [19] reported that the level of malignant pancreaticobiliary obstruction was correctly identified in about 80 % of cases using breath-hold MRCP. Hanninen et al. [20] also reported that the tumor status according to the Bismuth-Corlette classification was determined correctly in 27 of 30 patients by MRCP.

When the patient has not received any biliary decompression, multiplanar reconstructed images (MPR) were thought to have a superior ability to reveal tumor extensions, both longitudinally and vertically. In an undrained dilated bile duct, the tumor extension clearly depicts as a thickened duct

W.Y. Lau (ed.), *Hilar Cholangiocarcinoma*,
DOI 10.1007/978-94-007-6473-6_6, © Springer Science+Business Media Dordrecht and People's Medical Publishing House 2013

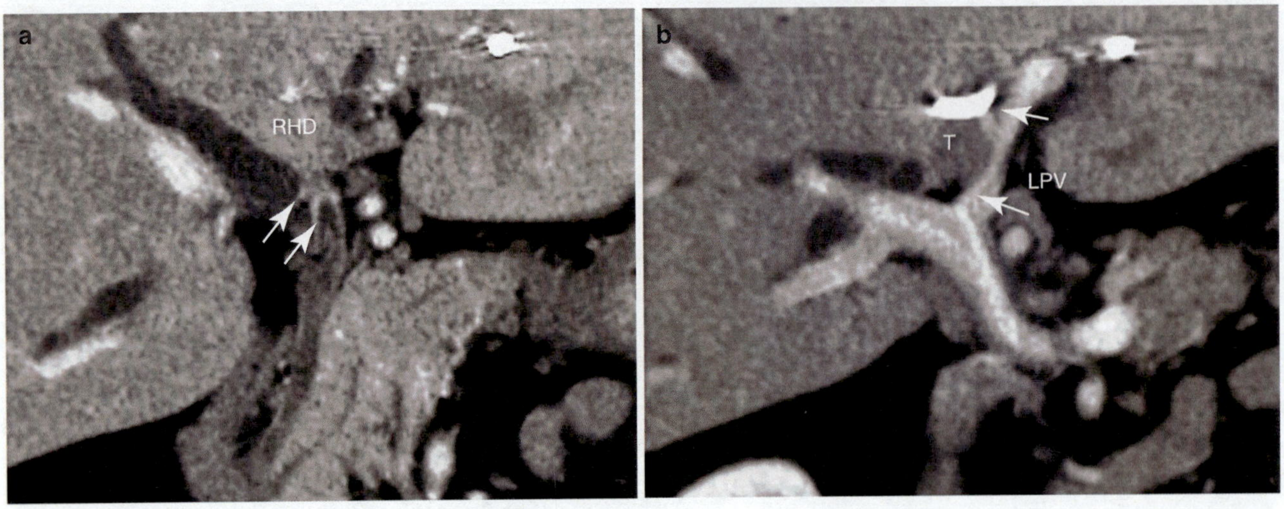

Fig. 6.1 (**a**) Multiplanar reconstructive image. Undrained dilated right hepatic duct (*RHD*) clearly depicts tumor extension as a thickened duct wall with tapering (*arrow*). (**b**) The tumor adjacent to the left portal vein which does not have a wall with a thin, low density layer. Direct invasion is suspected

wall with tapering (Fig. 6.1). In a tumor which is adjacent to surrounding vessels such as the hepatic artery or the portal vein, direct invasion is suspected when there is an absence of a thin, low density layer on MPR images. In such instances, these vessels should be subjected to a combined resection.

6.3 Image Processing

The number of software used to create 3D images and preoperative hepatectomy simulation is increasing in recent years. We use the Liver Explorer 2 software for image analysis [8]. Our routine procedures for CT images are obtained with a 16-detector row CT scanner (Somatom Sensation 16; Siemens, Forchheim, Germany). With the patient supine, a 1:5 dilution of nonionic contrast material (meglumine sodium amidotrizoate, Urografin 60 %; Schering, Berlin, Germany) mixed with normal saline is injected gently through the PTBD or ENBD tube, with the volume based on the results from antecedent cholangiography, and the biliary drainage tube is clamped. A scout image is obtained to identify the bile duct before full-scale CT scanning. Patients who do not have external biliary drainage tubes receive drip cholangiography. One hundred millilitre of meglumine iotroxate (Biliscopin, Schering, Berlin, Germany) are administered by intravenous drip infusion. Infusion takes 30 min. The MDCT scan is started 30 min after the infusion is completed.

The multi-detector row CT protocol creates four-image sets (choledochal, arterial, portal venous, and hepatic venous phases) of the liver that are collected in succession using the following variables: 140 kV; 150 mA s; section thickness/collimation, 5/0.75 mm; feed/rotation, 12 mm; rotation time, 0.5 s; reconstruction increment, 1 mm for the arterial scan and 2 mm for the venous scans. Subsequently, 120 ml of the nonionic contrast material iohexol (Omnipaque 300; Daiichi Pharmaceutical Co., LTD., Tokyo, Japan) are infused at a rate of 3.5 m/s with power injector. To display portal and hepatic venous anatomy, the second and third CT-image sets are acquired 10 and 40 s after the arterial phase.

6.4 Preoperative Evaluation for Anatomical Variations

Advances in radiological techniques has allowed three-dimensional (3D) hepatic modeling from CT images, which provides detailed hepatic vascular anatomy [21–23]. 3D imaging is thought to be useful in the determination of vascular anatomy and the decision on the line of transection in donor hepatectomy [2]. The surgeon can perform selective control of sectoral liver vascular branches to prevent bleeding as well as to delineate the extent of resection [24–26]. The virtual reality allows the surgeon to confirm preoperatively the anatomical distribution of arteries and portal branches and resect the hepatic lobe. Kanazawa et al. [2] stated that 3D images is helpful to avoid intraoperative injuries to the hepatic vasculature because it can accurately demonstrate anatomical variations preoperatively. In hilar cholangiocarcinoma, anatomical variation is especially important. It helps the decision-making in operative procedures. Since the hepatic artery runs through the hilar region close to the tumor, it is often involved by hilar tumors. If the hepatic artery is involved by tumor, the surgeon has to make a decision on how to reconstruct the arterial flow to the remnant liver, although the significance of a combined resection of the hepatic artery is still controversial [27–29].

It is well known that there is a great deal of variations in the arterial supply to the liver. The hepatic artery arises from

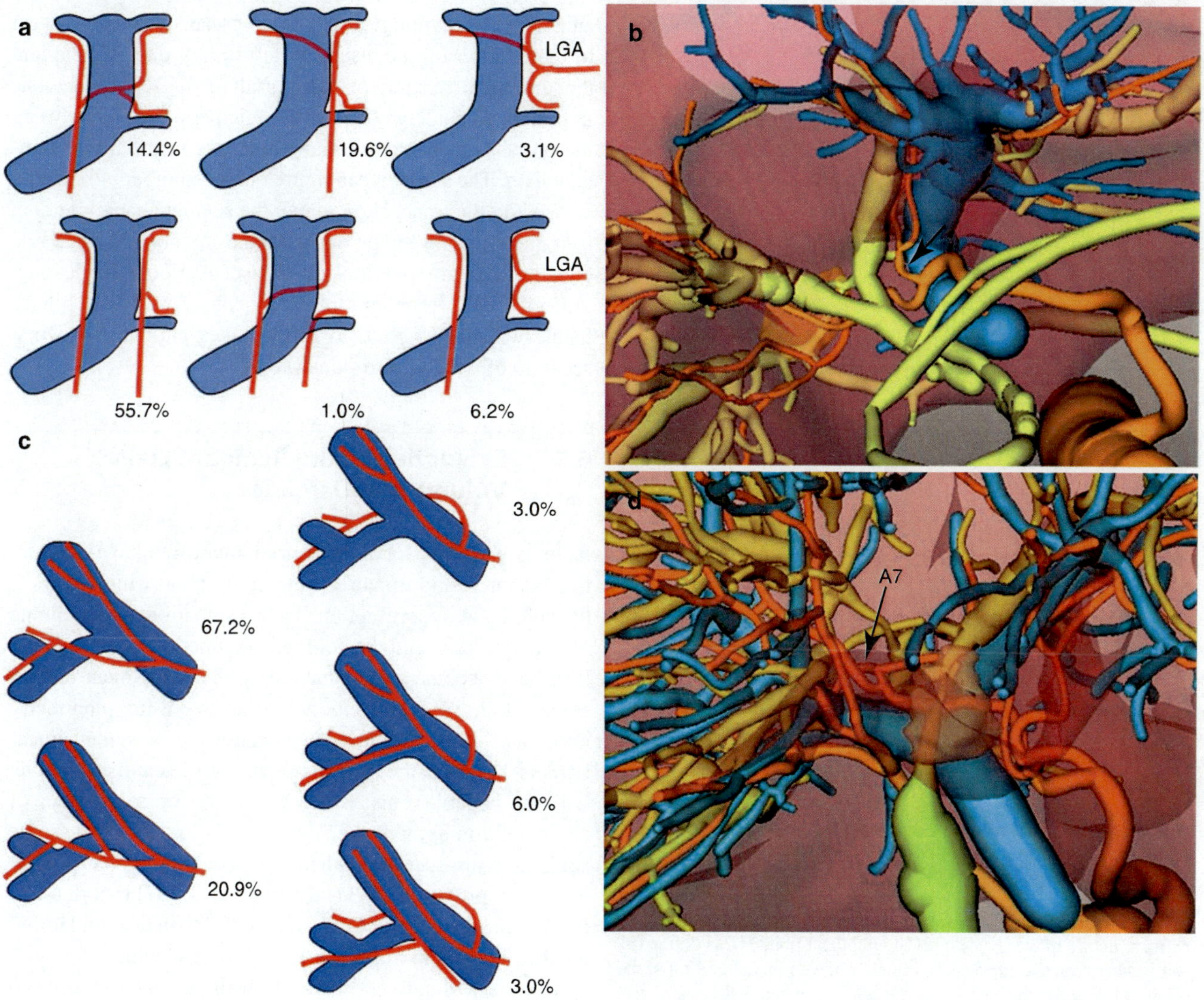

Fig. 6.2 (**a**) Branching patterns of the left and middle hepatic artery based on 3D images of 97 patients. As can be seen on the *lower row*, two hepatic arteries enter the left liver in around 60 % of cases. In such instances, the middle hepatic artery can be resected with the tumor if it is involved. On the other hand, as can be seen on the *upper row*, a single hepatic artery should be preserved, or otherwise reconstructed. There were nine patients with aberrant left hepatic artery arising from the left gastric artery. (**b**) 3D reconstructive image shows the subtle narrowing of the left hepatic artery (*arrow*). Since intraoperative findings also suggested that the left hepatic artery was involved by tumor, in concomitant with a right hemihepatectomy, the artery was resected and reconstructed. The patient is alive and without tumor recurrence 4 years after the operation. (**c**) Branching patterns of the right hepatic artery based on 3D images from 67 patients. There were ten patients with a replaced right hepatic artery arising from the superior mesenteric artery. While the branch to the posterior sector passes across in front of the right portal vein in around 90 % of the patients, it goes around the right portal vein in 10 % of patients as can be seen on the *right column*. In such instances, the posterior branch runs behind the right hepatic duct. Thus, it can be involved by the tumor. For left hemihepatectomy with caudate lobectomy, the surgeon should pay attention to the artery when the right hepatic duct is dissected. It seems almost impossible to visualize this kind of variation of the hepatic artery without the assistance of a 3D reconstructive image. (**d**) A rare case with an independent A7 arising from the middle hepatic artery. There was a replaced right hepatic artery which included A6 arising from the superior mesenteric artery. The middle hepatic artery seems to be involved by the tumor. Since it looks difficult to reconstruct the middle hepatic artery, right hemihepatectomy with caudate lobectomy was carried out

the celiac axis, but it may be entirely replaced by a common hepatic artery which takes origin from the superior mesenteric artery in one-fourth of patients. It is widely accepted that a replaced hepatic artery is susceptible to operative injury if it is not recognized. While the relatively proximal branches are important, the more distal branches such as the segmental branches originating from the left, middle or right hepatic artery are also important (Fig. 6.2). These arterial variations can sometimes preclude surgical resection. If such variations are not noticed before laparotomy, it can seriously mislead the surgeon. It is nearly impossible to visualize in the surgeon's mind the branching patterns of the hepatic arteries at the segmental branch levels by 2D-CT alone. Angiography was routinely used for hilar cholangiocarcinoma. However, 3D reconstructive image almost completely replaces angiography because of its less invasive nature.

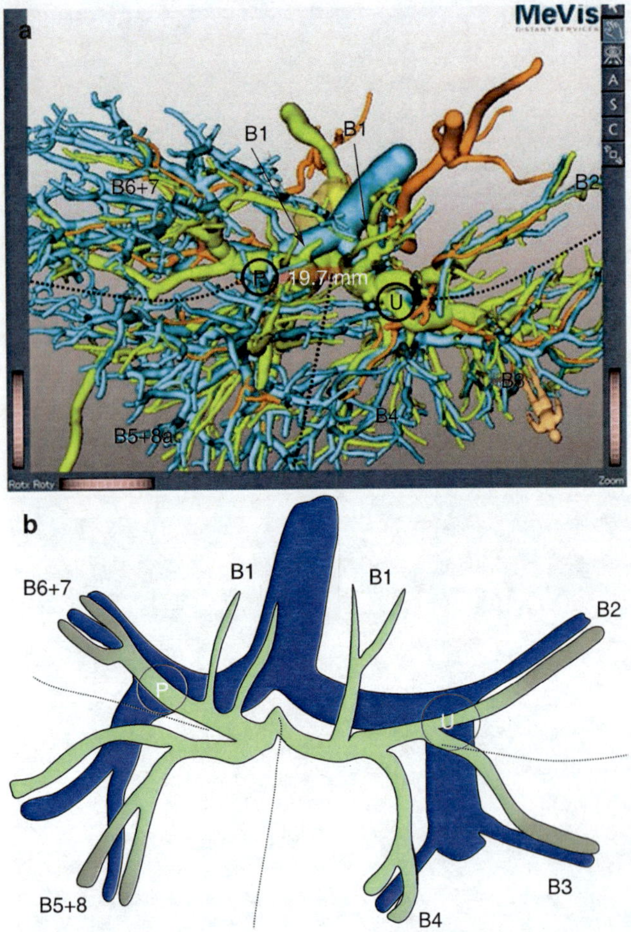

Fig. 6.3 (**a**) The dorsal aspect of the liver which demonstrates the symmetric structure of the liver [51]. The Umbilical-point (*U*) is defined as the bend between the transverse portion and the umbilical portion of the left portal vein, i.e. bifurcation of the left lateral sectoral branch (*B2*) and the left paramedian sectoral branch (*B3+4*). The Posterior-point (*P*) is defined as the bifurcation of the anterior branch and the posterior branch of the right portal vein, i.e. the bifurcation of the right lateral sectoral branch (*B6+7*) and the right paramedian sectoral branch (*B5+8*). U and P-points can be identifiable both on preoperative 3D reconstructive images and intraoperative inspection. (**b**) A schematic figure demonstrates both the symmetry of the liver and the relative positions of the bile duct and *U* and *P*-point. It gives a concrete and readily understandable picture

Anatomical variations of the biliary ducts is another important issue for the hepatobiliary surgeons. Most segmental bile ducts bifurcates within the hilar plate (Fig. 6.3). Thus, multiple bile duct orifices emerge at the transection plane at the hilar plate [30]. Usually, the number of these sectoral or segmental branches are three to four. Some investigators emphasize the usefulness of 3D cholangiography [13, 14]. It is more than just simple visualization of the biliary tract alone which is important for the surgeon. When an operative procedure is planned by 3D imaging, the planned transection line of the bile duct can be planned in relationship to the Umbilical or Posterior point (U or P-point) of the portal vein. Cho et al. stated that discrepancies between anatomic and radiologic study findings can exist with respect to the relationship between the left biliary duct system and the umbilical portion of the portal vein [31]. Thus, it is important to perceive the correct relative positions between the portal branches and biliary branches in the future remnant liver. The surgeon can figure out the number of bile duct orifices on the transection plane, the segment each bile duct is draining and he can be free from the anxiety that small bile duct orifices are overlooked. These overlooked bile duct orifices in the remnant liver can cause persistent biliary fistula which may need to further interventions, the worst scenario of which is a re-laparotomy.

6.5 Evaluation of the Remnant Liver Volume by 3D Images

Patients with hilar cholangiocarcinoma often have obstructive jaundice, and impaired hepatic function which restricts the volume of liver resection. Thus, estimation of the volume of liver resection and the volume and function of the residual liver have become a fundamental part of assessment in liver surgery [32, 33]. Conventional volumetry using planimetry introduces considerable error because the presumed linear borders between the liver segments are established along with the hepatic veins, which are shown on axial slices of computed tomography (CT) scans [34–36]. Recently, some studies of an operation planning system for liver surgery have been proposed [2, 37]. Lamade et al. [37] reported that the 3D reconstruction system was useful to understand tumor localization and to make a proposal for resection.

A variety of software is used for these analyses. In most applications, it allows an accurate evaluation of liver volume as well as identification of the vascular branches of the liver. The software is based on an algorithm to define the vascular perfusion area according to the direction and diameter of the portal veins. The algorithm includes major portal veins down to the peripheral portal branches; therefore, the whole liver can be examined along each portal tract. This virtual hepatectomy simulation is programmed to recognize a tumor-bearing portal branch and to quantify the perfusion area by clipping the corresponding branch. Thus, this software can be applied to any type of liver resection, which varies from lobectomy to partial resection.

We have expanded the software to analyze the drainage areas of the hepatic veins to determine the possibility of liver injury due to congestion by dividing the hepatic veins. Estimation of the hepatic venous drainage is essential to avoid liver graft and residual donor liver congestion [38].

The need for hepatic vein branch reconstruction or preservation should be assessed preoperatively (Fig. 6.4). The surgeon can modify the operative procedure in accordance to the individual's anatomy and liver function. Consequently, it

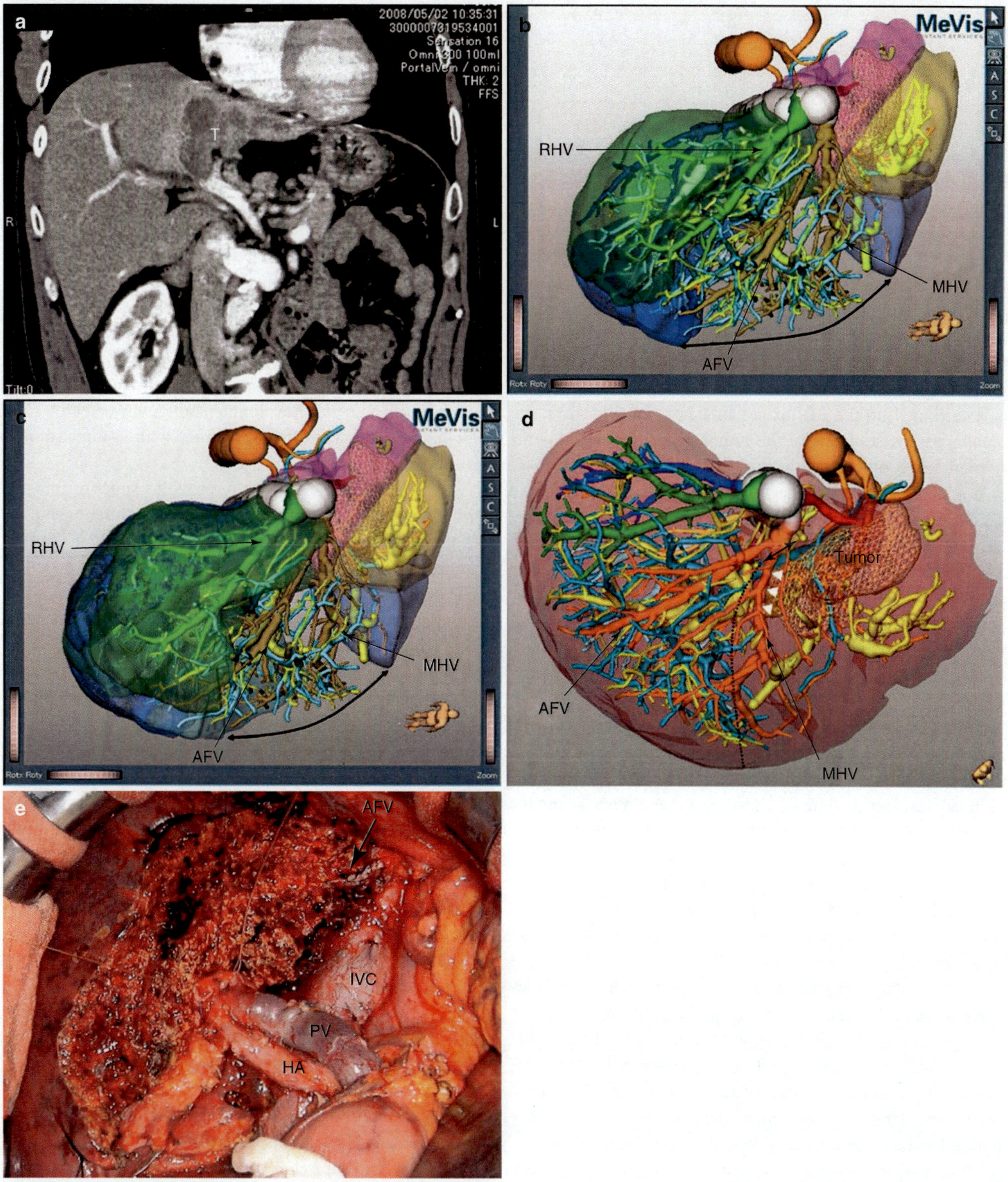

Fig. 6.4 (**a**) Intrahepatic cholangiocarcinoma invading the hilar region. The right hepatic duct is dilated. T: tumor. (**b**) Cranio-dorsal view of the liver. Each portal segment is colored except the anterior segment (*arrow*). A thick anterior fissural vein (*AFV*) passes through the center of the anerior segment. Right hepatic vein (*RHV*) is placed at the *left edge* of the portal segmentation of the posterior segment. (**c**) The drained area of the RHV is overlaid on Fig. 6.5b. More than 70 % of the anterior segment drains into the *AFV* and the middle hepatic vein (*MHV*). This area may be congested if the MHV is resected at its root. (**d**) Based on these findings, we decided on the line of transection (*dotted line*) of the MHV resection and preserved the branch from segment 8 (*AFV*). AFV can be preserved because it runs away from the tumor (*white short arrow*). This kind of modification might improve the short-term results of the operation such as blood loss, postoperative complications, and hospital stay. (**e**) Left hemihepatectomy with caudate lobectomy was carried out. *AFV* is preserved. No obvious congested area is observed on the surface of the remnant liver. The patient was discharged 10 days after the operation. The (*arrow*) points to the anteior fissural vein (*AFV*) which was preserved

improves safety in operative procedures even in patients with impaired liver function.

6.6 Operative Planning and Simulation

Based on the location of the tumor, left or right hemihepatectomy concomitant with caudate lobe resection should usually be selected. Knowing the anatomic relationships between the tumor and the surrounding vessels, particularly the portal vein and hepatic artery, is essential [39]. Liver resection is planned preoperatively based on the longitudinal tumor spread and vertical invasion of the adjacent major vessels. Longitudinal spread is determined by MPR or direct cholangiography. Vertical invasion is determined by MPR. This can be interpreted on the 3D images interactively (Fig. 6.5). A preoperative assessment of the tumor extent should be performed based on the landmarks which can be recognizable on both the preoperative imaging study and on intraoperative visual inspection. Then, an appropriate operative planning becomes possible.

In the left liver, the Umbilical-point is defined as the point at the turn bend from the transverse portion to the umbilical portion of the left portal vein, and the line of transection of the left hepatic duct in right hepatic lobectomy is restricted by the right border of the umbilical portion of the left portal vein.

For right-sided hepatectomy, when the longitudinal spread is limited to the right side of the U-point, the left hepatic duct is planned to be excised just to the right of the U-point. The planned transection line of the liver parenchyma is made along the Cantlie line to the right of the MHV. After ducking under the MHV, the line of transection is angled to the U-point through the Alantian duct (Fig. 6.6).

When the longitudinal invasion extends beyond the right border of the U-point, a right trisectionectomy is considered.

In the right liver, the Posterior-point is defined as the bifurcation of the anterior branch and the posterior branch of the right portal vein, and the line of transection of the right hepatic duct in left hemihepatectomy is restricted by the left border of the anterior branch of the right portal vein. Also, the left border of the posterior branch corresponds with the border between the caudate lobe and the posterior segment.

For left-sided hepatectomy, when the longitudinal spread is limited to the left of the P-point, the right hepatic duct is planned to be excised just to the left of the P-point. The planned line of transection of the liver parenchyma begins along the Cantlie line to the left of the MHV. After ducking under the MHV, the line of transection is angled to the P-point and then through to the right border of the IVC (Fig. 6.6). When the longitudinal invasion extends to the left of the P-point, a left trisectionectomy is considered. When the tumor extends beyond both the left border of the U-point and the right border of the P-point, it is deemed unresectable.

6.7 Operative Curatibility

Results of surgical treatment of hilar cholangiocarcinoma have improved during the recent two decades, in parallel with developments in surgical techniques, better knowledge of surgical anatomy and advances in radiologic imaging. Several authors have emphasized that curative resection remains the most important prognostic factor. Apart from a few exceptions, the curative resection rates remain unsatisfactory [40–43].

Recent progress in imaging of hepatobiliary pancreatic disease has led to the development of multi-detector row computed tomography (MDCT) [44] with 3-dimensional (3D) imaging.

Although 3D cholangiography provides superior images of intraluminal tumor spread, it has a flaw in relationship to extraluminal infiltration to the surrounding tissues. On the other hand, multiplanar reconstructed images have better diagnostic power for extraluminal, i.e., vertical invasion of the tumor, than 3D images and conventional axial 2D images alone. Thus, 3D imaging with a complimentary use of MPR have led to a better topologic understanding of the relationship of the tumor to the vascular system in an individual patient. It is expected that the introduction of 3D reconstructive imaging together with MPR will lead to an increase in the rate of resection with negative tumor margin.

6.8 Mortality and Morbidity

Complex biliary and hepatic resections are required to achieve a complete resection, the perioperative morbidity and mortality are significant [45]. Although recent reports have suggested a decrease in morbidity and mortality with the use of preoperative portal vein embolization, in major liver resections including extended right/left hepatectomy, the morbidity and mortality rates still ranges 14–76 % and 0–19 %, respectively.

Several authors reported that 3D images help to reduce postoperative complications in living-donor liver transplantation [3, 4]. Hiroshige et al. reported that 3D images reduced blood loss during donor operation due to lowered risk in blood vessel injury [35]. Preoperative 3D-CT has also been found to be useful for the determination of vascular anatomical variations and the decision on the line of transection in donor hepatectomy [3].

Extrapolating these studies on donor hepatectomy, 3D imaging may be useful in the reduction of intraoperative blood loss in surgery for hilar cholangiocarcinoma.

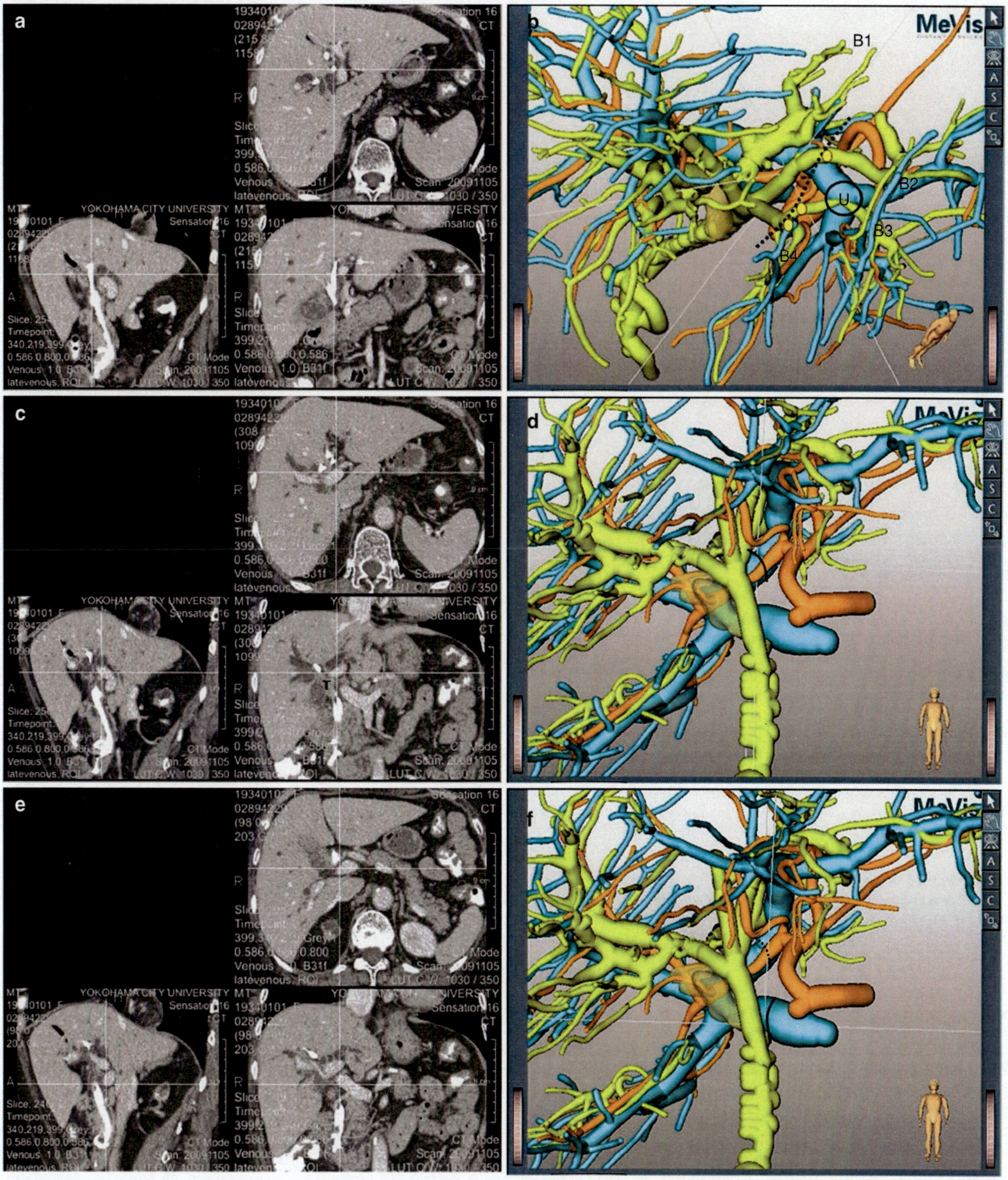

Fig. 6.5 Linkage of 2D multiplanar reconstructive images and 3D images. (**a**) The surgeon puts a marker on the site to where the tumor extended on a 2D multiplanar image. Simultaneously, a marker appears on the 3D reconstructive image (**b**). Thus, the findings on 2D images can be reflected on the 3D images. (**b**) When the hilar plate is dissected at the right border of the U-point (*dotted line*), three bile duct orifices should appear on the transection line of the hilar plate. The surgeon can estimate the segment to which each bile duct is draining. In this case B4, B3, and B2 orifices should appear on the transection plane on the ventral side. (**c**) When the surgeon puts a marker on the site where the tumor is adjacent to the left portal vein on a 2D multiplanar image, simultaneously a marker appears on the 3D reconstructive image (**d**). (**e**) When the surgeon puts a marker on the site to where the tumor is adjacent to the main portal vein on a 2D multiplanar image, simultaneously a marker appears on the 3D reconstructive image (**f**). (**f**) From these results, portal vein resection can be planned from the solid line on the main portal vein to the *dotted line* on the left portal vein

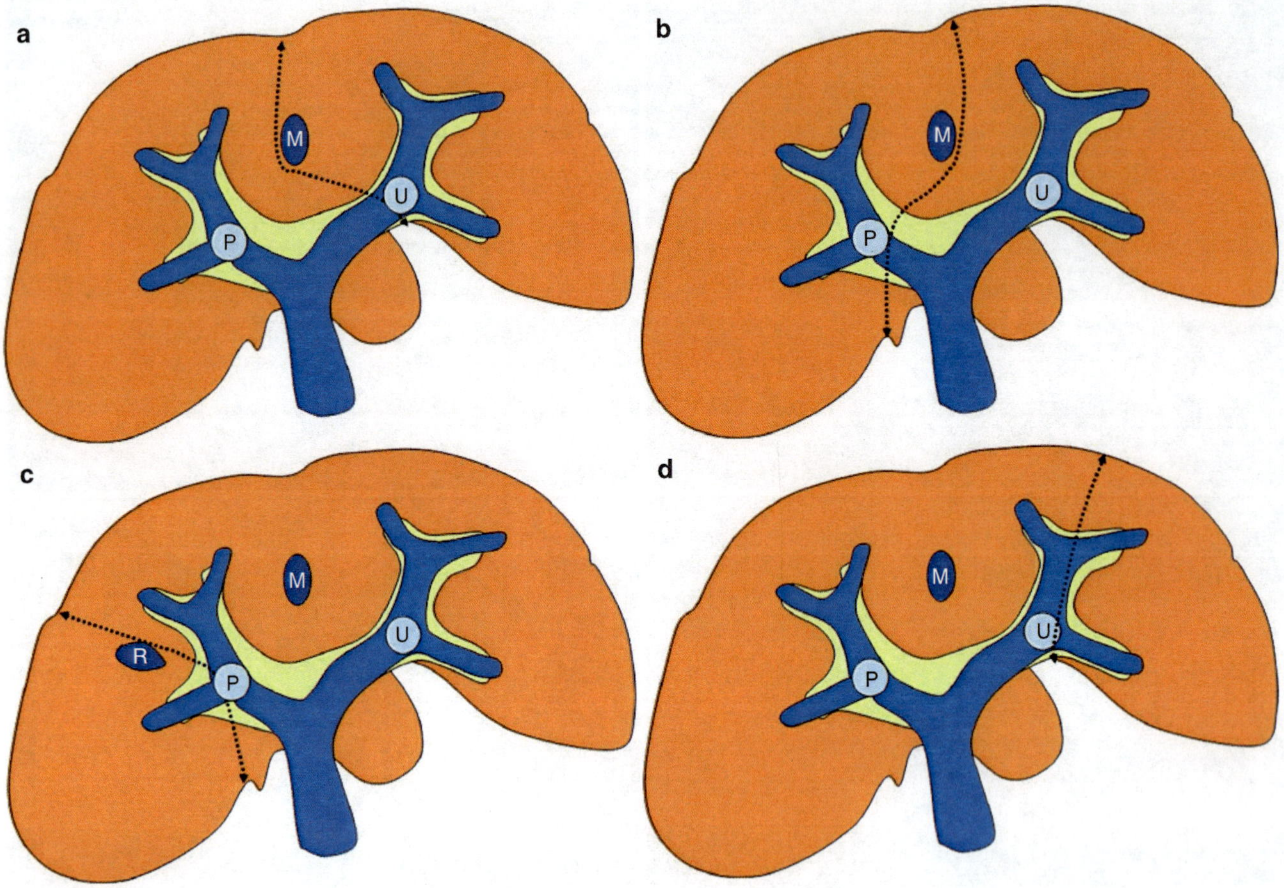

Fig. 6.6 U and P-point oriented hepatectomy by 3D reconstructive imaging. (**a**) Usually, making a virtual transection line on the 3D images, there are three landmarks, the middle hepatic vein, umbilical point, and posterior point. For right hemihepatectomy with caudate lobectomy, the planned transection line of liver parenchyma begins along with the Cantlie line to the right of the MHV. After ducking under the MHV, the transection line is angled to the U-point through the Arantian duct. (**b**) For left hemihepatectomy with caudate lobectomy, the planned transection line of liver parenchyma begins along with the Cantlie line to the left of the MHV. After ducking under the MHV, the transection line is angled to the P-point, and then to the right border of the IVC. (**c**) When longitudinal invasion extends to the left border of the P-point, left trisectionectomy should be considered. The liver parenchyma is transected along the portal segmentation of the anterior sector and the posterior sector toward the right hepatic vein. After passing through the RHV, the transection line is angled to the right border of the P-point, and then to the right border of the IVC. (**d**) When longitudinal tumor invasion extends to the right border of the U-point, right trisectionectomy should be considered. The liver parenchyma is transected just to the left of the umbilical portion of the left portal vein. When the tumor extends beyond both the left border of the U-point and the right border of the P-point, it is deemed unresectable

Our preliminary data demonstrated that intraoperative blood loss in patients evaluated by 2D-CT only and those evaluated by 3D-CT and MPR were 2,949 ± 2,306 ml and 1,454 ± 988 ml ($P = 0.0001$), respectively.

Biliary fistula is the most frequent morbidity after liver resection with biliary reconstruction. 3D images help to avoid injury of the biliary branch during parenchymal transection of the liver. Thus, it may decrease the incidence of postoperative morbidity. Postoperative morbidity is known to affect long-term outcomes after hepatic resection [45]. Several studies suggested that perioperative blood loss or transfusions have a negative impact on postoperative outcomes [46, 47].

If 3D imaging can reduce blood loss during surgery and postoperative complications, the long-term results of hilar cholangiocarcinoma are expected to improve in the near future.

6.9 Navigation Surgery for Hilar Cholangiocarcinoma

Computer-assisted navigation systems for rigid anatomical regions have been highly developed and used clinically. The obstacle that stands in the way of introducing 3D navigation surgery in HPB surgery is visceral plasticity. The shape of the liver and biliary tract can easily be changed during laparotomy. Beller et al. [48] demonstrated the feasibility of navigated resection using intraoperative 3-dimensional ultrasonography. They used a Polaris optical tracking system for position measurement. A tracker was attached to both the ultrasound probe and surgical instruments. After calibration and registration of the surgical instruments on the operative table, they can be visualized on the monitor with virtual environment of the registered 3D images. New direction in this field is the introduction of 3D imaging into laparoscopic surgery [49, 50]. Distortion of the liver is relatively less than under laparotomy. Mutter et al. stated that this facilitated the intraoperative identification of vascular anatomy and control of the left lateral sectional arteries and veins, thus preventing intraoperative bleeding [49]. With more advanced surgical simulators, surgeons may be able to work out the best operative procedure for each patient and to learn to use each individual step to improve the technique. 3D virtual reality can also be applied in robotic surgery. In the near future, intraoperative 3D navigation surgery may be used in hilar cholangiocarcinoma surgery as well.

Conclusions

3D images can estimate the extent of ductal infiltration of the tumor and anatomical variations of the hilar structures in an individual patient. These 3D images help to correlate the preoperative and intraoperative findings by identifying reliable anatomic landmarks, such as the U and P points, and thus allowing preoperative simulation. Consequently, the preoperative and intraoperative use of three-dimensional images may increase the proportion of potentially curable resection and also make the operative procedures less-invasive. In the future, 3D planning and simulation of operative procedures will become standard procedures for hilar cholangiocarcinoma.

References

1. Togo S, Shimada H, Kanemura E, et al. Usefulness of three-dimensional computed tomography for anatomic liver resection: sub-subsegmentectomy. Surgery. 1998;123(1):73–8.
2. Saito S, Yamanaka J, Miura K, et al. A novel 3D hepatectomy simulation based on liver circulation: application to liver resection and transplantation. Hepatology. 2005;41:1297–304.
3. Kanazawa A, Hirohashi K, Tanaka H, et al. Usefulness of three-dimensional computed tomography in a living-donor extended right lobe. Liver Transpl. 2002;8(11):1076–9.
4. Hiroshige S, Nishizaki T, Soejima Y, et al. Benefitial effects of 3-dimensional visualization on hepatic vein reconstruction in living donor liver transplantation using right lobe graft. Transplantation. 2001;72:1993–6.
5. Soyer P, Bluemke DA, Choti MA, et al. Variations in the intrahepatic portions of the hepatic and portal veins: findings on helical CT scans during arterial portography. Am J Roentgenol. 1995;164:103–8.
6. Ahrendt SA, Cameron JL, Pitt HA. Current management of patients with perihilar cholangiocarcinoma. Adv Surg. 1997;30:427–52.
7. Stain SC, Baer HU, Dennison AR, et al. Current management of hilar cholangiocarcinoma. Surg Gynecol Obstet. 1992;175:579–88.
8. Endo I, Shimada H, Sugita M, et al. Role of three-dimensional imaging in operative planning for hilar cholangiocarcinoma. Surgery. 2007;142(5):666–75.
9. Soto JA, Barish MA, Yucel EK, et al. Magnetic resonance cholangiography: comparison with endoscopic retrograde cholangiopancreatography. Gastroenterology. 1996;110:589–97.
10. Morimoto K, Shimoi M, Shirakawa T, et al. Biliary obstruction: evaluation with three-dimensional MR cholangiography. Radiology. 1992;183:578–80.
11. Vogl TJ, Schwarz WO, Heller M, et al. Staging of Klatskin tumors (hilar cholangiocarcinomas): comparison of MR cholangiography, MR imaging, and endoscopic retrograde cholangiography. Eur Radiol. 2006;16(10):2317–25.
12. Jarnagin WR, Fong Y, DeMatteo RP, et al. Staging and outcome in 225 patients with hilar cholangiocarcinoma. Ann Surg. 2001;234:507–19.
13. Furukawa H, Sano K, Kosuge T, et al. Analysis of biliary drainage in the caudate lobe of the liver: comparison of three-dimensional CT cholangiography and rotating cine cholangiography. Radiology. 1997;204:113–7.
14. Kim HJ, Kim AY, Hong SS, et al. Biliary ductal evaluation of hilar cholangiocarcinoma: three-dimensional direct multi-detector row CT cholangiographic findings versus surgical and pathologic results – feasibility study. Radiology. 2006;238:300–8.
15. Fulcher AS, Turner MA. Hasten MR cholangiography in the evaluation of hilar cholangiocarcinoma. AJR Am J Roentgenol. 1997;169:1501–5.
16. Figueras J, Llado L, Valls C, et al. Changing strategies in diagnosis and management of hilar cholangiocarcinoma. Liver Transpl. 2000;6:786–94.
17. Otto G, Romaneehsen B, Hoppe-Lotichius M, et al. Hilar cholangiocarcinoma: resectability and radicality after routine diagnostic imaging. J Hepatobiliary Pancreat Surg. 2004;11:310–8.
18. Nesbit GM, Johnson CD, James EM, et al. Cholangiocarcinoma: diagnosis and evaluation of resectability by CT and sonography as procedures complementary to cholangiography. AJR Am J Roentgenol. 1988;151:933–8.
19. Schwartz LH, Lefkowitz RA, Panicek DM, et al. Breath-hold magnetic resonance cholangiopancreatography in the evaluation of malignant pancreaticobiliary obstruction. J Comput Assist Tomogr. 2003;27:307–14.
20. Hanninen EL, Pech M, Jonas S, et al. Magnetic resonance imaging including magnetic resonance cholangiopancreatography for tumor localization and therapy planning in malignant hilar obstructions. Acta Radiol. 2005;46:462–70.
21. Marescaux J, Clement J, Tassetti V, et al. Virtual reality applied to hepatic surgery simulation: the next recolution. Ann Surg. 1998;228:627–34.
22. Wigmore SJ, Redhead DN, Yan XJ, et al. Virtual hepatic resection using three-dimensional reconstruction of helical computed tomography angioportograms. Ann Surg. 2000;233:221–6.
23. Rau HG, Schauer R, Helmberger T, et al. Impact of virtual reality imaging on hepatic liver tumor resection: calculation of risk. Langenbecks Arch Surg. 2000;385:162–70.
24. Makuuchi M, Hasegawa H, Yamazaki S. Ultrasonically guided subsegmentectomy. Surg Gynecol Obstet. 1985;161(4):346–50.
25. Launois B, Jamieson GG. The importance of Glisson's capsule and its sheaths in the intrahepatic approach to resection of the liver. Surg Gynecol. 1992;174:7–10.
26. Billingsley KG, Jarnagin WR, Fong Y, et al. Segment-oriented hepatic resection in the management of malignant neoplasms of the liver. J Am Coll Surg. 1998;187:471–81.
27. Shimada H, Endo I, Sugita M, et al. Hepatic resection combined with portal vein or hepatic artery reconstruction for advanced carcinoma of the hilar bile duct and gallbladder. World J Surg. 2003;27(10):1137–42.

28. Miyazaki M, Kato A, Ito H, et al. Combined vascular resection in operative resection for hilar cholangiocarcinoma: does it work or not? Surgery. 2007;141(5):581–8.
29. Nagino M, Nimura Y, Nishio H, et al. Hepatectomy with simultaneous resection of the portal vein and hepatic artery for advanced perihilar cholangiocarcinoma: an audit of 50 consecutive cases. Ann Surg. 2010;252(1):115–23.
30. Masunari H, Shimada H, Endo I, et al. Surgical anatomy of hepatic hilum with special reference of the plate system and extrahepatic duct. J Gastrointest Surg. 2008;12(6):1047–53.
31. Cho A, Okazumi S, Yoshinaga Y, et al. Relationship between left biliary duct system and left portal vein: evaluation with three-dimensional portocholangiography. Radiology. 2003;228:246–50.
32. Okamoto E, Kyo A, Yamanaka N, et al. Prediction of the safe limits of hepatectomy by combined volumetric and functional measurements in patients with impaired hepatic function. Surgery. 1984;95: 586–91.
33. Nagino M, Nimura Y, Hayakawa N, et al. Logistic regression and discriminant analyses of hepatic failure after liver resection for carcinoma of the biliarytract. World J Surg. 1993;17:250–5.
34. Kubota K, Makuuchi M, Kusaka K, et al. Measurement of liver volume and hepatic functional reserve as a guide to decision-making in resectional surgery for hepatic tumors. Hepatology. 1997;26:1176–81.
35. Hiroshige S, Shimada M, Harada N, et al. Accurate preoperative estimation of liver-graft volumetry using three-dimensional computed tomography. Transplantation. 2003;75:1561–4.
36. Müller SA, Bläuer K, Kremer M, et al. Exact CT-based liver volume calculation including nonmetabolic liver tissue in three-dimensional liver reconstruction. J Surg Res. 2010;160(2):236–43.
37. Lamade W, Glombitza G, Fischer L. The impact of 3-dimensional reconstructions on operation planning in liver surgery. Arch Surg. 2000;135:1256–61.
38. Sano K, Makuuchi M, Miki K, et al. Evaluation of hepatic venous congestion: proposed indication criteria for hepatic vein reconstruction. Ann Surg. 2002;236:241–7.
39. Kondo S, Hirano S, Ambo Y, et al. Forty consecutive resections of hilar cholangiocarcinoma with no postoperative mortality and no positive ductal margins. Results of a prospective study. Ann Surg. 2004;240:95–101.
40. Neuhaus P, Jonas S, Bechstein WO, et al. Extended resections for hilar cholangiocarcinoma. Ann Surg. 1999;230:808–18.
41. Nimura Y, Kamiya J, Kondo S, et al. Aggressive preoperative management and extended surgery for hilar cholangiocarcinoma: Nagoya experience. J Hepatobiliary Pancreat Surg. 2000;7:155–62.
42. Lee SG, Lee YJ, Park KM, et al. One hundred and eleven liver resections for hilar bile duct cancer. J Hepatobiliary Pancreat Surg. 2000;7:135–41.
43. Kawasaki S, Imamura H, Kobayashi A, et al. Results of surgical resection for patients with hilar bile duct cancer. Application of extended hepatectomy after biliary drainage and hemihepatic portal vein embolization. Ann Surg. 2003;238:84–92.
44. Denecke T, Degutyte E, Stelter L, et al. Minimal intensity projections of the biliary system using 16-channel multidetector computed tomography in patients with biliary obstruction: comparison with MRCP. Eur Radiol. 2006;16:1719–26.
45. Laurent C, Sa Cunha A, Couderc P, et al. Influence of postoperative morbidity on long-term survival following liver resection for colorectal metastases. Br J Surg. 2003;90(9):1131–6.
46. Ito H, Are C, Gonen M, et al. Effect of postoperative morbidity on long-term survival after hepatic resection for metastatic colorectal cancer. Ann Surg. 2008;247(6):994–1002.
47. de Boer MT, Molenaar IQ, Porte RJ. Impact of blood loss on outcome after liver resection. Dig Surg. 2007;24(4):259–64.
48. Beller S, Hünerbein M, Eulenstein S, et al. Feasibility of navigated resection of liver tumors using multiplanar visualization of intraoperative 3-dimensional ultrasound data. Ann Surg. 2007; 246(2):288–94.
49. Mutter D, Dallemagne B, Bailey C, et al. 3D virtual reality and selective vascular control for laparoscopic left hepatic lobectomy. Surg Endosc. 2009;23(2):432–5.
50. Yamanaka J, Okada T, Saito S, et al. Minimally invasive laparoscopic liver resection: 3D MDCT simulation for preoperative planning. J Hepatobiliary Pancreat Surg. 2009;16(6):808–15.
51. Couinaud C. Le Foie: etudes anatomiques et chirurgicales. Paris: Masson; 1957.

7 Assessment of Liver Function

D.V. Mann

7.1 Introduction

The selection and timing of management options for cholangiocarcinoma must necessarily be informed by the function of the liver. The consideration of major resectional hepatic surgery is predicated on the ability of that organ to sustain and recover adequate hepatocyte function and mass, whereas individuals presenting with biliary obstruction may benefit from axial or segmental restoration of bile egress prior to planned therapy. Assessment of liver physiological status therefore guides treatment options for cholangiocarcinoma whether arising in the extrahepatic or intrahepatic components of the biliary system. Ideally, an evaluation of liver function should assess not only ambient homeostatic performance but also the recuperative and regenerative capacity of that organ (the functional reserve) since these restorative processes are less efficient in the severely parenchymal-depleted, diseased or cholestatic state [1, 2]. It should be appreciated however, that when the malignant process is confined to one hemi-liver (or segmental components) there may be no measurable disturbance in serum biochemistry or test-substance handling due to compensation by the unaffected liver, and in this situation techniques that assess hepatocyte status per se may be more informative. In addition to those estimations used for initial evaluation prior to planned therapy, serial or longitudinal studies can be used to monitor hepatic status after intervention and to detect deviation from expected patterns of recovery before these become clinically manifest.

The term liver function encompasses a whole host of the biologic roles of that organ including not only diverse metabolic tasks, but also the physiological response to injury (acute phase reaction) and capability for restoration of lost liver mass (regeneration). Although many of the commonly used traditional peripheral blood "liver function tests" do not directly measure actual function, and changes in most are not specific to that organ, these analyses (particularly in combination) have generally proven robust in the prediction of outcomes following hepatectomy [3]. Estimations of liver volume are often used to predict physiological capacity and reserve. However, parenchymal mass and function may be dissociated in the diseased or regenerating condition and therefore probing of some other dimension of hepatic performance may be desirable for more complete representation.

The assessment of liver physiology can be considered according to the following conceptual framework of four main types of test (Table 7.1):

1. Homeostatic: traditional "liver function tests"; biochemical analyses of blood reflecting the balance between production and disappearance of bile metabolites, hepatic enzymes and plasma proteins. These may be combined with clinical evaluations to produce composite clinico-biochemical scoring systems (e.g., Child-Pugh grading)
2. Radiological: image based assessments of liver parenchymal volume and quality;

Table 7.1 Taxonomy of liver function tests

Type	Examples
Homeostatic	Bilirubin
	Transaminases
	Alkaline phosphatase
	Albumin
	Prothrombin time
	Clinico-laboratory scoring (e.g., Child-Pugh score)
Radiological	Computer tomography volumetry
	Hepatic steatosis measurement
Bioenergetic	Redox state
	Adenine nucleotide/mitochondrial analysis
	Magnetic resonance spectroscopy
Dynamic	Clearance tests e.g., indocyanine green, aminopyrine, MEGX
	Hexose sugar handling capacity
	Hepatic scintigraphy
	Portal vein embolization

D.V. Mann, MS, FRCS
8/F Hang Wai Building, 231 Queens Road East,
Wanchai, Hong Kong
e-mail: darrenmann@biznetvigator.com

W.Y. Lau (ed.), *Hilar Cholangiocarcinoma*,
DOI 10.1007/978-94-007-6473-6_7, © Springer Science+Business Media Dordrecht and People's Medical Publishing House 2013

3. Bioenergetic: measures of hepatic energy state (in plasma and at tissue level);
4. Dynamic tests: in which some aspect of liver physiology is assessed in a time dependent manner (e.g., tracer excretion) or repeated measures of any of the above tests used to assess the longitudinal response to a provocation such as metabolic stress or portal vein embolization.

This chapter will describe these tests, with greatest emphasis on those that have become clinically established in the management of patients with cholangiocarcinoma. Emerging technologies poised to contribute to clinical advancements in the future or that provide new insights with which to interpret currently used tests will also be discussed.

7.2 Homeostasis

The term liver function is used to describe the diverse biological duties of that organ, which include intermediary metabolism of carbohydrates, protein and fat, production of bile, synthesis of plasma proteins and clotting factors, metabolic handling and excretion of endo- and xenobiotics and urea synthesis. In addition, the cellular integrity of hepatocytes and bile canaliculi can be inferred from circulating levels of enzymes normally confined to the intracellular domain. A common biochemical panel of "liver function tests" comprises estimation of the serum level of bilirubin, transaminases, alkaline phosphatase, albumin level and clotting factor analysis. Each of these elements is reflective of a different element of liver physiology and its disorder.

7.2.1 Bilirubin

The plasma concentration of the chemical tetrapyrrole bilirubin, the main degradation product of heme-protein metabolism, reflects the aggregate processes of production by the reticulo-endothelial system, and subsequent hepatic extraction, conjugation and excretion by an active anionic transport mechanism. When rate of generation is constant, the circulating level is taken to represent overall bile pigment "handling" by the liver. However, bilirubin levels may be influenced by non-hepatic factors, for example increased production by haemolysis and sepsis, and decreased clearance due to mechanical obstruction to bile flow, and therefore may not reflect hepatocyte function per se in these instances. Although independently predictive of morbidity following hepatic resection [4], plasma bilirubin concentration is most commonly combined with other laboratory and clinical factors such as Child-Pugh scoring system or Model for End-stage Liver Disease (MELD) (see below). A pattern of progressive increase in bilirubin after liver resection may herald the onset of organ dysfunction, although sepsis, drug reaction, biliary obstruction and portal vein thrombosis may also present in this way.

7.2.2 Transaminases

Serum activities of amino-transferase enzymes are reflective of hepatic cellular integrity, although specificity may be reduced by contributions from other organs, particularly striated muscle. Alanine transferase (ALT) is purely cytosolic in origin (and more specific), whilst aspartate transferase (AST) is of mixed mitochondrial and cytosolic provenance (and more sensitive). Elevated preoperative transaminase levels have been found to be associated with increased risk of complications and death after liver resection in cirrhotic patients [5]. A markedly elevated transaminase level is suggestive of ongoing hepatic necrosis, for example active viral or alcoholic hepatitis, ischemia or sepsis (particularly of biliary tract). The relative weighting of these enzymes for risk is comparatively weak, and they do not routinely feature in composite preoperative scores.

7.2.3 Alkaline Phosphatase

Alkaline phosphatases are a group of hydrolase enzymes responsible for removing phosphate groups in the 5- and 3-positions from many types of molecules, including nucleotides, proteins, and alkaloids. They are distributed in liver, bile ducts, bone, kidney and placenta. Hepatic-origin alkaline phosphatase levels are elevated in the presence of liver disease with hepatic cell injury or biliary obstruction, mechanistically due to increased enzyme synthesis as well as plasma spill-over. Preoperative serum activity of alkaline phosphatase may be predictive of risk of hepatic failure following hepatectomy [6]. Liver regeneration following hepatectomy is associated with an elevation of alkaline phosphatase levels, and failure of regeneration may be presaged when levels of this enzyme do not increase in the post-hepatectomy period.

7.2.4 Albumin

This plasma protein is synthesized exclusively by the liver. The circulating half-life is 20 days, and assay can be used to interpret steady state synthetic function (although starvation and protein losing conditions also influence levels). An acute reduction in plasma concentration more likely reflects change in volume of distribution due to capillary leakage rather than diminished synthesis. Albumin has prognostic value for risk of liver surgery as part of the Child-Pugh score.

Table 7.2 Child-Pugh score

Measure	1 point	2 points	3 points	Units
Bilirubin (total)	<34 (<2)	34–50 (2–3)	>50 (>3)	umol/l (mg/dL)
Serum albumin	>35	28–35	<28	g/L
INR	<1.7	1.71–2.20	>2.20	No unit
Ascites	None	Suppressed with medication	Refractory	No unit
Hepatic encephalopathy	None	Grade I–II (or suppressed with medication)	Grade III–IV (or refractory)	No unit

7.2.5 Prothrombin Time

The liver is the predominant site for the manufacture of blood clotting cascade proteins. Derangements in liver function may therefore be detected by disturbed laboratory measures of clotting times, or reduced amounts of individually assayed clotting factors. The commonest measurement is that of prothrombin time, which is indicative of the extrinsic pathway of coagulation involving factors II, V, VII, X and fibrinogen. The prothrombin time is predominantly affected by factor VII which has the shortest half life (4–6 h) and is vitamin K dependent (so abnormalities may arise from vitamin K insufficiency states such as biliary obstruction as well as protein-synthetic deficits). Prothrombin time is a component of the Child-Pugh score.

7.2.6 Prognostic Clinico-Laboratory Scoring

A common method for evaluation of hepatic function is the use of a composite prognostication system based on laboratory measures and selected clinical criteria. These components reflect different core aspects of liver physiology including endobiotic handling and excretion, protein synthesis and clinical estimates of degree of established portal hypertension, which can be combined into an overall score. In general the scores are formulated by multivariate logistic regression methods, and the advantage is that a greater degree of overall liver function is represented (parallel testing enhances sensitivity) and the predictive power goes beyond that of any individual component test. Although initially devised for risk assessment in the setting of liver cirrhosis, the use of scoring systems is often extended in clinical practice to evaluate suitability for liver surgery in general. Such scores are predictive of natural history of liver disease, and may stratify risk of therapeutic interventions and prioritise selection for transplantation.

7.2.6.1 The Child-Pugh Score

The Child score (Pugh modification) is the most widely used system and is composed of bilirubin (excretion), albumin (synthetic function), prothrombin time (synthesis), ascites (portal hypertension) and encephalopathy (porto-systemic shunting) [7]. Components of the system and point allocation for scoring are shown in Table 7.2. Individuals are grouped onto Classes according to the number of points, as follows: Class A 5–6; Class B 7–9 and Class C 10–15 (there is some variation in the literature between authors on Class allocation). Since cholangiocarcinoma (and mixed cholangio-hepatocellular carcinoma) may occasionally arise in the setting of pre-existing liver disease, the Child-Pugh score is commonly used to evaluate operative risk. In particular, the outcomes of liver resectional surgery are numerically related to Child-Pugh score, with mortality rates being lower and survival rates higher in Child-Pugh Class A compared to Class B and C [8, 9]. Child-Pugh Class A, well-compensated cirrhosis, does not negatively impact on survival after hepatectomy [10].

7.2.6.2 Model for End-Stage Liver Disease (MELD)

The MELD score is a commonly used to rank patients for liver transplantation, and is mentioned here because this is a therapeutic option that can be selectively considered in the management of cholangiocarcinoma [11]. Scores are calculated according to the formula: MELD = 0.957 × log e (creatinine mg/dl) + 0.378 × log e (bilirubin mg/dl) + 1.120 log e (INR) + 0.643.

MELD has been examined as an alternative to Child-Pugh score for prediction of liver failure post hepatectomy. Although MELD score is correlated with risk of liver failure after resection, it is unclear whether the discriminant function is superior to Child-Pugh Class [3, 12].

7.3 Radiological Imaging and Qualitative Assessments

Volumetric analysis of the liver parenchyma forms an integral component of the assessment of functioning liver cell mass, and by extension predicted physiological reserve. Computed tomography liver volumetry can be used to assess the respective volumes of liver and tumour, and to estimate the parenchymal resection rate and so judge the suitability for resectional surgery [13, 14]. Estimates of postoperative liver volume can be used to guide selection of therapies for cholangiocarcinoma, in the context of the condition of the underlying liver [15]. For example, when inadequate post-operative parenchymal volume is anticipated, measures to increase hepatic cell mass such as portal vein embolization may be indicated, or non-resectional alternatives (transplantation, chemo-irradiation, local ablation, etc.) considered.

Volumetric estimations can be combined with functional analyses such as indocyanine green retention (see below) to provide composite scores of high accuracy for predicting complications and outcomes of liver surgery [16].

Hepatic steatosis (fatty liver) is a risk factor for complications and death after liver resection, and some authors advocate pre-operative identification prior to major hepatic resection: the fat content of the liver can be assessed by ultrasound, computed tomography or magnetic resonance imaging [17].

7.4 Bioenergetic Tests

The traditional liver function tests outlined above are used to identify disturbance in several of the possible biologic roles of the liver. However, results may be influenced by diverse non-hepatic factors and there is often variation in the degree of perturbation of different tests. A limitation common to these evaluations is that they are indirectly reflective of underlying liver physiology. Although these tests can be augmented by liver volumetry, it should be appreciated that in the diseased state there may be a dissociation between hepatocyte mass and performance, and therefore volumetric indices may not accurately reflect functional reserve. Conversely, serum biochemistry may be misleadingly normal in certain disease states, for example a biliary obstructed hemi-liver, due to compensatory processes. Because of these limitations, estimations of organ energy balance have intrinsic appeal since they may more reliably reflect the condition of hepatocytes.

Fundamentally, the key determinant of hepatic functional status and reserve is the energy state of the organ, which in turn is determined by the aggregate energy balance of individual hepatocytes. Energy transduction for maintenance of cellular integrity and function is achieved through the adenylate high-energy phosphate system, the principal mediator being adenosine triphosphate (ATP). In the liver, each individual hepatocyte may be considered as a self-recharging battery in which energy status is controlled according to energy charge $(\mathrm{ATP}+1/2\mathrm{ADP})/(\mathrm{ATP}+\mathrm{ADP}+\mathrm{AMP})$ or phosphorylation potential $(\mathrm{ATP}/\mathrm{ADP}\times\mathrm{Pi})$[18]. These key metabolic parameters govern the balance between energy-producing (exergonic) and energy-consuming (endergonic) processes, thereby maintaining the biochemical poise of the system.

A fall in energy state induces a curtailment of synthetic, secretory and storage reactions, while favouring energy-producing ones (and vice versa) thereby tending to restore equipoise when energy demands and supply (temporarily) dissociate (Fig. 7.1). When net energy consumption exceeds supply, whether due to increased physiologic demands or to limitations of ATP-generating ability secondary to disease (or some combination of the two) then a fall in energy state is produced. By the action of feedback modification, a compensatory suppression of ATP-consuming processes will result. This has widespread and varied consequences for liver function, but not all aspects of hepatocyte biology will necessarily be affected to the same degree for any given magnitude of energy state depression (Fig. 7.2 shows schematically the physiologic consequences of energy balance deficit after liver resection). Active anionic transport and protein synthesis are typical of energy-consuming processes that are curtailed during conditions of energy state depression, hence plasma bilirubin levels tend to rise and prothrombin and albumin levels fall. Other important energy-dependent processes such as nucleic acid synthesis may also be suppressed with important implications for mitotic capacity and regeneration. More extreme deviations

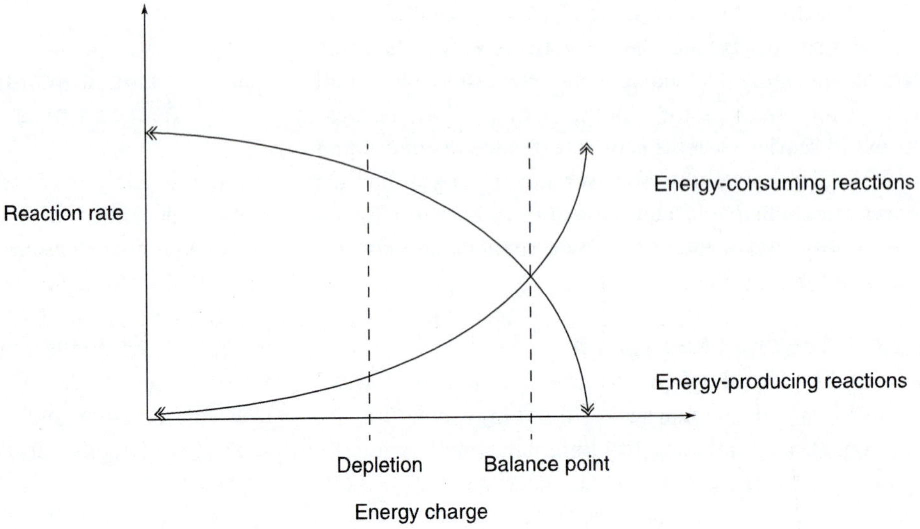

Fig. 7.1 Energy charge and metabolic control. The graph shows how a reduction in energy state at 'depletion' results in a decrease in energy-consuming reaction rates (secretion, synthesis, storage) and increase in energy-producing reaction rates, thereby restoring the system to the energy "balance point"

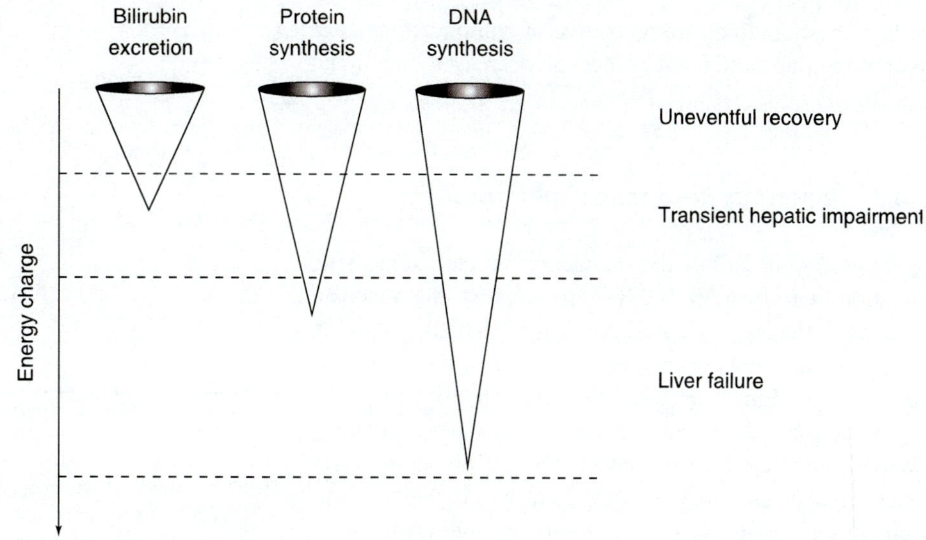

Fig. 7.2 Energy state and liver function after liver resectional surgery. A fall in hepatic energy charge necessarily results in some limitation of energy-consuming processes such as those for excretion of bilirubin, production of proteins and nucleic acid synthesis. The relative impairment varies, as does the tolerable degree of disturbance, which is reflected clinically in the different patterns of liver recovery seen after partial hepatectomy

from energy balance may result in metabolic decompensation and organ failure.

A variety of different methods are available with which to gauge hepatic energy balance, and determinations may be performed on peripheral blood or alternatively on the liver itself (by invasive and non-invasive means).

7.4.1 Peripheral Blood Redox State

Hepatic mitochondrial redox state can be estimated by measurement of the relative abundance of ketone bodies in peripheral blood. The ratio of acetoacetate to hydroxybutyrate (the arterial ketone body ratio, AKBR) is in equilibrium with that of oxidized to reduced nicotinamide-adenine dinucleotide ($NAD^+/NADH$) in mitochondria [19]:

$$\text{Acetoacetate} + \text{NADH} + \text{H}^+ \rightarrow 3-\text{hydroxybutyrate} + \text{NAD}^+$$

The balance between these states of NAD reflects the ATP synthesizing potential of the mitochondria. When electron acceptor (oxygen) availability is limited the ratio of $NAD^+/NADH$ falls, ATP generation is reduced and energy state declines: these changes are also reflected in a decrease acetoacetate/hydroxybutyrate ratio (and for biochemically analogous reasoning a decrease in the pyruvate to lactate ratio).

In the liver, acetoacetate is produced via the formation of 3-hydroxy-3-methylglutaryl-CoA (HMGCoA) and also by the deacylase reaction from acetoacetyl-CoA; when conditions leading to accumulation of reducing equivalents prevail, conversion to hydroxybutyrate increases.

The liver is the predominant source of ketone bodies, although other tissues are involved in their subsequent metabolism. The ratio of acetoacetate to hydroxybutyrate in arterial blood has been shown to be related to hepatic mitochondrial redox state [20]. A fall in arterial ketone body ratio can be taken to represent a decline in hepatic mitochondrial redox (phosphorylating) potential, and hence attenuation of those aspects of liver function that are dependent on energy supply. Single pre-operative measures of arterial ketone body ratio are of limited use in predicting outcomes, although refinements based on dynamic response to glucose loading have been described (see below) [21]. Serial post-operative estimates of arterial ketone body ratio can identify individuals most likely to develop hepatic failure after liver resection [22].

7.4.2 Tissue Adenine Nucleotide and Mitochondrial Analysis

Because of the requirement for tissue biopsy these measurements have principally been used in a research setting. Nevertheless, the information has proved valuable for proof of concept of novel, non-invasive methods for estimating energy state (see below). Assays of tissue-level metabolism are often based on chemical analysis of biopsy specimens for high-energy phosphate compounds. The relative concentrations of adenosine mono-phosphate (AMP), adenosine di-phosphate (ADP) and adenosine tri-phosphate (ATP) are used to determine the cellular energy charge (or equivalently the phosphorylation potential). As discussed earlier, these parameters are central to regulation of metabolism by constraining the balance between energy-producing and energy-consuming reactions. Alternative techniques involve analysis of mitochondrial phosphorylative activity and cytochrome chain component redox state. In general, the diseased liver (whether by dint of biliary obstruction or parenchymal pathology) displays altered energy-chain activity with negative influence on ATP-synthesizing ability: these findings are predictive of complications after liver resection as a consequence of decreased functional reserve [23–25].

7.4.3 Magnetic Resonance Spectroscopy

Spectroscopy describes the interaction of electromagnetic radiation with matter, and in this context the resonant exchange of energy by nuclei in a magnetic field. This is an emerging technique which allows non-invasive assay of hepatic intracellular metabolism in vivo. The measurements can be performed on standard magnetic resonance imaging (MRI) systems after suitable adaptation, and are increasingly being used in the modern clinical arena. The basis of the technique is similar to that of the more familiar magnetic resonance (hydrogen nucleus) imaging except that the information is obtained from a different chemical nucleus (usually 31-phosphorus, but also 13-carbon and 23-sodium amongst others). The principle of the measurement is that atomic nuclei have electrical charge and spin, and hence a magnetic moment (by Faraday's laws). If a sample of the tissue to be studied (or indeed a whole organ in vivo) is placed within an external magnetic field, nuclei with odd-quantum spin numbers will align themselves in one of a number of possible quantum states with a slight preponderance of nuclei aligned along the field (low-energy state) according to the Boltzman constant. Within this field, the nuclei precess at a specific rotational rate, the Larmor frequency (analogous to the way in which a spinning gyroscope precesses in the earth's magnetic field). When a radiowave pulse oscillating at the same (Larmor) frequency is applied perpendicular to the original field, the nuclei will absorb energy (the resonance condition) and change their quantum state: a greater proportion are now in the higher energy condition, which can be measured by electromagnetic induction of current in a detector. Different nuclei can be assayed by varying the frequency of the radiowave probing pulse. The signal obtained is mathematically treated (Fourier transformation) to produce a spectrum of concentration against frequency, with nuclei of the same type but within different chemical species, being resolved.

A typical liver spectrum obtained by resonating on the 31-phosphorus nucleus (31-phosphorus magnetic resonance spectroscopy, 31P-MRS) using a 1.5 T clinical MRI system is shown in Fig. 7.3 31-phopshorus magnetic resonance spectroscopy is particularly appealing for the study of liver metabolism in vivo, because this naturally occurring phosphorus isotope is central to biological energy transduction and ubiquitous in cell membrane phospholipids. Using 31-phosphorus magnetic resonance spectroscopy it is possible to measure the energy state of the liver and to appreciate changes in cell membrane composition.

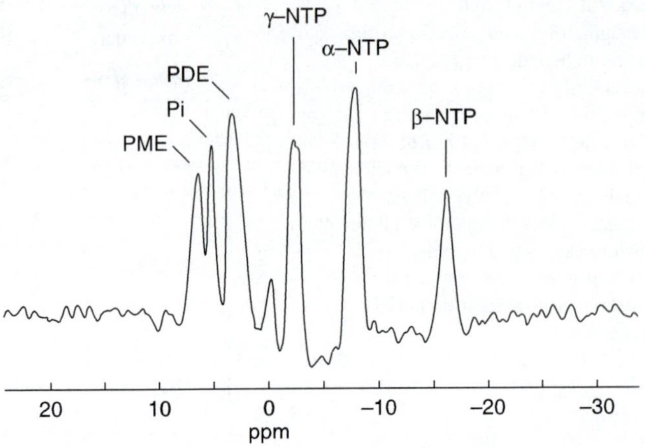

Fig. 7.3 31-phosphorus magnetic resonance spectrum of human liver. Peak area is proportional to amount of metabolite. Peaks labeled on scan: *PME* phosphomonoesters (mainly phospholipids precursors and sugar phosphates), *Pi* inorganic phosphate (product of adenosine triphosphate hydrolysis, which yields adenosine diphosphate and inorganic phosphate: ATP ↔ ADP + Pi), *PDE* phosphodiesters (principally phospholipid catabolites with some contribution from cell membranes), and γ-, α-, β-phosphates of nucleotide triphosphates, *NTP* (high-energy phosphate compounds). By convention, the [β-P] NTP peak is taken practically to represent adenosine triphosphate, ATP. Unlabeled peak at zero parts per million (ppm), is phosphocreatine contamination from muscle. Data are conventionally presented as ratios of peak areas, comprising energy status (ATP/Pi) and phosphoester metabolites (PME/PDE) respectively. Alternatively, individual peak areas may be expressed as a function of total visible phosphate (TP). These measures are independent of the volume of liver from which the signals are obtained

With respect to hepatic energy balance, two relevant phosphate-compounds are assayed: ATP and it's hydrolytic breakdown product inorganic phosphate (Pi)

$$\text{ATP} \leftrightarrow \text{ADP} + \text{Pi}.$$

The ratio of ATP/Pi is an estimate of energy state, analogous to cellular energy charge or phosphorylation potential [26]. Clinical 31P-MRS studies have shown, in general, that in the steady state condition, liver energy balance is often preserved in compensated parenchymal disease [27]. However, under conditions of changing metabolic stress, fluctuations in energy state can be detected. For example, serial measurements of ATP/Pi in the regenerating human liver after partial hepatectomy have revealed patterns of high-energy phosphate depletion and recovery [28]. In the clinical setting of obstructive jaundice, biliary decompression has been shown to enhance liver energy status as measured by this technique, a finding which may guide the selection and optimum timing of therapy [29]. This is important because the risks of liver resection are greater when biliary obstruction is present since this is associated with deficient regeneration [2].

The relative proportions of phospholipid compounds detectable by 31-phosphorus magnetic resonance

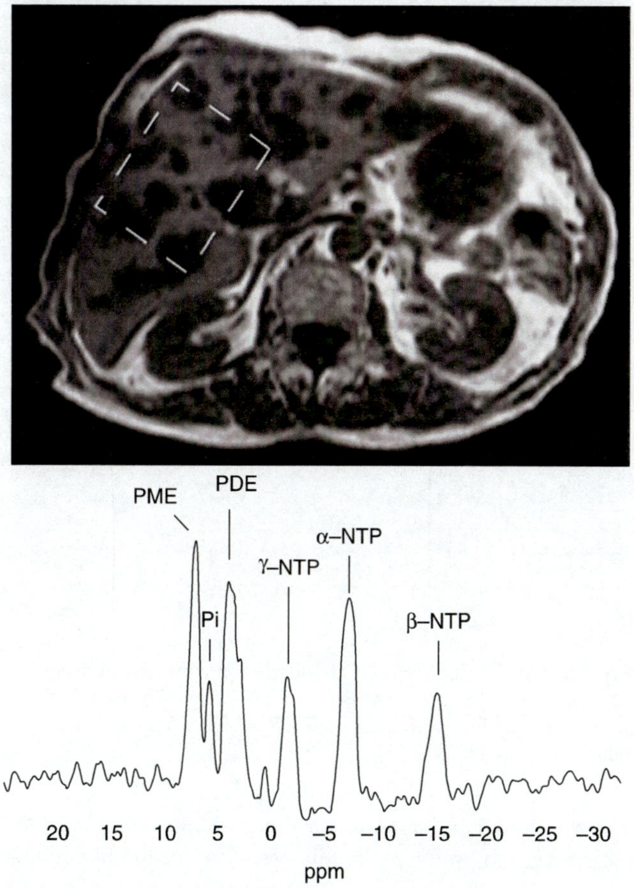

Fig. 7.4 MRI of liver from a patient with obstructive jaundice due to hilar cholangiocarcinoma showing grossly dilated intrahepatic biliary system. The corresponding 31 phosphorus magnetic resonance spectrum is shown. There are readily visible differences in the relative amounts of phospholipids in the PME (phospholipid precursor) and PDE (phospholipid catabolite) peaks when compared to the spectrum from normal liver shown in Fig. 7.3

spectroscopy are reflective of hepatocyte membrane phospholipid composition and metabolism. Two broad peaks representing phospholipids metabolites are generally observed. The phosphomonoester (PME) peak mainly consists of phospholipids precursors, while the phosphodiester peak (PDE) comprises phospholipid catabolites. Changes in the relative abundance of these compounds characterized by a relative excess of phospholipid precursors with respect to catabolites have been interpreted to reflect redirection of phospholipid turnover with generation of secondary messengers and sometimes true amplification of membrane synthesis. In the human liver this pattern of change has been observed in neoplasia, in the maturing neonatal organ, in benign parenchymal disease (including cirrhosis and hepatitis) and in biliary obstruction [27, 29–31]. Figure 7.4 shows a clinical 31-P magnetic resonance spectrum illustrating membrane phospholipid alterations in a patient with obstructive jaundice due to hilar cholangiocarcinoma. In general, disturbance of phospholipid balance correlates with grade of parenchymal disease in hepatic fibrosis and cirrhosis and it is likely that such measurements will find a role in the assessment of hepatic status in the future [32]. Changes in hepatic membrane phospholipid composition can also be detected after non-hepatic surgery, and in this context the changes appear to represent biochemical alterations during hepatocyte activation and acute phase physiology [28].

An appealing feature of magnetic resonance spectroscopy is that it can be used serially in the clinical setting to monitor in vivo liver function non-invasively, in addition to providing conventional imaging information on hepatic volume recovery, vessel patency and biliary tract morphology (see Sect. 7.6 Longitudinal Evaluation After Hepatectomy).

7.5 Dynamic Tests

These tests generally examine one or more aspects of liver physiology in a time dependent manner or in response to some provocation such a metabolic stress. The advantage of these assessments is that they can quantify hepatic function and when repeated can be used to assess changes in functional status over time. Traditionally, the commonest techniques are tracer excretion studies (clearance tests), although metabolic and bioenergetic measurements and sophisticated nuclear medicine studies are also available to the clinician. The response to portal vein embolization may be considered as a special case of dynamic testing of hepatic functional reserve.

7.5.1 Clearance Tests

These estimate hepatic extraction, handling and excretion of test substances. Depending on the compound selected, the process examined is variably specific but generally reflects the number of hepatocytes (liver cell mass), the functional ability of those hepatocytes and, for very high efficiency elimination, some dependence on hepatic blood flow. The most commonly used are the indocyanine green (ICG) test which measures an energy-dependent transport mechanism, and the aminopyrine test which is reflective of microsomal function. Some tests of metabolic function consequent upon sugar handling, such as galactose elimination capacity, are of practical and theoretical interest.

7.5.1.1 Indocyanine Green Test

This is probably the commonest quantitative liver function test in clinical use. Indocyanine green (ICG) is a tricarbocyanic green coloured dye, which when administered into the circulation rapidly combines with plasma proteins (albumin, lipo-proteins, etc.) and the volume of distribution is therefore the blood volume. ICG is taken up selectively by the liver, and is excreted unaltered into the bile by an energy (ATP) dependent carrier mediated mechanism. The carrier is a member of the canalicular multiple organic anion transporter (cMOAT) group, which is also responsible for the excretion of bilirubin. The disappearance of ICG from the blood is therefore a measure of an energy-dependant process. ICG exhibits a maximum absorbance at wavelength of 805 nm (near infrared region of the electromagnetic spectrum) and the principle of the measurement is one of photoabsorbance, using pulse densitometry based on pulse oximetry. The test is usually performed by administering ICG intravenously in a dose of 0.5 ml per kg, and monitoring the blood concentration by means of a non-invasive transcutaneous probe (with diodes emitting in the near infrared 805 and 905 nm wavelength) and photocell sensor. Since 805 nm also comprises an isobestic point at which absorption of oxyhaemoglobin intersects with that of deoxyhaemoglobin, the measurement of ICG is independent of oxygen saturation of the blood. ICG distributes uniformly in the blood within 2–3 min after intravascular injection, and the blood level then falls exponentially for about 20 min thereafter, by which time about 97 % is excreted. Because the physical nature of clearance is a natural exponential function, the measurements can be mathematically interpreted to produce values for: plasma half-life (T1/2), decay and time constants, and hence plasma disappearance rate and derived retention rate.

The exponential decay function of ICG concentration is converted by logarithmic transformation into a straight line to derive a half-life and decay constant (or its inverse, the time constant). The plasma disappearance rate (PDR, which equates to the decay constant of units 1/time) of the dye in the plasma is calculated from: $PDR = \ln 2 / T1/2 * 100 = 0.693 / T1/2 * 100$ and expressed as %/min with normal range between 18 and 25. ICG retention value is conventionally measured after 15 min (ICGR15) and is calculated by measurement of the plasma concentration after 15 min expressed as a ratio of that at time zero (calculated by backwards extrapolation of the transformed decay curve) according to the formula: $ICGR15 = [ICG\ t = 15 min] / [ICG\ t = 0] * 100 (\%)$, with normal range of the order of 0–10 %. An example of a typical ICG clearance test elimination curve is shown in Fig. 7.5.

The ICG test has been shown to be of value in predicting the risk of liver failure and death after hepatic resectional surgery, and is of particular value in patients with liver disease [33, 34]. Discriminant function analysis has shown that an ICG 15 min retention value of 14 % to be a useful predictor of risk, conferring a relative risk of three fold for mortality [35]. Refinements in the estimation of the extent of tolerable parenchymal resection can be made on the basis of ICG testing [36]. ICG testing can be combined with volumetric assessment of parenchymal hepatic resection rate (PHRR, given by Okamoto's formula: PHRR=resected volume−tumor volume/liver volume−tumor volume), and patient age, to produce a predictive score for the likelihood of developing liver failure after hepatectomy [13, 16]. ICG clearance estimation of the future liver remnant has been validated in predicting outcome after resection for biliary cancer [37]. Combined volumetric and functional evaluations of this type have the potential to reduce deaths related to excessive resection in individuals with impaired liver function. Postoperative (remnant liver) recovery of ICG elimination has also been shown to be predictive of the development of complications [38].

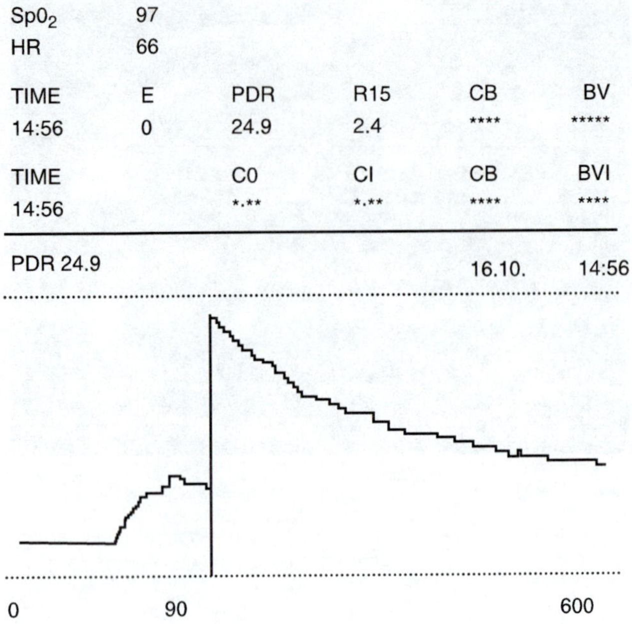

Fig. 7.5 Indocyanine green (ICG) elimination curve in a human subject. The graph shows an exponential decay curve. The derived values are for plasma disappearance rate (PDR)=24.9 %/min and retention value at 15 min (R15)=2.4 %

It is relevant to the management of patients with cholangiocarcinoma that plasma clearance of ICG is diminished in obstructive jaundice, and in this context it is preferable to measure plasma ICG after the relief of biliary obstruction [37, 39]. Alternatively, when external biliary drainage has been employed, measurement of ICG excretion in bile may more accurately reflect underlying liver energy state, and has been shown to correlate more closely with hepatic ATP levels than plasma ICG clearance [40]. An interesting area of ongoing research is in the use of near infrared spectroscopy for direct measurement of ICG clearance from hepatic parenchyma [41].

7.5.2 Microsomal Capacity Tests

These evaluations probe the capacity of the microsomal cytochrome P450 system, and are in essence an assessment of liver cell mass. This system of monooxygenases is responsible for the metabolism of a wide range of xenobiotic (and endobiotic) compounds using enzymatic hydroxylation. For any given compound, R, the reaction catalysed is:

$$R + 0_2 + NADPH + H^+ \rightarrow R\text{-}OH + H_2 0 + NADP$$

A number of test substances can be used for the purposes of testing liver microsomal function, including aminopyrine, caffeine, lidocaine and the lidocaine metabolite monoethylglycinexylidide (MEGX). A significant limitation of these tests is that the enzyme system is inducible by ethanol and influenced by many commonly used drugs, e.g. phenytoin (inductive potentiation) and omeprazole (inhibition).

7.5.2.1 Aminopyrine

The aminopyrine (dimethyl aminoantipyrine) test is the most commonly used, since the progress of metabolic conversion (N-demethylation) can be measured after oral administration by a breath test. The principle of the assay is that a dose of aminopyrine with radioactive (14C) or stable heavy isotope (13C) labelled methyl groups is given. The labelled methyl groups are cleaved by the hydrolytic action of microsomal P450, and subsequently converted to labelled carbon dioxide which is exhaled. The breath may then be analysed by radiation counter or isotope ratio mass spectrometry accordingly, and the result is expressed as percentage of the dose expired in a given time. Despite the potential for confounding outlined above, the aminopyrine breath test has been shown to be a sensitive and quantitative indicator of liver dysfunction, with the ability to stratify surgical risk in patients with liver disease [42]. A composite score, the Liver Resection Index (LRI), has been devised which combines aminopyrine breath test (ABT) with volumetric measures of parenchymal hepatic resection rate (PHRR) and tumor to liver volume ratio to formulate a preoperative risk assessment for fatal post-hepatectomy complications LRI $= ABT(\%) * 100 / PHRR * age(years) * tumour / liver$ volume ratio which has a reported sensitivity of 75 %, specificity of 83 % [43].

7.5.2.2 Lidocaine and MEGX

Lidocaine is a commonly used local anaesthetic and antiarrythmic agent. Lidocaine is metabolised in the liver by the cytochrome P450 pathway, with formation of monoethylglycinexylidide (MEGX). In the setting of chronic liver disease, the hepatic clearance of lidocaine is reduced with prolongation of its half-life. The generation of MEGX (a build-up or positive exponential process) is consequently reduced and it is the determination of this metabolite that forms the quantitative basis of the liver function test. Clinical studies indicate that this test is of value in assessing the likelihood of development of complications for cirrhotic patients undergoing liver resection [44].

7.5.3 Hexose Sugar Metabolic Capacity

Handling and metabolism of hexose sugars (glucose, galactose and fructose) by the liver involves energy dependent processes. Dynamic liver function tests using galactose and fructose have been described, together with the effect of glucose loading on ketone body ratio.

7.5.3.1 Galactose Elimination Capacity

The rate-limiting step in the metabolism of galactose within the liver is that catalysed by galactokinase which phosphorylates galactose to galactose-1-phosphate. The reaction is an energy dependent one, consuming ATP, and the phosphorylated galactose is then converted to glucose which is then oxidised in the standard way. The test is performed by administering galactose and then monitoring serial blood levels, or alternatively by a breath test which measures conversion of either radioactive 14C or mass spectrometric detection of 13C, in expired carbon dioxide. The test has been shown to predict complications and survival after hepatic resection [45].

7.5.3.2 Glucose Load: Redox Tolerance Test

The redox tolerance test quantifies the potentiation of hepatic mitochondrial energy metabolism (measured by arterial ketone body ratio, AKBR) in response to an oral glucose loading. The redox tolerance index is derived from the change in ketone body ratio as a function of change in blood glucose level: the lower the index the higher postoperative morbidity and mortality associated with major hepatic resections [21].

7.5.3.3 Fructose Tolerance Test

Fructose is phosphorylated in the liver by fructokinase, a reaction which consumes ATP. A bolus dose of fructose can deplete the liver of inorganic phosphate by trapping within fructose-1-phopshate and thereby limiting the regeneration of ATP from ADP within the cell. These changes can be followed by 31-phosphorus magnetic resonance spectroscopy which can measure the accumulation of fructose-1-phosphate, depletion of inorganic phosphate and decline in ATP levels [46]. When the liver is diseased, a reduced rate of fructose-1-phosphate formation is found following fructose loading, which may be explained by impaired fructose delivery to, transport into and handling by hepatocytes. These findings are of interest in view of the non-invasive way in which detailed bioenergetic information is obtained. However, the theoretical risk of precipitating lactic acidosis

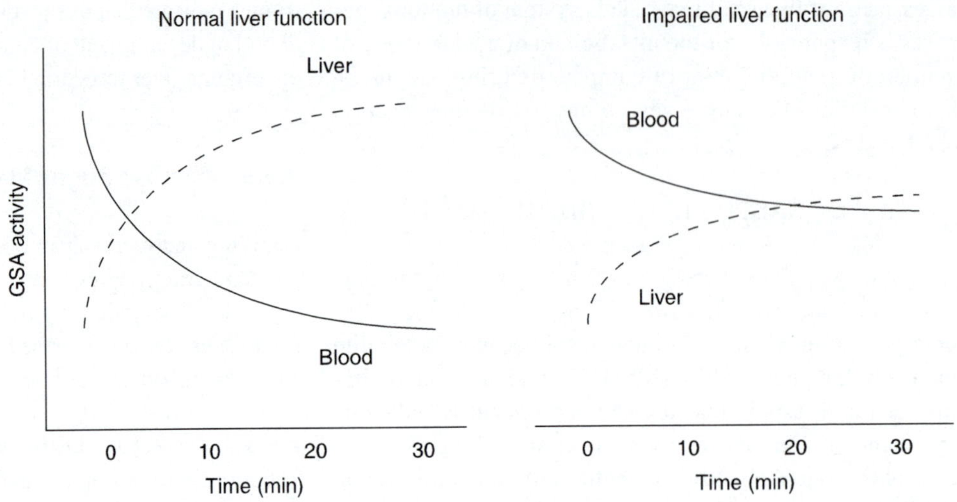

Fig. 7.6 Schematic 99m-Tc-GSA dynamic scintigraphy curves showing disappearance from blood (heart trace) and accumulation in liver. The effect of liver impairment is evidenced by inefficient plasma clearance and hepatic uptake of the tracer

warrants caution in the application of such tests outside of carefully controlled environments.

7.5.4 Hepatobiliary Uptake and Excretion Scintigraphy

7.5.4.1 Iminodiacetic Acid

Isotope-labelled organic anions such as 99m technetium-iminodiacetic acid (IDA) permit simultaneous evaluation of total and regional hepatocyte uptake (cell mass estimate) as well as excretory kinetics (functional evaluation). The biliary excretion mechanism is common to that of the energy-dependent organic anion transporter system, and hence the findings of dynamic testing correlate with those of indocyanine green clearance studies [47].

7.5.4.2 Asialoglycoprotein Receptor Scintigraphy

Naturally occurring asialoglycoproteins (ASGP), for example ceruloplasmin, are removed from the circulation by a mechanism that involves adherence to specific receptors in the sinusoidal membrane of hepatocytes (asialoglycoprotein receptor, ASGPR). When the liver is diseased the number of such receptors is reduced which is associated with accumulation of the glycoprotein in the blood. A manufactured scintigraphy agent which binds to ASGPR on hepatocytes, technetium-99m-galactosyl-human serum albumin (99mTc-GSA) can be used to probe the dynamics of clearance from blood, hepatic uptake and overall receptor complement. Schematic scintigraphs are shown in Fig. 7.6. Using a radiopharmacokinetic model, hepatic uptake and blood disappearance rates can be measured, and a quantitative index for receptor binding (typically indexed at 15 min) obtained [48, 49]. This value has been shown to be useful for the prediction of liver failure in high-risk patients. The technique is of interest because it is mechanistically distinct from other measures of liver function such as organic anion, hexose-sugar or microsomal-based clearance tests, and appears to more accurately reflect histological findings. Preoperative regional maximal removal rate of 99mTc-GSA in the predicted residual liver after hepatectomy has been proposed as a useful test for judging the safety and extent of liver resection [50].

7.5.5 Regenerative Capacity: Portal Vein Embolization

When a tumour is technically suitable for resection but there are concerns about the adequacy of residual hepatic parenchyma (and its functional reserve), one possibility that may be considered is portal vein embolization. Typical indications for portal vein embolization are when predicted remnant liver volume is 25 % or less of total liver volume for normal liver, and 40 % or less when liver function is compromised [51]. The principle of the technique is that when one lobe of the liver is deprived of portal blood flow it undergoes relative atrophy, and a hypertrophic (regenerative) compensatory response is induced within the contra-lateral lobe. In essence this represents a therapeutic trial of regenerative potential: if the hypertrophic response is adequate then formal resectional surgery may be entertained. However if the augmentation of hepatic cell mass is deficient, surgery would likely result in decompensation of an inadequate liver remnant with failure of regeneration. In this sense, the response to portal vein embolization can be considered as a dynamic test of liver function.

The growth of the non-embolized lobe is usually monitored by serial computed tomographic volumetry. In the commonest application, a right portal vein will be embolized to produce left lobe hypertrophy. The average growth of non-embolized tissue that can be anticipated is of the order of 30 %, with mean increase of the order of 10–15 % in total liver volume.

In addition to volumetric measurement (which is a surrogate for liver cell mass), the functional response of the non-embolized lobe can also be assessed. After a successful regenerative response, biliary excretion of indocyanine green by the non-embolized lobe is increased and energy charge is maintained within normal limits [52, 53]. Compensatory accrual of asialoglycoprotein receptor complement can also be monitored in the non-embolized regenerative lobe [54].

7.6 Longitudinal Evaluation After Hepatectomy

An accurate appraisal of liver status is important for the identification of individuals most at risk of developing liver failure after resectional surgery. Recovery from hepatectomy requires a metabolic compromise between differentiated function and parenchymal regrowth, and the likelihood of liver failure ensuing is determined by complex interplay involving liver-specific and general clinical parameters. Liver-specific factors include the current state of liver physiology and reserve, the presence and degree of underlying liver disease (and inherent regenerative potential), the magnitude of parenchymal resection and the size of the remnant liver (and its viability) [1].

Post-operative liver failure has not been uniformly defined, but clinical features include jaundice, ascites, hepatorenal syndrome and onset of encephalopathy. Derangements in commonly used biochemical tests, plasma proteins and coagulation profiles are characteristic, but there is no consensus on when these constitute liver failure, and moreover similar patterns (albeit with less extreme deviations) are noted after liver resection when the recovery proves to be uneventful. Clinical and laboratory experience has shown that events pivoting around the fifth post-operative day are of predictive value for eventual outcome [55, 56]. It is apposite to question what is happening to hepatocytes at this critical time after liver resection, and what types of measurement can inform interpretations and therapeutic decision making.

Preservation of liver function after resection requires that the remaining hepatocytes meet the inherited demands of baseline-differentiated activity. The average cellular workload will however be increased in direct proportion to the number of liver cells lost. Moreover, the remnant liver is also required to host an acute phase reaction characterized by a major redirection of protein synthesis designed to restore bodily equilibrium. The metabolic burden on hepatocytes is increased further by widespread mitosis to replenish lost cell mass. Indirect measures of cell cycling in humans have confirmed the regenerative process to be maximal 4–5 days after hepatectomy [57].

At the hepatocyte level, the metabolic kinetics underlying these events can be studied in a number of direct and indirect

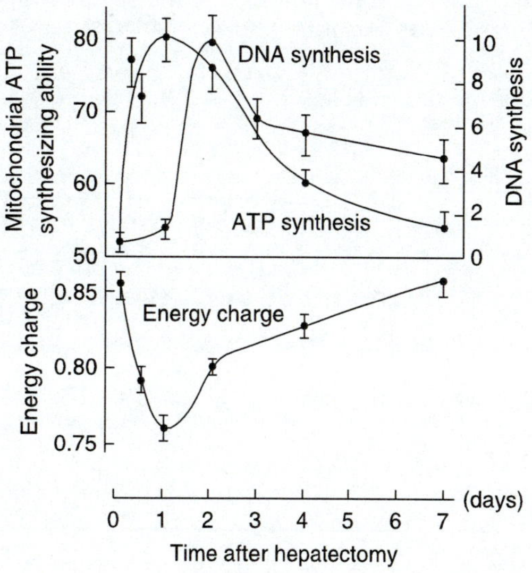

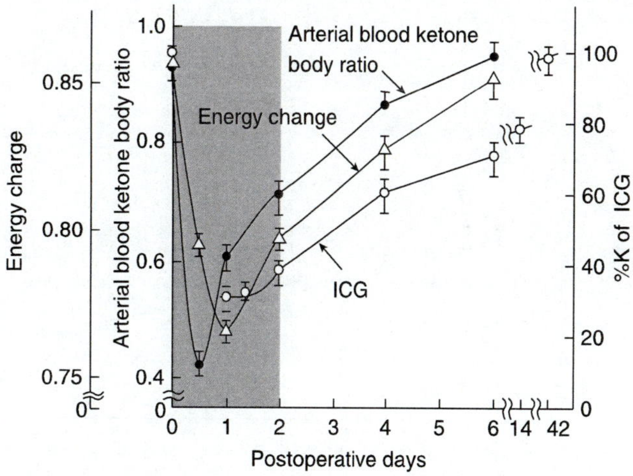

Fig. 7.7 Serial changes in ATP production, energy charge, DNA synthesis, ketone body ratio and ICG clearance after hepatectomy (Adapted and reproduced after Ozawa [62])

ways according to the techniques discussed earlier. Liver regeneration following hepatic resection is associated with a decline in cellular energy charge (with a compensatory increase in net hepatocyte ATP production) which produces a fall in both ketone body ratio and ICG clearance, and these changes normalise when volume recovery is complete [20, 58–61]. Figure 7.7 illustrates the time course of these events. Development of liver failure is reflected in increasing derangements of metabolic indices and can be shown by serial measurement of ketone body ratio and ICG elimination rates [22, 63].

In the modern clinical arena, 31-P MRS can be used for the non-invasive study of hepatic metabolism and regeneration after liver resection [28]. In one such study, the Fig. 7.8 shows that in the remnant normal liver, metabolic balance appears to be initially achieved by diverting energy away

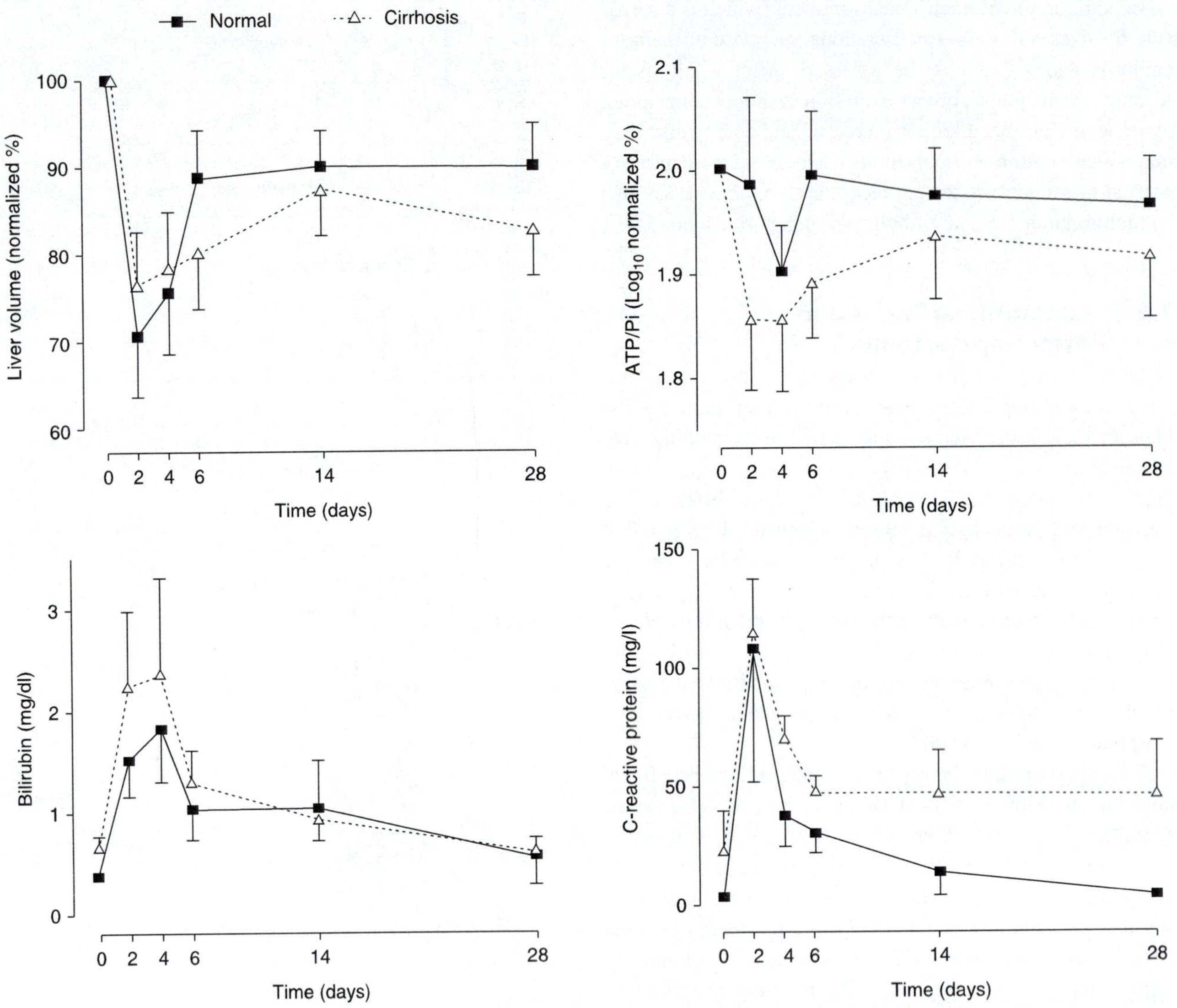

Fig. 7.8 Changes in liver volume (by MRI), energy state (ATP/Pi by 31-P MRS), function (bilirubin level) and acute phase reaction (C-reactive protein) after liver resection; comparison of normal and cirrhotic livers (data are mean ± SE; n=9 in each group) (Reproduced after Mann et al.)

from quiescent hepatic functions (such as bilirubin excretion) whilst also rechanneling resources for acute phase requirements. During the maximal growth phase between the fourth and sixth days after hepatectomy, energy expenditure exceeds ATP availability, inducing a decline in energy state. Accordingly, derangements in differentiated function tend to reach their extremes at this time when energy charge is at its nadir, around the fourth post-operative day. As organ regrowth progresses, the distribution of cellular metabolic load becomes more equitable so that energy balance and organ function are restored. This pattern of recovery is disturbed when the liver is diseased. In the cirrhotic liver the early demands of inherited workload and stress reaction are not matched by compensatory changes in energy usage and supply, and a sustained fall in energy state occurs, evident in greater degree of dysfunction. The regenerative response is retarded (most volume regain occurring between the sixth and fourteenth days) and incomplete, because the depressed energy state restricts protein and nucleic acid synthesis.

How can these findings explain the mechanisms of metabolic control and maintenance of hepatic function during liver regeneration, and can they be used to predict the development of post-resectional liver failure? A useful analogy here is the concept of a liver energy economy, which is comprised of the sum and distribution of reactions for energy-generation and energy-consumption. The metabolic demands on the remaining hepatocytes after liver resection can be apportioned into three vectors: (a) maintenance of differentiated function; (b) acute phase reaction and (c) cellular regeneration. These synchronous competing factors can be combined to produce a representation of hepatic energy economy after partial hepatectomy (Fig. 7.9). Successful

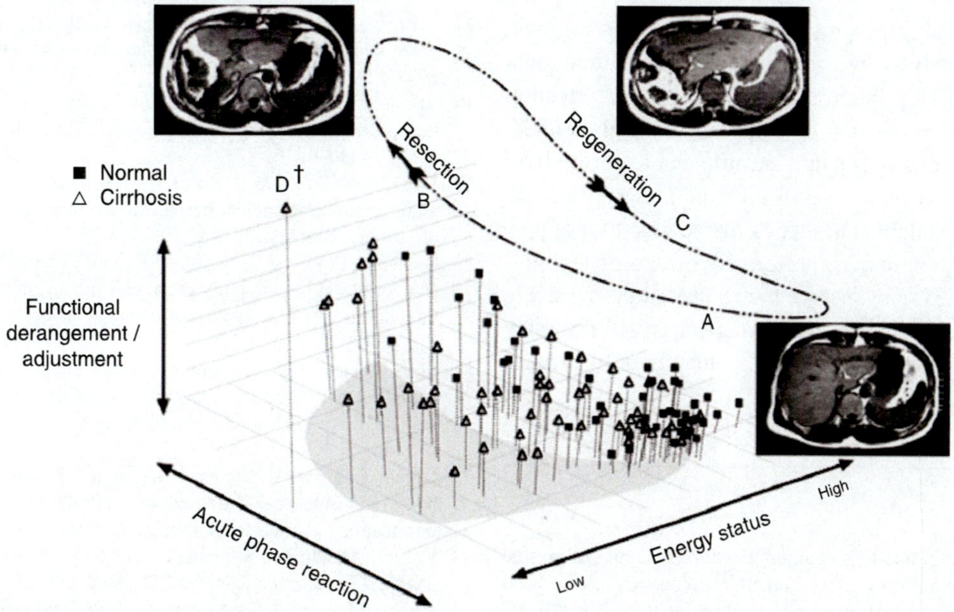

Fig. 7.9 Hepatic energy economy after partial hepatectomy. Three dimensional plot for patients undergoing hepatectomy with normal and cirrhotic livers. *A* Starting conditions. *B* Resection: liver cell mass is lost and acute phase reaction (x-axis) is initiated; DNA synthesis in preparation for mitosis follows. This condition is associated with a fall in energy state (z-axis) and compensatory adjustment (permissible derangement) in differentiated function (which for example could be prothrombin time prolongation on the y-axis). *C* Regeneration: recovery of liver cell mass and restitution of energy balance and functional status occurs within the framework of the integrated response loop shown here for survivors. The trajectory coordinates for cirrhotic liver (*darker shading*) are more extreme, indicating greater departure from equilibrium and strain on homeostatic recovery mechanisms when the organ is diseased. *D* Departure of an individual from these physiologic boundaries, as a result of inadequate energy production, will result in decompensation of liver function and failure of the organ. This is evident from the coordinates of a patient who died of post-operative liver failure

regeneration of human liver after partial hepatectomy involves modulation of hepatic energy economy in response to changing work demands. The efficiency of this process is influenced by the histopathologic state of the organ, and in turn governs physiologic reserve. Functional derangements after hepatectomy can therefore be regarded as adjustments according to energy status: these may occur within permitted limits, but if energy deficit is excessive then progression to liver failure ensues. The mechanism and timing of post-hepatectomy liver failure can be conceptually explained by an inability to maintain organ energy balance during recovery. This concept can also account for the well known clinical phenomenon of post-operative sepsis precipitating liver failure after hepatectomy [16]. In this instance, the infection induces a second-hit acute phase stress on the liver, which if it occurs at or around the critical regenerative growth spurt may be sufficient to induce metabolic decompensation. This framework can also be used to interpret the therapeutic role of portal vein embolization: in this case, the metabolic burden of regeneration is selectively dissociated from the demands of acute phase reaction, allowing a temporal separation (staging) of the metabolic load such that a critical threshold of energy-balance is not exceeded, and thereby stewarding successful recovery [64]. Pre-growing the remnant liver levers bioenergetic advantage over postoperative regrowth. With these insights in mind, organ monitoring based on intracellular metabolism after hepatectomy has the potential to provide for the early detection of impending liver failure, and has potential to guide the development and application of novel hepatic support strategies [65].

7.7 Summary and Synthesis

In general, clinical evaluation and standard liver blood tests, combined in a clinico-laboratory scoring system (usually Child-Pugh), provide a reliable means of gauging hepatic function and its reserve. Despite the biologic complexity of liver function, clinicians are able to identify healthy status and to discriminate between well-, moderately- and poorly-compensated liver disease with considerable accuracy using this assessment. Additional testing is usually performed when liver function is judged borderline (or potentially so), or when a major resection is under consideration in an otherwise apparently normal liver. The most useful supportive information is derived from computed tomography volumetric estimation of the anticipated magnitude of loss of hepatocyte cell mass and the size of the liver remnant. Dynamic testing of some component of performance such as substance-clearance (most popularly ICG) or receptor uptake (commonly by asialoglycoprotein scintigraphy) can augment the volumetric analysis by adding a quantitative functional dimension. In this way the stratification of risk and selection and timing of therapeutic options can be increasingly refined. When functional reserve is judged insufficient to permit liver resection, and this would otherwise be the preferred course of action, then in suitable instances a therapeutic trial of portal vein embolization may be performed. Emerging technologies that measure organ-specific metabolism non-invasively such as magnetic resonance spectroscopy are poised to play an increasingly important role in the evaluation of liver function in the future.

References

1. Yamanaka N, Okamoto E, Kawamura E, et al. Dynamics of normal and injured human liver regeneration after hepatectomy as assessed on the basis of computed tomography and liver function. Hepatology. 1993;18:79–85.
2. Yokoyama Y, Nagino M, Nimura Y. Mechanism of impaired hepatic regeneration in cholestatic liver. J Hepatobiliary Pancreat Surg. 2007;14:159–66.
3. Schroeder R, Marroquin C, Bute B, et al. Predictive indices of morbidity and mortality after liver resection. Ann Surg. 2006;243:373–9.
4. Sitzmann J, Greene P. Perioperative predictors of morbidity following hepatic resection for neoplasm. Ann Surg. 1994;219:13–7.
5. Noun R, Jagot P, Farges O, et al. High preoperative serum alanine transferase levels: effect on the risk of liver resection in child grade A cirrhotic patients. World J Surg. 1997;21:390–5.
6. Didolkar M, Fitzpatrick L, Elias G, et al. Risk factors before hepatectomy, hepatic function after hepatectomy and computed tomographic changes as indicators of mortality from hepatic failure. Surg Gynecol Obstet. 1989;169:17–26.
7. Pugh R, Murray-Lyon I, Dawson J, et al. Transection of the oesophagus for bleeding oesphageal varices. Br J Surg. 1973;60:646–9.
8. Franco D, Capussotti L, Smadja C, et al. Resection of hepatocellular carcinomas. Gastroenterology. 1990;98:733–8.
9. Nonami T, Harada A, Kurokawa T, et al. Hepatic resection for hepatocellular carcinoma. Am J Surg. 1997;173:288–91.
10. Vauthey J, Klimstra D, Franceschi D, et al. Factors affecting long-term outcome after hepatic resection for hepatocellular carcinoma. Am J Surg. 1995;169:28–35.
11. Freeman R, Wiesner R, Roberts J, et al. Improving liver allocation: MELD and PELD. Am J Transplant. 2004;4:114–31.
12. Cucchetti A, Ercolani G, Vivarelli M, et al. Impact of model for end-stage liver disease (MELD) score on prognosis after hepatectomy for hepatocellular carcinoma on cirrhosis. Liver Transpl. 2006;12:966–71.
13. Okamoto E, Kyo A, Yamanaka N, et al. Prediction of the safe limits of hepatectomy by combined volumetric and functional measurements in patients with impaired hepatic function. Surgery. 1984; 95:586–92.
14. Soyer P, Roche A, Elias D, et al. Hepatic metastases from colorectal cancer: influence of hepatic volumetric analysis on surgical decision making. Radiology. 1992;184:695–7.
15. Belghiti J, Ogata S. Assessment of hepatic reserve for the indication of hepatic resection. J Hepatobiliary Pancreat Surg. 2005; 12:1–3.
16. Yamanaka N, Okamoto E, Oriyama T, et al. A prediction scoring system to select the surgical treatment of liver cancer. Ann Surg. 1994;219:342–6.
17. Behrns K, Tsiotos G, Desouza N, et al. Hepatic steatosis as a potential risk factor for major hepatic resection. J Gastrointest Surg. 1998;2:292–8.
18. Atkinson D. The energy charge of the adenylate pool as a regulatory parameter: interaction with feedback modifiers. Biochemistry. 1968;7:4030–4.
19. Williamson D, Lund P, Krebs H. The redox state of free nicotinamide-adenine dinucleotides in the cytoplasma and mitochondria of rat liver. Biochem J. 1967;103:514–27.
20. Ozawa K, Fujimoto T, Nakatani T, et al. Changes in hepatic energy charge, blood ketone body ratio, and indocyanine green clearance in relation to DNA synthesis after hepatectomy. Life Sci. 1982; 31:647–53.
21. Mori K, Ozawa K, Yamamoto Y, et al. Response of hepatic mitochondrial redox state to oral glucose load: redox tolerance test as a new predictor of surgical risk in hepatectomy. Ann Surg. 1990;211: 438–46.
22. Kiuchi T, Ozawa K, Yamamoto Y, et al. Changes in arterial ketone body ratio in the phase immediately after hepatectomy: prognostic implications. Arch Surg. 1990;125:655–9.
23. Komura M, Chijiwa K, Naito T, et al. Sequential changes of energy charge, lipoperoxide level, and DNA synthesis rate of the liver following biliary obstruction in rats. J Surg Res. 1996;61:503–8.
24. Jikko A, Taki Y, Nakamura N, et al. Adenylate energy charge and cytochrome a(+a3) in the cirrhotic rat liver. J Surg Res. 1984;37: 361–8.
25. Sakai Y, Tanaka A, Ikai I, et al. Cytochrome c oxidase activity in human liver specimens: an index of prognosis for hepatic resection. Arch Surg. 1990;125:632–5.
26. Gadian D. Nuclear magnetic resonance and its applications to living systems. Oxford: Clarendon; 1982.
27. Menon D, Sargentoni J, Taylor-Robinson S, et al. Effect of functional grade and etiology on in vivo hepatic phosphorus-31 magnetic resonance spectroscopy in cirrhosis: biochemical basis of spectral appearances. Hepatology. 1995;21:417–27.
28. Mann D, Lam W, Hjelm N, et al. Metabolic control patterns in acute phase and regenerating human liver determined in vivo by 31-phosphorus magnetic resonance spectroscopy. Ann Surg. 2002; 235:408–16.
29. Mann D, Lam W, Hjelm N, et al. Biliary drainage for obstructive jaundice enhances hepatic energy status in humans: a 31-phosphorus magnetic resonance spectroscopy study. Gut. 2002;50:118–22.
30. Maris J, Evans A, McLaughlin A, et al. 31P nuclear magnetic resonance spectroscopic investigation of human neuroblastoma in situ. N Engl J Med. 1985;312:1500–5.
31. van Wassenaer-van Hall H, van der Grond J, van Hattum J, et al. 31P magnetic resonance spectroscopy of the liver: correlation with standardized serum, clinical, and histological changes in diffuse liver disease. Hepatology. 1995;21:443–9.
32. Jalan R, Sargentoni J, Coutts G, et al. Hepatic phosphorus-31 magnetic resonance spectroscopy in primary biliary cirrhosis and its relation to prognostic models. Gut. 1996;39:141–6.
33. Hemming A, Scudamore C, Shackleton C, et al. Indocyanine green clearance as a predictor of successful hepatic resection in cirrhotic patients. Am J Surg. 1992;163:515–8.
34. Fan S, Lai C, Lo C, et al. Hospital mortality of major hepatectomy for hepatocellular carcinoma associated with cirrhosis. Arch Surg. 1995;130:198–203.
35. Lau H, Man K, Fan S, et al. Evaluation of preoperative hepatic function in patients with hepatocellular carcinoma undergoing hepatectomy. Br J Surg. 1997;84:1255–9.
36. Kawasaki S, Makuuchi M, Miyagawa S, et al. Results of hepatic resection for hepatocellular carcinoma. World J Surg. 1995;19:31–4.
37. Yokoyama Y, Nishio H, Ebata T, et al. Value of indocyanine green clearance of the future liver remnant in predicting outcome after resection for biliary cancer. Br J Surg. 2010;97:1260–8.

38. Matsumata T, Kanematsu T, Yoshida Y, et al. The indocyanine green test enables prediction of postoperative complications after hepatic resection. World J Surg. 1987;11:678–81.
39. Stockmann M, Malinowski M, Lock J, et al. Factors influencing the indocyanine green (ICG) test: additional impact of acute cholestasis. Hepatogastroenterology. 2009;56:734–8.
40. Chijiiwa K, Watanabe M, Nakano K, et al. Biliary indocyanine green excretion as a predictor of hepatic adenosine triphosphate levels in patients with obstructive jaundice. Am J Surg. 2000;179: 161–6.
41. Jiao L, El-Desoky A, Seifalian A, et al. Effect of liver blood flow and function on hepatic indocyanine green clearance measured directly in a cirrhotic animal model. Br J Surg. 2000;87:568–74.
42. Gill R, Goodman M, Golfus G, et al. Aminopyrine breath test predicts surgical risk for patients with liver disease. Ann Surg. 1983;198:701–4.
43. Cohnert T, Rau H, Buttler E, et al. Preoperative risk assessment of hepatic resection for malignant disease. World J Surg. 1997;21: 396–401.
44. Ercolani G, Grazi G, Calliva R, et al. The lidocaine (MEGX) test as an index of hepatic function: its clinical usefulness in liver surgery. Surgery. 2000;127:464–71.
45. Redaelli C, Dufour J, Wagner M, et al. Preoperative galactose elimination capacity predicts complications and survival after hepatic resection. Ann Surg. 2002;235:77–85.
46. Sakuma H, Itabashi K, Takeda K, et al. Serial P-31 MR spectroscopy after fructose infusion in patients with chronic hepatitis. J Magn Reson Imaging. 1991;1:701–4.
47. Bennink R, Dinant S, Erdogan D, et al. Preoperative assessment of postoperative remnant liver function using hepatobiliary scintigraphy. J Nucl Med. 2004;45:965–71.
48. Kwon A-H, Ha-Kawa S, Uetsuji S, et al. Preoperative determination of the surgical procedure for hepatectomy using technetium-99m-galactosyl human serum albumin (99mTc-GSA) liver scintigraphy. Hepatology. 1997;25:426–9.
49. Satoh K, Yamamoto Y, Nishiyama Y, et al. 99mTc-GSA liver dynamic SPECT for the preoperative assessment of hepatectomy. Ann Nucl Med. 2003;17:61–7.
50. Kwon A-H, Matsui Y, Kaibori M, et al. Preoperative regional maximal removal rate of technetium-99m-galactosyl human serum albumin (GSA-Rmax) is useful for judging the safety of hepatic resection. Surgery. 2006;140:379–86.
51. Abdalla E, Hicks M, Vauthey J. Portal vein embolization: rationale, technique and future prospects. Br J Surg. 2001;88:165–75.
52. Uesaka K, Nimura Y, Nagino M. Changes in hepatic lobar function after right portal vein embolization: an appraisal by biliary indocyanine green excretion. Ann Surg. 1996;223:77–83.
53. Chijiiwa K, Saiki S, Noshiro H, et al. Effect of preoperative portal vein embolization on liver volume and hepatic energy status of the nonembolized liver lobe in humans. Eur Surg Res. 2000; 32:94–9.
54. Kubo S, Shiomi S, Tanaka H, et al. Evaluation of the effect of portal vein embolization on liver function by 99mTc-galactosyl human serum albumin scintigraphy. J Surg Res. 2002;107:113–8.
55. Balzan S, Belghiti J, Farges O, et al. The "50-50 Criteria" on postoperative day 5: an accurate predictor of liver failure and death after hepatectomy. Ann Surg. 2005;242:824–9.
56. Cucchetti A, Ercolani G, Cescon M, et al. Recovery from liver failure after hepatectomy for hepatocellular carcinoma in cirrhosis: meaning of the model for end-stage liver disease. J Am Coll Surg. 2006;203:670–6.
57. Francavilla A, Panella C, Polimeno L, et al. Hormonal and enzymatic parameters of hepatic regeneration in patients undergoing major liver resections. Hepatology. 1990;12:1134–8.
58. Ove P, Takai S, Umeda T, et al. Adenosine triphosphate in liver after partial hepatectomy and acute stress. J Biol Chem. 1967; 242:4963–71.
59. Kamiyama Y, Ozawa K, Honjo I. Changes in mitochondrial phosphorylative activity and adenylate energy charge of regenerating rabbit liver. J Biochem. 1976;80:875–81.
60. Rikkers L, Moody F. Estimation of functional hepatic mass in resected and regenerating rat liver. Gastroenterology. 1974;67: 691–9.
61. Okochi O, Kaneko T, Sugimoto H, et al. ICG pulse spectrophotometry for perioperative liver function in hepatectomy. J Surg Res. 2002;103:109–13.
62. Ozawa K. Liver surgery approached through the mitochondria. Tokyo: Medical Tribune; 1992.
63. Sugimoto H, Okochi O, Hirota M, et al. Early detection of liver failure after hepatectomy by indocyanine green elimination rate measured by pulse dye-densitometry. J Hepatobiliary Pancreat Surg. 2006;13:543–8.
64. Mann D, Lam W, Hjelm N, et al. Human liver regeneration: hepatic energy economy is less efficient when the organ is diseased. Hepatology. 2001;34:557–65.
65. Demetriou A, Brown R, Busuttil R, et al. Prospective, randomized, multicenter, controlled trial of a bioartificial liver in treating acute liver failure. Ann Surg. 2004;239:660–70.

8 Diagnosis

X.Y. Yin

The diagnosis of hilar cholangiocarcinoma is suspected clinically, but it is usually made with serum tumor markers and on medical imaging. Cytological and molecular techniques help in the diagnosis of difficult cases.

8.1 Clinical Manifestations

Hilar cholangiocarcinoma is usually asymptomatic, or occasionally associated with non-specific symptoms such as abdominal discomfort, anorexia and even weight loss in the early stage [1]. These symptoms are often vague and neglected, hence it is rarely detected at this stage. As the tumor grows and obstructs the common hepatic duct and/or biliary confluence, jaundice gradually develops. Most patients with hilar cholangiocarcinoma seek medical advice because of jaundice, which is commonly painless, progressive, and is accompanied by pruritus, clay-colored stool and dark urine [2]. Fever is uncommon and is due to acute cholangitis which happens in about 10 % of patients with hilar cholangiocarcinoma [3]. Patients then present with fever, chills and abdominal pain, in addition to jaundice.

Physical examination often reveals hepatomegaly with a firm consistency, but the gallbladder is usually impalpable. An enlarged gallbladder suggests a more distal biliary obstruction rather than at the hepatic hilum. In patients with pruritus, multiple excoriations of skin are frequently found.

In liver function tests, a markedly elevation of serum total bilirubin is usually shown, with the conjugated bilirubin being predominant. Simultaneous elevations of alkaline phosphatase (ALP) and gamma glutamyltransferase (GGT) are frequent [4].

X.Y. Yin, MD, PhD
Department of Hepatobiliary Surgery,
First Affiliated Hospital, Sun Yat-Sen University,
Guangzhou, China
e-mail: yinxy@medmail.com.cn

These clinical manifestations suggest obstructive jaundice. The differential diagnosis for obstructive jaundice is broad, and it includes a long list of hilar cholangiocarcinoma, ampullary carcinoma, duodenal carcinoma, pancreatic carcinoma, gallbladder carcinoma, choledocholithiasis, benign biliary stricture, etc. The presumptive diagnosis of hilar cholangiocarcinoma is usually based on serum tumor markers and medical imaging investigations. Brush cytology or forceps biopsy can offer a definite diagnosis. Its low sensitivity, however, limits its clinical role. Currently, a definitive diagnosis of hilar cholangiocarcinoma before an operation still remains a major challenge.

8.1.1 Serum Tumor Markers

Some serum tumor markers may be helpful in the diagnosis of hilar cholangiocarcinoma. Carbohydrate antigen 19-9 (CA19-9) and carcinoembryonic antigen (CEA) are the most widely used markers. They may be elevated in hilar cholangiocarcinoma, but they are non-specific and inadequately sensitive. CA19-9 and CEA can also be raised in many other malignancies, including gastric carcinoma, colorectal carcinoma, pancreatic carcinoma and gynecological carcinomas. In addition, CA19-9 can be elevated in some benign conditions, like cholangitis, choledocholithiasis and benign biliary stricture [5].

Patel et al. [6] compared the levels of CA19-9 in 36 cholangiocarcinomas without primary sclerosing cholangitis (PSC), 41 non-malignant liver diseases and 26 benign biliary strictures and found that a cutoff value of CA19-9 >100 U/ml had a sensitivity of 53 % for the diagnosis of cholangiocarcinoma, and a true negative rate of 76 % for non-malignant liver diseases and 92 % for benign biliary stricture. Other studies show in patients with PSC, CA19-9 at a cutoff value of >100 U/ml has a sensitivity of 75–89 % and a specificity of 80–86 % for the detection of cholangiocarcinoma [7–9]. A higher cutoff value improves its specificity [10], but impairs its sensitivity. Recently, Juntermanns et al. [11]

W.Y. Lau (ed.), *Hilar Cholangiocarcinoma*,
DOI 10.1007/978-94-007-6473-6_8, © Springer Science+Business Media Dordrecht and People's Medical Publishing House 2013

analyzed retrospectively the CA19-9 level in 136 patients with hilar cholangiocarcinoma, and found that it was closely related to the tumor staging, being 253±561 U/ml for UICC stage I, 742±1,572 U/ml for stage II, 906±1,708 U/ml for stage III and 1,707±3,053 U/ml for stage IV.

CEA alone has an unsatisfactorily low sensitivity and specificity for the diagnosis of cholangiocarcinoma [12]. Koea et al. [5] reported that CEA was elevated in only 2 out of 28 patients with hilar cholangiocarcinoma. Juntermanns et al. [11] found that the CEA level in patients with hilar cholangiocarcinma was related to the tumor staging, being 2.9±3.8 U/ml for UICC stage I, 4.6±6.5 U/ml for stage II, 18.1±29.6 U/ml for stage III and 22.7±53.9 U/ml for stage IV. A combination of CEA and CA19-9 improves the capability to detect cholangiocarcinoma. Siqueira and his associates reported that CEA>5.2 ng/mL in combination with CA19-9>180 U/ml had a sensitivity of 100 % and a specificity of 78.4 % for the detection of cholangiocarcinoma in patients with PSC [13].

New markers, such as the human mucin subtypes A and C (mucin-5AC), trypsinogen and soluble fragment of cytokeratin 19, are now being investigated [14]. Bamrungphon et al. reported that mucin-5AC at a cutoff value of 0.074 had a sensitivity of 71 % and a specificity of 90 % for the diagnosis of cholangiocarcinoma [15]. The diagnostic values of these new markers still need to wait for large-scale clinical trials to assess.

8.1.2 Imaging Investigations

Imaging investigations play an essential role in the diagnosis and management of hilar cholangiocarcinoma. The commonly used imaging modalities include ultrasound, computed tomography (CT), magnetic resonance imaging (MRI)/ magnetic resonance cholangiopancreatography (MRCP), direct cholangiographies and positron emission tomography (PET).

8.1.3 Ultrasound

The widespread availability, convenience and low cost have made duplex ultrasound (DUS) of liver, biliary system and pancreas to be the most common first-step imaging study for patients with jaundice. DUS provides valuable diagnostic clues for hilar cholangiocarcinoma: firstly, DUS is sensitive and accurate in identifying biliary dilatation. Based on the distribution of biliary dilatation, the location of biliary obstruction can be precisely defined. Dilatation of intrahepatic bile ducts alone indicates a proximal biliary obstruction, and dilatation of both intra-hepatic and extra-hepatic bile ducts indicates a distal biliary obstruction. In a series of 429 patients with obstructive jaundice, the sensitivity and specificity of DUS in defining the location of biliary obstruction were 94 and 96 %, respectively [16].

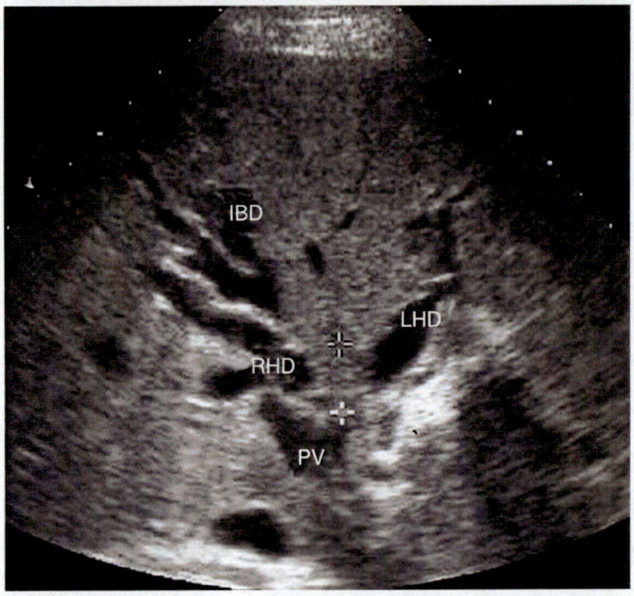

Fig. 8.1 A 49-year-old male with a hilar cholangiocarcinoma. Ultrasound examination reveals a mass inside the hepatic duct confluence (T) with dilatation of the intrahepatic bile ducts (*IBD*). Both the right hepatic duct (*RHD*) and the left hepatic duct (*LHD*) are not involved by the tumor, and the portal vein (*PV*) has an intact wall. The imaging features suggest a Bismuth-Corlett type II hilar cholangiocarcinoma

In the identification of etiology of the obstructive jaundice, DUS may directly show the bile duct tumor and its extention (Fig. 8.1). Hann et al. [17] reported in 39 patients with hilar cholangiocarcinoma, DUS detected bile duct tumors in 87 % of patients: as intra-ductal polypoid masses in 18 %, infiltrative lesions in 26 % and nodular mural thickening in 56 %. At the same time, it correctly evaluated the tumor extension in the bile duct in 87 %. Recently, contrast-enhanced ultrasound (CEUS) has been used in the diagnosis of hilar cholangiocarcinoma. The enhancement patterns of lesions are useful for the diagnosis and differential diagnosis of cholangiocarcinoma. In 30 patients with hilar cholangiocarcinoma, CEUS made a correct diagnosis in 93.8 % [18]. More large-scale clinical trials are still needed to assess its true role in the diagnosis of hilar cholangiocarcinoma.

Furthermore, DUS can accurately assess the status of the portal vein. In the study by Hann et al. [17], DUS correctly predicted the involvement of portal veins in 86 % of the 21 portal veins which were invaded by tumor in 16 patients. In another study, Bach et al. compared the accuracy of DUS and angiography combined with CT during arterial portography (CTAP) for the evaluation of portal vein involvement by tumor. The results showed that DUS detected 38 of 41 involved portal veins in 63 patients who received hepatectomy, with a sensitivity of 93 %, specificity of 99 %, positive predictive value of 97 % and negative predictive value of 98 %. The results were similar to those obtained by angiography combined with CTAP [19].

The role of DUS in the diagnosis of hilar cholangiocarcinoma has been well established. However, its sensitivity, specificity and accuracy are operator-dependent. Hence, other imaging investigations are usually needed following ultrasound examination.

8.1.4 Computed Tomography (CT)

Triple-phase CT scanning plays an important role in the diagnosis and staging of hilar cholangiocarcinoma, since it can provide information regarding to the location of the biliary obstruction, tumor extension along the bile duct axis, vascular invasion, hepatic lobar atrophy, lymph node involvement and distant metastases. Its accuracy has been remarkably improved with the application of high-resolution multidetector-row CT scanners.

On Triple-phase CT scanning, hilar cholangiocarcinoma appears as an hyperattenuating intra-ductal mass, focal mural thickening or lumen obliteration at the hilar bile duct with dilatation of the intra-hepatic bile ducts (Fig. 8.2). The sensitivity of triple-phase CT for the diagnosis of hilar cholangiocarcinoma reaches up to 90–100 % [4], with an accuracy of 92.3–95 % [20, 21]. However, it has a tendency to underestimate the horizontal extension of tumor along the bile duct axis, with an accuracy of 77–80.9 % [21, 22].

CT is accurate in assessing the status of the portal vein and hepatic artery (Fig. 8.2). In 18 patients with hilar

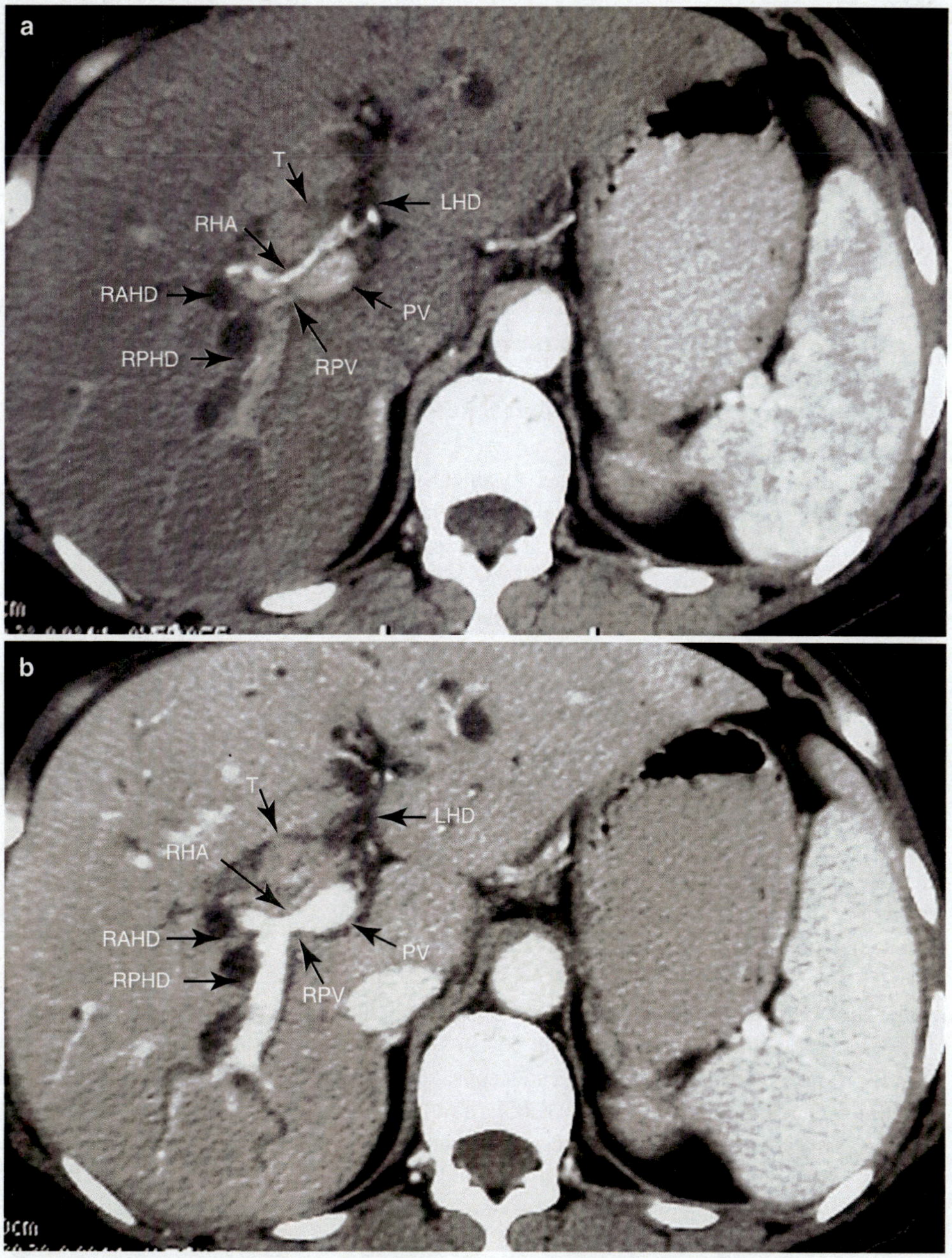

Fig. 8.2 A 56-year-old female with hilar cholangiocarcinoma. Triple-phase CT scanning shows a contrast-enhanced mass (*T*) inside the hepatic duct confluence at the arterial phase (**a**). The tumor presents with washout at the portal phase (**b**). The right hepatic duct is invaded by the tumor up to the confluence of the right anterior sectoral duct (*RAHD*) and right posterior sectoral duct (*RPHD*), and the left hepatic duct (*LHD*) remains intact (**a** and **b**). Part of the wall of the right hepatic artery (*RHA*) is not clear (as shown by an *arrow* in **a**), and the right portal vein (*RPV*) is markedly stenotic (as shown by an *arrow* in **b**), suggesting that both of these vessels have been invaded by the tumor. *PV* portal vein

cholangiocarcinoma, it correctly detected portal vein involvement in 47 of 51 invaded portal veins, with a sensitivity of 92.3 % and a specificity of 90.2 %. Its sensitivity and specificity for the detection of hepatic artery involvement were 100 and 90 %, respectively [23]. In another study involving 55 patients with hilar cholangiocarcinoma, CT had an accuracy of 85.5 % in detecting portal vein invasion and 92.7 % in detecting hepatic artery invasion [24].

Additionally, CT is useful in detecting hepatic lobar atrophy, lymph node involvement and distant metastases. Atrophy of one liver lobe is usually accompanied with hypertrophy of the contra-lateral lobe. This condition presents in hilar cholangiocarcinoma when the tumor invades one portal branch and causes atrophy of the ipsilateral liver lobe. Compensatory hypertrophy causes the contra-lateral liver lobe to enlarge. In the detection of lymph node involvement, CT has a sensitivity of 35–63 % [21, 25] and a specificity of 75–95 % [21, 24]. CT is also useful in detecting distant metastases, such as liver metastases and peritoneal metastases, but it is not sensitive enough to detect sub-centimeter metastatic lesions.

Overall, the resectability of hilar cholangiocarcinoma as assessed by preoperative CT has a sensitivity of 94–100 %, a specificity of 48–79 %, and an accuracy of 60–88 % [26].

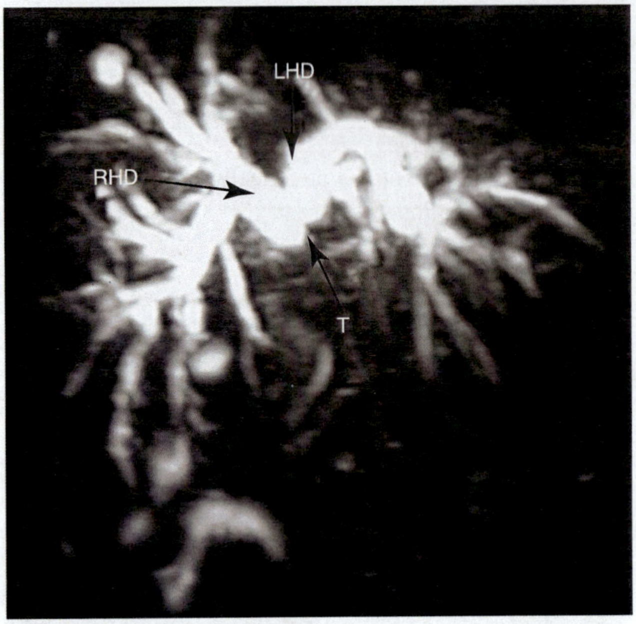

Fig. 8.3 A 50-year-old female with a hilar cholangiocarcinoma. MRCP shows a complete biliary obstruction at the confluence of the hepatic ducts (*T*), but both the right hepatic duct (*RHD*) and the left hepatic duct (*LHD*) are intact. The features suggest a Bismuth-Corlett type II hilar cholangiocarcinoma

8.1.5 Magnetic Resonance Imaging (MRI)/Magnetic Resonance Cholangiopancreatography (MRCP)

MRI combined with MRCP is another excellent imaging modality for the diagnosis and staging of hilar cholangiocarcinoma. Like CT scanning, MRI/MRCP provides reliable information regarding the level of biliary obstruction, extent of biliary ductal involvement, vascular invasion, hepatic lobar atrophy, lymph node involvement and distant metastases.

MRI has an accuracy of 66 % for the detection of lymph node involvement [27], a sensitivity of 78 % and a specificity of 91 % for portal vein involvement, a sensitivity of 58–73 % [28] and a specificity of 93 % for hepatic arterial involvement [29]. In addition, MRCP offers a two-dimensional or three-dimensional reconstruction of the entire biliary tree, which is valuable for precisely defining the longitudinal tumor extension within the bile duct (Fig. 8.3). The accuracy of MRCP in defining the extent of biliary ductal involvement in hilar cholangiocarcinoma reaches 71–96 % [25]. Compared with direct cholangiographies, including percutaneous transhepatic cholangiography (PTC) and endoscopic retrograde cholangiopancreatography (ERCP), MRCP has a similar diagnostic accuracy in hilar cholangiocarcinoma but with the advantages of non-invasiveness, convenience and no risk of procedure-related cholangitis [4].

Park et al. [30] compared MRI/MRCP versus CT with direct cholangiographies in the evaluation of 27 patients with bile duct cancer. The accuracies of MRI/MRCP or CT with direct cholangiography were 90.7 % vs. 85.1 % in defining the involvement of bilateral secondary biliary confluence, and 87 % vs. 87 % in defining the involvement of intra-pancreatic common bile duct. Both had a similar accuracy in assessing vascular invasion and lymph node metastases.

Overall, MRI/MRCP has been extensively used in the diagnosis and staging of hilar cholangiocarcinoma, with an accuracy of 72–83 % in predicting its resectability [26].

8.1.6 Direct Cholangiographies

PTC and ERCP are the two commonly used direct cholangiographies carried out by direct injection of contrast media into the biliary system. Both provide a clear delineation of the biliary tree and demonstrate precisely the location and extent of biliary obstruction. An abrupt, irregular and eccentric biliary stenosis with proportional dilatation of the proximal biliary tree usually implies malignancy (Fig. 8.4). The sensitivity, specificity and accuracy of ERCP/PTC for the diagnosis of malignant biliary obstruction are 58–85 % [31–33], 70–75 % and 72–81 % [32, 33], respectively. Compared with ERCP, PTC is more reliable to demonstrate the complex intrahepatic biliary tree in patients with hilar

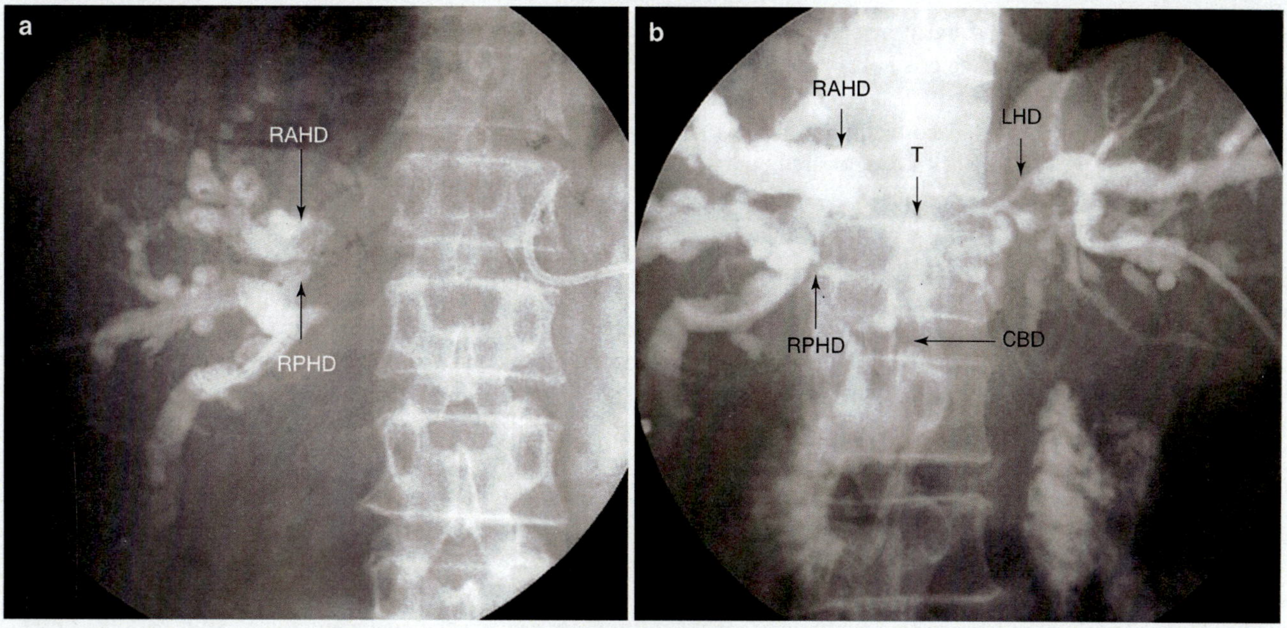

Fig. 8.4 A 60-year-old male with a hilar cholangiocarcinoma. Right PTC only delineated dilatation of the right anterior sectoral ducts (*RAHD*) and the right posterior sectoral duct (*RPHD*) with no visualization of the right hepatic duct (**a**). Subsequent left PTC shows dilatation of the left intrahepatic bile ducts with visualization of part of the left hepatic duct (*LHD*) and the common bile duct (*CBD*) (**b**). The features suggest the biliary obstruction (*T*) to involve the right hepatic duct, the hepatic confluence and part of the LHD (**b**)

cholangiocarcinoma, which is a pivotal factor for surgical planning. Hence, PTC is preferred than ERCP in most centers [34].

One limitation of ERCP/PTC is their failure to display the full biliary tree in some patients with complete biliary obstruction. In such cases, PTC can only display the proximal intrahepatic biliary tree but not the distal biliary system. On the contrary, ERCP can only depict the distal biliary system but not the proximal intraheptic biliary tree. Neither can accurately assess the full extent of biliary involvement under such circumstances.

Another limitation is that they are invasive procedures and have their risks of associated complications, which include bile leakage, cholangitis, bleeding, pancreatitis and duodenal perforation [4, 12]. The PTC-related mortality ranges between 0.6 and 5.6 % [12].

Because of these limitations, ERCP/PTC has largely been replaced by MRCP in many centers [1]. However, ERCP/PTC has potential advantages. They can be used therapeutically for biliary drainage as well as for the collection of bile for cytological and molecular analysis.

8.1.7 Positron Emission Tomography (PET)

Positron emission tomography, using the radionucleotide tracer 18-fluorodeoxyglucose (FDG-PET), has been evaluated for the diagnosis and staging of hilar cholangiocarcinoma. An intensive focal accumulation of FDG at the hepatic hilum suggests hilar cholangiocarcinoma, but sometimes it is difficult to distinguish between malignancy from chronic biliary inflammation.

Preliminary studies show that the sensitivity of FDG-PET in the detection of hilar cholangiocarcinoma ranges between 59 and 100 % [35–38], with an accuracy of 67–100 % [35, 38]. FDG-PET shows no superiority to conventional triple-phase CT scanning in the detection of primary lesion of hilar cholangiocarcinoma [36]. FDG-PET is disappointing in identifying lymph node metastases, with a sensitivity between 13 and 42 % [36, 39, 40]. However, FDG-PET has been shown to be a promising modality to detect occult distant metastases. It is more accurate than conventional CT to identify distant metastases, with a sensitivity between 56 and 100 % [36, 40], and a specificity of 88 % [36]. FDG-PET leads to a change in the management in 17–24 % patients with cholangiocarcinoma [35, 40, 41]. More large-scale clinical trials are needed to evaluate the role of FDG-PET in the diagnosis and staging of hilar cholangiocarcinoma.

8.2 Cytological and Molecular Diagnosis

8.2.1 Brush Cytology and Forceps Biopsy

Currently the diagnosis of hilar cholangiocarcinoma is primarily based on imagings. The imaging-orientated diagnosis for hilar cholangiocarcinoma has some limitations. Sometimes it is difficult for imagings to discriminate a malignant biliary stricture from a benign one when the imaging features are not characteristic. Moreover, even in patients with characteristic imaging features the diagnosis is only presumptive and not always correct [5, 42]. Hence, the imaging-based diagnosis for hilar cholangiocarcinoma is not adequate. To achieve a definite diagnosis of hilar cholangiocarcinoma, although clinically important, remains a major challenge.

Brush cytology and forceps biopsy via ERCP or PTC are the two most commonly used techniques to provide a definite diagnosis of hilar cholangiocarcinoma. Compared with forceps biopsy, brush cytology is less technically-demanding, less time-consuming and safer, and hence it is applied more widely. The detection of malignant cells in tissue specimens is diagnostic for malignancy. However, both brush cytology and forceps biopsy have a low sensitivity for diagnosing hilar cholangiocarcinoma since the tumor is usually abundant in fibrous stroma with only few cancerous cells [43]. The sensitivity of brush cytology and forceps biopsy for cancer detection in malignant biliary strictures ranges from 9 to 60 %, and 43 to 81 %, respectively [12, 44]. For hilar cholangiocarcinoma, the diagnostic sensitivity is between 41 and 50 % for brush cytology [42, 45], and 53 % for forceps biopsy [45]. A combination of brush cytology and forceps biopsy improves the diagnostic sensitivity to 60 % [45].

8.2.2 Endoscopic Ultrasonography-Guided Fine Needle Aspiration (EUS-Guided FNA)

In patients with a negative brush cytology and forceps biopsy, EUS-guided FNA is an alternative technique to provide a definite diagnosis of hilar cholangiocarcinoma. Good results have been reported in two small series of proximal biliary stricture, with a sensitivity of 77–89 % and a specificity of 100 %, for the detection of hilar cholangiocarcinoma [46, 47]. However, its negative predictive value was only 29 % [47]. This implies that a negative EUS-FNA does not necessarily exclude the possibility of hilar cholangiocarcinoma. EUS-guided FNA has other limitations that are technically demanding, and it is only feasible in patients with a focal mass or else its sensitivity sharply declines.

8.2.3 Fluorescence In Situ Hybridization (FISH) and Digitized Image Analysis (DIA)

Recently, sophisticated cytological techniques, including FISH and DIA, have been used to improve the sensitivity of brush cytology in cancer detection for malignant biliary strictures. FISH assay detects malignant cells by using fluorescent probes to identify chromosomal polysomy, and DIA detects malignant cells by using special stains to quantitate nuclear DNA and to identify aneuploidy [4]. Kipp et al. [48] compared the sensitivity and specificity of FISH and routine brush cytology for the detection of malignancy in 131 patients with biliary strictures, including 66 malignant and 65 benign biliary strictures. Compared with routine brush cytology, FISH markedly improved the sensitivity from 15 to 34 %. There was no significant difference in the specificity between FISH and routine brush cytology, being 91 % vs. 98 %, respectively. In another prospective study consisting of 100 patients with biliary stirctures, including 56 malignant and 44 benign biliary strictures, the sensitivity and specificity of DIA and routine brush cytology for the detection of malignancy were compared. DIA significantly improved the sensitivity from 18 to 39 %, but it simultaneously impaired the specificity from 98 to 77 % when compared with routine brush cytology [49]. However, these two studies were conducted on heterogeneous bilio-pancreatic carcinomas. The usefulness of FISH and DIA for the detection of hilar cholangiocarcinoma still awaits further evaluation.

8.2.4 DNA Hypermethylation

DNA hypermethylation of genes, such as the tumor suppressor genes and cell cycle regulation genes, is a common epigenetic change in malignancies, including cholangiocarcinomas. Hence, analysis the DNA methylation status of some important genes in the exfoliated cells of the bile provides diagnostic evidences for malignancy in patients with biliary strictures. We prospectively analyzed the methylation status of P16 and APC gene promoters of the exfoliated cells in the bile aspirates from 70 patients with biliary obstruction using methylation-specific PCR. Forty-eight of these patients were diagnosed to have malignant biliary obstruction (bile duct carcinomas in 36, pancreatic carcinoma in 8 and duodenal carcinoma in 4) by pathological examination, and 22 had benign biliary obstruction caused by cholelithiasis. Hypermethylation of P16 promoter was present in 72.9 % (35/48) of patients with malignant biliary obstruction, and in 9 % (2/22) of patients with benign obstruction ($P<0.05$). Hypermethylation of APC promoter was present in 56.2 % (27/48) of patients with malignant biliary obstruction, and in 9 % (2/22) of patients with benign obstruction ($P<0.05$). For malignant biliary obstruction, the sensitivity, specificity, positive predictivity and negative predictivity for the P16 gene were 72.9, 90.9, 94.6 and 60.6 %, respectively, and they were 56.2, 90.9, 93.1, 48.8 %, respectively, for the APC gene. Our results suggested that the methylation status of the P16 and APC gene promoters in the bile aspirate was valuable in the diagnosis of malignant biliary obstruction. The specificity was excellent. The P16 gene had a higher sensitivity than the APC gene [50]. The role of the DNA methylation status in the diagnosis of hilar cholangiocarcinoma needs to be further assessed in large-scale clinical trials.

8.3 Summary

Despite improvements in diagnostic modalities in the past decade, differentiation between malignant and benign hilar biliary obstruction still remains a challenge. An accurate preoperative diagnosis is important for hilar biliary stricture to avoid inappropriately extensive resection. Although brush cytology and forceps biopsy are able to make a definite diagnosis, their sensitivity is low. EUS-guided FNA has a greater sensitivity for cancer detection, but it is only feasible for patients with a focal mass and it is technically demanding. Identification of molecular changes of the exfoliated cells in the bile, such as DNA methylation, may represent a novel approach for the diagnosis of hilar cholangiocarcinoma.

References

1. Jarnagin WR, Saldinger PF, Blumgart LH. Cancer of the bile ducts: the hepatic ducts and common bile duct. In: Blumgart LH, Fong Y, editors. Surgery of the liver and biliary tract. 3rd ed. Philadelphia: W. B. Saunders; 2000. p. 1017–40.
2. Khan SA, Davidson BR, Goldin R, et al. Guidelines for the diagnosis and treatment of cholangiocarcinoma: consensus document. Gut. 2002;51 Suppl 6Suppl 6:VI1–9.
3. Washburn WK, Lewis WD, Jenkins RL. Aggressive surgical resection for cholangiocarcinoma. Arch Surg. 1995;130:270–6.
4. Aljiffry M, Walsh MJ, Molinari M. Advances in diagnosis, treatment and palliation of cholangiocarcinoma: 1990–2009. World J Gastroenterol. 2009;15:4240–62.
5. Koea J, Holden A, Chau K, et al. Differential diagnosis of stenosing lesions at the hepatic hilus. World J Surg. 2004;28:466–70.
6. Patel AH, Harnois DM, Klee GG, et al. The utility of CA 19-9 in the diagnoses of cholangiocarcinoma in patients without primary sclerosing cholangitis. Am J Gastroenterol. 2000;95:204–7.
7. Maestranzi S, Przemioslo R, Mitchell H, et al. The effect of benign and malignant liver disease on the tumor markers CA19-9 and CEA. Ann Clin Biochem. 1998;35(Pt 1):99–103.
8. Chalasani N, Baluyut A, Ismail A, et al. Cholangiocarcinoma in patients with primary sclerosing cholangitis: a multicenter case-control study. Hepatology. 2000;31:7–11.
9. Nichols JC, Gores GJ, LaRusso NF, et al. Diagnostic role of serum CA 19-9 for cholangiocarcinoma in patients with primary sclerosing cholangitis. Mayo Clin Proc. 1993;68:874–9.
10. Nehls O, Gregor M, Klump B. Serum and bile markers for cholangiocarcinoma. Semin Liver Dis. 2004;24:139–54.
11. Juntermanns B, Radunz S, Heuer M, et al. Tumor markers as a diagnostic key for hilar cholangiocarcinoma. Eur J Med Res. 2010;15:357–61.
12. Weber A, Schmid RM, Prinz C. Diagnostic approaches for cholangiocarcinoma. World J Gastroenterol. 2008;14:4131–6.
13. Siqueira E, Schoen RE, Silverman W, et al. Detecting cholangiocarcinoma in patients with primary sclerosing cholangitis. Gastrointest Endosc. 2002;56:40–7.
14. Alvaro D. Serum and bile biomarkers for cholangiocarcinoma. Curr Opin Gastroenterol. 2009;25:279–84.
15. Bamrungphon W, Prempracha N, Bunchu N, et al. A new mucin antibody/enzyme-linked lectin-sandwich assay of serum MUC5AC mucin for the diagnosis of cholangiocarcinoma. Cancer Lett. 2007; 247:301–8.
16. Sharma MP, Ahuja V. Aetiological spectrum of obstructive jaundice and diagnostic ability of ultrasonography: a clinician's perspective. Trop Gastroenterol. 1999;20:167–9.
17. Hann LE, Greatrex KV, Bach AM, et al. Cholangiocarcinoma at the hepatic hilus: sonographic findings. AJR Am J Roentgenol. 1997; 168:985–9.
18. Xu HX, Chen LD, Xie XY, et al. Enhancement pattern of hilar cholangiocarcinoma: contrast-enhanced ultrasound versus contrast-enhanced computed tomography. Eur J Radiol. 2010;75:197–202.
19. Bach AM, Hann LE, Brown KT, et al. Portal vein evaluation with US: comparison to angiography combined with CT arterial portography. Radiology. 1996;201(1):149–54.
20. Watadani T, Akahane M, Yoshikawa T, et al. Preoperative assessment of hilar cholangiocarcinoma using multidetector-row CT: correlation with histopathological findings. Radiat Med. 2008; 26:402–7.
21. Akamatsu N, Sugawara Y, Osada H, et al. Diagnostic accuracy of multidetector-row computed tomography for hilar cholangiocarcinoma. J Gastroenterol Hepatol. 2010;25:731–7.
22. Unno M, Okumoto T, Katayose Y, et al. Preoperative assessment of hilar cholangiocarcinoma by multidetector row computed tomography. J Hepatobiliary Pancreat Surg. 2007;14:434–40.
23. Okumoto T, Sato A, Yamada T, et al. Correct diagnosis of vascular encasement and longitudinal extension of hilar cholangiocarcinoma by four-channel multidetector-row computed tomography. Tohoku J Exp Med. 2009;217:1–8.
24. Lee HY, Kim SH, Lee JM, et al. Preoperative assessment of resectability of hepatic hilar cholangiocarcinoma: combined CT and cholangiography with revised criteria. Radiology. 2006;239:113–21.
25. Choi JY, Kim MJ, Lee JM, et al. Hilar cholangiocarcinoma: role of preoperative imaging with sonography, MDCT, MRI, and direct cholangiography. AJR Am J Roentgenol. 2008;191:1448–57.
26. Vilgrain V. Staging cholangiocarcinoma by imaging studies. HPB (Oxford). 2008;10:106–9.
27. Hänninen EL, Pech M, Jonas S, et al. Magnetic resonance imaging including magnetic resonance cholangiopancreatography for tumor localization and therapy planning in malignant hilar obstructions. Acta Radiol. 2005;46:462–70.
28. Masselli G, Manfredi R, Vecchioli A, et al. MR imaging and MR cholangiopancreatography in the preoperative evaluation of hilar cholangiocarcinoma: correlation with surgical and pathologic findings. Eur Radiol. 2008;18:2213–21.
29. Lee MG, Park KB, Shin YM, et al. Preoperative evaluation of hilar cholangiocarcinoma with contrast-enhanced three-dimensional fast imaging with steady-state precession magnetic resonance angiography: comparison with intraarterial digital subtraction angiography. World J Surg. 2003;27:278–83.
30. Park HS, Lee JM, Choi JY, et al. Preoperative Evaluation of bile duct cancer: MRI combined with MR cholangiopancreatography versus MDCT with direct cholangiography. AJR Am J Roentgenol. 2008;190:396–405.
31. Yeh TS, Jan YY, Tseng JH, et al. Malignant perihilar biliary obstruction: magnetic resonance cholangiopancreatographic findings. Am J Gastroenterol. 2000;95:432–40.
32. Rösch T, Meining A, Frühmorgen S, et al. A prospective comparison of the diagnostic accuracy of ERCP, MRCP, CT, and EUS in biliary strictures. Gastrointest Endosc. 2002;55:870–6.
33. Park MS, Kim TK, Kim KW, et al. Differentiation of extrahepatic bile duct cholangiocarcinoma from benign stricture: findings at MRCP versus ERCP. Radiology. 2004;233:234–40.
34. Anderson CD, Pinson CW, Berlin J, et al. Diagnosis and treatment of cholangiocarcinoma. Oncologist. 2004;9:47–53.

35. Fritscher-Ravens A, Bohuslavizki KH, Broering DC, et al. FDG PET in the diagnosis of hilar cholangiocarcinoma. Nucl Med Commun. 2001;22:1277–85.
36. Li J, Kuehl H, Grabellus F, et al. Preoperative assessment of hilar cholangiocarcinoma by dual-modality PET/CT. J Surg Oncol. 2008;98:438–43.
37. Moon CM, Bang S, Chung JB, et al. Usefulness of 18F-fluorodeoxyglucose positron emission tomography in differential diagnosis and staging of cholangiocarcinomas. J Gastroenterol Hepatol. 2008;23:759–65.
38. Reinhardt MJ, Strunk H, Gerhardt T, et al. Detection of Klatskin's tumor in extrahepatic bile duct strictures using delayed 18F-FDG PET/CT: preliminary results for 22 patient studies. J Nucl Med. 2005;46:1158–63.
39. Kluge R, Schmidt F, Caca K, et al. Positron emission tomography with [(18)F]fluoro-2-deoxy-D-glucose for diagnosis and staging of bile duct cancer. Hepatology. 2001;33:1029–35.
40. Petrowsky H, Wildbrett P, Husarik DB, et al. Impact of integrated positron emission tomography and computed tomography on staging and management of gallbladder cancer and cholangiocarcinoma. J Hepatol. 2006;45:43–50.
41. Corvera CU, Blumgart LH, Akhurst T, et al. 18F-fluorodeoxyglucose positron emission tomography influences management decisions in patients with biliary cancer. J Am Coll Surg. 2008;206:57–65.
42. Kloek JJ, van Delden OM, Erdogan D, et al. Differentiation of malignant and benign proximal bile duct strictures: the diagnostic dilemma. World J Gastroenterol. 2008;14:5032–8.
43. Lazaridis KN, Gores GJ. Cholangiocarcinoma. Gastroenterology. 2005;128:1655–67.
44. Harewood GC, Baron TH, Stadheim LM, et al. Prospective, blinded assessment of factors influencing the accuracy of biliary cytology interpretation. Am J Gastroenterol. 2004;99:1464–9.
45. Weber A, von Weyhern C, Fend F, et al. Endoscopic transpapillary brush cytology and forceps biopsy in patients with hilar cholangiocarcinoma. World J Gastroenterol. 2008;14:1097–101.
46. Fritscher-Ravens A, Broering DC, Knoefel WT, et al. EUS-guided fine-needle aspiration of suspected hilar cholangiocarcinoma in potentially operable patients with negative brush cytology. Am J Gastroenterol. 2004;99:45–51.
47. DeWitt J, Misra VL, Leblanc JK, et al. EUS-guided FNA of proximal biliary strictures after negative ERCP brush cytology results. Gastrointest Endosc. 2006;64:325–33.
48. Kipp BR, Stadheim LM, Halling SA, et al. A comparison of routine cytology and fluorescence in situ hybridization for the detection of malignant bile duct strictures. Am J Gastroenterol. 2004;99:1675–81.
49. Baron TH, Harewood GC, Rumalla A, et al. A prospective comparison of digital image analysis and routine cytology for the identification of malignancy in biliary tract strictures. Clin Gastroenterol Hepatol. 2004;2:214–9.
50. Yin XY, Yan G, Peng JX, et al. The clinical values of methylation status of P16, APC genes in bile in diagnosis of malignant obstructive jaundice. Gastrointestinal cancer symposium proceedings; San Francisco, California, USA. 2011. p. 91.

Differential Diagnosis

9

W. Kassahun, P. Stumpp, A. Hoffmeister, and S. Jonas

9.1 Introduction

The differential diagnosis of hilar cholangiocarcinoma (HCCA) that include primary malignancies, metastatic disease and benign lesions is challenging and presents a diagnostic dilemma in surgery. Generally, biliary tumors are accompanied by painless jaundice with evidence of biliary obstruction [1, 2]. Currently, this presentation by itself is usually enough to raise a strong suspicion of neoplastic biliary obstruction. The clinical findings and laboratory values including tumor markers are non-specific and cannot correctly identify the exact cause of the stricture. Thus, preoperative differential diagnosis, which is desirable to confirm surgical indication and to advise patients about the disease and their respective prognosis, is extremely difficult. Although the assessment of patients with obstructive jaundice has greatly improved by the currently available noninvasive, and invasive imaging modalities, all these techniques cannot always be relied upon to provide a definitive diagnosis, in particular in the absence of a visible tumor mass [3]. In addition, it is well known that not all hilar obstructions are due to HCCA and alternative diagnosis that mimic HCCA may count for up to 25 % of all hilar obstructions [4–7]. Benign strictures for example, occasionally manifest as focal areas of wall thickening that obstruct the lumen and, thus, mimic malignant strictures. Approximately 16 % (range, 3.4–58.6 %) of patients initially diagnosed with hilar cholangiocarcinoma proved to have a benign stricture [3–20]. Biopsy is so often nondiagnostic that decisions about therapy are usually made on the basis of the imaging tests and lack of evidence for some other disease [3, 4, 21–26]. Although specific radiographic features, such as absence of tumor mass, smooth concentric pattern or tapering of the bile duct, can be associated with benign lesions, none can unequivocally exclude the presence of malignancy [6]. As a result, differentiating HCCA related biliary obstructions (Fig. 9.1) from obstructions caused by other malignant (Figs. 9.2 and 9.3) and benign (Figs. 9.4 and 9.5) lesions remains a challenge. Because the majority of biliary strictures at the liver hilum in the absence of previous surgery are usually malignant in nature and presumed to be due to HCCA, a reasonable approach is to assume the presence of HCCA until proved otherwise [15, 27–29]. However, surgeons should always be aware of the possibility of other disease particularly a benign disease and advise their patients appropriately. The diagnosis is much less specific than is generally thought, so there is considerable opportunity for mismanaging such patients. Although it has always been clear that basing the diagnosis on indirect evidence would occasionally be incorrect, a 25 % rate of false diagnosis by a team of highly specialized clinicians who encounter many such complicated cases is higher than most would have expected. Alternative diagnosis with proximal biliary obstruction mimicking HCCA is present in such a proportion of patients that it really deserves a place in the differential diagnosis of biliary obstruction. Differentiating HCCA from other causes of obstructive jaundice is important because of the differences in treatment. Curative surgical therapy for HCCA requires bile duct resection with concomitant major hepatectomy and caudate lobe resection or neoadjuvant chemoradiation, followed by liver transplantation in highly selected patients [30, 31]. This type of surgery is generally not necessary for benign conditions and generally not warranted for metastatic

W. Kassahun, MD • S. Jonas, MD (✉)
Faculty of Medicine, Department of Abdominal, Transplantation, Thoracic and Vascular Surgery, University of Leipzig, Leipzig, Germany
e-mail: sven.jonas@medizin.uni-leipzig.de

P. Stumpp, MD
Faculty of Medicine, Department of Radiology, University of Leipzig, Leipzig, Germany

A. Hoffmeister, MD
Faculty of Medicine, Department of Gastroenterology and Rheumatology, University of Leipzig, Leipzig, Germany

W.Y. Lau (ed.), *Hilar Cholangiocarcinoma*,
DOI 10.1007/978-94-007-6473-6_9, © Springer Science+Business Media Dordrecht and People's Medical Publishing House 2013

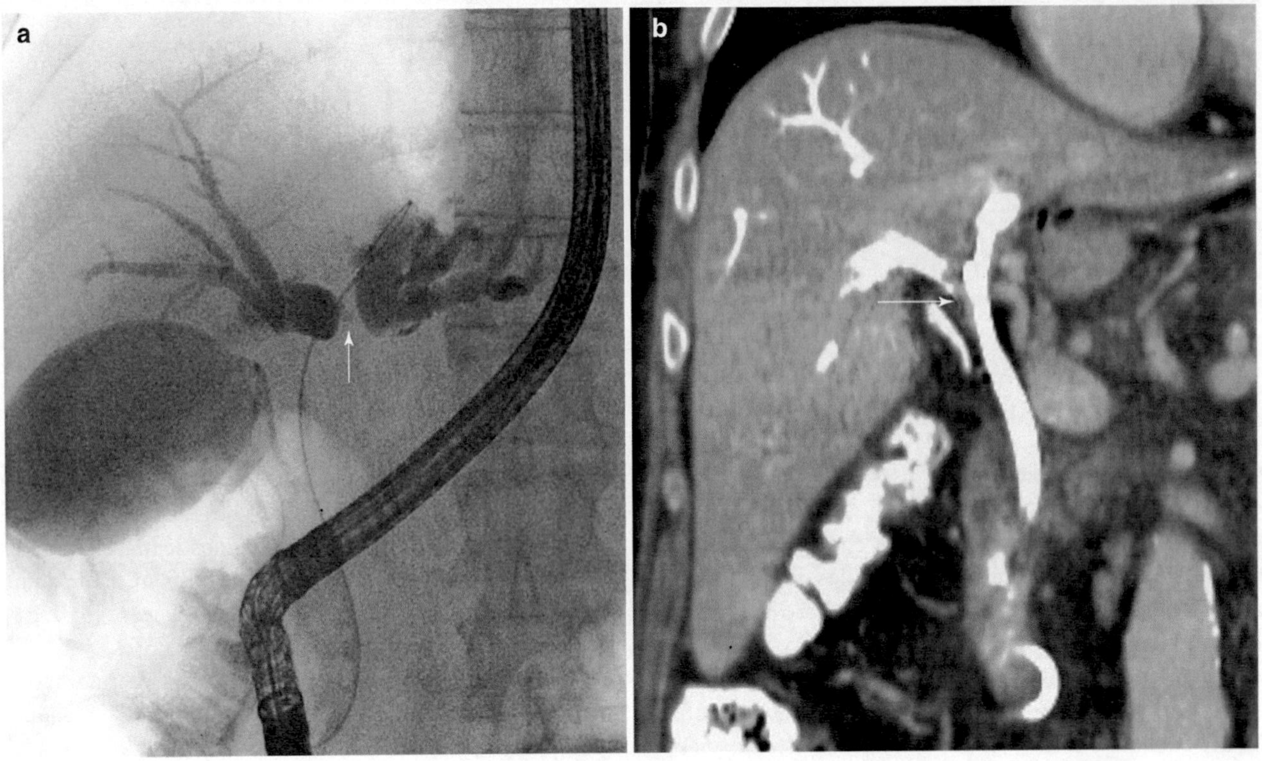

Fig. 9.1 (**a**) ERCP image from a patient with obstructive jaundice caused by histologic proved HCCA demonstrating complete obstruction at the hilar confluence level (*arrow*) with upstream ductal dilatation; (**b**) multiplanar reconstructed CT image of the same patient demonstrating intrahepatic biliary dilatation with a mass-forming lesion (*arrow*) at the confluence and stent placed across the lesion

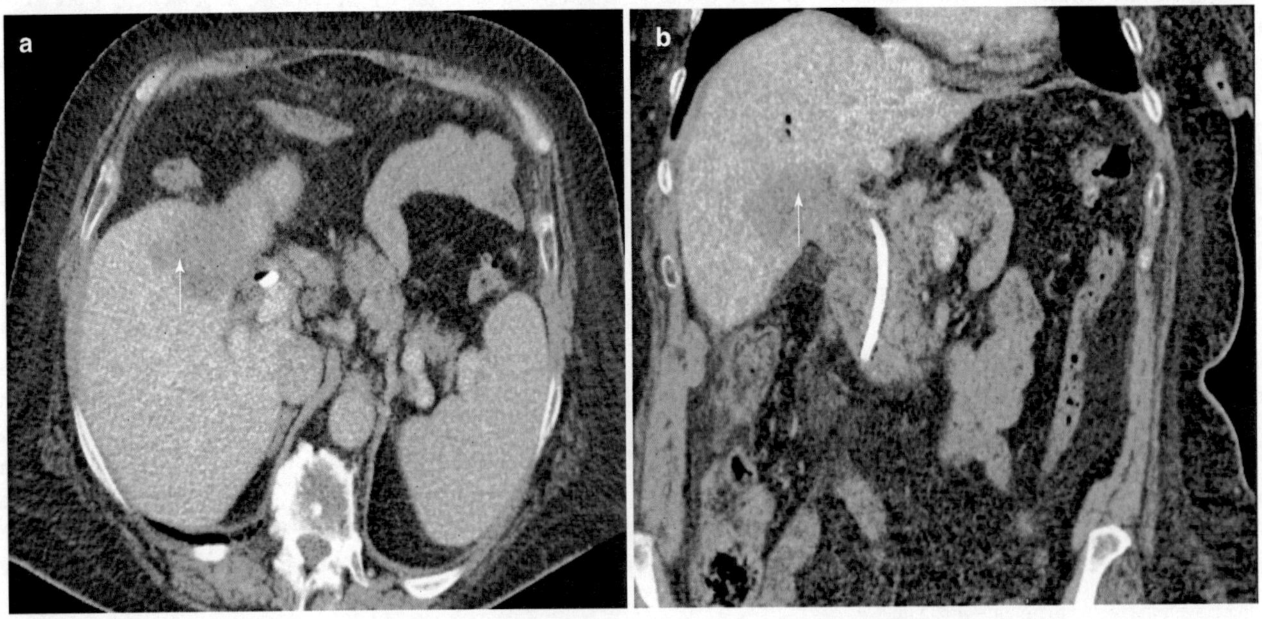

Fig. 9.2 Computed tomographic (CT) scans in the axial (**a**) and multiplanar reconstruction in the coronal plane (**b**) from a patient with carcinoma of the gallbladder (*arrow*) filling the entire gallbladder and invading the liver hilum and adjoining right lobe

or other non-HCCA malignancies. Thus, preoperative precise characterization of obstructive jaundice due to hilar obstruction has important clinical implications. It would potentially improve planning for surgery and may prevent subjecting some patients to major and risky surgical interventions unnecessarily.

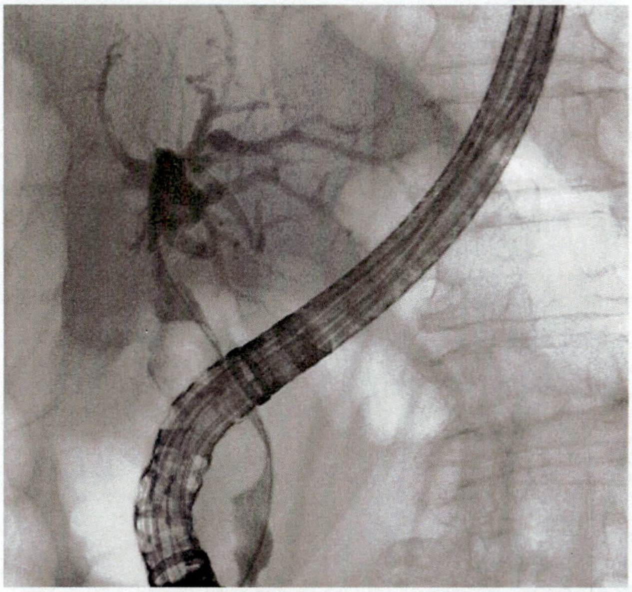

Fig. 9.3 ERCP of the same patient shows intrahepatic ductal dilatation indicating invasion of the common bile duct und thus resembles HCCA. An ERCP stent is placed across the lesion in to the left duct as this provides drainage of the future remnant liver following resection

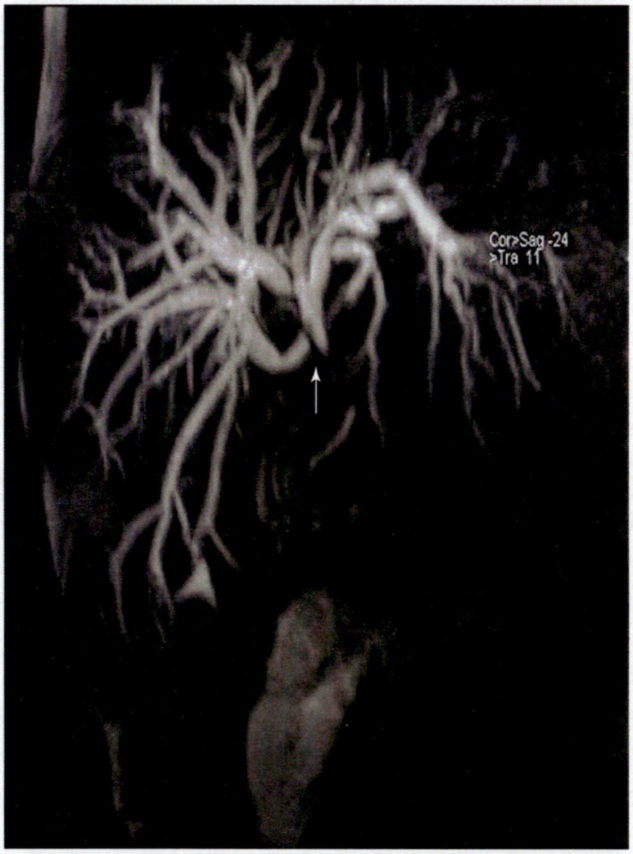

Fig. 9.4 Coronal image from color-coded 3D T2-weighted MRCP image from a 22-year-old patient with progressive jaundice demonstrating complete obstruction at the hilar confluence (*arrow*) with intrahepatic biliary dilatation in both the left and right lobes of the liver. Hilar cholangiocarcinoma was suspected. The patient was treated with extended right hepatic lobectomy with removal of the biliary confluence. Histology revealed a chronic inflammatory stricture of the Confluence including the right duct with no evidence of malignancy

9.2 Type of Malignant Lesions Mimicking Hilar Cholangiocarcinoma (HCCA)

9.2.1 Carcinoma of the Gallbladder

Because of the intimate anatomic relationship of the biliary confluence to the gallbladder, carcinoma of the gallbladder in some cases involves the hepatic hilum, either through direct extension or from metastatic spread. In some studies it was the most common non-HCCA malignancy involving the biliary confluence, accounting for more than 50 % of alternative diagnosis [15]. While 45 % of patients with carcinoma of the gallbladder present with jaundice as a marker of advanced disease [32], the number of patients with HCCA that develop jaundice exceeds 90 % [33]. Normally, the presence of a mass on imaging originating from the gallbladder wall and invading the liver with or without involvement of the biliary tree indicates toward gallbladder cancer. In addition, gallbladder cancer-related stricture of the biliary tree is localized mostly at a more distal location below the biliary confluence. Unfortunately, such clear-cut diagnostic findings are not uniformly present. Thus, clinical features, laboratory values and imaging studies including ERCP are helpful in only a small proportion of patients differentiating advanced stage gallbladder cancer from HCCA.

9.2.2 Malignant Melanoma of the Biliary Tract

Malignant melanoma of the biliary tract is a rare entity arising primarily from the biliary epithelium [34]. It can also result from systemic dissemination of a primary location elsewhere as it exhibits a remarkable ability to metastasize to diverse locations [35]. When it does occur as a primary or metastatic disease, it usually presents with obstructive jaundice and an intraluminal polypoid soft tissue mass on imaging, thus simulating and further complicating the diagnosis of HCCA [36]. Features at multiple, complimentary imaging techniques such as ultrasonography, CT, MRI and ERCP are nonspecific. Thus, accurate differentiation of obstructive jaundice related to melanoma from that of HCCA is almost impossible.

9.2.3 Neuroendocrine Neoplasia of the Bile Ducts

Neuroendocrine neoplasia of the biliary tract are extremely rare with only few cases being reported to date [34]. These tumors may arise anywhere along the intrahepatic or extrahepatic biliary tree. Approximately 50–60 % of neuroendocrine neoplasia of the biliary tree occur at the common bile duct, and the remainder occur in the perihilar region (28 %), cystic

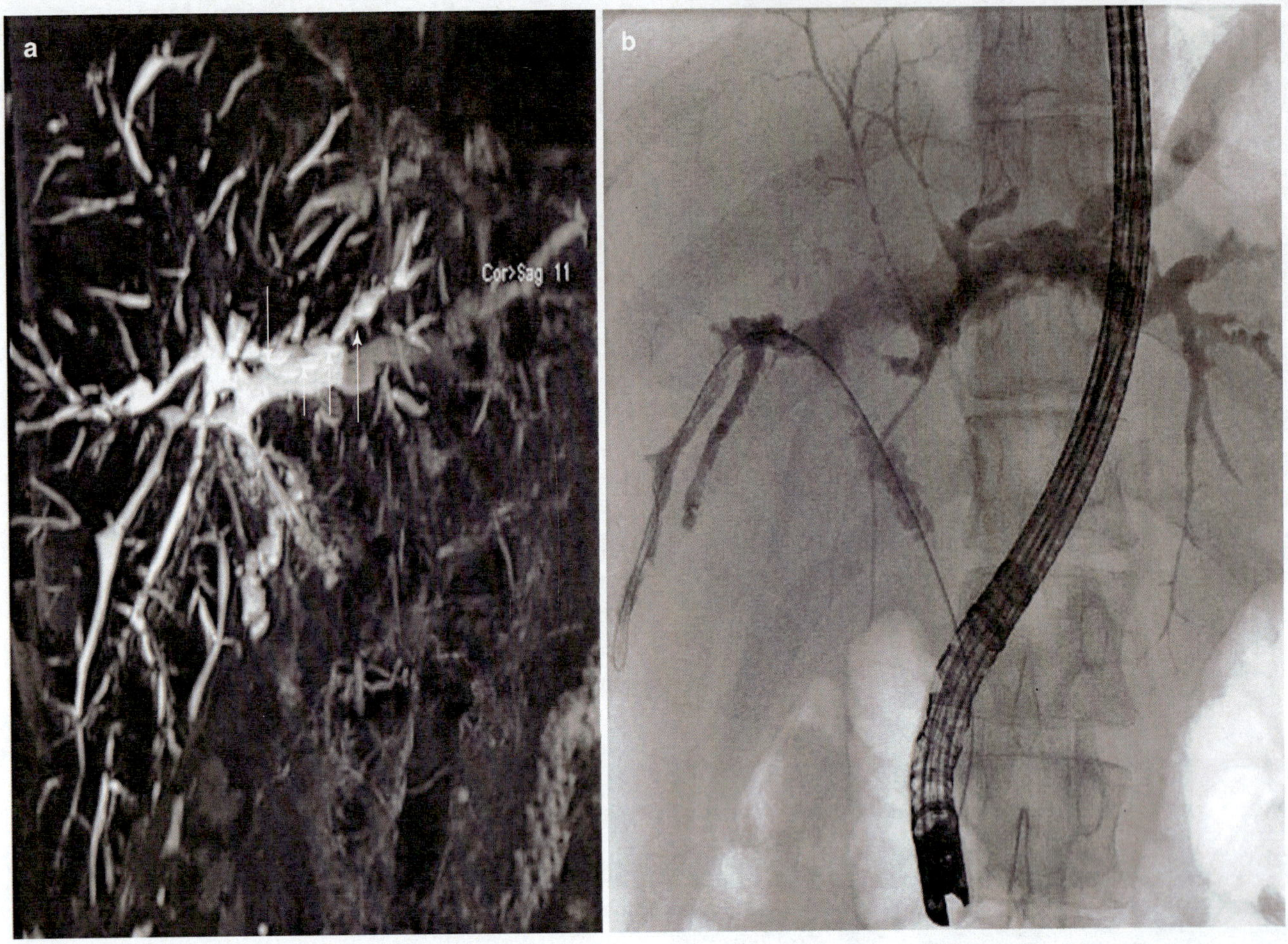

Fig. 9.5 (**a**) Coronal image from color-coded 3D T2-weighted MRCP in a patient with primary sclerosing cholangitis showing segmental strictures (*thin arrows*) and dilatation (*thick arrow*) of the bile ducts as a classic imaging finding; (**b**) ERCP image reveals bile duct strictures with upstream ductal dilatation simulating infiltrating cholangiocarcinoma

duct (11 %) or the hepatic duct bifurcation (3 %) [37]. Patients are usually young and present with painless jaundice from biliary obstruction and related symptoms including clay-colored stools and dark urine. Although radiologic findings of these tumors are diverse and nonspecific, they may appear as long segment biliary stricture with wall thickening with or without mass formation, thus simulating HCCA.

9.2.4 Lymph Node Metastases

Metastatic processes in the liver including the liver hilum, in particular from cancers of the gastrointestinal tract, are responsible for most cancer related deaths in the world [38, 39]. The liver is the most common site of colorectal cancer metastases and frequently the only affected organ. Up to 35 % of patients with colorectal cancer will have hepatic metastases at the time of surgery for the primary lesion, and further, 8–25 % will develop metachronous hepatic metastases after primary resection [40]. Furthermore, colorectal adenocarcinoma, on account of its proclivity to spread along epithelial surfaces, shows an increased predilection to involve the biliary ducts and cause obstructive jaundice as well [41]. Lymph node bearing metastatic deposits at the liver hilum may be enlarged to many times their normal size, often exceeding even the diameter of the primary lesion and causing obstructive jaundice. Therefore, a history of malignancy, cholestasis and a mass lesion at the hepatic hilum should also raise the suspicion of metastatic lymphadenopathy as differential diagnosis of HCCA.

9.2.5 Primary Hematolymphoid Malignancies Involving the Hepatic Hilum

Obstructive jaundice is a common consequence of malignancy but only rarely has been reported as a presenting manifestation of primary hematolymphoid malignancies [42, 43]. The majority of cases involve secondary infiltration of the biliary tree including the hepatic hilum from systemic dissemination of extrahepatic wide spread disease [44]. However, the existence of primary hematolymphoid malignancies of the biliary tract characterized by obstructive jaundice has been recognized for many years [45, 46]. It includes non-Hodgkin lymphomas, plasmocytomas, non-leukemic granulocytic sarcomas and others. These malignancies of the bile duct are extremely rare and ill defined. Clinical symptoms and signs such as abdominal pain, fever and weight loss are common in those patients. However, these symptoms are nonspecific and patients with HCCA can also present with such symptoms too. In addition, there are no laboratory and radiologic findings that help differentiate these malignancies of the bile duct accurately from HCCA. As a result their exact diagnosis as a cause of cholestasis could only be established with certainty retrospectively. Owing to the above mentioned diagnostic difficulties, and in particular their rarity, this kind of malignancies of the bile duct causing obstructive jaundice often are not included in the differential diagnosis of HCCA and rather mistakenly being attributed to it. On the other hand, differentiating HCCA from primary hematolymphoid malignancies causing obstructive jaundice is important because of the differences in treatment. Extensive surgery, which is the main stay of therapy in HCCA, is rarely indicated in primary hematolymphoid malignancies. Most of these malignancies can be treated safely and effectively with multiple agent chemotherapy alone without the need for extensive and risky surgical procedures [47]. Surgery is indicated only when lesions produce complications, that are not amenable to non-surgical treatment, or chemotherapy fails to eradicate localized disease [43].

9.3 Type of Benign Lesions Mimicking Hilar Cholangiocarcinoma (HCCA)

9.3.1 Primary Sclerosing Cholangitis (PSC)

PSC is an idiopathic, chronic cholestatic disease of possible autoimmune origin characterized by periductal inflammation, resulting in multifocal strictures of the intrahepatic and extrahepatic bile ducts [48, 49]. This disorder is the commonest known predisposing condition for cholangiocarcinoma in the west [50, 51]. Cholangiocarcinoma rates of 8–40 % (follow-up studies, autopsy and explant specimens) have been reported in patients with PSC, making cholangiocarcinoma the most dreaded complication of PSC [50–53]. Cholangiocarcinoma in such patients tends to present earlier, in the fourth or fifth decade, than in sporadic cases [50, 54]. Its natural history is variable, and the true incidence of cholangiocarcinoma is unclear. However, the highest incidence of developing cholangiocarcinoma is reported in the first 2 years of diagnosis of PSC and the risk of cholangiocarcinogenesis seems unrelated to the duration of the inflammatory disease [50, 55]. Distinguishing benign from malignant strictures is challenging in the setting of PSC particularly in the presence of localized bile duct stricture. Pool data composed of 190 patients with obstructing benign lesions of the common bile duct whose initial clinical and imaging diagnosis was hilar cholangiocarcinoma showed 1.6 % PSC at final histology [4–15, 18].

9.3.2 Secondary Sclerosing Cholangitis Syndromes (SSCS)

Secondary sclerosing cholangitis syndromes are a heterogeneous group of chronic cholestatic disorders that are morphologically similar to PSC but differ in pathological processes [56, 57]. The clinical and cholangiographic features of these disorders may mimic PSC and HCC, yet its natural history may be more favourable if recognition is prompt and appropriate treatment is introduced. The wide spectrum of these entities includes inflammatory pseudotumor (IPT), autoimmune pancreatocholangitis (AIP), recurrent pyogenic cholangitis (RPC), portal biliopathy, AIDS cholangiopathy, eosinophilic cholangitis, mast cell cholangitis, ischemic cholangitis and other conditions.

9.3.3 Inflammatory Pseudotumor (IPT)

Inflammatory pseudotumor is an idiopathic entity that regroups benign lesions of the extrahepatic bile duct with inflammatory components [56, 57]. At histologic analysis, a heterogeneous population of inflammatory cells-predominantly plasma cells, eosinophils, macrophags, and fibroblasts-as well as areas of fibrosis and/or necrosis characterizes this disorder [4–7, 11, 13, 15, 58, 59]. Associations with PSC, Crohn's disease and phlebitis have been described [60–62]. Next to the lungs of young adults the hepatobiliary system is the second most common target location of IPT [34, 63]. Its aetiology remains obscure and there are neither specific signs on imaging, nor conclusive diagnostic biochemical tests. Although its incidence is not exactly known, about 4–20 % of bile duct strictures mimicking hilar cholangiocarcinoma are IPT [4–11, 13]. These lesions appear on imaging as masses that may show delayed and persistent enhancement due to the fibrous content; and biliary strictures of intra- or extrahepatic ducts on cholangiography, findings remarkably similar to those of cholangiocarcinoma [64, 65]. Furthermore, associations between IPT and RPC that leads to biliary stricture formation and thus mimic HCCA have been described [60]. There is also evidence that its histologic findings are quite similar to autoimmune pancreatocholangitis (AIP) and feature many IgG4-positive plasma cells, thereby suggesting a shared pathogenic mechanism [66].

9.3.4 Recurrent Pyogenic Cholangitis

Recurrent pyogenic cholangitis (RPC) also known as Hong Kong disease and oriental cholangiohepatitis, is a condition that most commonly affects patients with East Asian descent [67]. Although most prevalent in the East, it is seen increasing in the West mainly owing to immigration [68]. This disorder is characterized by recurrent episodes of bacterial cholangitis that occur in association with biliary obstruction from strictures and pigmented stones [69, 70]. RPC peaks in the third and fifth decades of life with no specific sex predilection. Patients most often present with abdominal pain, fever and jaundice [71]. It is thought to occur in patients suffering from chronic infestation of the biliary tree by Ascaris lumbricoides, Clonorchis sinensis, Opisthorchis viverrini, Fasciola hepatica and Opisthorchis felineus that may obstruct the biliary tract with resultant bile stasis, pigment stone formation and bacterial super infection [69, 72]. Although sepsis is the major threat to life in these patients, approximately 10 % will develop cholangiocarcinoma [73, 74]. Imaging may identify biliary strictures, ductal wall thickening secondary to fibrosis, and hepatolithiasis [75, 76]. The ductal wall thickening and enhancement may not be distinguished from cholangiocarcinoma with imaging studies alone [34].

9.3.5 AIDS Cholangiopathy

AIDS cholangiopathy is a syndrome of biliary duct obstruction caused by infection-related strictures [77–79]. The clinical spectrum of disease includes papillary stenosis, sclerosing cholangitis, combined sclerosis of the duct and papillary stenosis, and long strictures of the extrahepatic bile ducts [56, 80]. The large intrahepatic ducts are preferentially affected [56]. It typically manifests as biliary strictures associated with wall thickening and mural stenosis [81]. Among those four distinct cholangiographic abnormalities, which have been demonstrated by endoscopic retrograde cholangiopancreatography (ERCP), the combination of sclerosing cholangitis and papillary stenosis is the most common and occurs in 50 % of patients [82]. This disorder, once considered to have extremely poor prognosis, is now rarely fatal, in part due to the wide spread use of antiretroviral drugs. The current incidence is not known but remains significant in areas where access to retroviral drugs is limited. Its aetiology is multifactorial. Opportunistic infections such as Cryptosporidium and Cytomegalovirus are the most common causes of AIDS cholangiopathy [83]. However, no definite organism is identified in up to 50 % of patients [34]. Patients typically present in the advanced stage of the HIV spectrum, when their CD4 counts are below 135/mm^3 [84]. The presentation of AIDS cholangiopathy varies from features of cholangitis to isolated right upper quadrant abdominal pain. Sometimes the only abnormality is an elevated serum alkaline phosphatase, generally five to seven times above the normal limit [80, 83].

9.3.6 Autoimmune Sclerosing Pancreatocholangitis

Autoimmune pancreatitis (AIP) is a type of chronic pancreatitis characterized by an autoimmune inflammatory process in which prominent lymphocyte infiltration with associated fibrosis of the pancreas causes organ dysfunction [85]. In addition to findings specific to the pancreas, about 49 % of patients with this disorder can have extrapancreatic manifestations including sclerosing inflammation of the intrahepatic or extrahepatic bile duct system or the gallbladder [86]. It can mimic malignancy and is commonly named autoimmune pancreatocholangitis [87]. The pathogenesis of AIP is uncertain, and no gold standard exists for its diagnosis. The estimated prevalence of AIP is 5–11 % of all patients with chronic pancreatitis [88, 89]. It is twice as common in men as in women, and most patients are older than 50 years, an age at which pancreatic carcinoma occurs [88, 90]. Immunohistochemical studies demonstrate prominent lymphocyte and Immunglobulin G4-positive plasma cell infiltration and fibrosis [91]. Imaging studies show diffuse or homogeneous enlargement of the pancreas with a moderate enhancement, and a peripheral rim of hypoattenuation [85]. Regarding ductal structures, it is characterized by focal or diffuse strictures of the pancreatic and bile ducts. Narrowing of the intrahepatic bile duct and bile duct strictures with upstream ductal dilatation can also be seen, which may mimic the periductal infiltrating type of cholangiocarcinoma [85].

9.3.7 Portal Biliopathy

The term portal biliopathy (PB) refers to the morphologic abnormalities of the entire biliary tract including extrahepatic and intrahepatic bile ducts in patients with portal hypertension [92]. Chronic thrombotic obstruction of the extrahepatic portal vein is usually followed by the formation of bridging hepatopetal collaterals which drain splanchnic venous blood from the splenic, superior mesenteric and coronary veins to the porta hepatis in an attempt to bypass the obstruction. This results in the formation of a venous network known as portal cavernoma or cavernous transformation [93, 94]. Although extrahepatic portal vein thrombosis is the most common cause of PB, liver cirrhosis, portal vein fibrosis without cirrhosis and congenital hepatic fibrosis can also cause the disorder [92]. Mechanical protrusion of the paracholedochal veins in the lumen of the bile duct and a secondary ischemic vascular bile duct injury with or without cholangitis is believed to lead to the development of significant strictures. It may lead to asymptomatic cholestasis in more than 50 % of patients; and rarely, it can cause symptomatic biliary obstruction [95]. Symptomatic patients are usually adults, indicating that PB is a slowly progressive disease, because most are thought to have acquired their portal vein thrombosis in early childhood [56]. Direct cholangiographic findings include segmental upstream dilation, calibre irregularity, filling defects that may be interpreted as common bile duct calculi, stricture and extrinsic impression on the bile duct due to collaterals [96]. These cholangiographic appearances may mimic bile duct cancer, with the cavernoma appearing as a solid tumor, the so-called "pseudocholangiocarcinoma sign" [97].

9.3.8 Mirizzi Syndrome

Mirizzi described in 1948 a functional hepatic syndrome that consisted of a common hepatic duct obstruction secondary to compression by a gallstone impacted at the gallbladder neck or cystic duct [98]. The current definition of this syndrome that now bears his name includes four components [99–101]: anatomic arrangement of the cystic duct at the gallbladder neck such that it runs parallel to the common hepatic duct; impaction of a stone in the cystic duct or neck of the gallbladder; mechanical obstruction of the common hepatic duct by a stone itself or by secondary inflammation; and intermittent or constant jaundice causing possible recurrent cholangitis and, if long-standing, secondary biliary cirrhosis. Based on the severity of the disease Csendes et al. classified this syndrome into four types [99]. Type I lesion is a simple pressure on the common hepatic duct due to an extrinsic stone impacted at the neck of the gallbladder or at the cystic duct. Type II lesion is a more severe disease with cholecystobiliary fistula that involves less than one-third of the circumference of the common bile duct. Type III lesion is a cholecystobiliary fistula with erosion of the wall of the common duct that involves two-thirds of the ductal wall. Type IV lesion is a more severe disease with cholecystobiliary fistula, which involves the entire circumference of the ductal wall. This syndrome is rare and occurs in 0.3–3 % of all cholecystectomies performed [100–102].

Recently, a number of methods for the diagnosis of biliary tract disease have been introduced. Ultrasound, endoscopic retrograde cholangiopancreatography (ERCP), percutaneous transhepatic cholangiography (PTC), magnetic resonance cholangiopancreatography (MRCP), magnetic resonance imaging (MRI), and computed tomography (CT) are all useful. Despite these advances in medical technology the diagnosis of Mirizzi's syndrome is still difficult. The imaging findings are not always specific [103]. For example, gallstones are not always visible at CT, thereby making conclusive diagnosis difficult. Obstruction of the common bile duct leads to chronic, recurrent episodes of cholangitis and stricture formation which may resemble the periductal-infiltrating type of cholangiocarcinoma.

9.3.9 Biliary Adenomas

These are rare benign epithelial tumors, with few cases reported in the literature. About 90 % of all patients with symptomatic biliary adenomas present with obstructive jaundice as a cardinal presenting sign [104]. Less common symptoms include right upper quadrant abdominal pain, weight loss, fever, and nausea [105]. Most lesions are localized in the common bile duct, particularly in the distal common duct and ampulla of Vater [105]. However, biliary adenomas within the cystic duct have also been described [106]. Although it has been suggested that adenomas of the biliary tract may result from a focal, reactive process to injury, possibly post-inflammatory or post-traumatic, the cause of these lesions in the majority of patients appears to be idiopathic [107]. The radiographic features of these lesions are often difficult to distinguish from cholangiocarcinoma. Small or solitary lesions are usually difficult to detect by CT scan [108]. Sonography indicates a non-shadowing intraluminal mass, occasionally with a pedicle [109]. The occasionally correct preoperative diagnosis of biliary adenomas may be provided by ERCP, cholangiography or cholangioscopy [109, 110]. In addition to mimicking cholangiocarcinoma, these lesions are considered premalignant with a definite risk of recurrence and progression to cholangioncarcinoma if left untreated [111].

9.3.10 Hepatobiliary Sarcoidosis

Sarcoidosis is a chronic, multisystem granulomatous disorder of unknown cause that is pathologically characterized by noncaseating granulomas [112]. It present most frequently in young adults with bilateral hilar adenopathy and pulmonary infiltrates. More than 50 % of patients with sarcoidosis have hepatobiliary involvement, varying from asymptomatic granulomatosis to portal hypertension and severe liver diseases [113]. Most patients with hepatobiliary sarcoidosis are asymptomatic. Although 50–65 % of patients with sarcoidosis show hepatobiliary involvement at liver biopsy, only 5–15 % of patients show signs and symptoms of the disease [113]. The clinical manifestations of hepatobiliary sarcoidosis are protean and include multifocal micronodular granulomas, macronodular granulomas, liver cirrhosis, portal hypertension and granulomatous cholangitis. Granulomatous cholangitis is an extremely rare disease characterized by insidious onset and chronic progression to biliary cirrhosis [34]. The formation of granulomas in bile ducts in this disorder leads to strictures and ductopenia [114]. This seems to be the underlying mechanism of chronic cholestasis syndrome featuring jaundice, pruritus, hepatomegaly, and marked elevation in serum alkaline phosphatise [115]. In patients with hepatobiliary sarcoidosis featuring biliary strictures and hilar lymphadenopathy, it can be very difficult to exclude a diagnosis of hilar cholangiocarcinoma. The imaging findings are sometimes indistinguishable from those of cholangiocarcinoma [116].

9.3.11 Xanthogranulomatous Cholecystitis and Cholangitis

Xanthogranulomatous cholecystits (XGC) is an unusual and destructive form of severe, chronic cholecystitis characterized by multiple, yellow-brown, intramural nodular formations, proliferative fibrosis, and foamy histiocytes [117, 118]. The incidence of this disease have been reported to range from 1 to 13 %, with a slight predominance in women and almost all patients presenting with gallstones [117–119]. Although the exact pathogenesis of XGC is unknown, study results suggest that XGC may begin as an acute inflammation of the gallbladder and obstruction [118, 120]. Pathologic changes occur primarily in the gallbladder wall and can extend into the surrounding structures. Imaging studies show gallbladder wall thickening associated with extra gallbladder changes such as pericholecystic infiltration, hepatic involvement, biliary obstruction with inflammatory strictures and hilar lymphadenopathy. Thus, there is much overlap between adenocarcinoma of the gallbladder and XGC to reliably differentiate between the two entities [121]. Moreover, xanthogranulomatous cholangitis may occur in isolation or association with XGC [122]. It appears as a biliary stricture with wall thickening and may simulate hilar cholangiocarcinoma [123].

9.3.12 Chemotherapy-Induced Sclerosing Cholangitis

Unlike hepatic parenchyma, which depends on a dual blood supply from the portal vein and hepatic artery, the biliary system drives its vascular supply almost exclusively from branches of the hepatic arteries and is more susceptible to injury if arterial flow is reduced [124]. Arterial occlusion may result in bile duct ischemia and fibrosis without causing significant parenchymal infarction. Possible mechanisms include toxic vasculitis and drug-induced intravascular thrombosis leading to ischemic insult and stricture formation [56]. Chemotherapy-induced sclerosing cholangitis results as a complication of hepatic arterial infusion of chemotherapeutic agents, particularly floxuridine and fluorouracil [56, 125], widely used chemotherapeutic agents for the treatment of liver metastases from colorectal cancer. It has a reported incidence of 8–55 % [126–128]. Floxuridine, fluorouracil and other agents have been used in the last decades as intravenous or intraarterial infusion for both resectable and unresectable disease [129, 130]. It has been suggested that intraarterial application of these agents causes ischemic cholangitis ultimately leading to biliary stricture formation. Ischemic cholangitis is not known to occur from intravenous systemic chemotherapy indicating local vascular inflammation from hepatic arterial chemotherapy but not hepatocellular toxicity of the drug that leads to biliary injury [131].

References

1. Ohsawa M, Aosaza K, Horiuchi K, et al. Malignant lymphoma of the liver: report of 5 cases and review of the litrature. Dig Dis Sci. 1992;37:1105–9.
2. Eliason SC, Grosso LE. Primary biliary malignant lymphoma clinically mimicking cholangiocarcinoma: a case report and review of the literature. Ann Diagn Pathol. 2001;5:25–33.
3. Principe A, Ercolani G, Bassi F, et al. Diagnostic dilemmas in biliary strictures mimicking cholangiocarcinoma. Hepatogastroenterology. 2003;50:1246–9.
4. Hadjis NS, Collier NA, Blumgart LH. Malignant masquerade at the hilum of the liver. Br J Surg. 1985;72:659–61.
5. Wetter LA, Ring EJ, Pellegrini CA, et al. Differential diagnosis of sclerosing cholangiocarcinomas of the common hepatic duct (Klatskin tumors). Am J Surg. 1991;161:57–63.
6. Gerhards MF, Vos P, van Gulik TM, et al. Incidence of benign lesions in patients resected for suspicious hilar obstruction. Br J Surg. 2001;88:48–51.
7. Koea J, Holden A, Chau K, et al. Differential diagnosis of stenosing lesions at the hepatic hilus. World J Surg. 2004;28:466–70.
8. Standfield NJ, Salsbury JR, Howard ER. Benign non-traumatic inflammatory strictures of the extrahepatic biliary system. Br J Surg. 1989;76:849–52.
9. Verbeek PCM, van Leeuwen DJ, de Wit LT, et al. Benign fibrosing disease at the hepatic confluence mimicking Klatskin tumors. Surgery. 1992;112:866–71.
10. Nakayama A, Imamura H, Shimada R, et al. Proximal bile duct stricture disguised as malignant neoplasm. Surgery. 1999;125: 514–25.
11. Knoefel WT, Prenzel KL, Peiper M, et al. Klatskint tumors and Klatskin mimicking lesions of the biliary tree. Eur J Surg Oncol. 2003;29:658–61.
12. Park MS, Kim TK, Kim KW, et al. Differentiation of extrahepatic bile duct cholangiocarcinoma from benign stricture: findings at MRCP versus ERCP. Radiology. 2004;233:234–40.
13. Corvera CU, Blumgart LH, Darvishian H, et al. Clinical and pathologic features of proximal biliary strictures masquerading as hilar cholangiocarcinoma. J Am Coll Surg. 2005;201:862–9.
14. Uhlmann D, Wiedmann M, Schmidt F, et al. Management and outcome in patients with Klatskin-mimicking lesions of the biliary tree. J Gastrointest Surg. 2006;10:1144–50.
15. Are C, Gonen M, DÁngelica M, et al. Differential diagnosis of proximal biliary obstruction. Surgery. 2006;140:756–63.

16. Saluja SS, Sharma R, Paul S, et al. Differentiation between benign and malignant hilar obstructions using laboratory and radiological investigations: a prospective study. HPB. 2007;9:373–82.
17. Kloek JJ, van Delden OM, Erdogan D, et al. Differentiation of malignant and benign proximal bile duct strictures: the diagnostic dilemma. World J Gastroenterol. 2008;14:5032–8.
18. Erdogan D, Kloek JJ, ten Kate FJW, et al. Immunoglobulin G4-related sclerosing cholangitis in patients resected for presumed malignant bile duct strictures. Br J Surg. 2008;95:727–34.
19. te Boekhorst DS, Gerhards MF, van Gulik TM, et al. Granular cell tumor at the hepatic duct confluence mimicking Klatskin tumor. Dig Surg. 2000;17:299–303.
20. Binkley CE, Eckhauser FE, Colleti LM. Unusual cases of benign biliary strictures with cholangiographic features of cholangiocarcinoma. J Gastrointest Surg. 2002;6:676–81.
21. Harell GS, Anderson MF, Berry PF. Cytologic bile examination in the diagnosis of biliary duct neoplastic strictures. Am J Roentgenol. 1981;137:1123–6.
22. Evander A, Ihse I, Lunderquist A, et al. Percutaneous cytodiagnosis of carcinoma of the pancreas and bile duct. Ann Surg. 1978;188: 90–2.
23. Cohan RH, Illscas FF, Newman GE, et al. Biliary cytodiagnosis. Bile sampling for cytology. Invest Radiol. 1985;20:177–9.
24. Ponchon T, Gagnon P, Berger F, et al. Value of endobiliary brush cytology and biopsies for the diagnosis of malignant bile duct stenosis: results of a prospective study. Gastrointest Endosc. 1995; 42:565–72.
25. van Gulik TM, Reeders JW, Bosma A, et al. Incidence and clinical findings of benign inflammatory disease in patients resected for presumed pancreatic head cancer. Gastrointest Endosc. 1997; 46:417–23.
26. Andersson R, Andren-Sandberg A, Lundstedt C, et al. Implantation metastasis from gastrointestinal cancer after percutaneous puncture or biliary drainage. Eur J Surg. 1996;162:551–4.
27. Klatskin G. Adenocarcinoma of the hepatic duct at its bifurcation within the porta hepatis. An unusual tumor with distinctive clinical and pathological features. Am J Med. 1965;38:241–56.
28. Longmire Jr WP, McArthur MS. The management of extrahepatic bile duct carcinoma. Jpn J Surg. 1973;3:1–8.
29. Cameron JL, Broe P, Zuidema GD. Proximal bile duct tumors: surgical management with silastic transhepatic biliary stents. Ann Surg. 1982;196:412–9.
30. Rea DJ, Heimback JK, Rosen CB, et al. Liver transplantation with neoadjuvant chemoradiation is more effective than resection for hilar cholangiocarcinoma. Ann Surg. 2005;242:451–61.
31. Ito F, Cho CS, Rikkers LF, et al. Hilar cholangiocarcinoma: current management. Ann Surg. 2009;250:210–8.
32. Perpetuo MD, Valdivieso M, Heilbrun LK, et al. Natural history study of gallbladder cancer. A review of 36 years experience at MD Anderson Hospital and Tumor Institute. Cancer. 1978;42:330–5.
33. De Groen PC, Gores GJ, LaRusso NF, et al. Biliary tract cancers. N Engl J Med. 1999;341:1368–78.
34. Menias CO, Surabhi VR, Prasad SR, et al. Mimics of cholangiocarcinoma: spectrum of disease. Radiographics. 2008;28:1115–29.
35. Dasgupta T, Brasfield R. Metastasic melanoma: a clinicopathologic study. Cancer. 1964;15:1323–39.
36. Medina V, Darnell A, Bejarano N, et al. Primary biliary tract malignant melanoma: US, CT, and MR findings. Abdom Imaging. 2003; 28:842–6.
37. El Rassi ZS, Mohsine RM, Berger F, et al. Endocrine tumors of the extrahepatic bile ducts: pathological and clinical aspects, surgical management and outcome. Hepatogastroenterology. 2004;51: 1295–300.
38. Penna C, Nordlinger B. Surgery and local treatments of liver metastases from colorectal cancer: how to improve results. Scand J Surg. 2003;92:90–6.
39. Saha S, Bardelli A, Buckhaults P, et al. A phosphatase associated with metastasis of colorectal cancer. Science. 2001;294:1343–6.
40. Jatzko GR, Lisborg PH, Stettner HM, et al. Hepatic resection for metastases from colorectal carcinoma: a survival analysis. Eur J Cancer. 1995;31A:41–6.
41. Riopel MA, Klimstra DS, Godellas CV, et al. Intrabiliary growth of metastatic colonic adenocarcinoma: a pattern of intrahepatic spread easily confused with primary neoplasia of the biliary tract. Am J Surg Pathol. 1997;21:1030–6.
42. Rivindra KV, Stringer MD, Prasad KR, et al. Non-Hodgkin lymphoma presenting with obstructive jaundice. Br J Surg. 2003;90:845–9.
43. Das K, Fisher A, Wilson DJ, et al. Primary non-Hodgkin's lymphoma of the bile ducts mimicking cholangiocarcinoma. Surgery. 2003;134:496–500.
44. Brouland JP, Molimard J, Nemeth J, et al. Primary T-cell rich B-cell lymphoma of the common bile duct. Virchows Arch A Pathol Anat Histopathol. 1993;423:513–7.
45. Van Slyck EJ, Schuman BM. Lymphocytic lymphosarcoma of the gallbladder. Cancer. 1972;30:810–6.
46. Nguyen GK. Primary extranodal non-Hodgkin's lymphoma of the extrahepatic bile ducts. Report of a case. Cancer. 1982;50:2218–22.
47. Page RD, Romaguera JE, Osborne B, et al. Primary hepatic lymphoma: favorable outcome after combination chemotherapy. Cancer. 2001;92:2023–9.
48. Chapman RWG, Arborgh BAM, Rohdes JM, et al. Primary sclerosing cholangitis: a review of its clinical features, cholangiography, and hepatic histology. Gut. 1980;21:870–7.
49. Thompson HH, Pitt HA, Tompkins RK, et al. Primary sclerosing cholangitis: a heterogeneous disease. Ann Surg. 1982;196:127–36.
50. Broome U, Olsson R, Loof L, et al. Natural history and prognostic factors in 305 Swedish patients with primary sclerosing cholangitis. Gut. 1996;38:610–5.
51. Shaib Y, El-Serag HB. The epidemiology of cholangiocarcinoma. Semin Liver Dis. 2004;24:115–25.
52. LaRussso NF, Shneider BL, Black D, et al. Primary sclerosing cholangitis: summary of a workshop. Hepatology. 2006;44:746–64.
53. Burak K, Angulo P, Pasha TM, et al. Incidence and risk factors for cholangiocarcinoma in primary sclerosing cholangitis. Am J Gastroenterol. 2004;99:523–6.
54. Pitt HA, Dooley WC, Yeo CJ, et al. Malignancies of the biliary tree. Curr Probl Surg. 1995;32:1–90.
55. Bergquist A, Glaumann H, Persson B, et al. Risk factors and clinical presentation of hepatobiliary carcinoma in patients with primary sclerosing cholangitis: a case-control study. Hepatology. 1998;27: 311–6.
56. Abdalian R, Heathcote EJ. Sclerosing cholangitis: a focus on secondary causes. Hepatology. 2006;44:1063–74.
57. Buc E, Lesurtel M, Belghiti J. Is preoperative histological diagnosis necessary before referral to major surgery for cholangiocarcinoma? HPB. 2008;10:98–105.
58. Sasahira N, Kawabe T, Nakamura A, et al. Inflammatory pseudotumor of the liver and peripheral eosinophilia in autoimmune pancreatitis. World J Gastroenterol. 2005;11:922–5.
59. Coffin CM, Hamphrey PA, Dehner LP. Extrapulmonary inflammatory myofibroblastic tumor: a clinical and pathological survey. Semin Diagn Pathol. 1998;15:85–101.
60. Nonomura A, Minato H, Shimizu K, et al. Hepatic hilar inflammatory pseudotumor mimicking cholangiocarcinoma with cholangitis and phlebitis: a variant of primary sclerosing cholangitis? Pathol Res Pract. 1997;193:519–25.
61. Amankonah TD, Strom CB, Vierling JM, et al. Inflammatory pseudotumor of the liver as the first manifestation of Chrohn's disease. Am J Gastroenterol. 2001;96:2520–2.
62. Horiuchi R, Uchida T, Kojima T, et al. Inflammatory pseudotumor of the liver. Clinicopathological study and review of the literature. Cancer. 1990;65:1583–90.

63. Pack GT, Baker HW. Total right hepatic lobectomy; reports of a case. Ann Surg. 1953;138:253–8.
64. Yan FH, Zhou KR, Jiang YP, et al. Inflammatory pseudotumor of the liver: 13 cases of MRI findings. World J Gastroenterol. 2001;7:422–4.
65. Tublin ME, Moser AJ, Marsh JW, et al. Biliary inflammatory pseudotumor: imaging features in seven patients. AJR Am J Roentgenol. 2007;188:W44–8.
66. Zen Y, Harada K, Sasaki M, et al. IgG4-related sclerosing cholangitis with and without hepatic inflammatory pseudotumor, and sclerosing pancreatitis-associated sclerosing cholangitis: do they belong to a spectrum of sclerosing pancreatitis? Am J Surg Pathol. 2004;28:1193–203.
67. Nakayma F, Solowa RD, Nakama T, et al. Hepatolithiasis in East Asia. Retrospective study. Dig Dis Sci. 1986;31:21–6.
68. Harris HW, Kumwenda ZL, Sheen-Chen S. Recurrent pyogenic cholangitis. Am J Surg. 1998;176:34–7.
69. Seel DJ, Park YK. Oriental inflectional cholangitis. Am J Surg. 1983;146:366–70.
70. Lim JH. Oriental cholagiohepatitis: pathologic, clinical, and radiologic features. AJR Am J Roentgenol. 1991;157:1–8.
71. RM S, Koch J, Sandhu JS, et al. Recurrent pyogenic cholangitis in Asian immigrants to the United States: natural history and role of therapeutic ERCP. Dig Dis Sci. 1997;42:865–71.
72. Reynolds WR, Brinkman JD, Haney BD, et al. Oriental cholangiohepatitis. Mil Med. 1994;159:158–60.
73. Park MS, Yu JS, Kim KW, et al. Recurrent pyogenic cholangitis: comparison between MR cholangiography and direct cholangiography. Radiology. 2001;220:677–82.
74. Kim MJ, Cha SW, Mitchel DJ, et al. MR imaging findings in recurrent pyogenic cholangitis. AJR Am J Roentgenol. 1999;173:1545–9.
75. Lim JH, Ko YT, Lee DH, et al. Oriental cholangiohepatitis: sonographic findings in 48 cases. AJR Am J Roentgenol. 1990;155:511–4.
76. Chan FL, Man SW, Leong LL, et al. Evaluation of recurrent pyogenic cholangitis with CT: analysis of 50 patients. Radiology. 1989;170:165–9.
77. Coppel MS. Hepatobiliary manifestations of the acquired immune deficiency syndrome. Am J Gastroenterol. 1991;86:1–15.
78. Cello JP. Human immunodeficiency virus associated biliary tract disease. Semin Liver Dis. 1992;12:213–28.
79. Margulis SJ, Honig CL, Soave R, et al. Biliary tract obstruction in the acquired immunodeficiency syndrome. Ann Intern Med. 1986;105:207–10.
80. Bouche H, Housset C, Dumont JL. AIDS-related cholangitis: diagnostic features and course in 15 patients. J Hepatol. 1993;17:34–9.
81. Dolmatch BL, Laing FC, Ferderle MP, et al. AIDS-related cholangitis: radiographic findings in 9 patients. Radiology. 1987;163:313–6.
82. Cello JP, Chan MF. Long-term follow up of endoscopic retrograde cholangiopancreatography sphincterotomy for patients with acquired immune deficiency syndrome papillary stenosis. Am J Med. 1995;99:600–3.
83. Nash JA, Cohen SA. Gallbladder and biliary tract disease in AIDS. Gastroenterol Clin North Am. 1997;26:323–35.
84. Pol S, Romana CA, Richard S, et al. Microsporadia infection in patients with the human immunodeficiency virus and unexplained cholangitis. N Engl J Med. 1993;328:95–9.
85. Finkelberg DL, Sahani D, Deshpande V, et al. Autoimmune pancreatitis. N Engl J Med. 2006;355:2670–6.
86. Krasinskas AM, Raina A, Khalid A, et al. Autoimmune pancreatitis. Gastroenterol Clin North Am. 2007;36:239–57.
87. Ectors N, Maillet B, Aerts R, et al. Non-alcoholic duct destructive chronic pancreatitis. Gut. 1997;41:263–8.
88. Kim KP, Kim MH, Song MH, et al. Autoimmune chronic pancreatitis. Am J Gastroenterol. 2004;99:1605–16.
89. Pearson RK, Longnecker DS, Chari ST, et al. Controversy in clinical pancreatology: autoimmune pancreatitis: does it exist? Pancreas. 2003;27:1–13.
90. Kamisawa T, Egawa N, Nakajima H, et al. Clinical difficulties in the differentiation of autoimmune pancreatitis and pancreatic carcinoma. Am J Gastroenterol. 2003;98:2694–9.
91. Kamisawa T, Funata N, Hayashi Y, et al. A new clinicopathological entity of IgG4-related autoimmune disease. J Gastroenterol. 2003;38:982–4.
92. Sarin SK, Bhatia B, Makawane U. Portal biliopathy in extrahepatic portal vein obstruction. Indian J Gastroenterol. 1992;2:A82.
93. Sarin SK, Agarwal SR. Extrahepatic portal vein obstruction. Semin Liver Dis. 2002;22:43–58.
94. Dumortier J, Vaillant E, Boillot O, et al. Diagnosis and treatment of biliary obstruction caused by portal cavernoma. Endoscopy. 2003;35:446–50.
95. Condat B, Vilgrian V, Asselah T, et al. Portal cavernoma-associated cholangiopathy: a clinical and MR cholangiography coupled with MR portography imaging study. Hepatology. 2003;37:1302–8.
96. Shin SM, Kim S, Lee JW, et al. Biliary abnormalities associated with portal biliopathy: evaluation on MR cholangiography. Am J Roentgenol. 2007;188:W341–7.
97. Bayrakatar Y, Balkanci F, Kayhan B, et al. Bile duct varices or "pseudocholangiocarcinoma sign" in portal hypertension due to cavernous transformation of the portal vein. Am J Gastroenterol. 1992;87:1801–6.
98. Mirizzi PL. Sindrome del conducto hepatico. J Int Chir. 1948;8:731–7.
99. Csendes A, Diaz JC, Burdiles P, et al. Mirizzi syndrome and cholecystobiliary fistula: a unifying classification. Br J Surg. 1989;76:1139–43.
100. Johnson LW, Sehon JK, Lee WC, et al. Mirizzi's syndrome: experience from a multi-institutional review. Am Surg. 2001;67:11–4.
101. Lai ECH, Lau WY. Mirizzi syndrome: history, present and future development. ANZ J Surg. 2006;76:251–7.
102. Baer HU, Matthews JB, Schweizer WP, et al. Management of the Mirizzi syndrome and the surgical implication of cholecystocholedochal fistula. Br J Surg. 1990;77:743–5.
103. Becker CD, Hassler H, Terrier F. Preoperative diagnosis of the Mirizzi syndrome: limitations of sonography and computed tomography. AJR Am J Roentgenol. 1984;143:591–6.
104. Kunisaki SM, Hertl M, Bodner BE, et al. Mirizzi syndrome secondary to an adenoma of the cystic duct. J Hepatobiliary Pancreat Surg. 2005;12:159–62.
105. Loh A, Kamar S, Dickson GH. Solitary benign papilloma (papillary adenoma) of the cystic duct: a rare cause of biliary colic. Br J Clin Pract. 1994;48:167–8.
106. Satoh H, Hirano T, Ogawa Y, et al. Adenoma arising from the cystic duct and extending to the confluence of the extrahepatic biliary tract. J Hepatobiliary Pancreat Surg. 1999;6:186–9.
107. Allaire GS, Rabin L, Ishak KG, et al. Bile duct adenoma. A study of 152 cases. Am J Surg Pathol. 1988;12:708–15.
108. Kawakatsu M, Vilgrain V, Zins M, et al. Radiologic features of papillary adenoma and papilomatosis of the biliary tract. Abdom Imaging. 1997;22:87–90.
109. Buckley JG, Salimi Z. Villous adenoma of the common bile duct. Abdom Imaging. 1993;18:245–6.
110. Jennings PE, Rode J, Coral A, et al. Villous adenoma of the common hepatic duct: the role of ultrasound in management. Gut. 1990;31:558–60.
111. Burhans R, Meyers RT. Benign neoplasms of the extrahepatic biliary ducts. Am Surg. 1971;37:161–6.
112. Cox CE, Davis-Allen A, Judson MA. Sarcoidosis. Med Clin North Am. 2005;89:817–28.

113. Judson MA. Extrapulmonary sarcoidosis. Semin Respir Crit Care Med. 2007;28:83–101.
114. Pungpapong S, Steers JL, Wallace MB, et al. Hepatobiliary sarcoidosis mimicking Klatskin's cholangiocarcinoma. Gastrointest Endosc. 2006;64:124–5.
115. Ishak KG. Sarcoidosis of the liver and bile ducts. Mayo Clin Proc. 1998;73:467–72.
116. Alam I, Levenson SD, Ferrell LD, et al. Diffuse intrahepatic biliary strictures in sarcoidosis resembling sclerosing cholangitis. Case report and review of the literature. Dig Dis Sci. 1997;42: 1295–301.
117. Howard TJ, Bennion RS, Thompson Jr JE. Xanthogranulomatous cholecystitis: a chronic inflammatory pseudotumor of the gallbladder. Am Surg. 1991;57:821–4.
118. Kwon AH, Matsui Y, Uemura Y. Surgical procedures and histopathologic findings for patients with xanthogranulomatous cholecystitis. J Am Coll Surg. 2004;199:204–10.
119. Dixit VK, Prakash A, Gupta A, et al. Xanthogranulomatous cholecystitis. Dig Dis Sci. 1998;43:940–2.
120. Benbow EW. Xanthogranulomatous cholecystitis. Br J Surg. 1990;77:255–6.
121. Shuto R, Kiyosue H, Komatsu E, et al. CT and MR imaging findings of xanthogranulomatous cholecystitis: correlation with pathologic findings. Eur Radiol. 2004;14:440–6.
122. Kawate S, Ohawada S, Ikota H, et al. Xanthogranulomatous cholangitis causing obstructive jaundice: a case report. World J Gastroenterol. 2006;12:4428–30.
123. Krishna RP, Kumar A, Singh RK, et al. Xanthogranulomatous inflammatory strictures of extrahepatic biliary tract: presentation and surgical management. J Gastrointest Surg. 2008;12: 836–41.
124. Batts KP. Ischemic cholangitis. Mayo Clin Proc. 1998;73:380–5.
125. Alazmi WM, McHenry L, Watkins JL, et al. Chemotherapy-induced sclerosing cholangitis: long-term response to endoscopic therapy. J Clin Gastroenterol. 2006;40:353–7.
126. Barnett KT, Malafa MP. Complications of hepatic artery infusion: a review of 4580 reported cases. Int J Gastrointest Cancer. 2001; 30:147–60.
127. Lorenz M, Muller HH. Randomized multicenter trial of fluorouracil plus leucoverin administered either via hepatic arterial or intravenous infusion versus fluorodeoxyuridine administered via hepatic arterial infusion in patients with non-resectable liver metastases from colorectal carcinoma. J Clin Oncol. 2000;18: 243–54.
128. Martin RC, Edwards MJ, McMasters KM. Morbidity of adjuvant hepatic arterial infusion pump chemotherapy in the management of colorectal cancer metastatic to the liver. Am J Surg. 2004;188: 714–21.
129. Kerr DJ, McArdle SC, Ledermann J, et al. Intrahepatic arterial versus intravenous fluorouracil and folinic acid for colorectal cancer liver metastases: a multicenter randomized trial. Lancet. 2003; 361:368–73.
130. Kemeny N, Huang Y, Cohen AM, et al. Hepatic arterial infusion of chemotherapy after resection of hepatic metastases from colorectal cancer. N Engl J Med. 1999;341:2039–48.
131. Hohn D, Melnick J, Stagg R, et al. Biliary sclerosis in patients receiving hepatic arterial infusion of floxuridine. J Clin Oncol. 1985;3:98–102.

Molecular Markers of Cholangiocarcinoma

10

J.Y.H. Chan, K.K.H. Lee, and Y.L. Chui

10.1 Introduction

Bile is a fluid that helps us to digest food and its main function is to break down fats in food. Bile is made by the liver and stored in the gall bladder. Bile ducts are tubes that carry bile and they connect the liver and the gall bladder to the duodenum and the small intestine. In people who have had their gall bladders removed, bile flows directly from the liver into the duodenum and the small intestine. The bile ducts and gall bladder are known as the biliary system (Fig. 10.1). Cholangiocarcinoma (CC) is a malignant tumor arising from the bile duct epithelium. They start in mucus glands that line the bile ducts. If cancer starts in the part of the bile ducts within the liver it is known as intra-hepatic. If it starts in bile ducts outside the liver it is known as extra-hepatic. It may arise from the right and left hepatic ducts at or near their junction (hilar cholangiocarcinoma) which are considered as carcinoma of the extrahepatic bile ducts (for a review, please see Refs. [1–8]). Cancers of the biliary system are almost always adenocarcinomas. The incidence of cholangiocarcinoma reveals wide geographic variations: the highest incidence is reported in areas suffering from endemic infestation with liver fluke. The liver flukes, *Opisthorchis viverrini* and *Clonorchis sinensis*, which induce cholangiocarcinomas, are common in Africa and Asia, especially in Thailand and Laos in Southeast Asia, and in some parts of China. Intrahepatic cholangiocarcinoma is the second most prevalent intrahepatic primary cancer. Hilar cholangiocarcinoma is the fourth most common gastrointestinal malignancy.

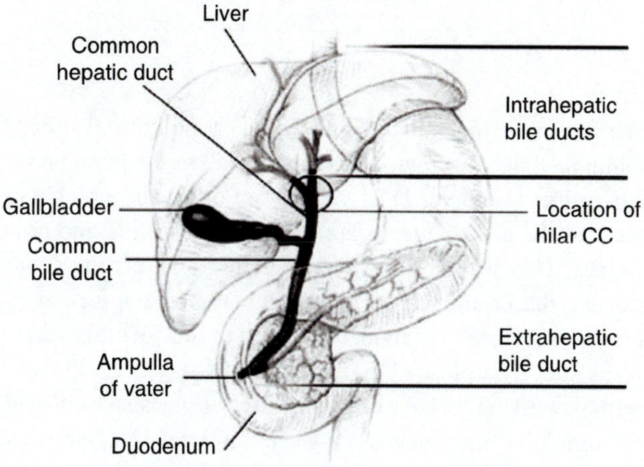

Fig. 10.1 The Biliary systems (Bile duct). Bile ducts are tubes that carry bile and they connect the liver and the gall bladder to the duodenum as shown

10.2 Molecular Carcinogenesis of Cholangiocarcinoma

The development of cholangiocarcinoma, similar to other types of cancer, can be divided into at least three stages, namely, Initiation, Promotion and Progression [9, 10]. A molecular scheme of cholangiocarcinoma development, and the various factors that affect the development of cholangiocarcinoma are shown in Fig. 10.2. The etiological factors of cholangiocarcinoma can be broadly divided into genetic/epigenetic factors and environmental factors. The Initiation stage of carcinogenesis involves damages and genetic/epigenetic alterations of the genome. Increased carcinogenic nitroso-compounds as a result of regional dietary factors or environmental contaminants, are thought to produce genetic

J.Y.H. Chan, PhD (✉)
Joint JNU-CUHK Key Laboratories of Regenerative Medicine, Ministry of Education, Jinan University, Guangzhou, China
e-mail: chanjyh01@hotmail.com

K.K.H. Lee, PhD
Stem Cell & Regeneration Thematic Research Program, School of Biomedical Sciences, The Chinese University of Hong Kong, Shatin, New Territories, Hong Kong

Y.L. Chui, PhD
Department of Chemical Pathology, The Chinese University of Hong Kong, Shatin, New Territories, Hong Kong

W.Y. Lau (ed.), *Hilar Cholangiocarcinoma*,
DOI 10.1007/978-94-007-6473-6_10, © Springer Science+Business Media Dordrecht and People's Medical Publishing House 2013

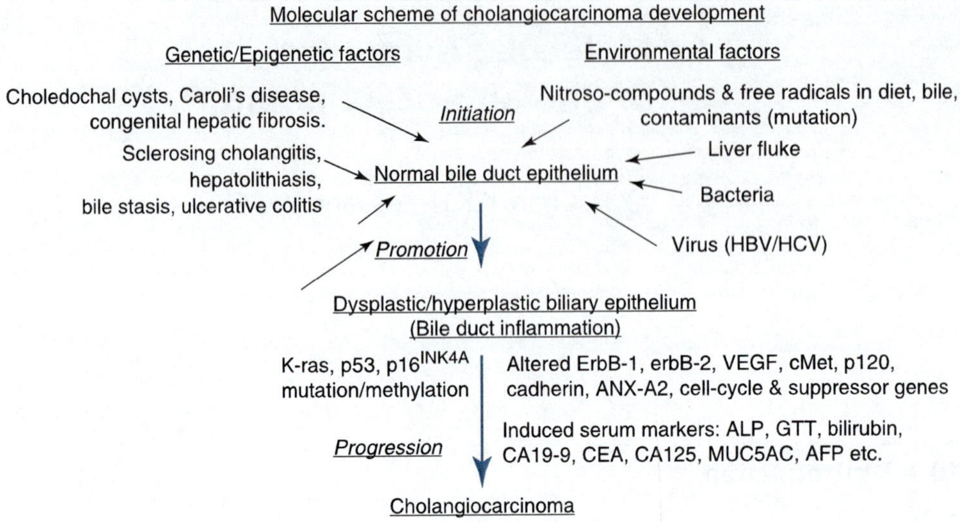

Fig. 10.2 A molecular scheme of cholangiocarcinoma development. The various factors that affect the development of cholangiocarcinoma are presented. The etiological factors of cholangiocarcinoma can be divided broadly as genetic/epigenetic factors and environmental factors. The developmental process can be divided into three stages, namely 1st stage: Initiation, 2nd stage: Promotion, and 3rd stage: Progression

changes including mutations in DNA of the normal biliary epithelial cells. The mutations are "fixed" in the genome by subsequent rounds of DNA replication or repair, which can occur as the bile duct cells are stimulated to divide and proliferate. This becomes the second step of the carcinogenic process, the Promotion stage, which may proceed further as a result of chronic inflammation of the tissues. At this stage, dysplastic/hyperplastic biliary epithelium may develop from normal epithelial cells. Liver fluke infestation causes chronic inflammation and enhances susceptibility of the bile duct epithelium to carcinogens/free radicals, leading to genetic and epigenetic changes in cells.

Hepatolithiasis, the presence of stones in the bile ducts of the liver, is associated with a high-risk for intrahepatic cholangiocarcinoma because of recurrent bacterial infections and bile stasis. It is more frequently seen in East Asian than in Western countries. Hepatitis virus infection has also been reported as a risk factor for cholangiocarcinoma. Infection by hepatitis virus may contribute to the stage of promotion by inducing chronic inflammation, cell-death and cell-proliferation. However, the relationship between HBV/HCV and cholangiocarcinoma formation is not unequivocally established. Recent reports indicated that hepatitis C and hepatitis B nucleic acids as well as viral proteins are present in intrahepatic cholangiocarcinomas [11–13].

In addition, primary sclerosing cholangitis (PSC), another risk factor, is a chronic liver condition producing progressive inflammation and scarring of the bile ducts of the liver [6]. The inflammation impedes flow of bile to the gut, which can ultimately lead to liver cirrhosis, liver failure and liver cancer. The underlying cause of inflammation is believed to be due to autoimmunity. Patients with primary sclerosing cholangitis have a tendency to develop bile duct carcinoma. Moreover, inflammatory bowel disease (IBD), such as ulcerative colitis, is a chronic inflammatory bowel condition. People with this disease are also at an increased risk of developing cholangiocarcinoma. It is of interest to note that patients with congenital abnormal bile duct diseases, such as choledochal cysts, Caroli's disease and congenital hepatic fibrosis, are more at risk of developing cholangiocarcinoma. Other genetic/epigenetic defects that may contribute to the development of cholangiocarcinoma include drug detoxification defect (MGMT), DNA repair defect (hMLH1) and excessive production of pro-inflammatory cytokines.

The third stage of development of cholangiocarcinoma is the Progression stage, which involves the transition of dysplastic/hyperplastic biliary epithelium to become carcinoma of the bile-duct. At this stage, many critical genes that have been altered can be detected, especially the proto-oncogenes and tumor suppressor genes, for example, p53 [14–16], p16^{INK4A} [17–22], ErbB-1, erbB-2, VEGF [23–27], K-ras [28–31], cMet, p120, Cadherin and many Cell-cycle genes. Induced serum markers such as ALP, GTT, bilirubin, Ca19-9, CA125, CEA, MUC5AC are found. Cholangiocarcinomas can arise in the absence of any known etiological factors.

10.3 "Yin-Yang" Negative- and Positive-Control Hypothesis of Cholangiocarcinoma Cell Development

Similar to other kinds of cancer including hepatocellular carcinoma [9], the development of cancer cells of the bile-duct epithelium may be considered as Yin-Yang or negative-positive control of cell-growth and cell-death. As shown in Fig. 10.3, the "Yang" factors usually refer to the growth factors, receptors, cellular signal transducers and nuclear transcriptional factors which are mostly proto-oncogenes that promote cellular proliferation and survival. On the other hand the "Yin" factors are molecules that suppress cell-growth

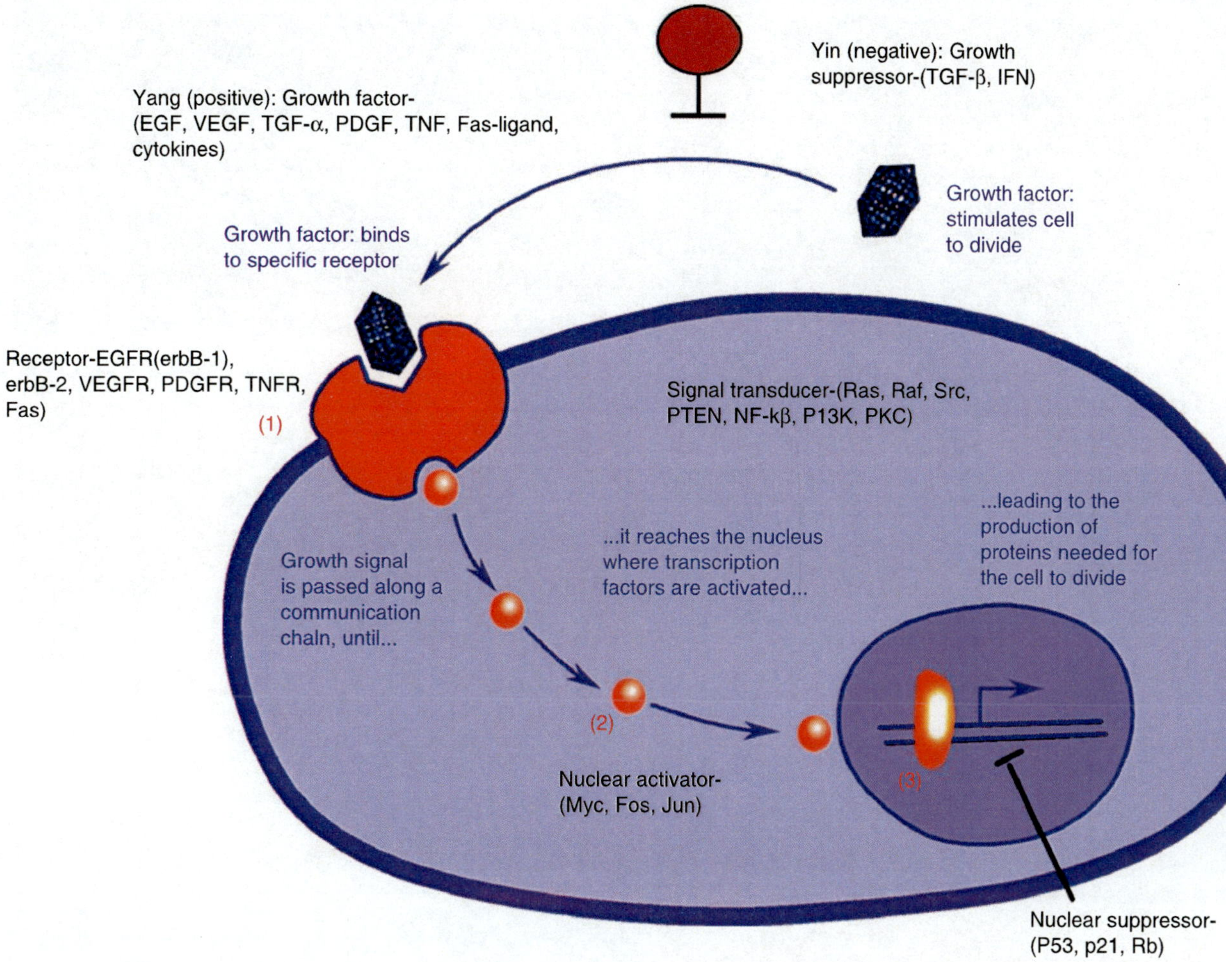

Fig. 10.3 "Yin-Yang" Negative- and positive-control hypothesis of cholangiocarcinoma cell development. The development of cancer cells of the bile-duct epithelium may be considered as Yin-Yang or negative-positive control of cell-growth and cell-death

and facilitate cell-death including apoptosis. It is the delicate interplay and regulation of expression and action of these positive and negative modulators that result in the control-growth of a normal cell. Mutations and/or altered expression in proto-oncogenes and suppressor genes lead to aberrant functions of proteins, which in turn may induce abnormal growth and differentiation of the cells.

10.4 Molecular Markers of Cholangiocarcinoma

The histology of cholangiocarcinoma with H and E staining is shown in Fig. 10.4a, b. Figure 10.4a shows a typical cholangiocarcinoma (glandular type with numerous fibrous stromal-regions), and Fig. 10.4b shows a papillary type with mucous and intraluminal papillary masses. The expressions of several important molecular markers such as K-ras (Fig. 10.4c), CK19 (Fig. 10.4d, e), and tumor suppressor p16INK4A (Fig. 10.4f), are also shown [21].

10.5 Tumor Suppressor Gene P53 Mutation

The wild-type p53 plays an important role in the regulation of the cell cycle process, cell growth, and apoptosis in the event of DNA damage. It is also known as the gate-keeper for these important cellular events. P53 encodes a phosphorylated protein with a molecular weight of 53 kD. It is the most commonly mutated tumor suppressor gene associated with human cancer, being abnormal in over 50 % of known human cancers [14–16]. The suppressor p53 protein is involved in many pathways by interacting with many gene products including transcription, DNA repair, cell cycling and genomic stability. DNA damages stabilize p53 which binds to p53 control elements in genes and activate transcription. These p53 modulating genes include cell-cycle genes such as p21CIP/WAF1, a cyclin kinase inhibitor, BAX and Fas for apoptosis, and GADD45 for DNA repair. Alternatively, p53 may form protein-protein complexes with proteins of DNA synthesis and repair such as RPA, topoisomerase I and XPD helicase. Mutated p53 is also more stable and render

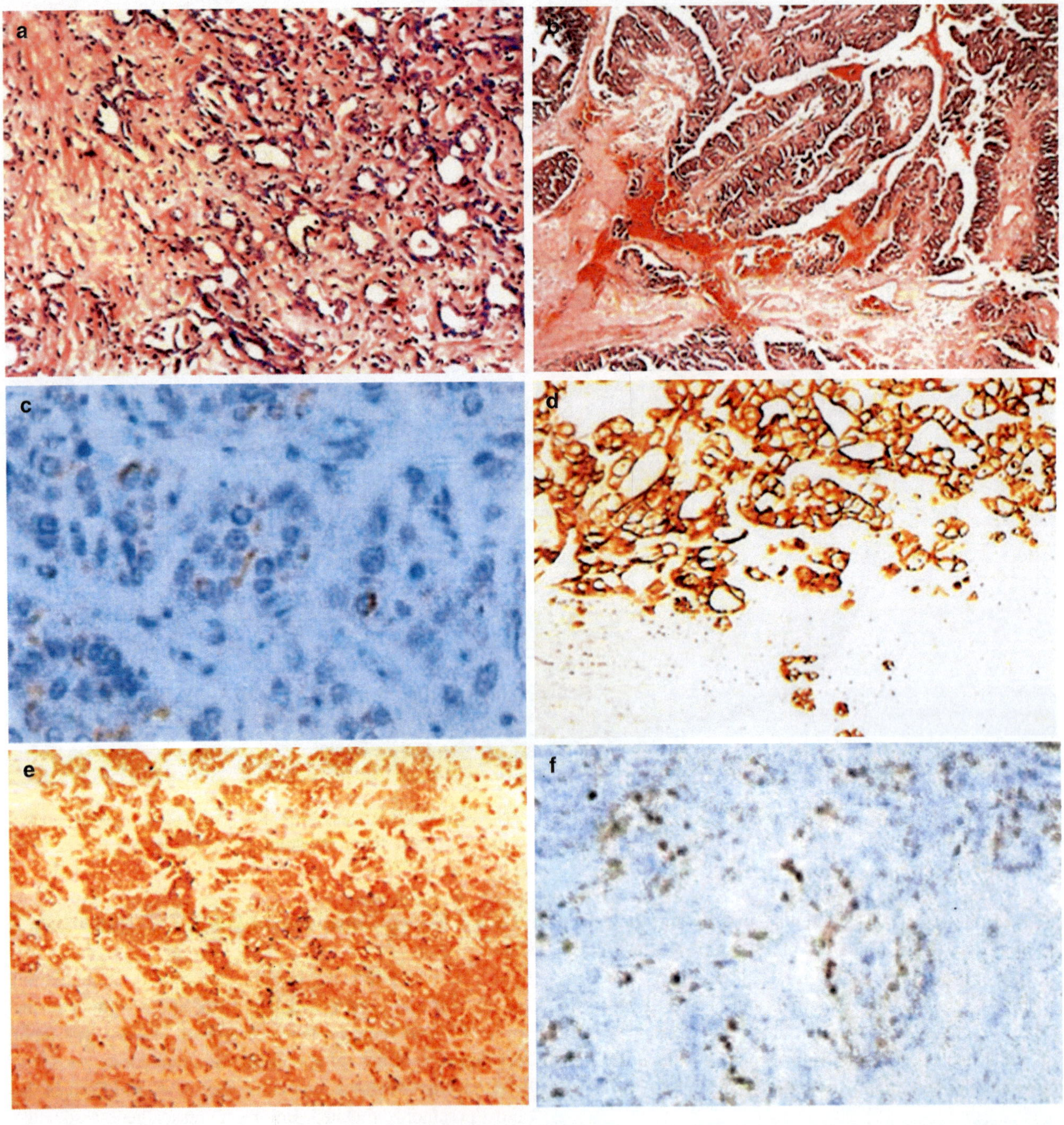

Fig. 10.4 The histology and molecular markers of cholangiocarcinoma H and E staining and markers of cholangiocarcinoma are shown. Cholangiocarcionoma (**a**, **b**: H&E), (**a**) is an adenocarcinoma with numerous fibrous stromal regions, and (**b**) is a papillary cholangiocarcinoma with intraluminal papillary masses. The expressions (immunohistochemical stainings) of K-ras (**c**), CK19 (**d**, **e**), and p16 (**f**) are also shown [21]

cells to escape from cell-cycle arrest, delay in S-phase synthesis, and apoptosis.

The p53 gene is resided on the short arm of chromosome 17 (17p13.1). Inactivation of the p53 gene by missense or nonsense mutations and by loss of chromosome 17p, induces disruption of critical growth-regulating mechanisms and may have a crucial role in carcinogenesis. The reported incidence of p53 mutation is 11–37 % in intrahepatic cholangiocarcinomas [14]. It has been reported that loss of chromosome 17p was present in 38 % of intrahepatic cholangiocarcinomas [9]. It has also been documented that there are over 90 different types of p53 mutations found in cholangiocarcinoma p53 database, by the International Agency for Research on Cancer (IARC). The codon distribution and mutation pattern is described in Figs. 10.5 and 10.6. The spectrum of mutations for p53 apparently is specific for the populations in different regions and presumably for the carcinogens. Over 50 % of mutated p53 in

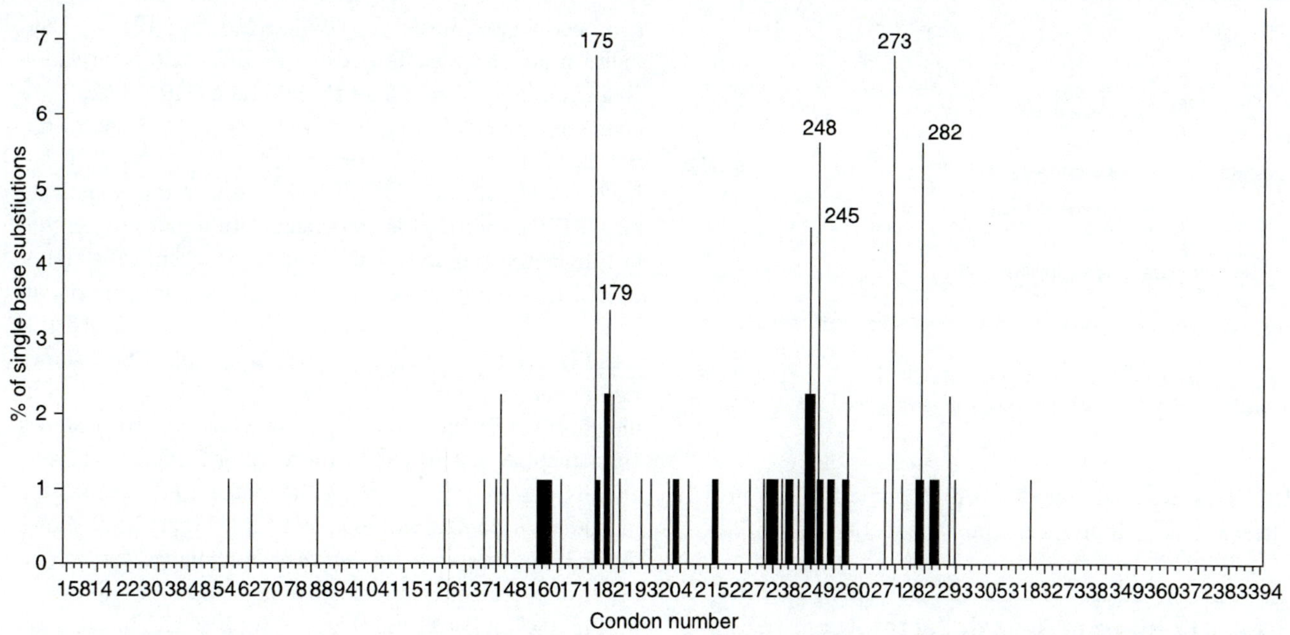

Fig. 10.5 Tumor suppressor gene P53 mutation distribution in cholangiocarcinoma. Codon distribution of p53 single base substitutions in cholangiocarcinoma. The bar chart shows the proportion of all reported single base substitutions at each codon of p53 in cholangiocarcinoma which is the number of single base substitutions at each codon divided by the total number of single base substitutions [14]

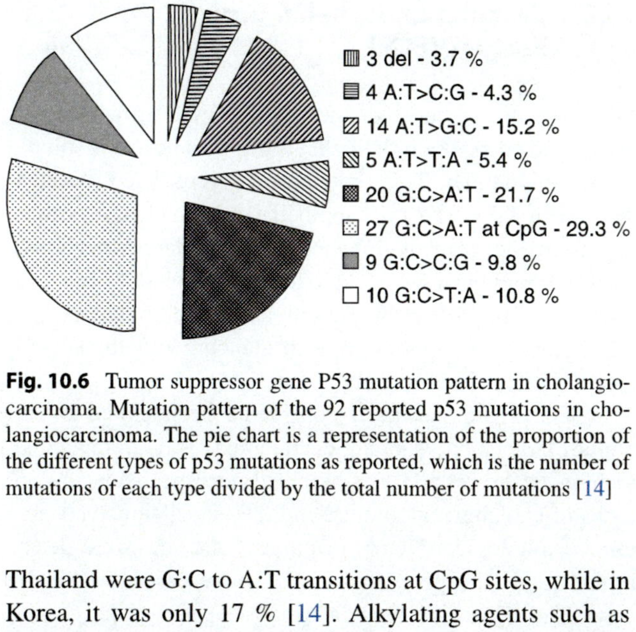

Fig. 10.6 Tumor suppressor gene P53 mutation pattern in cholangiocarcinoma. Mutation pattern of the 92 reported p53 mutations in cholangiocarcinoma. The pie chart is a representation of the proportion of the different types of p53 mutations as reported, which is the number of mutations of each type divided by the total number of mutations [14]

Thailand were G:C to A:T transitions at CpG sites, while in Korea, it was only 17 % [14]. Alkylating agents such as N-nitroso compounds, tend to induce G:C to A:T transitions in genes via the formation of O-6-methylguanine. Mutation in p53 is apparently dependent on environmental factors and carcinogens exposed, which may vary in different populations and locations. Figure 10.5 shows the mutation distribution of p53 in cholangiocarcinoma. The codon distribution of p53 single base substitutions in cholangiocarcinoma indicates that the mutation hotspots are at codons 175, 179, 245, 248, 273 and 282 respectively [14]. In Fig. 10.6, the mutation pattern of the 92 reported p53 mutations in cholangiocarcinoma is shown. This is the proportion of the different types of p53 mutations as reported, which is the number of mutations of each type divided by the total number of mutations [14]. The most commonly reported type of mutation is at CpG sites (29.3 %), which was found in over 50 % of p53 mutations in Thai patients. Alkylating agents such as N-nitroso compounds tend to induce G:C-A:T transitions in p53 via the formation of O-6-methylguanine [14]. It is apparently dependent on environmental factors including differences in nature or dose of exposure, which vary in different populations.

10.6 Tumor Suppressor P16^{INK4A} Alteration and Methylation

p16^{INK4A} is a regulatory protein in the cell cycle and a cyclin-dependent kinase (cdk4/cdk6) inhibitor. The tumor suppressor gene p16 is commonly inactivated in many neoplasms. Three distinct mechanisms of p16 inactivation have been reported in biliary neoplasms: deletion and point mutations of the p16 gene, and hypermethylation of 5′ regulatory regions of p16 [17–22]. As shown in Fig. 10.7, the methylation pattern of the promoter region of p16 shows increased methylation in the tumor tissues as compared to the non-tumor tissues. The increased methylation is a mechanism for down-regulating the expression of the gene. A study of intrahepatic cholangiocarcinomas reports that no p16 gene mutations are present but alterations of p16 gene are frequent: methylation of CpG island is present in the 5′ region of the gene (54 %), allelic loss at the p16 locus on chromosome 9p21 (20 %), and homozygous deletion (5 %). Therefore, the p16 gene may possibly be crucial for intrahepatic biliary carcinogenesis and progression. This is somewhat similar to

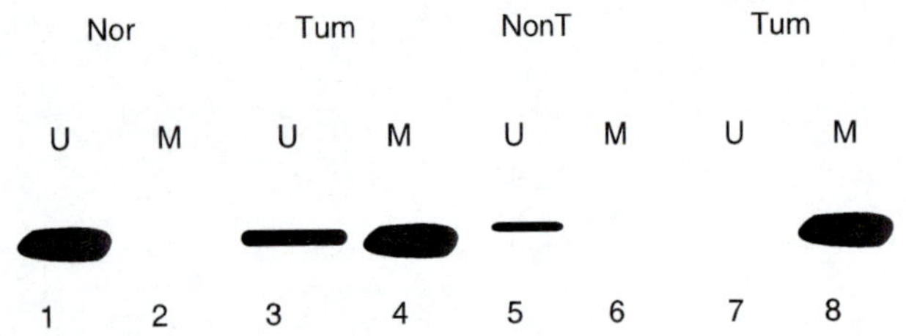

U: unmethylated, M: methylated

Fig. 10.7 Tumor suppressor p16[INK4A] methylation in cholangiocarcinoma. Methylation analysis of p16 promoter region in normal, non cholangiocarcinoma. Methylation specific PCR results are expressed as unmethylated p16 specific bands (*U*) and methylated bands (*M*) [21]

HCCs as we had reported which contain multiple p16 alternations including deletions and methylations [22].

10.7 Epidermal Growth Factor Receptor (EGFR) Family ErbB-1 and ErbB-2

This is the family of the avian erythroblastic leukemia viral (v-erb-b) oncogene homolog. They are members of the Epidermal growth factor receptor subfamily (EGFR), which are typeItyrosine kinase receptors, and can bind EGF and TGF-α. ErbB-1 (HER1) and ErbB-2 (HER2) share approximately 40 % homology in their extracellular binding domains. On the other hand, ErbB-2 has no ligand binding domain of its own and therefore cannot bind growth factors. However, it does bind tightly to other ligand-bound EGF receptor family members to form a heterodimer, stabilizing ligand binding and enhancing kinase-mediated activation of downstream signalling pathways. Amplification and overexpression of c-erbB-2 are frequently seen in cancers of the biliary tract [23–26]. It has been reported that a high incidence of cholangiocarcinomas (intrahepatic and extrahepatic) and gallbladder cancers developed in transgenic mice overexpressing ErbB-2. Reported values of the frequency of tumors overexpressing ErbB-2 varies from 0 to 73 %.

In another report, 44 % of intrahepatic cholangiocarcinoma are ErbB-1-positive and that ErbB-1 expression is correlated with grade and proliferative index [26]. Immunohistochemical expression of these molecules was assessed retrospectively in 236 cases of cholangiocarcinoma, as well as the associations between the expression of these molecules and clinicopathological factors or clinical outcome. The proportions of positive cases for EGFR and HER2 overexpression were 27.4, and 0.9 % in intrahepatic cholangiocarcinoma (IHCC), and 19.2 and 8.5 % in extrahepatic cholangiocarcinoma (EHCC), respectively. EGFR overexpression was associated with macroscopic type ($P=0.0120$), lymph node metastasis ($P=0.0006$), tumor stage ($P=0.0424$), lymphatic vessel invasion ($P=0.0371$), and perineural invasion ($P=0.0459$) in EHCC, and multivariate analysis showed that EGFR expression was a significant prognostic factor [hazard ratio (HR), 2.67; 95 % confidence interval (CI), 1.52–4.69; $P=0.0006$] and also a risk factor for tumor recurrence (HR, 1.89; 95 % CI, 1.05–3.39, $P=0.0335$) in IHCC. These results strongly indicate that EGFR expression is associated with tumor progression in cholangiocarcinoma. The immunohistochemical staining of EGFR family members in cholangiocarcinoma is shown in Fig. 10.8. Figure 10.8a is EGFR, Fig. 10.8b is HER2, and Fig. 10.8c is VEGF. In addition, Fig. 10.8d shows Epidermal growth factor receptor tends to be expressed in the poorly differentiated component while Fig. 10.8e shows Human epidermal growth factor receptor 2, which is preferentially expressed in more differentiated areas such as the glandular or papillary component [26]. Figure 10.9 shows the EGFR expression and survival in cholangiocarcinoma. Survival curves of EGFR-positive and -negative expression in (Fig. 10.9a), IHCC and (Fig. 10.9b), EHCC. The outcome of EGFR-positive cases was significantly worse than that of EGFR-negative cases in both IHCC and EHCC [26].

10.8 Vascular Endothelial Growth Factor (VEGF)

This gene is a member of the PDGF/VEGF growth factor family and encodes a protein that is often found as a disulfide linked homodimer. This protein is a glycosylated mitogen that specifically acts on endothelial cells and has various effects, including mediating increased vascular permeability, inducing angiogenesis, vasculogenesis and endothelial cell growth, promoting cell migration, and inhibiting apoptosis. VEGF plays an important role in inducing endothelial cell growth and in promoting angiogenesis.

VEGF which has been considered as potential therapeutic targets in cholangiocarcinoma and immunohistochemical expression was assessed retrospectively in 236 cases of cholangiocarcinoma, and the associations between clinicopathological factors or clinical outcome were determined [26]. The proportions of positive cases for VEGF were 53.8 % overexpression in intrahepatic cholangiocarcinoma (IHCC), and 59.2 % in extrahepatic cholangiocarcinoma (EHCC), respectively. Clinicopathologically, VEGF overexpression was related to intrahepatic metastasis ($P=0.0224$) in IHCC. These results suggest that VEGF expression may be involved in haematogenic metastasis in cholangiocarcinoma. Another report showed that VEGF A expression was more frequently encountered in peripheral cholangiocarcinoma (69 % vs. 25 %, $P<0.0001$) and correlated with increased vascular density [27]. Thus, VEGF is a potentially useful marker in predicting metastasis and angiogenesis in cholangiocarcinoma.

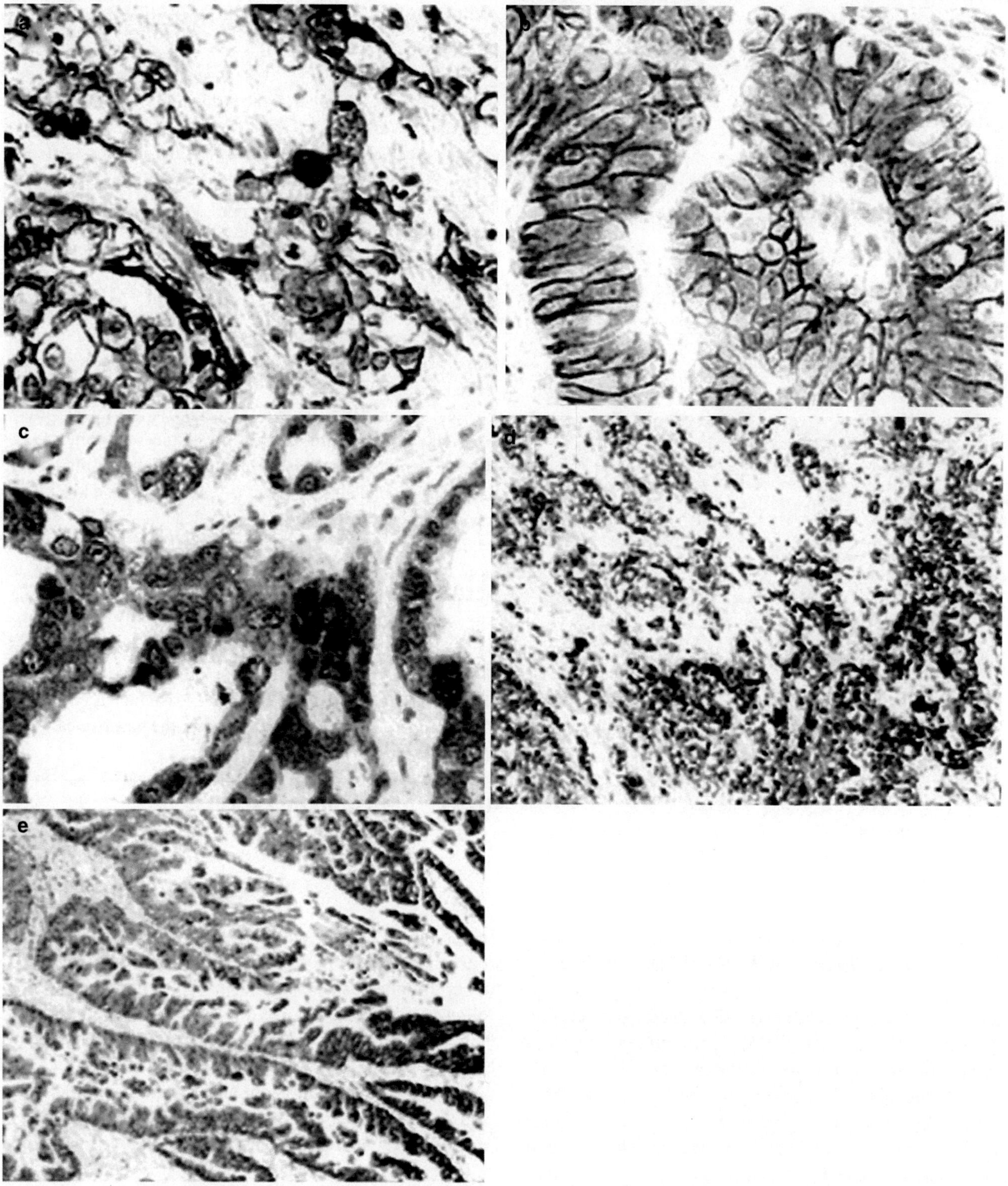

Fig. 10.8 EGFR immunohistochemical staining in cholangiocarcinoma. Immunohistochemical staining of (**a**) EGFR, (**b**) HER2, and (**c**) VEGF in cholangiocarcinoma. (**d**) Epidermal growth factor receptor tends to be expressed in the poorly differentiated component. (**e**) Human epidermal growth factor receptor 2 is preferentially expressed in more differentiated areas such as the glandular or papillary component [26]

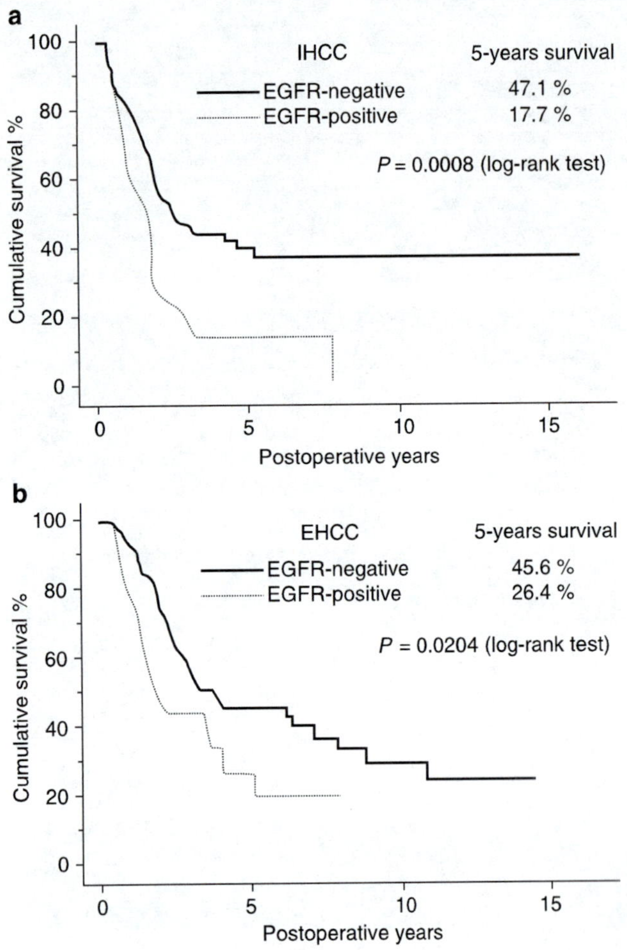

Fig. 10.9 EGFR expression and survival in cholangiocarcinoma. Survival curves of EGFR-positive and -negative expression in (**a**), IHCC and (**b**), EHCC. The outcome of EGFR-positive cases was significantly worse than that of EGFR-negative cases in both IHCC and EHCC (26)

10.9 Proto-Oncogene K-ras Mutation

K-ras is a proto-oncogene of GTP-GDP binding protein family with GTPase activity. The K-ras proto-oncogene is thought to exert control over the mechanisms of cell growth and differentiation. This gene is converted to an active oncogene by point mutations, significantly concentrated in codons 12, 13 or 61, similar to the H-ras mutations in other tumors. The reported rates of K-ras mutations in intrahepatic cholangiocarcinomas vary widely (28–32]. Variations are caused by racial and geographic variations, and the use of different assay techniques, for example, a mutation rate of 50–56 % was found in Japanese patients versus 0–8 % in Thai patients. It has been reported that mutation rates are higher in periductal and spicular-forming tumors than mass-forming ones. The expression of K-ras in cholangiocarcinoma is shown in Fig. 10.4c.

10.10 Reduced Expression of P120 Catenin and Cadherin

P120-catenin is a member of the Armadillo (ARM)/β-catenin gene family and is essential for mesenchymal cadherin-mediated regulation of cell motility and invasiveness. Altered expression of beta-catenin was reported in intrahepatic cholangiocarcinoma [32]. On the other hand, Cadherin, one of the transmembrane cell-cell adhesion receptors involved in development, and morphogenesis of intrahepatic cholangiocarcinoma (ICC), is necessary and sufficient for P120 targeting cell-cell junctions. P120 is to stabilize cadherins at the cell membrane by regulating cadherin turnover and degradation. P120 may stabilize cell junctions or regulate membrane trafficking machinery. Down-regulated expression of E-cadherin and P120 occurs frequently in ICC which may contribute to the progression and development of tumor [33]. Both of them may be valuable biologic markers for predicting tumor invasion, metastasis and patients' survival, and P120 is an independent prognostic factor for ICC [34]. In Fig. 10.10, reduced E cadherin (A–C) and p120 catenin (D–F) expression by immunohistochemistry in cholangiocarcinoma is shown. Figure. 10.10a, d are the preserved type, while Fig. 10.10b, e are the reduced type, and Fig. 10.10c, f are the complete absent type [33]. Figure 10.11 shows the correlation of survival of patients against the expression of p120 catenin (Fig. 10.11a) and E-cadherin (Fig. 10.11b). Increased survivals were found in the positive cases, vs. the negative cases.

10.11 Up-Regulated Expression of the Multi-Functional Receptor Annexin A2 (ANXA2) and its Ligand Tenascin

In one recent study, membrane protein was extracted from four cholangiocarcinoma (CC) cell lines with different tumor forming capabilities [35]. Two-dimensional-PAGE followed by MALDI-TOF-MS was used to identify differentially expressed proteins. Among 20 up-regulated membrane proteins identified in the CC cell lines was ANXA2, a participant in tumor invasion and metastasis in other cancers. ANXA2 expression was verified in human subjects by probing, using monoclonal antibody and a tissue microarray of CC (301 diagnosed cases), where it was found to associate with one of several tumor progression stages as reflected by lymphatic invasion ($P=0.014$) and metastasis ($P=0.026$). Patients with high expressions of ANXA2 had a significantly shorter survival time ($P=0.011$). ANXA2 expression in tumors may be useful for predicting the poor outcome of CC patients. We also had found that the expression of ANXA2 was up-regulated in hepatocellular carcinoma (Chan et al., unpublished data). These results indicated that

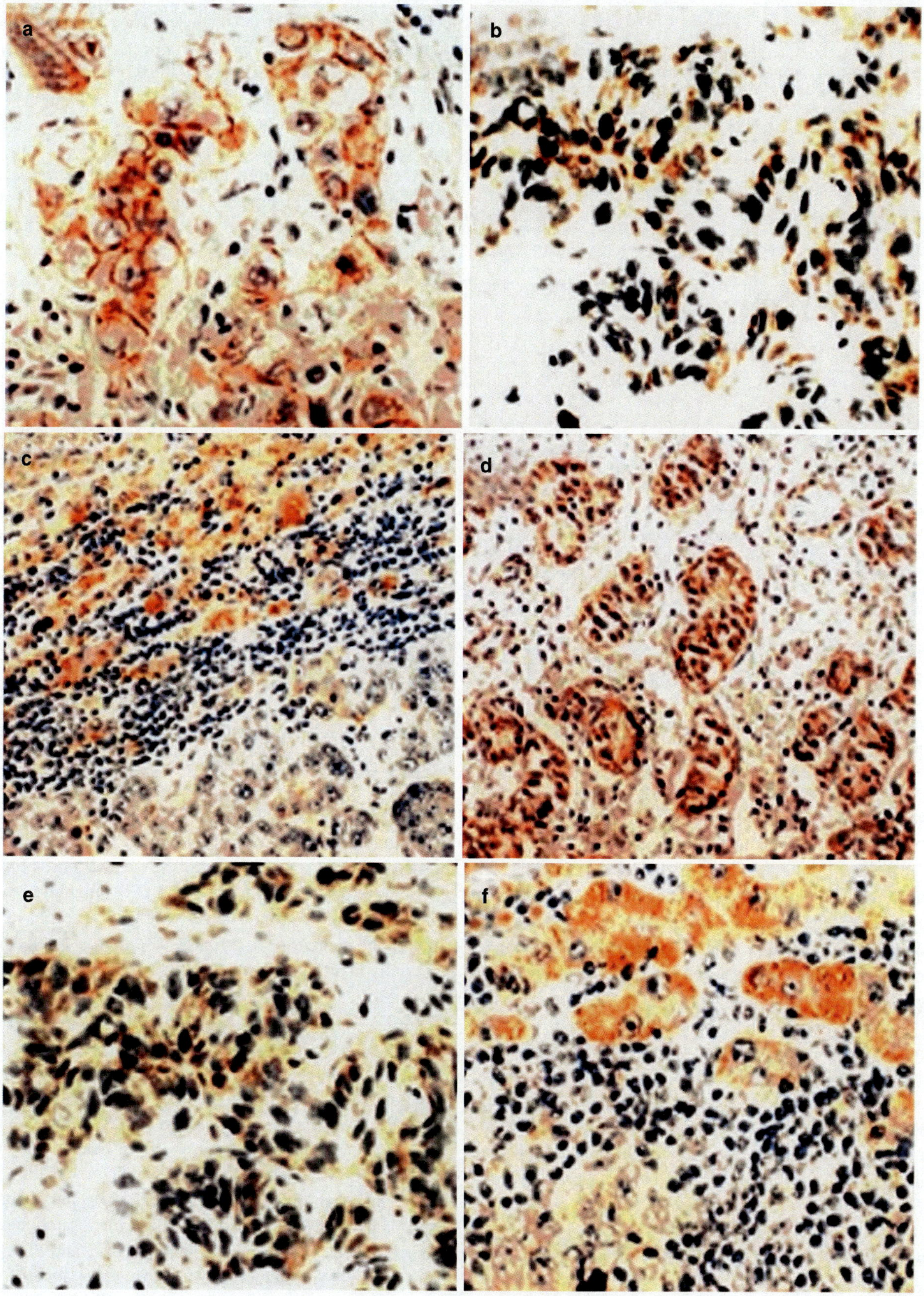

Fig. 10.10 Reduced p120 and cacherin expression in cholangiocarcinoma. Immunostaining of E-cadherin and p120 catenin in intrahepatic cholangiocarcinoma. (**a**, **d**) Preserved type, (**b**, **e**) reduced type, and (**c**, **f**) completely absent type [33]

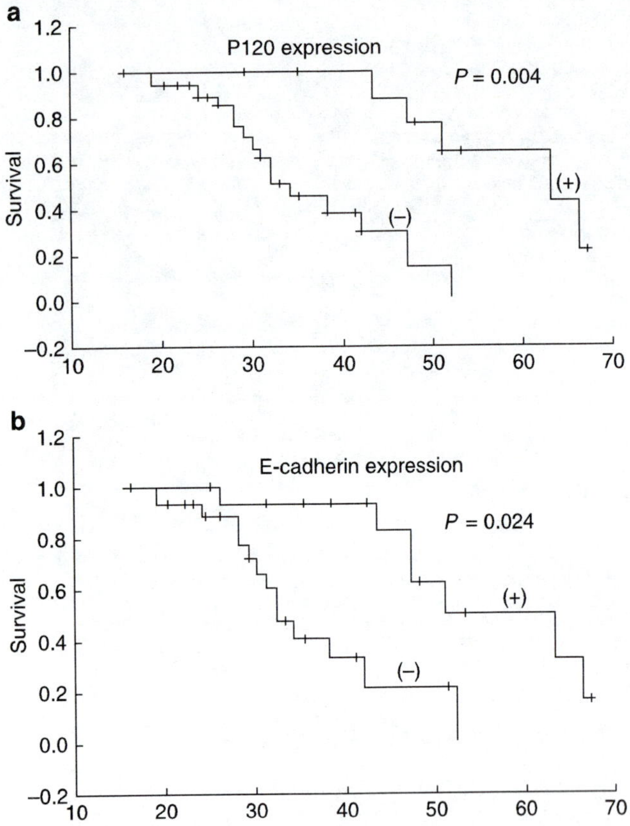

Fig. 10.11 Correlation of p120 cadherin expression and survival in cholangiocarcinoma. (**a**) Survival curve of p120-catenin positive and negative cholangiocarcinoma. (**b**) Survival curve of E-cadherin positive and negative cholangiocarcinoma [33]

ANXA2 could be a useful biomarker for different kinds of hepatic malignancies. In addition, one of the ligands of ANXA2, Tenascin, has been shown to express strongly at the invasive front of IHCC which was associated with poor prognosis in intrahepatic cholangiocarcinoma [36]. Figure 10.12 shows the enhanced ANXA2 expression in cholangiocarcinoma. The immunohistochemical staining of Annexin A2 (ANXA2) in normal liver tissue is shown in (Fig. 10.12A), in bile duct hyperplasia tissue (Fig. 10.12B), and in cholangiocarcinoma (CCA) tissues (Fig. 10.12C, D). Annexin A2-positive cells were clustered within bile duct hyperplasia (B) and CCA tissues (C and D), but not detected or expressed at very low levels in stroma, normal liver and bile duct cells (A). Annexin A2 was preferably membranous (D) in location of CCA tissues, although some cytoplasmic staining (C) was observed [35].

10.12 Cytokeratin 19 (CK19)

The keratins are intermediate filament proteins responsible for the structural integrity of epithelial cells. CK19 is also involved in the organization of myofibers and together with KRT8, it helps to link the contractile apparatus to dystrophin at the costameres of striated muscle [37, 38]. Cytokeratin immunostaining forms the bedrock of the immunohistochemical evaluation of tumors. CK19 belongs to a family of keratins, which are normally expressed in the lining of the gastroenteropancreatic and hepatobiliary tracts [37]. CK19 has been shown to be an independent prognostic factor for pancreatic neuroendocrine tumors, especially the insulin-negative tumors. CK19 positive tumors are associated with poor outcomes irrespective of the established pathologic parameters such as size, mitoses, lymphovascular invasion, and necrosis. CK19 is useful in the work-up of pancreatic endocrine tumors. CK19 is also positive in most neuroendocrine tumors occurring in the rest of the GIT, except rectal tumors, which are negative.

In the liver, CK19 is of prognostic value in hepatocellular carcinomas and is of use in distinguishing cholangiocarcinoma from hepatocellular carcinomas. It can also be used to highlight native ductules in the liver and helps separate conditions such as focal nodular hyperplasia from hepatic adenoma. The vast majority of adenocarcinomas in the GIT and pancreas are CK19 positive. In a study of the differences between hepatocellular carcinoma (HCC) and peripheral type of cholangiocarcinoma (CC) using cytokeratin (CK) and carcinoembryonic antigen (CEA) expressions, 50 % of HCCs were positive for CEA, presenting a canalicular staining pattern [38]. For CK7, all but one (which was focally positive), or 80 % of CHCs were diffusely positive, whereas only two HCCs were positive. For CK19, 80 % of CCs were diffusely positive, while all but two HCCs (a moderately and a poorly differentiated tumor) were negative. For CK, 8/18, or 70 % of HCCs were diffusely positive, whereas only 20 % of CHCs were positive. For CK17, 60 % of CHCs were positive, while all HCCs were negative. 80 % of CHCs were positive for AB1 anti-CKs complex, whereas only 50 % of HCCs were positive. Thus, CKs and CEA might be considered helpful, in addition to other diagnostic criteria, for the differential diagnosis of primary carcinomas of the liver, especially in difficult cases.

10.13 Other Molecular Markers

Other markers for cholangiocarcinoma that showed alterations are DNA repair proteins and repair defects such as Methyguanine methyl transferase [39], mismatch repair proteins MSH2, MLH1 [40, 41], and RAD51 associating protein-1 [42], oxo-dihydro-dG [43], nitrative and oxidative DNA damage [44], hTERT mRNA [45], microsatellite instability, stem cell factor and c-Kit [46], Cox-2 and PE2 [47], other epigenetic alteration [48], hedgehog ligand [49], Galectin-3 [50], Maspin and Bax [51], p27 [52], TGF-beta type II receptor [40], angiogenesis and lymphangiogenesis [5]. However, Glycine-N-methyltransferase was shown to be a favorable factor for cholangiocarcinoma [53].

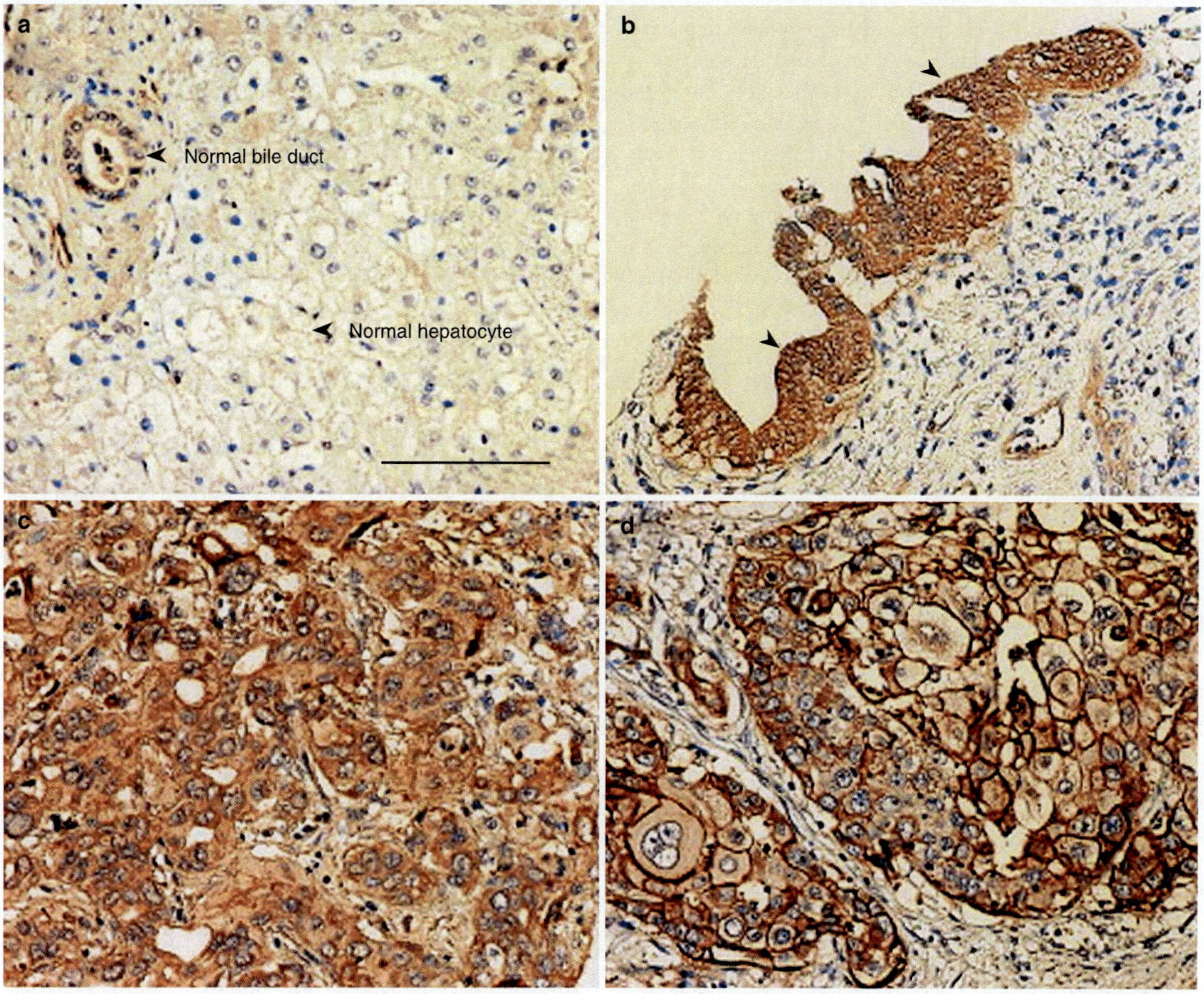

Fig. 10.12 Enhanced ANXA2 expression in cholangiocarcinoma. Immunohistochemical staining of Annexin A2 (ANXA2) in normal liver tissue (**a**), bile duct hyperplasia tissue (**b**) and cholangiocarcinoma (CCA) tissues (**c**, **d**). Annexin A2-positive cells were clustered within bile duct hyperplasia (**b**) and CCA tissues (**c**, **d**), but not detected or expressed at very low levels in stroma, normal liver and bile duct cells (**a**). Annexin A2 was preferably membranous (**d**) in location of CCA tissues, although some cytoplasmic staining (**c**) was observed [35]

10.14 Chromosomal Alteration

In intrahepatic cholangiocarcinoma, losses of heterozygosity at chromosomal loci 3p13-p21, 5q35-qter, 8p22, 17p13, and 18q have been reported [8]. These chromosomal alterations may contain other unidentified proto-oncogenes or tumor suppressor genes.

10.15 Serum Tumor Markers

For non-invasive diagnostic tests of cholangiocarcinoma, blood tests are probably the best at this juncture in time [54–56]. Serum biochemical tests usually support the clinical suspicion of CC but they are rarely diagnostic. Jaundice occurs if there is obstruction of the right and left hepatic ducts or the common bile duct. In these circumstances, elevation of serum levels of bilirubin and markers of biliary epithelial injury, such as alkaline phosphatase (ALP) and gamma glutamyltransferase (GTT) are common [56, 57]. However, in the presence of unilateral intrahepatic biliary obstruction, elevation of ALP or GTT may be present without any increase in the serum bilirubin level. Other abnormal laboratory findings include hypo-albuminemia and prolonged prothrombin time, which reflect the combination of diminished hepatic synthetic function, cachexia and malabsorption of vitamin.

Other tumor markers may support the diagnosis of CC, although none of them is sensitive enough to be used for screening purposes. The commonly used markers are carbohydrate antigen (CA19-9), carcinoembryonic antigen (CEA) and CA-125. CA19-9 is the most useful of these three [57–61]. CA19-9 is frequently upregulated in pancreatobiliary neoplasia. However, it may also be elevated in patients with jaundice due to biliary obstruction, but in the absence of a tumor, and in other non-hepato-pancreaticobiliary conditions. Thus, these tumor markers are not very specific as they can be elevated in the presence of other malignancies (e.g. pancreas and stomach) and with benign conditions such as cholangitis and hepatolithiasis. Serum CA19-9 levels above 100 U/ml in patients without PSC have a sensitivity of 53 % and a specificity of 75–90 % for the diagnosis of CC. In patients with PSC, serum CA19-9 levels above 100 U/ml have a sensitivity of 75–89 % and a specificity of 80–86 % for the diagnosis of CC. In a recent study the optimal cutoff value for serum CA19-9 in patients with PSC was 20 U/ml which provided a sensitivity of 78 %, a specificity of 67 %, a positive predictive value of 23 % and a negative predictive value of 96 % [60]. Nevertheless, serum CA19-9 combined with either ultrasonography, computed tomography, or magnetic resonance imaging provided a sensitivity of 91, 100 and 96 % respectively for CC diagnosis. The levels of CA19-9 appear to correlate with the stage of the disease. It was reported that the sensitivity of CA19-9 above 100 U/ml for the diagnosis of CC in patients with resectable tumors was 33 % compared to 72 % in patients with unresectable tumors [58]. Using more than one tumor marker for patients with PSC may improve the detection rate of CC. Thus, CA19-9 and CEA are helpful devices in the management of gastrointestinal malignancies and belong to clinical routine in surgical oncology. The validity of these parameters in terms of tumor extension and prognosis of bile duct malignancies still remains unclear. From 1998 to 2008, preoperative CA19-9 and CEA serum levels in 136 patients with hilar cholangiocarcinoma were obtained. In another correlative study, the tumor stage, resectability rate and survival were correlated with preoperative CA19-9 and CEA serum levels. CA19-9 and CEA levels increased significantly with rising tumor stages. Patients with pre-operative serum levels of CA19-9 (>1,000 U/ml) and CEA (>14.4 ng/ml) showed a significant poorer resectability rate and survival than patients with lower CA19-9 and CEA serum levels respectively. CA19-9 and CEA serum levels were associated with the tumor stage. If preoperatively obtained CA19-9 and CEA serum levels were highly elevated patients had an even worse survival and the frequency of irresectability was significantly higher. Several new markers are currently being investigated. The human mucin five, subtypes A and C (MUC5AC) are the most promising for future clinical use with a sensitivity and specificity of 71 and 90 %, respectively [62–64]. MMPs are also potentially useful serum makers for CC [65]. Alpha-fetal-protein is known to be a useful serum marker for HCC, but it can be expressed in intrahepatic cholangiocarcinoma as well [66, 67], which suggests probable cancer stem cell origin [67]. Figure 10.13 shows the correlation of CA19-9 with bilirubin and the sensitivity and specificity. Figure 10.13a is a plot of total bilirubin versus CA19-9 for benign diseases, while Fig. 10.13b is a plot of total bilirubin versus CA19-9 for malignant diseases. Figure 10.13c is a plot of sensitivity versus 1-Specificity for CA19-9 [60]. These data indicate that CA19-9 is positively correlated with bilirubin in benign diseases while it is randomly distributed in malignant diseases.

10.16 Molecular Markers as Target of Therapy

For therapy of cholangiocarcinoma, complete surgical resection is the only curative approach. This can be accomplished only in a minority of patients, since most of them present with an advanced disease. In addition, those patients who have undergone complete surgical resection experience a high tumor recurrence rate. Non-resectable biliary tract cancer is associated with a poor prognosis due to resistance of the tumor to chemotherapy agents and radiotherapy. It is essential to search for new therapeutical approaches. Clinical study data with molecular therapy are now starting to be available for this tumor [68–73]. Inhibitors of the epidermal growth factor receptor (EGFR) family, such as erlotinib, cetuximab, and lapatinib were recently investigated [68]. Furthermore, bortezomib, an inhibitor of proteasome, imatinib mesylate, an inhibitor of c-kit-R, bevacizumab, an inhibitor of vascular endothelial growth factor (VEGF), and sorafenib (BAY 43-9006), a multiple kinase inhibitor that blocks not only receptor tyrosine kinases but also serine/threonine kinases along the RAS/RAF/MEK/ERK pathway, have been tried. Although early evidence of antitumor activity was seen, the results are still too early and require further investigations. Another report indicated that biliary cancers overexpress epidermal growth factor receptor (EGFR), and angiogenesis has been correlated with a poor outcome. Erlotinib, an EGFR tyrosine kinase inhibitor, and bevacizumab, a vascular endothelial growth factor (VEGF) inhibitor have been shown to have activity in biliary cancer. Patients with advanced cholangiocarcinoma or gallbladder cancer were treated with bevacizumab (5 mg/kg) and erlotinib (150 mg). In 53 eligible patients, 6 had a confirmed partial response while stable disease was documented in another 25 patients (51 %) [69]. The median overall survival (OS) was 9.9 months, and the time to progression (TTP) was 4.4 months. Combination chemotherapy with bevacizumab and erlotinib showed clinical activity with infrequent adverse effects. Thus, the combination of bevacizumab and erlotinib may be a therapeutic alternative in patients with advanced biliary cancer.

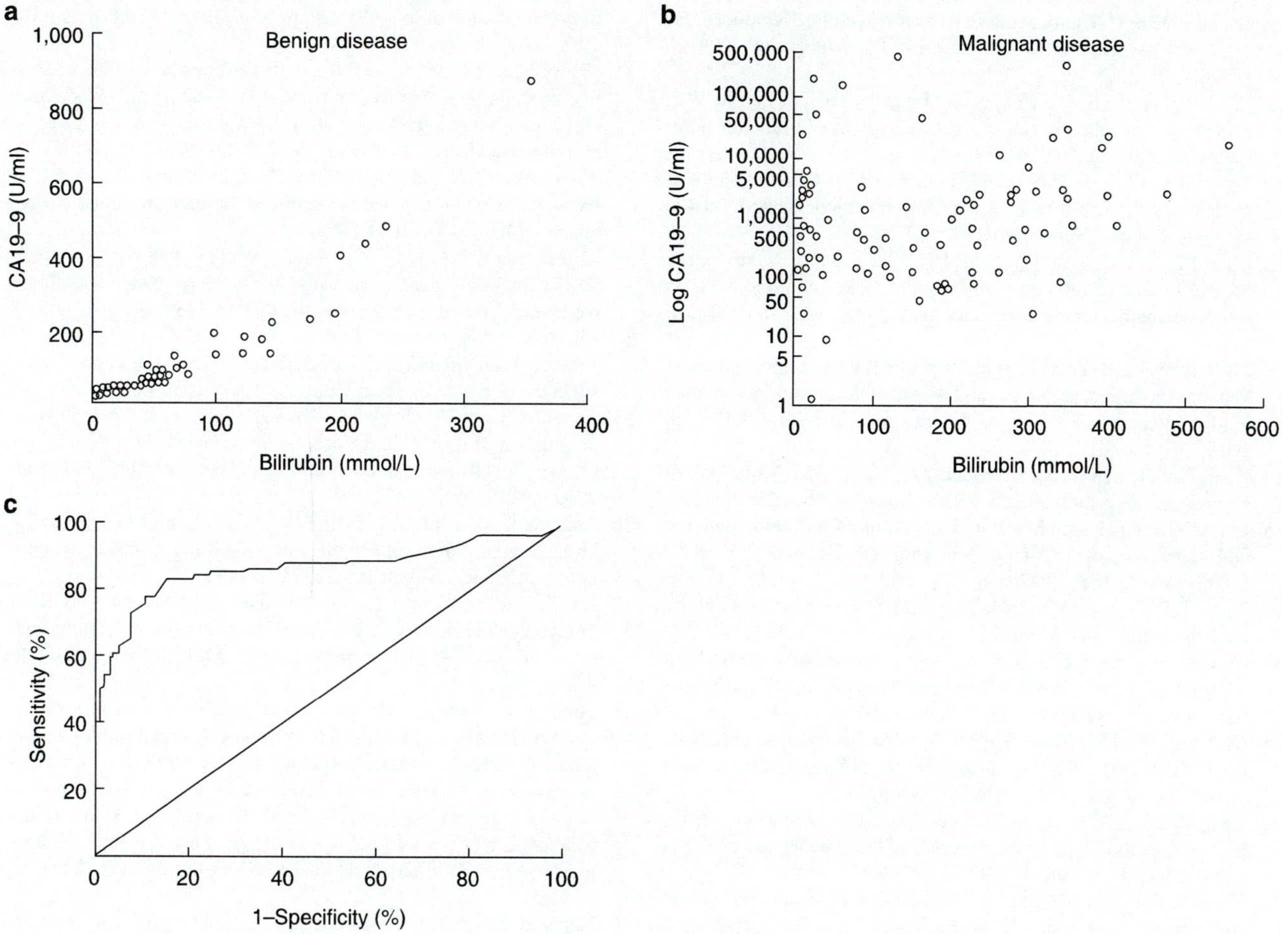

Fig. 10.13 Serum tumor marker CA19-9 in cholangiocarcinoma. (**a**) Plot of total bilirubin versus CA19-9 for benign diseases. (**b**) Plot of total bilirubin versus CA19-9 for malignant diseases. (**c**) Plot of sensitivity versus 1-Specificity for CA19-9 [60]

Conclusion

Cholangiocarcinomas are epithelial neoplasms that originate from cholangiocytes. They can occur at any level of the biliary tree and they are classified into intrahepatic tumors, (extrahepatic) hilar tumors and (extrahepatic) distal bile duct tumors. A better understanding of the predispositions, risk factors and the molecular pathways for cholangiocarcinoma development will provide new insights in the management of this cancer. The environmental factors and genetic/epigenetic factors can be eliminated, neutralized or avoided. The diagnosis can be established much earlier and accurately with new molecular markers and improved non-invasive imaging. Advanced cytological and chromosomal analysis may aid early diagnosis. Biological therapy basing on the molecular markers discovered (including proto-oncogenes and tumor suppressor genes) may be very useful for patients with unresectable cholangiocarcinoma. These, together with neoadjuvant chemo-irradiation, can be used as therapeutic alternatives in patients with advanced or recurrent biliary cancers.

References

1. Ben-Menachem T. Risk factors for cholangiocarcinoma. Eur J Gastroenterol Hepatol. 2007;19:615–7.
2. Malhi H, Gores GJ. Review article: the modern diagnosis and therapy of cholangiocarcinoma. Aliment Pharmacol Ther. 2006;23:1287–96.
3. Aljiffry M, Walsh MJ, Molinari M. Advances in diagnosis, treatment and palliation of cholangiocarcinoma: 1990–2009. World J Gastroenterol. 2009;15:4240–62.
4. Meza-Junco J, Montano-Loza AJ, Ma M, et al. Cholangiocarcinoma: has there been any progress? Can J Gastroenterol. 2010;24:52–7.
5. Thelen A, Scholz A, Weichert W, et al. Tumor-associated angiogenesis and lymphangiogenesis correlate with progression of intrahepatic cholangiocarcinoma. Am J Gastroenterol. 2010;105:1123–32.
6. Karlsen TH, Schrumpf E, Boberg KM. Genetic epidemiology of primary sclerosing cholangitis. World J Gastroenterol. 2007;13:5421–31.
7. Shen WF, Zhong W, Xu F, et al. Clinicopathological and prognostic analysis of 429 patients with intrahepatic cholangiocarcinoma. World J Gastroenterol. 2009;15:5976–82.
8. Rashid A. Cellular and molecular biology of biliary tract cancers. Surg Oncol Clin N Am. 2002;11:995–1009.

9. Chan JY, Wang Z. Tumor markers. In: Lau WY, editor. Hepatocellular carcinoma. Singapore: World Scientific Publishing Co; 2008. p. 159–82.
10. Chan JY, Lee KKH, Chui YL, et al. Molecular aspects. In: Lau WY, editor. Hepatocellular carcinoma. Singapore: World Scientific Publishing Co; 2008. p. 243–78.
11. Perumal V, Wang J, Thuluvath P, et al. Hepatitis C and hepatitis B nucleic acids are present in intrahepatic cholangiocarcinomas from the United States. Hum Pathol. 2006;37:1211–6.
12. Chen RF, Li ZH, Zou SQ, et al. Effect of hepatitis C virus core protein on modulation of cellular proliferation and apoptosis in hilar cholangiocarcinoma. Hepatobiliary Pancreat Dis Int. 2005;4: 71–4.
13. Zhou H, Wang H, Zhou D, et al. Hepatitis B virus-associated intrahepatic cholangiocarcinoma and hepatocellular carcinoma may hold common disease process for carcinogenesis. Eur J Cancer. 2010;46:1056–61.
14. Khan SA, Thomas HC, Toledano MB, et al. p53 Mutations in human cholangiocarcinoma: a review. Liver Int. 2005;25:704–16.
15. Liu XF, Zhang H, Zhu SG, et al. Correlation of p53 gene mutation and expression of P53 protein in cholangiocarcinoma. World J Gastroenterol. 2006;12:4706–9.
16. Tullo A, D'Erchia AM, Honda K, et al. New p53 mutations in hilar cholangiocarcinoma. World J Surg. 2004;28:995–1000.
17. Caca K, Feisthammel J, Klee K, et al. Inactivation of the INK4a/ARF locus and p53 in sporadic extrahepatic bile duct cancers and bile tract cancer cell lines. Int J Cancer. 2002;97:481–8.
18. Klump B, Hsieh CJ, Dette S, et al. Promoter methylation of INK4a/ARF as detected in bile-significance for the differential diagnosis in biliary disease. Clin Cancer Res. 2003;9:1773–8.
19. Kang YK, Kim WH, Jang JJ. Expression of G1-S modulators (p53, p16, p27, cyclin D1, Rb) and Smad4/Dpc4 in intrahepatic cholangiocarcinoma. Hum Pathol. 2002;33:877–83.
20. Taniai M, Higuchi H, Burgart LJ, et al. p16INK4a promoter mutations are frequent in primary sclerosing cholangitis (PSC) and PSC-associated cholangiocarcinoma. Gastroenterology. 2002;123:1090–8.
21. Tannapfel A, Benicke M, Katalinic A, et al. Frequency of p16(INK4A) alterations and K-ras mutations in intrahepatic cholangiocarcinoma of the liver. Gut. 2000;47:721–7.
22. Liew CT, Li HM, Lo KW, et al. High frequency of p16INK4A gene alterations in hepatocellular carcinoma. Oncogene. 1999;18: 789–95.
23. Zheng J, Zhu YM. Expression of c-erbB-2 proto-oncogene in extrahepatic cholangiocarcinoma and its clinical significance. Hepatobiliary Pancreat Dis Int. 2007;6:412–5.
24. Nakazawa K, Dobashi Y, Suzuki S, et al. Amplification and overexpression of c-erbB-2, epidermal growth factor receptor, and c-met in biliary tract cancers. Hum Pathol. 2003;34:902–10.
25. Treekitkarnmongkol W, Suthiphongchai T. High expression of ErbB2 contributes to cholangiocarcinoma cell invasion and proliferation through AKT/p70S6K. World J Gastroenterol. 2010;16: 4047–54.
26. Yoshikawa D, Ojima H, Iwasaki M, et al. Clinicopathological and prognostic significance of EGFR, VEGF, and HER2 expression in cholangiocarcinoma. Br J Cancer. 2008;98:418–25.
27. Guedj N, Zhan Q, Perigny M, et al. Comparative protein expression profiles of hilar and peripheral hepatic cholangiocarcinomas. J Hepatol. 2009;51:93–101.
28. Tada M, Omata M, Ohto M. High incidence of ras gene mutation in intrahepatic cholangiocarcinoma. Cancer. 1992;69:1115–8.
29. Kiba T, Tsuda H, Pairojkul C, et al. Mutations of the p53 tumor suppressor gene and the ras gene family in intrahepatic cholangiocellular carcinomas in Japan and Thailand. Mol Carcinogen. 1993;8:312–8.
30. Tsuda H, Satarug S, Bhudhisawasdi V, et al. Cholangiocarcinomas in Japanese and Thai patients: difference in etiology and incidence of point mutation of the c-Ki-ras proto-oncogene. Mol Carcinogen. 1992;6:266–9.
31. Chen CY, Shiesh SC, Wu SJ. Rapid detection of K-ras mutations in bile by peptide nucleic acid-mediated PCR clamping and melting curve analysis: comparison with restriction fragment length polymorphism analysis. Clin Chem. 2004;50:481–9.
32. Sugimachi K, Taguchi K, Aishima S, et al. Altered expression of beta-catenin without genetic mutation in intrahepatic cholangiocarcinoma. Mod Pathol. 2001;14:900–5.
33. Zhai B, Yan HX, Liu SQ, et al. Reduced expression of P120 catenin in cholangiocarcinoma correlated with tumor clinicopathologic parameters. World J Gastroenterol. 2008;14:3739–44.
34. Riener MO, Vogetseder A, Pestalozzi BC, et al. Cell adhesion molecules P-cadherin and CD24 are markers for carcinoma and dysplasia in the biliary tract. Hum Pathol. 2010;41:1558–65.
35. Yonglitthipagon P, Pairojkul C, Chamgramol Y, et al. Up-regulation of annexin A2 in cholangiocarcinoma caused by Opisthorchis viverrini and its implication as a prognostic marker. Int J Parasitol. 2010;40:1203–12.
36. Aishima S, Taguchi K, Terashi T, et al. Tenascin expression at the invasive front is associated with poor prognosis in intrahepatic cholangiocarcinoma. Mod Pathol. 2003;16:1019–27.
37. Jain R, Fischer S, Serra S, et al. The use of Cytokeratin 19 (CK19) immunohistochemistry in lesions of the pancreas, gastrointestinal tract, and liver. Appl Immunohistochem Mol Morphol. 2010;18: 9–15.
38. Stroescu C, Herlea V, Dragnea A, et al. The diagnostic value of cytokeratins and carcinoembryonic antigen immunostaining in differentiating hepatocellular carcinomas from intrahepatic cholangiocarcinomas. J Gastrointestin Liver Dis. 2006;15:9–14.
39. Koga Y, Kitajima Y, Miyoshi A, et al. Tumor progression through epigenetic gene silencing of O6-methylguanine-DNA methyltransferase in human biliary tract cancers. Ann Surg Oncol. 2005;12: 354–63.
40. Nagai M, Kawarada Y, Watanabe M, et al. Analysis of microsatellite instability, TGF-beta type II receptor gene mutations and hMSH2 and hMLH1 allele losses in pancreaticobiliary maljunction-associated biliary tract tumors. Anticancer Res. 1999;19(3A): 1765–8.
41. Obama K, Satoh S, Hamamoto R, et al. Enhanced expression of RAD51 associating protein-1 is involved in the growth of intrahepatic cholangiocarcinoma cells. Clin Cancer Res. 2008;14: 1333–9.
42. Liengswangwong U, Karalak A, Morishita Y, et al. Immunohistochemical expression of mismatch repair genes: a screening tool for predicting mutator phenotype in liver fluke infection-associated intrahepatic cholangiocarcinoma. World J Gastroenterol. 2006;12:3740–5.
43. Thanan R, Murata M, Pinlaor S, et al. Urinary 8-oxo-7,8-dihydro-2′-deoxyguanosine in patients with parasite infection and effect of antiparasitic drug in relation to cholangiocarcinogenesis. Cancer Epidemiol Biomarkers Prev. 2008;17:518–24.
44. Pinlaor S, Sripa B, Ma N, et al. Nitrative and oxidative DNA damage in intrahepatic cholangiocarcinoma patients in relation to tumor invasion. World J Gastroenterol. 2005;11:4644–9.
45. Leelawat K, Leelawat S, Ratanachu-Ek T, et al. Circulating hTERT mRNA as a tumor marker in cholangiocarcinoma patients. World J Gastroenterol. 2006;12:4195–8.
46. Mansuroglu T, Ramadori P, Dudás J, et al. Expression of stem cell factor and its receptor c-Kit during the development of intrahepatic cholangiocarcinoma. Lab Invest. 2009;89:562–74.
47. Han C, Wu T. Cyclooxygenase-2-derived prostaglandin E2 promotes human cholangiocarcinoma cell growth and invasion through EP1 receptor-mediated activation of the epidermal growth factor receptor and Akt. J Biol Chem. 2005;280: 24053–63.

48. Tischoff I, Wittekind C, Tannapfel A. Role of epigenetic alterations in cholangiocarcinoma. J Hepatobiliary Pancreat Surg. 2006;13:274–9.
49. Jung Y, McCall SJ, Li YX, et al. Bile ductules and stromal cells express hedgehog ligands and/or hedgehog target genes in primary biliary cirrhosis. Hepatology. 2007;45:1091–6.
50. Dechaphunkul A, Kanngurn S, Dechsukhum C, et al. The significance of galectin-3 immunohistochemistry, clinical characteristics and liver imaging in differentiating intrahepatic cholangiocarcinoma from adenocarcinoma liver metastasis. J Med Assoc Thai. 2010;93:523–8.
51. Romani AA, Soliani P, Desenzani S, et al. The associated expression of Maspin and Bax proteins as a potential prognostic factor in intrahepatic cholangiocarcinoma. BMC Cancer. 2006;6:255–8.
52. Fiorentino M, Altimari A, D'Errico A, et al. Low p27 expression is an independent predictor of survival for patients with either hilar or peripheral intrahepatic cholangiocarcinoma. Mod Pathol. 2001;14: 900–5.
53. Huang YC, Chen M, Shyr YM, et al. Glycine N-methyltransferase is a favorable prognostic marker for human cholangiocarcinoma. J Gastroenterol Hepatol. 2008;23:1384–9.
54. Nuzzo G, Giuliante F, Ardito F, et al. Intrahepatic cholangiocarcinoma: prognostic factors after liver resection. Updates Surg. 2010; 62:11–9.
55. Zhang F, Chen XP, Zhang W, et al. Combined hepatocellular cholangiocarcinoma originating from hepatic progenitor cells: immunohistochemical and double-fluorescence immunostaining evidence. Histopathology. 2008;52:224–32.
56. Charatcharoenwitthaya P, Enders FB, Halling KC, et al. Utility of serum tumor markers, imaging, and biliary cytology for detecting cholangiocarcinoma in primary sclerosing cholangitis. Hepatology. 2008;48:1106–17.
57. Juntermanns B, Radunz S, Heuer M, et al. Tumor markers as a diagnostic key for hilar cholangiocarcinoma. Eur J Med Res. 2010; 20(15):357–61.
58. Patel AH, Harnois DM, Klee GG, et al. The utility of CA 19-9 in the diagnoses of cholangiocarcinoma in patients without primary sclerosing cholangitis. Am J Gastroenterol. 2000;95:204–7.
59. Hatzaras I, Schmidt C, Muscarella P, et al. Elevated CA 19-9 portends poor prognosis in patients undergoing resection of biliary malignancies. HPB (Oxford). 2010;12:134–8.
60. Morris-Stiff G, Teli M, Jardine N, et al. CA19-9 antigen levels can distinguish between benign and malignant pancreaticobiliary disease. Hepatobiliary Pancreat Dis Int. 2009;8:620–6.
61. Furmanczyk PS, Grieco VS, Agoff SN. Biliary brush cytology and the detection of cholangiocarcinoma in primary sclerosing cholangitis: evaluation of specific cytomorphologic features and CA19-9 levels. Am J Clin Pathol. 2005;124:355–60.
62. Yuan SF, Li KZ, Wang L, et al. Expression of MUC1 and its significance in hepatocellular and cholangiocarcinoma tissue. World J Gastroenterol. 2005;11:4661–6.
63. Bamrungphon W, Prempracha N, Bunchu N, et al. A new mucin antibody/enzyme-linked lectin-sandwich assay of serum MUC5AC mucin for the diagnosis of cholangiocarcinoma. Cancer Lett. 2007;247:301–8.
64. Boonla C, Sripa B, Thuwajit P, et al. MUC1 and MUC5AC mucin expression in liver fluke-associated intrahepatic cholangiocarcinoma. World J Gastroenterol. 2005;11:4939–46.
65. Leelawat K, Sakchinabut S, Narong S, et al. Detection of serum MMP-7 and MMP-9 in cholangiocarcinoma patients: evaluation of diagnostic accuracy. BMC Gastroenterol. 2009;9:30–3.
66. Zhou YM, Yang JM, Li B, et al. Clinicopathologic characteristics of intrahepatic cholangiocarcinoma in patients with positive serum a-fetoprotein. World J Gastroenterol. 2008;14:2251–4.
67. Ishikawa K, Sasaki A, Haraguchi N, et al. A case of an alpha-fetoprotein-producing intrahepatic cholangiocarcinoma suggests probable cancer stem cell origin. Oncologist. 2007;12:320–4.
68. Wiedmann MW, Mössner J. Molecular targeted therapy of biliary tract cancer–results of the first clinical studies. Curr Drug Targets. 2010;11:834–50.
69. Lubner SJ, Mahoney MR, Kolesar JL, et al. Report of a multicenter phase II trial testing a combination of biweekly bevacizumab and daily erlotinib in patients with unresectable biliary cancer: a phase II Consortium study. J Clin Oncol. 2010;28:3491–7.
70. Qun W, Tao Y. Effective treatment of advanced cholangiocarcinoma by hepatic arterial infusion chemotherapy combination with sorafenib: one case report from China. Hepatogastroenterology. 2010;57:426–9.
71. Francis H, Alpini G, DeMorrow S. Recent advances in the regulation of cholangiocarcinoma growth. Am J Physiol Gastrointest Liver Physiol. 2010;299:G1–9.
72. Tonini G, Virzì V, Fratto ME, et al. Targeted therapy in biliary tract cancer: 2009 update. Future Oncol. 2009;5:1675–84.
73. Zhang Z, Oyesanya RA, Campbell DJ, et al. Preclinical assessment of simultaneous targeting of epidermal growth factor receptor (ErbB1) and ErbB2 as a strategy for cholangiocarcinoma therapy. Hepatology. 2010;52:975–86.

Laparoscopy and Laparoscopic Ultrasound

11

N.J. Peel and O.J. Garden

11.1 Introduction

Hilar cholangiocarcinoma usually presents late with a poor prognosis that results in diagnostic and therapeutic challenges for the clinician. For individuals diagnosed with cholangiocarcinoma, surgery currently offers the only potential curative option, however a laparotomy and surgical resection of localized disease is itself associated with significant morbidity and mortality [1–3]. For patients diagnosed with advanced disease, life expectancy is short and survival in those who have incomplete tumour resection is identical to patients who receive palliative therapy alone for non resectable illness [1]. The benefits of avoiding laparotomy can therefore not be overemphasized and include less pain and morbidity, decreased hospital stay, decreased overall cost and earlier initiation of palliative therapy [2, 3]. Consequently, adequate staging is of utmost importance to prevent unnecessary laparotomy in those with advanced illness not suitable for potentially curative surgery. Whenever surgical palliation is preferred, laparotomy is indicated, regardless of tumour resectability. Nevertheless, despite improvements in imaging, the incidence of non therapeutic laparotomies remains high, up to 46 % in some studies [1].

Laparoscopy has been used as a diagnostic staging tool for some years in hepato-pancreato-biliary tumours. Its main function is to further stage those patients deemed suitable for surgical resection after undergoing conventional radiological assessment. Hilar cholangiocarcinomas are often small and tend not to form a bulky mass. For this reason they are difficult to visualise and therefore stage accurately on any standard imaging modality [4]. CT and MRI imaging are usually accurate in identifying portal vein occlusion, however, more discrete tumour invasion is often missed [4]. Even with the most sophisticated radiological imaging, the false-negative rate for identifying small liver (Fig. 11.1), omental or peritoneal (Fig. 11.2) deposits is approximately 10–30 % [5]. Hilar cholangiocarcinoma in particular tends to be unresectable and the surgeon is often faced with major

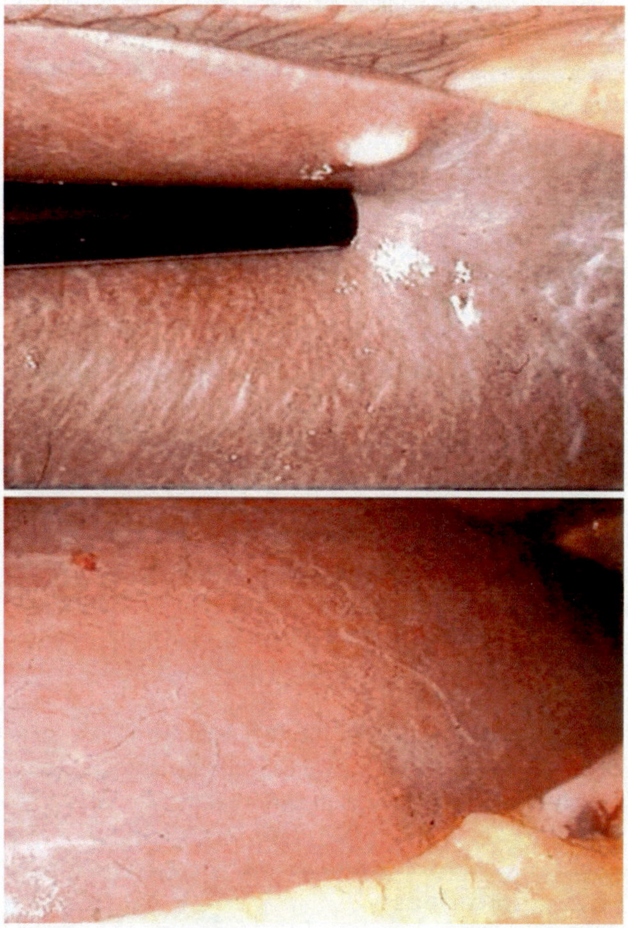

Fig. 11.1 Small liver metastasis on under surface of left lobe of liver

N.J. Peel, MBChB, BSc, MRCS(Glas)
Clinical Research Fellow, University of Edinburgh,
Royal Infirmary of Edinburgh, Edinburgh, UK

O.J. Garden, BSc, MBChB, MD, FRCS(Glasg), FRCS(Ed), FRCP(Ed), FRACS(Hon), FRCSC(Hon) (✉)
Clinical and Surgical Sciences (Surgery),
University of Edinburgh, Royal Infirmary of Edinburgh,
Edinburgh, UK
e-mail: o.j.garden@ed.ac.uk

W.Y. Lau (ed.), *Hilar Cholangiocarcinoma*,
DOI 10.1007/978-94-007-6473-6_11, © Springer Science+Business Media Dordrecht and People's Medical Publishing House 2013

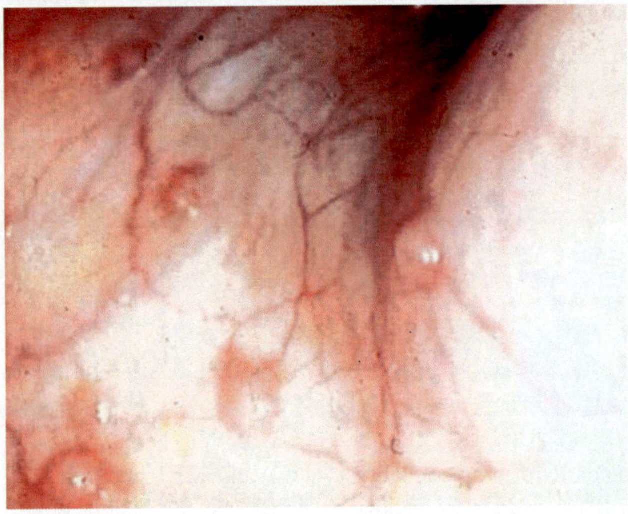

Fig. 11.2 Peritoneal dissemination of cholangiocarcinoma

discrepancies between staging performed by radiological imaging alone, and actual findings at laparotomy [4]. Therefore, the main benefits of laparoscopy include the increased likelihood of visualizing small metastatic tumour deposits on the surface of the liver and peritoneum which would otherwise go undetected by conventional radiological techniques alone.

There are limited studies on the added benefits of incorporating this modality into the staging of hilar cholangiocarcinoma and the outcomes appear to be influenced by a multitude of factors including the quality of the conventional radiological imaging, the timing of the laparoscopy in the staging process and the expertise of the surgeon performing the procedure [4–7]. Adding laparoscopic ultrasound (LUS) may further aid staging and increase the yield of laparoscopy by highlighting radiologically undetectable intrahepatic metastases and localized vascular invasion [4, 7]. Again the chief limitation of LUS is that it is highly operator dependent and, even in the hands of the most experienced of operator, biopsies are difficult to obtain [8].

The low yield of laparoscopy in identifying patients unsuitable for laparotomy is the primary reason that it has not been accepted as universal practice in all centres [3–7, 9, 10]. It is also likely that as non-invasive radiological imaging techniques improve, the yield of staging laparoscopy will decrease. Furthermore, it has been postulated that laparoscopy could be useful in guiding palliative treatment by identifying patients with locally advanced disease suitable for chemoradiation from those with metastatic disease suitable for chemotherapy alone [4].

11.2 Indications

Staging laparoscopy is recommended for patients who have been diagnosed with cholangiocarcinoma that has been demonstrated to be potentially curable by surgical excision after a full battery of radiological investigations. A second indication to perform a laparoscopy would be to confirm the presence of locally advanced disease as opposed to metastatic, in order to guide neo-adjuvant palliative treatment although evidence for this is less robust [11]. Contra-indications to laparoscopy are signs of duodenal obstruction as the patient will require definitive surgery to relieve the obstruction.

11.3 Technique

In our institution, staging laparoscopy and laparoscopic ultrasound are generally performed separately to subsequent laparotomy. This is mainly due to logistical reasons relating to anaesthetic planning and patient preference but in some centres both procedures are performed at a single sitting. Although this may present challenges with effective theatre time management, carrying out staging laparoscopy and laparotomy in a single session may be more beneficial to the individual patient as it would prevent two procedures and two hospital visits.

Staging laparoscopy is performed under general anaesthetic with the patient placed supine and the principle operating surgeon positioned on the left side of the patient. Pneumoperitoneum is established in the standard fashion, gaining access using an open "Hassan" technique and insufflating with CO_2 at a pressure of 12–15 mmHg through a 12 mm infra-umbilical port [12]. A second 12 mm port is placed in the right mid quadrant.

A 30° scope is inserted through the infra-umbilical port and the abdominal cavity is visualized. A careful inspection of the peritoneum is undertaken to identify any tumour deposits. Intraabdominal organs are inspected in turn, the visceral peritoneum, the liver including the undersurface, the anterior aspect of the stomach, the lesser and greater omentum, the diaphragm and porta are inspected. By retracting the greater omentum superiorly, the small bowel and root of the mesentery can be identified [12]. Suspicious lesions should be biopsied at the end of the procedure using a biopsy forcep or a biopsy needle [4]. The biopsies should be taken under direct laparoscopic vision or by laparoscopic ultrasound guidance [4, 12].

Laparoscopic ultrasound is best performed using a high-resolution flexible tip linear array transducer [12]. Isotonic saline can be introduced to the peritoneal cavity if required to provide an acoustic window, and decreasing the abdominal pressure to 7–8 mmHg has been shown to improve contact with the liver surface [4, 12]. The ultrasound probe should be inserted through both ports to allow imaging in two planes. The probe is normally sterilized or can be wrapped in a sterile cover sheet, filled with sterile ultrasonic gel. A systematic approach should be taken to examine the liver starting with the identification of standard landmarks. The liver parenchyma should be investigated for signs of intrahepatic metastatic lesions, which can appear as hyper-, iso-, or hypo-echoic

[12]. Furthermore, the portal triad should be examined and its relationship to the primary tumour should be considered [12]. The portal structures are viewed by inserting the probe through the sub umbilical port and placing it on the hepatoduodenal ligament [12]. This allows the surgeon to view the inferior vena cava posteriorly [12]. If the probe is then rotated clockwise, the portal vein, bile duct, and hepatic artery may be inspected [12].

Withdrawing the probe allows the portal vein to be followed to the spleno-portal confluence and continues down the SMV [12]. A loss of tissue planes between the primary tumour and the surrounding vessels suggests vascular invasion [12]. This part of the procedure is particularly operator dependent as placing too much pressure on the probe can create images consistent with that of vascular involvement. A further indication of vascular involvement that can be demonstrated by laparoscopic ultrasound is a fixed stenosis of the vessel in more than one plane [4]. For hilar cholangiocarcinoma in particular it is important to assess the primary lesion in order to determine its proximal and distal extent, radial extension and lymph node metastases [12]. Involved lymph nodes appear as hyper-echoic, less well circumscribed nodes. Suspicious nodes should be confirmed by biopsy [12]. After biopsies have been taken, the wounds are inspected for excess bleeding, the ports are removed and the wounds are closed in the usual fashion.

11.4 Safety and Complications of Staging Laparoscopy

Staging laparoscopy is an established safe procedure. It has a low morbidity with complications reported in 0.15–3 % of cases, and the mortality is negligible (0.05 %) [4, 13].

The introduction of the infra umbilical trocar is the most hazardous part of any laparoscopic procedure. This is due to the risk of injury to the abdominal aorta or other vulnerable parts of the vascular tree and the risk of injury to the bowel. Penetrating vascular injuries can be catastrophic and mortality in these patients have been reported to be up to 17 % however the incidence of such events remains low (0.001–0.005 %) [14]. Similarly, the mortality associated with a bowel injury during staging laparoscopy has been reported in some studies to be 3.6 % although the incidence is low at 0.13 % [15]. Obviously, if a patient has undergone previous abdominal surgery then the incidence of complications rises. In our unit, a Hasson open technique is used to gain access to the peritoneum. Using this technique does not remove the risk of delayed injury to the bowel from injury by diathermy, however, we believe that it does reduce the risk of penetrating injury to the bowel and vasculature and increases the chance of any injury being directly visualized and therefore identified early.

van Dijkum and colleagues studied prospectively a series of 420 patients undergoing staging laparoscopy for upper gastrointestinal cancers [16]. Following the procedure, 1 % of patients had major complications which included anaphylactic shock, small bowel injury and bile leakage following a liver biopsy [16]. A further 3 % of patients suffered minor complications such as wound infections, wound haematomas, post operative pain, aspiration pneumonia, post operative urinary retention and incisional hernia [16]. All patients survived the procedure and the mean discharge time was 1.5 days [16]. Shoup and his colleagues in New York corroborated these findings in a similar study with a comparable group of patients [17].

Port site metastases are often sited as a major complication of staging laparoscopy and are much feared as the consequences for the patient may be devastating. The expected risk, however, is probably overestimated and is not supported by present evidence [4]. In the study of van Dijkum, port site metastasis occurred in 2 % of patients all of whom had metastatic disease at the time of staging laparoscopy and had evidence of very advanced disease when the port site lesions were identified [16]. Shoup et al. reported an even lower incidence (0.8 %). However, although small, the risk of port site metastasis should still be respected and it is recommended that attempts at biopsy of hilar cholangiocarcinoma should be restricted to suspected metastases at staging laparoscopy to pathologically confirm a diagnosis [4]. The risk of unnecessary laparotomy significantly outweighs that of port site metastasis which does not influence the outcome for the patient if metastatic disease is already present [4].

11.5 Peritoneal Washings

Cytological analysis of peritoneal washings, obtained during staging laparoscopy has been established as a means of increasing laparoscopic yield in many solid organ malignancies [18–22]. Peritoneal lavage has been shown to identify occult disease in both gastric and pancreatic cancers that were otherwise deemed resectable [18]. Burke and colleagues demonstrated that patients with seemingly resectable gastric cancer but positive peritoneal cytology had a similar prognosis to patients diagnosed with metastatic disease [18]. Similarly, for pancreatic cancer, patients found to have malignant cells in peritoneal lavage fluid despite having no overt signs of metastatic deposits have a similar prognosis to those diagnosed with disseminated disease [20, 21].

On the basis of this knowledge, Martin and colleagues examined peritoneal washings of 26 patients with confirmed hilar cholangiocarcinoma that were deemed suitable for resection by radiological staging [22]. Malignant cells were identified in only two of the patients who were also found to have gross peritoneal deposits at laparoscopy. Interestingly nine other patients were found to have metastatic disease present at laparoscopy but had negative washings. It would therefore seem that unlike pancreatic and gastric cancers, peritoneal lavage does not provide any useful additional information in the staging of hilar cholangiocarcinoma and should not be routinely practiced.

11.6 Literature Review

There have been a small number of studies in recent years that have examined the benefits of staging laparoscopy and laparoscopic ultrasound in patients with hilar cholangiocarcinoma. At the Memorial Sloan-Kettering Cancer Centre, Weber et al. conducted a large study to investigate the use of staging laparoscopy in patients with both gallbladder cancer and hilar cholangiocarcinoma [2]. Fifty-six patients who were diagnosed with potentially resectable hilar cholangiocarcinoma were included, 14 (25 %) of whom were identified as having metastatic disease at staging laparoscopy. Forty-two patients therefore proceeded to open laparotomy, but 19 were shown to have unresectable cancer at surgery. In this study, laparoscopy detected the majority (83 %) of patients with peritoneal or liver metastasis but failed to identify those with locally advanced tumours and most with nodal metastasis [23]. The yield of laparoscopy (i.e. the number of patients who were identified as unsuitable for resection) in the New York experience was 25 %, therefore the majority of patients did not benefit from the procedure. Weber and his colleagues attempted to identify patients most at risk of occult metastatic disease to target the use of staging laparoscopy more effectively. They analysed the yield of laparoscopy with respect to the MSKCC T staging system (Table 11.1) that assesses local tumour-related factors present on preoperative imaging [24]. This staging system has previously been shown to predict survival, resectability, and the likelihood of metastatic disease [24]. They found that as T stage advanced so too did laparoscopic yield. The yield increased from 9 % in patients with T1 tumours to 36 % in those with T2/T3 tumours. The authors concluded that staging laparoscopy should be targeted at those diagnosed with T2/T3 tumours as this group had the greatest yield. It is unclear however if T staging was based on preoperative imaging alone or was modified after intra operative findings. Laparoscopic ultrasound was carried out in 23 patients as part of their staging assessment. No additional patients with unresectable disease were identified solely using this investigation, it is uncertain therefore if the laparoscopic yield would have been increased had all 56 patients been investigated with laparoscopic ultrasound.

Our own group studied patients with suspected hilar cholangiocarcinoma over 11 years (1992–2003) [8, 23]. Eighty-four patients deemed potentially suitable for resection after standard radiological investigations underwent staging by laparoscopy and laparoscopic ultrasound. Twenty of the 84 patients (24 % yield) were felt to be unresectable after staging laparoscopy alone as 15 patients were found to have metastatic peritoneal or liver deposits and 5 had histologically confirmed nodal disease outside the resection field. The yield was increased to 42 % after laparoscopic ultrasound was added and identified a further 14 patients, 1 of whom had an intra hepatic metastasis and 13 who were found to have locally advanced disease. Despite the addition of laparoscopic ultrasound and its apparent ability to detect locally advanced disease, 10 of the 19 patients undergoing resection were found to have positive resection margins, indicating that in practice, identifying patients with local invasion continues to represent a significant challenge.

Table 11.1 MSKCC revised preoperative staging system for patients with hilar cholangiocarcinoma

T Stage	Description
1	Tumour involving biliary confluence ± unilateral extension to 2° biliary radicles No liver atrophy or portal vein involvement
2	Tumour involving biliary confluence ± unilateral extension to 2° biliary radicles with ipsilateral portal vein involvement ± ipsilateral hepatic lobar atrophy No main portal vein involvement
3	Tumour involving biliary confluence + bilateral extension to 2° biliary radicles OR unilateral extension to 2° biliary radicles with contralateral portal vein involvement OR unilateral extension to 2° biliary radicles with contralateral hepatic lobar atrophy OR main or bilateral portal venous involvement

Adapted from Weber et al. [23]

The patients in the Edinburgh study were again graded according to the MSKCC T staging system. As in Weber and colleagues' study, it was also noted that laparoscopic yield increased with T stage. The yield for T1, T2, and T3 tumours was 26, 37 and 69 % respectively. Fourteen, 25 and 5 patients in the T1, T2 and T3 groups respectively were found to have resectable disease after staging however, at laparotomy, only eight, 11 and one patient in each T stage group did indeed have cancer that was potentially curable be surgery. Interestingly, the reasons for this differed between T stage groups. In the T1/T2 groups, metastatic disease was most likely to be the culprit, however in the T3 group local invasion was the primary reason for unresectability. This suggests that a different biological process is taking place in the T3 group.

The yield from staging laparoscopy and laparoscopic ultrasound in this study was 42 % with an overall accuracy of 53 %. These figures are higher than that of Weber et al. The Edinburgh study was conducted over a longer time period during which the quality of radiological imaging has undoubtedly varied and the selective approach to employing

Table 11.2 Studies on the value of staging laparoscopy and laparoscopic ultrasound for hilar cholangiocarcinoma and detection of unresectable disease at laparotomy

Author	Year	Patients	Study type	Unresectable found at laparoscopy (%)	Unresectable found at laparoscopic ultrasound (%)	Additional unresectable found at laparotomy (%)	Total unresectable patients (%)
Weber et al. [23]	2001	56	Prosp	25	0	34	60
Connor et al. [10]	2005	84	Prosp	24	16	12	52
Tillerman et al. [25]	2002	110	Prosp	41	1	27	67

laparoscopic ultrasound as a staging modality by the MSKCC team may have decreased their overall yield.

In a larger study carried out by Tilleman and colleagues in the Netherlands [25], 110 patients with cholangiocarcinoma were investigated between 1993 and 2000, for tumour that was deemed potentially resectable by standard radiological imaging [25]. In these patients who were staged using laparoscopy without laparoscopic ultrasound, the results were similar to that of the Edinburgh group. Laparoscopy revealed histologically proven incurable disease in 41 % of patients with an accuracy of 56 %. Again, the authors comment that radiological staging has substantially improved in recent years both with the introduction of spiral CT with 3 mm slides and with the improvements in endoscopic ultrasonography [25], thereby accounting for the high yield in this study. The findings of all three studies are summarised in Table 11.2.

Conclusion

Patients with hilar cholangiocarcinoma often have unresectable disease that is not evident on pre-operative radiological imaging. Laparoscopic staging can prevent unnecessary laparotomies in around 30 % of patients. It would appear that the addition of laparoscopic ultrasound, is useful, and significantly improves the yield. Although the yield of laparoscopic staging is reasonable, the accuracy remains poor and unfortunately the majority of patients who undergo laparoscopic staging do not benefit from it. Unresectable disease in patients that is not detected at laparoscopy is most often due to locally advanced disease. Detecting this remains the biggest challenge in improving the yield and accuracy of laparoscopic staging. It is likely, as radiological technology improves, that the yield of laparoscopic staging may decrease as the majority of patients with non resectable disease will be identified pre-operatively, but until then many centres will continue to include this modality in its investigative and staging algorithm.

References

1. Goere D, Wagholikar GD, Pessaux P, et al. Utility of staging laparoscopy in subsets of biliary cancers. Surg Endosc. 2006;20:721–5.
2. D'Angelica M, Fong Y, Weber S, et al. The role of staging laparoscopy in hepatobiliary malignancy: prospective analysis of 401 cases. Ann Surg Oncol. 2002;10(2):183–9.
3. Rumstadt B, Schwab M, Schuster K, et al. The role of laparoscopy in the pre-operative staging of pancreatic carcinoma. J Gastrointest Surg. 1997;1:245–50.
4. van der Gaag NA, Busch ORC, Bemelman WA, et al. Laparoscopy in staging and assessment of hepatobiliary disease. In: Garden OJ, editor. Hepatobillary and pancreatic surgery. 4th ed. Saunders: Elsevier; 2009. p. 37–53.
5. Carlos U, Covera MD, Sharon M, et al. Role of laparoscopy in the evaluation of biliary tract cancer. Surg Oncol Clin N Am. 2002; 11:877–91.
6. Brooks AD, Mallis MJ, Brennan MF, et al. The value of laparoscopy in the management of ampullary, duodenal and distal bile duct tumours. J Gastrointest Surg. 2002;62:139–45.
7. Jarnagin WR, Conlon KC, Bodniewicz J. A clinical scoring system predicts yield of diagnostic laparoscopy in patients with potentially resectable hepatic colorectal metastasis. Cancer. 2001;91:1121–8.
8. White R, Pappas TN. Laparoscopic staging for hepatobiliary carcinoma. J Gastrointest Surg. 2004;8:920–2.
9. D'Angelica M, Fong Y, Weber S. The role of staging laparoscopy in hepatobiliary malignancy: prospective analysis of 401 cases. Ann Surg Oncol. 2003;10:183–9.
10. Connor S, Barron E, Wigmore SJ, et al. The utility of laparoscopic assessment in the preoperative staging of suspected hilar cholangiocarcinoma. J Gastrointest Surg. 2005;9:476–80.
11. Gouma DJ, van Nieveen DEJM, de Wit LT, et al. Laparoscopic staging of biliopancreatic malignancy. Ann Oncol. 1999;10: s33–6.
12. Joseph S, Connor S, Garden OJ. Staging laparoscopy for cholangiocarcinoma. HPB. 2008;10:116–9.
13. Boyd WP, Nord HJ. Diagnostic laparoscopy. Endoscopy. 2000; 32:153–8.
14. Bateman BG, Kolp LA, Hoeger K. Complications of laparoscopy-operative and diagnostic. Fertil Steril. 1996;66:30–5.
15. van der Voort M, Heijnsdijk EA, Gouma DJ. Bowel injury as a complication of laparoscopy. Br J Surg. 2004;91:1253–8.
16. Niveen van Dijkum EJ, de Wit LT, van Delden OM, et al. Staging laparoscopy and laparoscopic ultrasound in more than 400 patients with upper gastrointestinal carcinoma. J Am Coll Surg. 1999;189: 459–65.
17. Shoup M, Brennan MF, Karpeh MS, et al. Port site metastasis after diagnostic laparoscopy for upper gastrointestinal tract malignancies: an uncommon entity. Ann Surg Oncol. 2002;9:632–6.
18. Burke EC, Karpeh MS, Conlon KC, et al. Peritoneal lavage cytology in gastric cancer: an independent predictor of outcome. Ann Surg Oncol. 1998;5:411–5.
19. Makary MA, Warshaw AL, Centeno BA, et al. Implications of peritoneal cytology for pancreatic cancer management. Arch Surg. 1998;133:361–5.
20. Leach SD, Rose JA, Lowy AM, et al. Significance of peritoneal cytology in patients with potentially resectable adenocarcinoma of the pancreatic head. Surgery. 1995;118:472–8.

21. Jimenez RE, Warshaw AL, Rattner DW, et al. Impact of laparoscopic staging in the treatment of pancreatic cancer. Arch Surg. 2000;135:409–14.
22. Martin II RCG, Fong Y, DeMatteo RP, et al. Peritoneal washings are not predictive of occult peritoneal disease in patients with hilar cholangiocarcinoma. J Am Coll Surg. 2001;193:620–5.
23. Weber SM, DeMatteo MD, Fong Y, et al. Staging laparoscopy in patients with extrahepatic biliary carcinoma. Ann Surg. 2001; 235:392–9.
24. Jarnagin WR, Fong Y, DeMatteo RP. Staging analysis of resectability and outcome in 225 patients with hilar cholangiocarcinoma. Ann Surg. 2001;234:540–8.
25. Tilleman EHBM, de Castro SMM, Busch ORC, et al. Diagnostic laparoscopy and laparoscopic ultrasound for staging of patients with malignant proximal bile duct obstruction. J Gastrointest Surg. 2002;6:426–30.

12 Preoperative Optimization of the Liver for Resection

J. Belghiti and D. Fuks

12.1 Introduction

Hilar cholangiocarcinoma (HCCC) usually presents with jaundice, indicating involvement of the right and/or left bile ducts at their confluence. Even when the tumor is small, it is often infiltrative and is difficult to be managed surgically. Its unique location frequently results in involvement of the portal vein, the hepatic artery and/or the parenchyma of the liver around the hepatic hilum. Long-term survival rates depend on complete tumor clearance with extensive hepatic resection, which is risky in jaundiced patients; several large series reported mortality rates up to 20 % and morbidity rates of up to 67 % [1–14]. Parenchymal transection in the cholestatic liver is associated with more bleeding and a high risk of biliary fistula, sepsis, and also results in impaired liver regeneration [3]. Therefore, preoperative preparation is necessary for a major hepatectomy in jaundiced patients [15]. In an attempt to improve perioperative outcomes, many centers have advocated preoperative biliary drainage (BD) and ipsilateral portal vein embolization (PVE) of the hemi-liver to be resected to improve the functions of the future liver remnant (FLR) [4, 7, 11, 12, 14]. In addition, early assessment to look for distant metastases or peritoneal involvement is worthwhile. Laparoscopic staging avoids extensive preparation for inoperable patients. In this chapter, we describe the surgical planning and preparation for major hepatectomy for HCCC, focusing on preoperative treatment such as BD, PVE and laparoscopic staging.

J. Belghiti, MD (✉)
Department of Surgery, Hospital Beaujon,
100 Boulevard du Général Leclerc, 92110 Clichy, France
e-mail: jacques.belghiti@bjn.aphp.fr

D. Fuks, MD
Department of Digestive Surgery,
Hospital Beaujon, Clichy, France

12.2 Preoperative Biliary Drainage

Liver resection in patients with obstructive jaundice is associated with increased risks of intraoperative bleeding, postoperative biliary fistula and liver failure. The aims of BD are: (a) to decrease bilirubin level, (b) to treat biliary infection, (c) to assess the intraductal extent of carcinoma and (d) to optimize hypertrophy of the liver if PVE is performed. The major risks of BD include: (a) tumor seeding which occurs in about 5 % of cases after percutaneous BD; (b) infection; and (c) bleeding. The risk of cholangitis caused by BD can be minimized by avoiding preoperative cholangiography [16]. As there have been no prospective randomized studies to evaluate the role of preoperative BD prior to extend liver resection, this practice is widely variable [17–19]. However, most centers would use BD under the following three situations: (a) when the FLR is less than 40 % of the total liver volume and when PVE is used; (b) when cholangitis caused by endoscopic injection of contrast media fails to respond to antibiotics; and (c) in the presence of malnutrition, renal failure or hypoalbuminemia. In principle, unilateral drainage of the future remnant lobe is sufficient [18].

The beneficial effects of BD should, however, be balanced with the prolongation of hospital stay and increase in cost [17]. Rarely, patients with HCCC with short duration of jaundice are directly referred to specialized surgical units for management. These patients can be subjected to curative surgical exploration without any preoperative optimization. In our experience, these patients have a good tolerance to major hepatectomy [15]. In a recent French nationwide study (2009) which included 595 HCCC patients, serum bilirubin level (SBL) was found to be correlated with the mortality which ranged from 9 % when the SBL was <50 U to 27 % when the SBL was >300 U. The mortality was higher in patients who had preoperative BD, particularly when the SBL was higher than 100 U. The mortality rate after extended

W.Y. Lau (ed.), *Hilar Cholangiocarcinoma*,
DOI 10.1007/978-94-007-6473-6_12, © Springer Science+Business Media Dordrecht and People's Medical Publishing House 2013

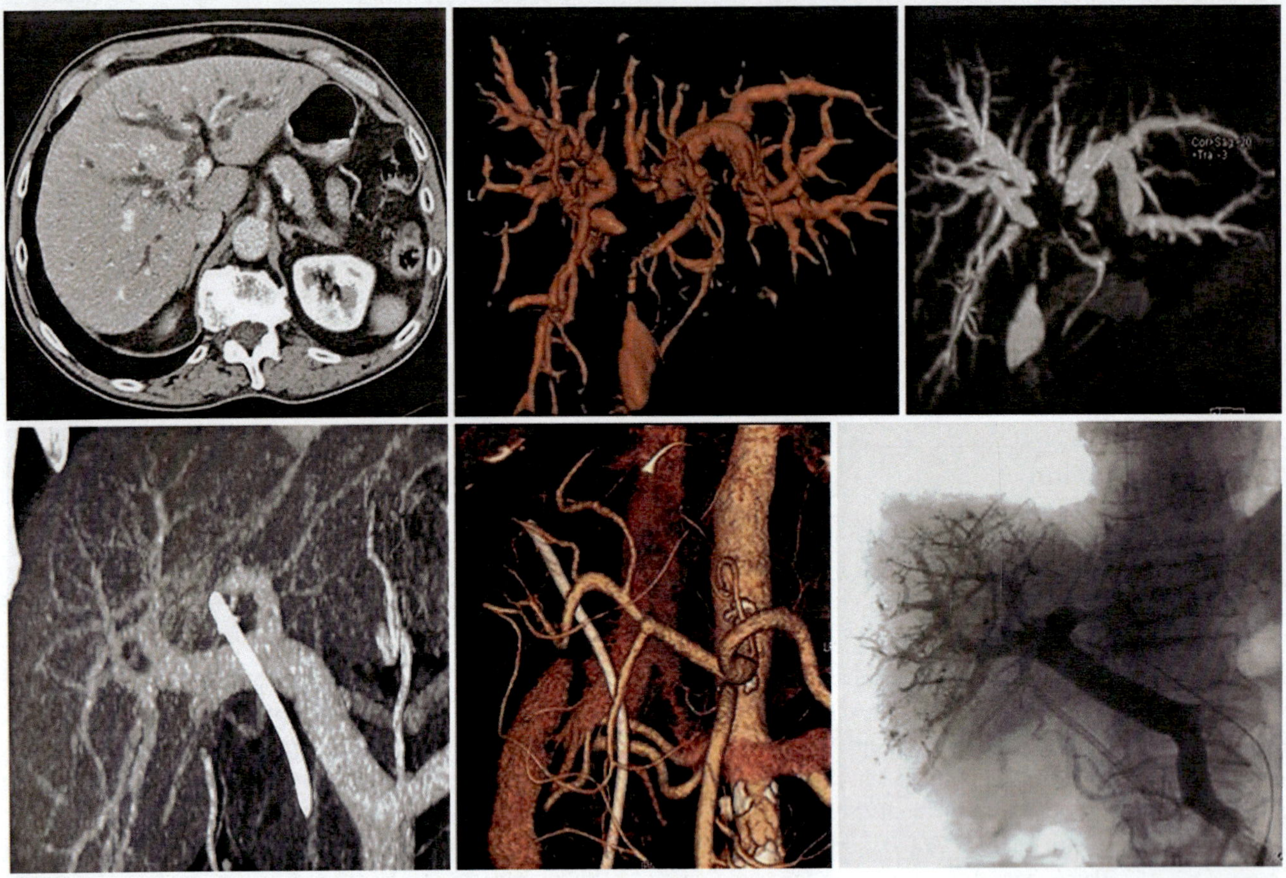

Fig. 12.1 CT and MRI reconstruction permits excellent visualization of hepatic parenchymal abnormalities, as well as visualization of the biliary tree and vascular structures

right hepatectomy was significantly lower in patients who had preoperative BD. The mortality in patients without BD increased exponentially with the SBL. However, the preoperative SBL was not related to the mortality in left hepatectomy. These unpublished results suggest that BD prior to surgery is useful only for right hepatectomy.

The choice of the route for preoperative BD has been debated controversial. A successful endoscopic retrograde biliary drainage (ERBD) using a plastic stent achieves an efficient drainage with a low morbidity and short hospital stay [20], and avoids the risk of tumor cell implantation in the percutaneous catheter tract [21]. However, the endoscopic approach is often technically difficult in patients with complete obstruction, especially when the left duct requires drainage. Regardless of the location of the biliary obstruction, either percutaneous transhepatic or endoscopic BD can be used and the choice depends on the availability of the local expertise. Cholestatic jaundice induces an increase in gut permeability due to altered villous morphology, activation of the gut components of the gut-associated lymphoid tissue and enterocytes, and a heightened acute phase response when exposed to endotoxin [22]. It has been shown that internal drainage is superior to external drainage by preventing bile loss from the gastrointestinal tract [23].

PTBD can be unilateral or bilateral, but most centers prefer a unilateral PTBD on the side of the FLR. If segmental cholangitis is not controlled after a technically successful hemi-hepatic BD, additional percutaneous BD can be used to drain the septic territory [9, 13, 16]. The duration of BD is not standardized but surgery is usually scheduled when the SBL is less than two or three times the upper limit of normal value (after 4–6 weeks) to restore the disturbances induced by jaundice. MRI permits excellent visualization of the hepatic parenchymal abnormalities, as well as the biliary tree and the vascular structures (Fig. 12.1) [24]. As MRI is non-invasive and it does not involve any radiation exposure, it may replace CT, angiography and cholangiography via PTBD.

12.3 Preoperative Portal Vein Embolization (PVE)

Extensive liver resection increases the chance of negative surgical resection margins [13]. However, chronic biliary obstruction restricts the tolerance of patients with HCCC to major parenchymal resection [11, 17]. Resection of more than 60 % of the total liver volume is associated with increased risks of major complications, postoperative liver failure, and mortality [25]. The aim of preoperative PVE is to initiate a compensatory hypertrophy of the FLR and thus minimizes postoperative liver dysfunction and liver failure [4, 11, 12, 26]. Although there has been no randomized controlled series to show the beneficial role of PVE in extended hepatectomy for HCCC, there are several arguments in favor of PVE before right extended resection, especially when vascular reconstruction is anticipated [26]. It has been shown that the mortality after liver resection for HCCC was significantly lower in patients with good hypertrophy of the FLR compared to patients without hypertrophy (3 % vs. 21 %) [1]. Also, hypertrophy of the FLR was more rapid when the SBL was lower than twofold of the normal value. Thus, for efficient hypertrophy of the FLR, PVE should be performed following BD and when the SBL has decreased to 50 IU. Liver resection can be performed between 2 and 3 weeks after PVE, although this wait is usually longer in Western countries [3–5, 15, 25]. Often, the FLR volume is overestimated due to the increase in volume of the biliary dilatation. Thus, the FLR volume should be measured only after sufficient biliary decompression.

The potential disadvantages of PVE are the risk of cholangitis in patients with extensive portal thrombosis, and sometimes the difficulty in determining the side of resection in patients with centrally placed tumor at the hilum. In extended right hepatectomy, supplemental embolization of segment 4 is not mandatory because the high part of segment 4 can be preserved. In addition, embolization of segment 4 is technically difficult and can result in migration of the thrombosis to the portal branches of the FLR. There have been some series which reported the experience of additional arterial embolization to improve the results of PVE [27]. This arterial embolization is performed 3–6 weeks after PVE and is more risky (infection) than PVE because the arterial branches are larger after PVE. Additional embolization of the hepatic vein was reported in very few series but it would increase the hypertrophy of the FLR [28].

In the French survey, about 33 % of right hepatectomy and 3 % of left hepatectomy received preoperative PVE. The mortality was lower in patients who underwent four or five segments of liver resection after PVE. Interestingly, in patients who underwent left hepatectomy after PVE, none died postoperatively suggesting that even in extended left hepatectomy, the risk of liver failure is very low.

12.4 Preoperative Staging Laparoscopy

It usually takes over 4 weeks for jaundice to resolve after BD, and sufficient hypertrophy of the FLR after PVE takes an additional 2 weeks. Unresectable HCCC can be formed at surgical exploration despite extensive preoperative evaluation including CT scan, ultrasonography, cholangio-MRI and cholangiography via PTBD. Peritoneal carcinomatosis and/or small intrahepatic metastases are not detectable by conventional preoperative investigations [29]. Of the patients who are surgically explored with a curative intent, only 40–50 % are ultimately resected. This has motivated the use of staging laparoscopy for patients with HCCC. The yield and accuracy of staging laparoscopy for patients with HCCC are between 25 and 42 %, and 42 and 53 %, respectively [30]. We perform staging laparoscopy before the above-mentioned preoperative preparation. Staging laparoscopy on patients who are initially assessed by conventional investigations to be resectable allowed us to discover peritoneal and distant metastasis in up to 20 % of patients. This policy of routine staging laparoscopy led to a shorter hospital stay and a more rapid and efficient treatment of these patients with metallic stents.

Recently, an innovative strategy has been described by German authors. The treatment involves a two-step procedure: transection of the liver parenchyma along with ligation of the biliary and portal branches while leaving the hepatic artery and vein intact. Liver resection is completed 1 week after regeneration of the FLR [31]. This novel technique dramatically shortened the long preparation of HCCC patients.

In conclusion, the resectability and the results of resection of HCCC can be improved with proper preoperative optimization of patients. Biliary drainage is indicated in patients with severe and prolonged jaundice. PVE improves resectability in patients with a marginal FLR and preoperative staging laparoscopy excludes patients who are not suitable for preoperative optimization (Fig. 12.2).

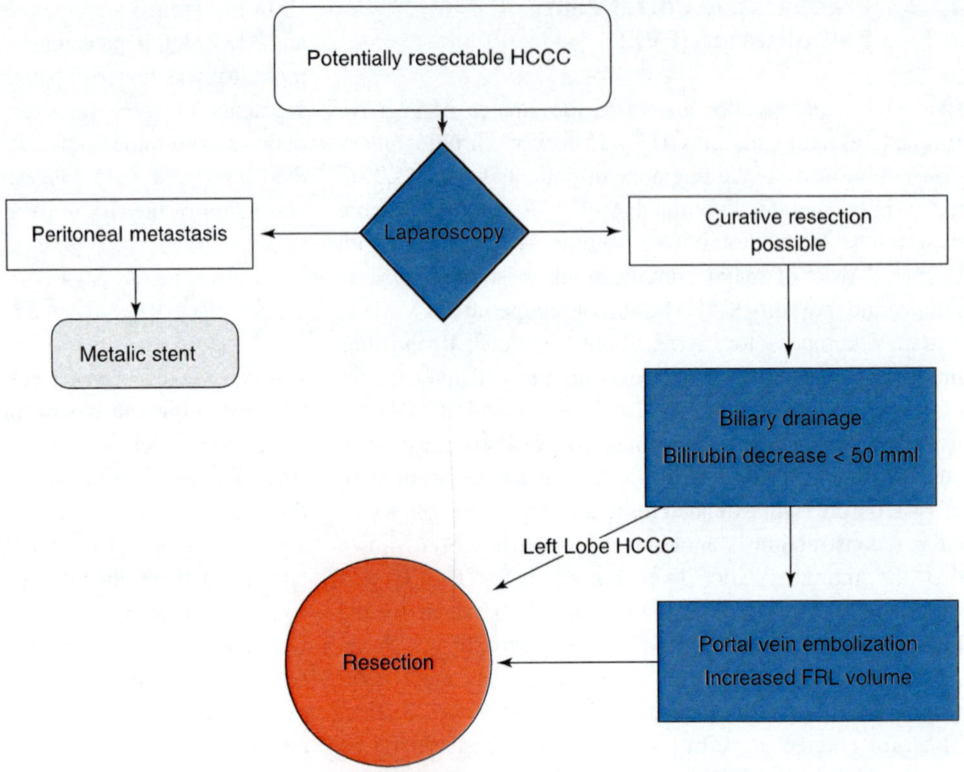

Fig. 12.2 Management protocol of HCCC requiring major hepatectomy

References

1. Hemming AW, Reed AI, Fujita S, et al. Surgical management of hilar cholangiocarcinoma. Ann Surg. 2005;241:693–9.
2. Neuhaus P, Jonas S, Bechstein WO, et al. Extended resections for hilar cholangiocarcinoma. Ann Surg. 1999;230:808–18.
3. Nimura Y, Kamiya J, Kondo S, et al. Aggressive preoperative management and extended surgery for hilar cholangiocarcinoma: Nagoya experience. J Hepatobiliary Pancreat Surg. 2000;7:155–62.
4. Sano T, Shimada K, Sakamoto Y, et al. One hundred two consecutive hepatobiliary resections for perihilar cholangiocarcinoma with zero mortality. Ann Surg. 2006;244:240–7.
5. Gerhards MF, Van Gulik TM, de Wit LT, et al. Evaluation of morbidity and mortality after resection for hilar cholangiocarcinoma-a single centre experience. Surgery. 2000;127:395–404.
6. Jarnagin WR, Bowne W, Klimstra DS, et al. Papillary phenotype confers improved survival after resection of hilar cholangiocarcinoma. Ann Surg. 2005;241:703–12.
7. Kawasaki S, Imamura H, Kobayashi A, et al. Results of surgical resection for patients with hilar bile duct cancer: application of extended hepatectomy after biliary drainage and hemihepatic portal vein embolization. Ann Surg. 2003;238:84–92.
8. Klempnauer J, Ridder GJ, von Wasielewski R, et al. Resectional surgery of hilar cholangiocarcinoma: a multivariate analysis of prognostic factors. J Clin Oncol. 1997;15:947–54.
9. Kosuge T, Yamamoto J, Shimada K, et al. Improved surgical results for hilar cholangiocarcinoma with procedures including major hepatic resection. Ann Surg. 1999;230:663–71.
10. Lee SG, Lee YJ, Park KM, et al. One hundred and eleven liver resections for hilar bile duct cancer. J Hepatobiliary Pancreat Surg. 2000;7:135–41.
11. Miyazaki M, Ito H, Nakagawa K, et al. Parenchyma-preserving hepatectomy in the surgical treatment of hilar cholangiocarcinoma. J Am Coll Surg. 1999;189:575–83.
12. Nagino M, Kamiya J, Arai T, et al. One hundred consecutive hepatobiliary resections for biliary hilar malignancy: preoperative blood donation, blood loss, transfusion, and outcome. Surgery. 2005;137:148–55.
13. Seyama Y, Kubota K, Sano K, et al. Long-term outcome of extended hemihepatectomy for hilar bile duct cancer with no mortality and high survival rate. Ann Surg. 2003;238:73–83.
14. Tabata M, Kawarada Y, Yokoi H, et al. Surgical treatment for hilar cholangiocarcinoma. J Hepatobiliary Pancreat Surg. 2000;7:148–54.
15. Ogata S, Belghiti J. Preoperative optimization of the liver for resection in patients with hilar cholangiocarcinoma. HPB (Oxford). 2005;7:252–3.
16. Grandadam S, Compagnon P, Arnaud A, et al. Role of preoperative optimization of the liver for resection in patients with hilar cholangiocarcinoma Type III. Ann Surg Oncol. 2010;17:3155–61.
17. Kennedy TJ, Yopp A, Qin Y, et al. Role of preoperative biliary drainage of liver remnant prior to extended liver resection for hilar cholangiocarcinoma. HPB. 2009;11:445–51.
18. Cherqui D, Benoist S, Malassagne B, et al. Major liver resection for carcinoma in jaundiced patients without preoperative biliary drainage. Arch Surg. 2000;135:302–8.
19. Nagino M, Takada T, Miyazaki M, et al. Preoperative biliary drainage for biliary tract and ampullary carcinomas. J Hepatobiliary Pancreat Surg. 2008;15:25–30.
20. Kawakami H, Kuwatani M, Onodera M, et al. Endoscopic nasobiliary drainage is the most suitable preoperative biliary drainage method in the management of patients with hilar cholangiocarcinoma. J Gastroenterol. 2011;46:242–8.
21. Takahashi Y, Nagino M, Nishio H, et al. Percutaneous transhepatic biliary drainage catheter tract recurrence in cholangiocarcinoma. Br J Surg. 2010;97:1860–6.
22. Welsh FK, Ramsden CW, MacLennan K, et al. Increased intestinal permeability and altered mucosal immunity in cholestatic jaundice. Ann Surg. 1998;227:205–12.

23. Saiki S, Chijiiwa K, Komura M, et al. Preoperative internal biliary drainage is superior to external biliary drainage in liver regeneration and function after hepatectomy in obstructive jaundiced rats. Ann Surg. 1999;230:655–62.
24. Choi JY, Kim MJ, Lee JM, et al. Hilar cholangiocarcinoma: role of preoperative imaging with sonography, MDCT, MRI, and direct cholangiography. AJR Am J Roentgenol. 2008;191:1448–57.
25. Abdalla EK, Barnett CC, Doherty D, et al. Extended hepatectomy in patients with hepatobiliary malignancies with and without preoperative portal vein embolization. Arch Surg. 2002;137:675–80.
26. Ebata T, Nagino M, Kamiya J, et al. Hepatectomy with portal vein resection for hilar cholangiocarcinoma: audit of 52 consecutive cases. Ann Surg. 2003;238:720–7.
27. Nagino M, Kanai M, Morioka A, et al. Portal and arterial embolization before extensive liver resection in patients with markedly poor functional reserve. J Vasc Interv Radiol. 2000;11:1063–8.
28. Hwang S, Lee SG, Ko GY, et al. Sequential preoperative ipsilateral hepatic vein embolization after portal vein embolization to induce further liver regeneration in patients with hepatobiliary malignancy. Ann Surg. 2009;249:608–16.
29. Weber SM, DeMatteo RP, Fong Y, et al. Staging laparoscopy in patients with extrahepatic biliary carcinoma. Analysis of 100 patients. Ann Surg. 2002;235:392–9.
30. Goere D, Wagholikar GD, Pessaux P, et al. Utility of staging laparoscopy in subsets of biliary cancers: laparoscopy is a powerful diagnostic tool in patients with intrahepatic and gallbladder carcinoma. Surg Endosc. 2006;20:721–5.
31. Baumgart J, Lang LH. A new method for induction of liver hypertrophy prior to right trisectionectomy: a report of 3 cases. HPB. 2011;13:71–2.

Preoperative Biliary Drainage 13

A.T. Ruys, E.A. Rauws, O.R.C. Busch, J.S. Lameris, D.J. Gouma, and T.M. van Gulik

13.1 Effects of Biliary Drainage

13.1.1 Introduction

Obstructive jaundice, clinically evident by jaundiced skin, nausea, pruritus, dark urine and discoloration of stool, is the most prevalent presenting symptom of hilar cholangiocarcinoma (HCCA). Obstructive jaundice is associated with a proinflammatory state, resulting from portal and systemic endotoxemia, increased permeability of the intestinal mucosal barrier, an altered reticuloendothelial system function of Kupffer cells in the liver, and increased concentrations of proinflammatory cytokines [1–3]. The exact link between jaundice and the development of infectious complications remains yet to be elucidated, but jaundice has been largely recognized as a major risk factor for performing pancreatic and liver surgery [4–6]. The presence of toxic substances such as bilirubin and bile salts, impaired liver function, and altered nutritional status have been proposed as responsible factors for increased infectious complications.

13.1.2 History

Already in 1935, the increased risk of surgery in jaundiced patients was acknowledged by Dr. Whipple [7]. He was the first to introduce the concept of preoperative biliary drainage (PBD) by performing a staged pancreatoduodenectomy. After a cholecystogastrostomy to reduce jaundice, a resection was performed at a later stage. In the mid 1960s, a preoperative less invasive biliary drainage method was developed, namely percutaneous transhepatic cholangiography (PTC) [8]. This was followed by the introduction of endoscopic retrograde cholangiopancreatography (ERCP) in the 70s of the previous century, which allowed endoscopists to leave a stent in the bile duct via the duodenum [9]. A variation of this endoscopic approach—the endoscopic nasobiliary drainage (ENBD)—was introduced in the beginning of the 80s [10]. With this technique, instead of leaving a stent through the stenosis, a tube is retracted from beyond the stenosis to the nose, where it is taped to the patient's cheek and attached to a drainage bag. The indication of biliary drainage, either by ERCP or PTC for pancreatic and liver surgery and the preferred method has been a matter of debate since the introduction of these techniques.

13.1.3 Differences in Drainage of Distal and Proximal Bile Duct Tumours

Since its introduction, ERCP has been widely used in patients with obstructive jaundice due to a tumour in the pancreatic head region, as a diagnostic tool as well as to drain the obstructed bile duct. However, the indispensability of a preoperative ERCP has slowly vanished over the years. Firstly, because today, state of- the-art radiological techniques offer a higher diagnostic accuracy than ERCP, are noninvasive, and have the advantage of assessing local tumour extension, as well as distant metastases. Therefore, nowadays ERCP is considered obsolete as a diagnostic tool. Secondly, complications of ERCP have been better assessed over the years, and consequently, the net benefit of the procedure is questioned. A large RCT in the USA concluded that PBD does not reduce operative risk, and does increase hospital cost and, therefore, should not be performed routinely [11]. In addition, a systematic review from our department

A.T. Ruys, MD • O.R.C. Busch, MD, PhD •
D.J. Gouma, MD, PhD • T.M. van Gulik, MD, PhD (✉)
Department of Surgery, Academic Medical Center,
University of Amsterdam, Amsterdam, The Netherlands
e-mail: t.m.vangulik@amc.uva.nl

E.A. Rauws, MD, PhD
Department of Gastroenterology and Hepatology,
Academic Medical Center, University of Amsterdam,
Amsterdam, The Netherlands

J.S. Lameris, MD, PhD
Department of Radiology, Academic Medical Center,
University of Amsterdam, Amsterdam, The Netherlands

W.Y. Lau (ed.), *Hilar Cholangiocarcinoma*,
DOI 10.1007/978-94-007-6473-6_13, © Springer Science+Business Media Dordrecht and People's Medical Publishing House 2013

summarized all retrospective and prospective studies until 2001, comparing PBD in jaundiced patients with patients that underwent direct surgical treatment [12]. Meta-analysis of both level I and level II studies showed no differences in mortality between patients who had PBD and those who had surgery without PBD. However, overall complication rate was significantly adversely affected by PBD compared with surgery without PBD. Furthermore, overall hospital stay was prolonged after PBD. The conclusion was that the potential benefit of PBD, in terms of postoperative rates of death and complications, does not outweigh the disadvantage of the drainage procedure and therefore should not be performed routinely, unless further improved PBD techniques would become available [12]. Finally, we conducted a large RCT in the Netherlands, in which patients were randomized between preoperative drainage and direct surgery [13]. A higher rate of serious complications was found in the drainage group, while mortality and hospital stay did not differ between the groups. Based on these findings, we concluded that routine PBD increases the rate of complications and thus should not be routinely performed. However, there remains an indication for PBD, when early surgery is not possible, due to logistics in terms of (local) referral patterns, waiting lists, extended diagnostic workup with laparoscopy (on indication), or scheduled neo-adjuvant chemotherapy.

While there is now evidence showing that PBD for distal (peripancreatic) tumours should not be routinely performed, this is not the case for the more proximal cholangiocarcinomas, i.e. HCCA. An important difference between distal tumours as compared with hilar tumours lies in the need for an (extended) liver resection in most patients with HCCA. Liver resections in jaundiced patients are associated with significantly increased rates of mortality and morbidity, resulting mainly from the development of postoperative complications such as sepsis, bleeding, and most importantly, liver failure [5]. Another important difference lies in the complexity of the procedure required to relieve jaundice. In distal tumours involving the common bile duct, complete drainage of the entire biliary tree can usually be accomplished by a single, well-placed catheter or stent because the obstruction is below the confluence of right and left bile ducts. In HCCA however, several segmental bile ducts are usually affected, rendering a single drainage catheter ineffective to completely drain the biliary tree.

13.2 Methods of Biliary Drainage

13.2.1 Endoscopic Biliary Drainage (ERCP)

13.2.1.1 Technique

Prior to stent insertion, crossectional studies such as CT or MRI, or ultrasound examinations are performed to assess biliary anatomy and to plan the most appropriate approach for intervention. In view of the high incidence of bacterial colonization of the obstructed biliary tree, broad-spectrum antibiotics are administered intravenously prior to the procedure to minimize the incidence of cholangitis. After a retrograde cholangiography is performed to localize the site of obstruction, the guidewire is maneuvered through and above the biliary stenosis followed by a catheter. The endoprosthesis is then pushed in position over the catheter (Fig. 13.1). It is important to reduce the risks of cholangitis by minimizing the amount of contrast injected and always draining ducts that have been opacified with significant amounts of contrast.

In addition to achieving imaging of the biliary system and adequate biliary drainage, ERCP is also used for tissue diagnosis. Tissue sampling during ERCP is however difficult and in case of using brush cytology, fine needle aspiration (FNA),

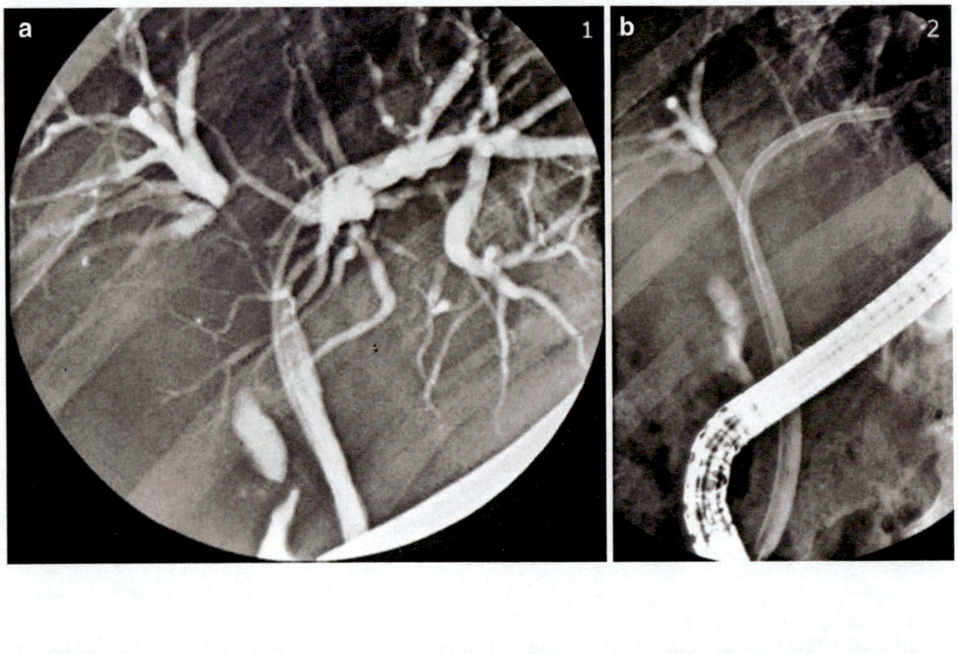

Fig. 13.1 ERCP in a patient with a Bismuth-Corlette type IIIa HCCA planned for hilar resection in combination with extended right hemihepatectomy. Cholangiography shows the anterior and posterior sectional obstruction on the *right side* and obstruction of the left hepatic duct (**a**); Stents are inserted in the right and left biliary systems (**b**)

fluoroscopically directed biopsy, or a combination of the above, a definitive diagnosis is only made in approximately 50 % of cases in most series [14, 15]. In a large study, ERCP brushings in 498 consecutive patients with pancreaticobiliary strictures were evaluated and compared with regard to diagnostic yield of routine cytology, addition of digital image analysis (DIA), and fluorescence in situ hybridization (FISH). None of the evaluated tests achieved a sensitivity above 43 % for detecting malignancy. Hence, clinical presentation and imaging studies (CT, PET-CT, MRCP, or ultrasound) remained the mainstay of diagnosis of HCCA.

Little evidence exists regarding the use of ERCP in preoperative drainage in potentially resectable patients with HCCA, while much more has been published about the results of ERCP in a palliative setting. Although in palliative drainage, different aspects are important as compared to the preoperative setting, several conclusions from studies in unresectable patients may also apply in resectable patients.

The major debate when using stent-directed biliary decompression has been the need for unilateral or bilateral drainage for anything more advanced than a Bismuth type II HCCA [16]. Bilateral stenting is technically challenging. The left system should be drained preferentially as a stent placed into the left main duct will usually produce more effective drainage than a stent in the right system. This is due to the longer length of the left main duct before branching leading to a larger volume of the liver being drained. The right system is more variable with earlier branching of the right hepatic duct; multiple segmental obstruction is more likely on the right side while a right sided stent more likely drains only a limited portion of the right system. Drainage of 25 % of the liver volume can achieve adequate palliation with improvement in biochemical parameters and relief of symptoms, with consequently improved quality of life [17]. No study comparing bilateral versus unilateral stenting for patients with resectable HCCA has been published. One RCT in unresectable patients showed a higher technical success rate of stent insertion and a significantly lower incidence of complications in patients who underwent unilateral drainage [18]. However, another study showed that mean survival, 30-day mortality, and deaths from sepsis were all significantly less with bilateral versus unilateral drainage [19]. In addition, a different group also found a better survival in patients who were drained bilaterally [20]. How this data should be extrapolated to the preoperative setting with curative intent remains to be determined. One additional factor should be acknowledged in the preoperative setting. Biliary drainage of the future remnant liver (FRL) promoted hypertrophy of the FRL after portal vein embolization, by which extended hemihepatectomy could be performed more safely [21].

Several studies have compared plastic with metal stents [22–24], and concluded that the patency rate of metal stents is superior. In order to further improve patency rates of the metal stents, covered metal stents were introduced. In contrast to patients with distal obstructions, patency rates did not improve with the use of covered stents in patients with proximal obstruction [25–27]. Due to the relatively short time to surgery, long patency is not essential for resectable patients, and metal stents may hamper hilar dissection and resection. Hence, although metal stents have advantages over plastic stents, this is not the case for resectable patients, and plastic stents are recommended in the preoperative work-up of patients with HCCA.

Finally, considering the difficulties in endoscopic management encountered in patients with HCCA, ERCP for hilar obstruction should only be undertaken in specialized centres with high success rates for endoscopic drainage of hilar obstruction. This is also supported by a study that evaluated 5,264 ERCP's in 66 centers, concluding that careful patient selection combined with skilled cannulation minimizes complications, while higher risk procedures should be performed in specialist centers [28].

13.2.1.2 Advantages and Complication

A major disadvantage of an endoscopic approach is contamination of the sterile environment of the biliary tree. This can lead to severe cholangitis, biliary sepsis, and even mortality of the procedure has been described. Several other complications of ERCP that have been reported include: cholangitis, acute cholecystitis, pancreatitis, duodenal perforation, post-papillotomy bleeding, biliary perforation, tube occlusion requiring re-intervention. A technical success rate of 81 % was found in a study including 90 patients who underwent ERCP for HCCA. The ERCP was accompanied by infectious complications in 43 patients, dislocation of the stent in 21 patients, pancreatitis in seven patients, duodenal perforation in one patient, and biliary perforation in another patient. Hence, complications or unsuccessful drainage attempts are encountered in the majority of patients.

Another disadvantage is that ERCP usually does not offer the possibility to perform selective biliary drainage, and typically, only part of the biliary system can be drained adequately. Lastly, ERCP is not feasible, or eventually not successful in a substantial part of patients with HCCA. Conversion of ERCP to PTBD or ENBD has been reported in 30–95 % of patients undergoing biliary drainage [29–32].

13.2.2 Percutaneous Transhepatic Biliary Drainage (PTBD)

13.2.2.1 Technique

Pre-procedural, broad spectrum antibiotic prophylaxis is given to all patients undergoing biliary drainage because transient bacteremia commonly occurs during the procedure, even in the absence of signs of infection. Biliary drainage is

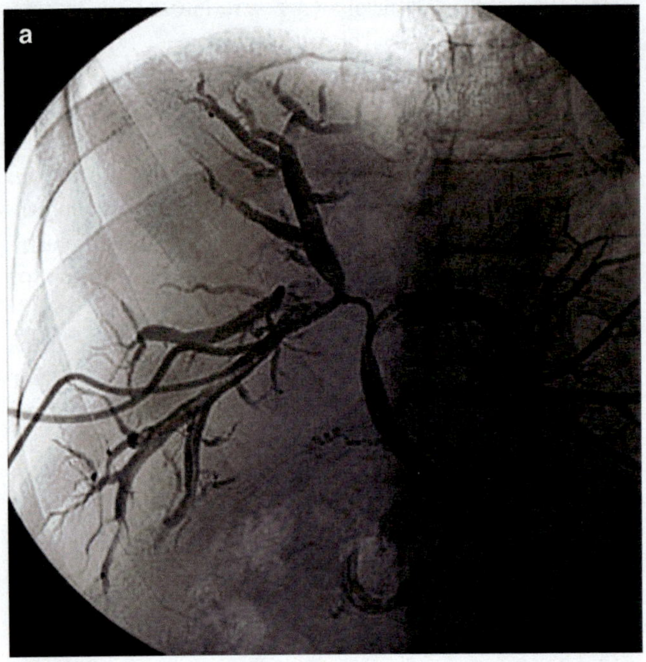

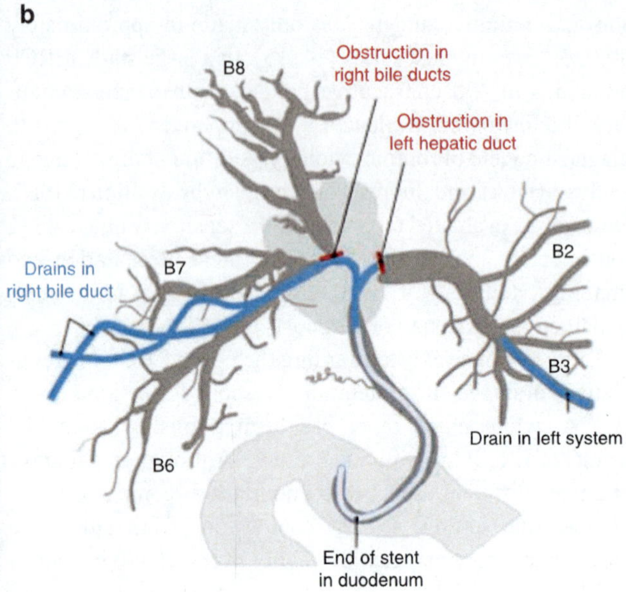

Fig. 13.2 Percutaneous cholangiogram of patient with a Bismuth-Corlette type IV tumour, in whom the right as well as the left bile duct system were drained separately. There is an obstruction of the first segmental bile ducts of the right system (B6, B7 and B8; B5 is not filled with contrast, due to obstruction), and an obstruction of the left hepatic duct, in which the segmental ducts (B2, B3, and B4) end. The B4 segmental duct has no connection with B2 and B3, and is therefore not filled with contrast. This patient underwent hilar resection in combination with extended right hemihepatectomy and resection of segment 1

performed with conscious sedation, often with short-acting benzodiazepines and narcotics. As with an endoscopic approach, PTCD is more challenging for a HCCA than for a distal bile duct tumour. Pre-procedural planning should involve evaluation of the exact level and extension of the stenosis or stenoses, selection of the most appropriate liver segments for drainage, and assessment of an appropriate access route, mostly by ultrasound guidance. This is particularly important when segmental bile duct obstruction is suspected, and every attempt should be made to avoid contaminating regions of the biliary tree that will not be drained.

Biliary drainage is most often performed using fluoroscopic guidance as shown in Fig. 13.2, after initial puncture of a bile duct using ultrasound guidance. Adequate drainage and stenting of one complete liver lobe is usually sufficient to relief the jaundice, but drainage of only one or two segments within one lobe is usually not enough. There is no consensus as to whether stents should be placed from the hilum all the way down the common bile duct through the papilla of Vater into the duodenum. Theoretically, preservation of function of the sphincter should lower the chance of developing ascending cholangitis. Although many authors advocate to stent through the papilla in distal obstructions, there is no evidence that this improves patency in proximal bile duct strictures. When one lobe is severely atrophied as a result of longstanding occlusion of the ipsilateral portal vein, it is usually not useful to stent the atrophied lobe, unless cholangitis is suspected to originate from this lobe. As hilar cholangiocarcinomas are often very rigid, it may in some cases be useful to pre-dilate the stricture to facilitate insertion of a stent. Dilating a self-expanding stent after insertion may also be required in selected cases.

13.2.2.2 Advantages, and Complications of PTBD

As for ERCP, most evidence regarding PTBD is available for application in a palliative setting, and large series reporting success rates and complications predominately deal with unresectable patients. PTBD has a distinct advantage over ERCP in that with ultrasound guidance one or more appropriate segments for drainage can be chosen and injection of contrast medium in segments that are too small to be drained can be prevented. Ultrasound guidance during PTBD is extremely useful in such patients. Furthermore, assessing hilar strictures and draining the appropriate segments can be very difficult with ERCP. Also, the extent of tumour infiltration into the proximal bile duct proximal to the obstruction is hardly assessable by ERCP, whereas proximal ductal extent can usually be precisely determined by PTCD.

Several complications after PTCD have been reported, including: occlusion, cholangitis, contralateral segmental cholangitis, portal vein injury and thrombosis, tube dislocation, cholecystitis, biliovenous fistula, biloma, hemobilia, and cancer dissemination.

Metastatic tumour seeding along the transhepatic biliary catheter was considered a very rare complication with only a few reported cases. But, recently several large series were reported on the incidence of catheter tract recurrence [30, 33]. The largest series containing 445 patients detected 23 patients (5 %) with catheter tract recurrence, and concluded that therefore, PTCD should no longer be performed in resectable patients. We use preoperative low dose radiation (3×3.5 Gy) to prevent this troublesome complication, and did not detect any recurrence after introduction of preoperative radiation [34]. In our department, standard preoperative low dose radiotherapy is instituted in all patients with HCCA planned for resection [34].

An additional advantage of the percutaneous route of biliary drainage is that the biliary tubes are an aid to locate the bile ducts proximal of the tumour in the liver parenchyma and that after the resection has taken place, the tubes can be used as transanastomotic drains to facilitate healing of the hepaticojejunostomies. The tubes are removed after control cholangiography via the tubes 3–6 weeks later.

Reported technical success of PTCD is more than 90 % in all series. Clinical success ranges from 80 to 100 %, procedure-related mortality ranges from 0 to 3 %, 30-day mortality ranges from 9 to 20 % and was usually related to the underlying disease. Procedure related complications range from 7 to 30 % and can be treated conservatively in the majority of cases. Recurrence of obstructive jaundice ranges from 15 to 25 % [29, 31, 35–39].

13.2.3 Endoscopic Nasobiliary Drainage (ENBD)

13.2.3.1 Technique

Although ENBD was introduced in the beginning of the 80s, very little information about this technique has been reported in literature. As was described already in 1984 [40], a guide wire is passed down the endoscope channel and through the stricture of the bile duct. The tip is advanced and looped high in the common hepatic duct or liver. A suitable drainage tube is then advanced through the endoscope to the tip of the wire. The guide wire is withdrawn, and the proximal end of the tube is rerouted from the mouth to the nose using temporary nasopharyngeal intubation. The tube is taped to the patient's cheek and attached to a drainage bag via a 3-way tap, so that the system can be closed, flushed, or aspirated as required. An anchorage system is necessary to avoid tube migration.

13.2.3.2 Advantages and Complications of ENBD

Advantages, disadvantages, and complications are similar to those of ERCP. Even though, due to the retrograde flow of duodenal fluid via the stent into the bile ducts, cholangitis occurs more frequently after ERCP. Furthermore, the availability of an external drain allows contrast cholangiography at any time via the nasobiliary tube. ENBD also permits evaluation of the volume and colour of biliary secretions. Enteral drainage in ERCP improves nutritional status and immune function by restoring enterohepatic recirculation to the digestive tract, and does not require a nasal tube. Clearly, internal drainage using a stent is a benefit for the patient as nasal intubation is a significant burden.

Until now, only three series have been published reporting the results of ENBD [29, 30, 41]. Complications were found in 13–38 % of patients who underwent ENBD, and included acute pancreatitis, segmental cholangitis, cholangitis with catheter obstruction, tube dislocation, and retroperitoneal perforation. Success rates of the initial procedure ranged from 74 to 78 % [29, 30].

13.3 Efficacy of ENBD, ERCP, and PTCD

Currently, the preferred technique of biliary drainage prior to surgery for a proximal bile duct tumour depends mainly on local expertise [42]. Controversy exists regarding the preferred technique of PBD, either by ERCP, PTBD, or ENBD. This is also illustrated by the report of a recent Japanese consensus meeting, stating that: "*Regardless of the location of the biliary obstruction, percutaneous transhepatic, endoscopic, or surgical drainage can be used*" [43].

Internal drainage by ERCP, although a less invasive technique, carries increased risk of developing cholangitis due to bacterial contamination from the duodenum and increased risk of procedure related complications such as duodenal perforation and post-ERCP, acute pancreatitis [44, 45]. Drainage by means of PTBD is associated with hemobilia, portal vein thrombosis, cancer cell seeding and potentially more patient discomfort. And lastly, ENBD has some advantages over ERCP, in particular less complications like stent occlusion and cholangitis. On the other hand, the external drainage of ENBD impairs nutritional status and immune function by undermining enterohepatic recirculation, while the nasal tube is a considerable burden for the patient. All mentioned advantages, and disadvantages are summarised in Table 13.1.

Three prospective, randomized controlled trials (RCTs) have been published comparing ERCP versus PTBD [46–48]. These RCTs included patients with unresectable bile duct tumours or carcinoma of the gallbladder and pancreas showing conflicting results. These studies addressed palliative treatment and although important in the context of biliary drainage, no distinction was made between distal and proximal bile duct obstruction. To date, no RCT has been performed regarding the optimal route of drainage in patients with a potentially resectable HCCA. Two retrospective studies, compared ERCP and PTBD in patients eligible for resection of a suspected HCCA [30, 31], and in one of these, ENBD was assessed as well. The studies showed conflicting results. The first study showed significantly less complications in the percutaneously treated patients, and advocated this technique for the future. The second study, found significantly more complications in the ERCP group, and comparable results for ENBD and PTCD. However, in the PTCD group as compared to the ENBD group, significantly more major complications (15 % vs. 2 %, $P<0.01$) were found, namely cancer dissemination and portal vein injury. In conclusion the authors highly recommended ENBD as the preferred method for PBD. Hence, with these conflicting results, it remains difficult to conclude what the preferred drainage method is. Both studies suffered from limitations, and especially the retrospective nature of these studies precludes a definitive conclusion. The results of other studies reporting on PTCD, ERCP, or ENBD are summarized in Table 13.2.

PTBD used to be the preferred method in Japan for relief of obstructive jaundice due to HCCA [42, 49]. In Europe and the USA, ERCP is usually performed as primary intervention and is followed by PTBD only when ERCP has failed, as shown in Fig. 13.3. Yet recently, Japanese authors published

Table 13.1 Advantages and complications of ENBD, ERCP, and PTCD

	Advantages	Disadvantages and complications
PTCD	Allows selective drainage	Drainage tract metastases
	Allows combined external/internal drainage	Bleeding complications
	Allows post-drainage cholangiography	
	High success rate	
	Useful as transanastomotic drain postoperatively	
ENBD	Less invasive than PTCD	Patient discomfort due to nasal tube
	Less stent obstruction than ERCP	Selective drainage is not always possible
	Allows post-drainage cholangiography	
ERCP	Internal drainage	Failure of complete drainage
	Non invasive	Stent obstruction
		Post-ERCP pancreatitis
		Post-drainage cholangiography is not feasible
		Selective drainage is not always feasible

Table 13.2 Outcome of ENBD, ERCP, and PTCD in HCCA

Author (year)	Method	Patients	Success rate	Complications (%)	Additional drainage (%)
Nimura (2000)	PTCD	133	–	23	–
Mansfield (2005)	PTCD	65	–	–	–
	ERCP	41	71		36 (88)
Maguchi (2007)	PTCD	9	67	–	3 (33)
	ENBD	12	25		9 (75)
	ERCP	4	0		4 (100)
Arakura (2009)	ENBD	62	74	13	16 (26)
Paik[a] (2009)	PTCD	41	93	32	42
	ERCP	44	72	30	38
Kawakami (2010)	PTCD	48	96	31	2 (4)
	ENBD	60	78	38	13 (22)
	ERCP	20	5	65	19 (95)
Kloek (2010)	PTCD	11	100	9	0
	ERCP	90	81	48	39 (43)

[a]RCT including unresectable HCCA patients

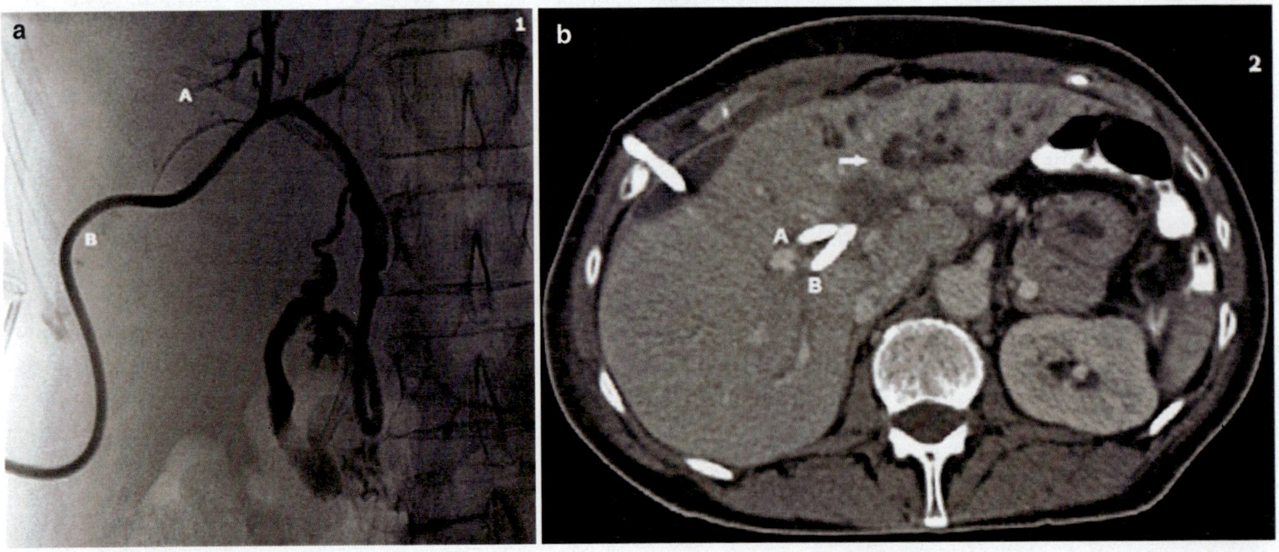

Fig. 13.3 Percutaneous transhepatic cholangiogram (**a**), and CT-scan (**b**) of a patient diagnosed with a Bismuth-Corlette type IV HCCA, referred with an ERCP-stent placed in the right anterior sectional bile duct. In preparation of hilar resection and extended left hemihepatectomy, the right posterior sectional ducts were drained using PTD. Only the future remnant liver is drained, and consequently the left bile duct system is still dilated (*arrow*). *A* ERCP-stent in right anterior sectional bile duct, *B* Percutaneous drain in right posterior sectional system

an article addressing the incidence of implantation metastases after PTCD and hereby pushed the pendulum back by recommending endoscopic drainage to prevent postoperative implantation metastases [33]. Hence, there is no evidence providing a clear-cut answer as to which method of PBD we should use.

Conclusions

The proper approach to jaundice in patients undergoing hepatobiliary and pancreatic surgery has been debated for several decades now. Although basic research on the mechanisms of the disease is progressing with time, the exact relation of jaundice and complications is still not fully understood. For distal bile duct tumours, evidence is nowadays fairly straight-forward, suggesting that PBD should not be routinely performed. For HCCA, high-quality evidence is still lacking, and consequently, the debate about the use of PBD for HCCA still continues. Nonetheless, mortality after extended liver resection in jaundiced patients is still highly significant, and therefore, most surgeons are in favour of PBD before undertaking extended hepatectomy, despite a lack of clear evidence based on RCTs.

The three usual drainage techniques, i.e. ERCP, ENBD and PTCD, all have their own pros, cons, and indications. These techniques are often used in combination with each other. Studies comparing PBD techniques, included different patient groups, are very outdated, or are retrospective in nature and are burdened by major methological flaws. In addition, these studies report conflicting results. Hence, solid advice regarding the recommended drainage technique to be used for PBD in HCCA cannot be given. Thus, until a well designed RCT proves otherwise, the preferred technique of biliary drainage prior to surgery for HCCA should mainly be contingent upon individual anatomy, and, in part, upon institutional expertise.

References

1. Greve JW, Gouma DJ, Buurman WA. Complications in obstructive jaundice: role of endotoxins. Scand J Gastroenterol Suppl. 1992; 194:8–12.
2. Kimmings AN, van Deventer SJ, Obertop H, et al. Inflammatory and immunologic effects of obstructive jaundice: pathogenesis and treatment. J Am Coll Surg. 1995;181(6):567–81.
3. Clements WD, McCaigue M, Erwin P, et al. Biliary decompression promotes Kupffer cell recovery in obstructive jaundice. Gut. 1996;38(6):925–31.
4. Sewnath ME, Birjmohun RS, Rauws EA, et al. The effect of preoperative biliary drainage on postoperative complications after pancreaticoduodenectomy. J Am Coll Surg. 2001;192(6):726–34.
5. Cherqui D, Benoist S, Malassagne B, et al. Major liver resection for carcinoma in jaundiced patients without preoperative biliary drainage. Arch Surg. 2000;135(3):302–8.
6. Sakata J, Shirai Y, Tsuchiya Y, et al. Preoperative cholangitis independently increases in-hospital mortality after combined major hepatic and bile duct resection for hilar cholangiocarcinoma. Langenbeck's Arch Surg. 2009;394(6):1065–72.
7. Whipple AO, Parsons WB, Mullins CR. Treatment of carcinoma of the ampulla of vater. Ann Surg. 1935;102(4):763–79.
8. Glenn F, Evans JA, Mujahed Z, et al. Percutaneous transhepatic cholangiography. Ann Surg. 1962;156:451–62.
9. Oi KS, Kondo T. Endoscopic pancreaticocholangiography. Endoscopy. 1970;2:103–6.
10. Cotton PB, Burney PG, Mason RR. Transnasal bile duct catheterisation after endoscopic sphincterotomy: method for biliary drainage, perfusion, and sequential cholangiography. Gut. 1979; 20(4):285–7.
11. Pitt HA, Gomes AS, Lois JF, et al. Does preoperative percutaneous biliary drainage reduce operative risk or increase hospital cost? Ann Surg. 1985;201(5):545–53.
12. Sewnath ME, Karsten TM, Prins MH, et al. A meta-analysis on the efficacy of preoperative biliary drainage for tumours causing obstructive jaundice. Ann Surg. 2002;236(1):17–27.
13. van der Gaag NA, Rauws EA, van Eijck CH, et al. Preoperative biliary drainage for cancer of the head of the pancreas. N Engl J Med. 2010;362(2):129–37.
14. Parsi MA, Li A, Li CP, et al. DNA methylation alterations in endoscopic retrograde cholangiopancreatography brush samples of patients with suspected pancreaticobiliary disease. Clin Gastroenterol Hepatol. 2008;6(11):1270–8.
15. Fritcher EG, Kipp BR, Halling KC, et al. A multivariable model using advanced cytologic methods for the evaluation of indeterminate pancreatobiliary strictures. Gastroenterology. 2009;136(7): 2180–6.
16. Kozarek RA. Inflammation and carcinogenesis of the biliary tract: update on endoscopic treatment. Clin Gastroenterol Hepatol. 2009;7(11 Suppl):S89–94.
17. Dowsett JF, Vaira D, Hatfield AR, et al. Endoscopic biliary therapy using the combined percutaneous and endoscopic technique. Gastroenterology. 1989;96(4):1180–6.
18. De Palma GD, Galloro G, Siciliano S, et al. Unilateral versus bilateral endoscopic hepatic duct drainage in patients with malignant hilar biliary obstruction: results of a prospective, randomized, and controlled study. Gastrointest Endosc. 2001;53(6):547–53.
19. Deviere J, Baize M, de Toeuf J, et al. Long-term follow-up of patients with hilar malignant stricture treated by endoscopic internal biliary drainage. Gastrointest Endosc. 1988;34(2):95–101.
20. Chang WH, Kortan P, Haber GB. Outcome in patients with bifurcation tumours who undergo unilateral versus bilateral hepatic duct drainage. Gastrointest Endosc. 1998;47(5):354–62.
21. Ishizawa T, Hasegawa K, Sano K, et al. Selective versus total biliary drainage for obstructive jaundice caused by a hepatobiliary malignancy. Am J Surg. 2007;193(2):149–54.
22. Kaassis M, Boyer J, Dumas R, et al. Plastic or metal stents for malignant stricture of the common bile duct? Results of a randomized prospective study. Gastrointest Endosc. 2003;57(2):178–82.
23. Prat F, Chapat O, Ducot B, et al. A randomized trial of endoscopic drainage methods for inoperable malignant strictures of the common bile duct. Gastrointest Endosc. 1998;47(1):1–7.
24. Soderlund C, Linder S. Covered metal versus plastic stents for malignant common bile duct stenosis: a prospective, randomized, controlled trial. Gastrointest Endosc. 2006;63(7):986–95.
25. Isayama H, Komatsu Y, Tsujino T, et al. A prospective randomised study of "covered" versus "uncovered" diamond stents for the management of distal malignant biliary obstruction. Gut. 2004;53(5): 729–34.
26. Kahaleh M, Tokar J, Conaway MR, et al. Efficacy and complications of covered Wallstents in malignant distal biliary obstruction. Gastrointest Endosc. 2005;61(4):528–33.

27. Yoon WJ, Lee JK, Lee KH, et al. A comparison of covered and uncovered Wallstents for the management of distal malignant biliary obstruction. Gastrointest Endosc. 2006;63(7):996–1000.
28. Williams EJ, Taylor S, Fairclough P, et al. Risk factors for complication following ERCP; results of a large-scale, prospective multicenter study. Endoscopy. 2007;39(9):793–801.
29. Arakura N, Takayama M, Ozaki Y, et al. Efficacy of preoperative endoscopic nasobiliary drainage for hilar cholangiocarcinoma. J Hepato-Biliary-Pancreat Surg. 2009;16(4):473–7.
30. Kawakami H, Kuwatani M, Onodera M, et al. Endoscopic nasobiliary drainage is the most suitable preoperative biliary drainage method in the management of patients with hilar cholangiocarcinoma. J Gastroenterol. 2010;46(2):242–8.
31. Kloek JJ, van der Gaag NA, Aziz Y, et al. Endoscopic and percutaneous preoperative biliary drainage in patients with suspected hilar cholangiocarcinoma. J Gastrointest Surg. 2010;14(1):119–25.
32. Rerknimitr R, Kladcharoen N, Mahachai V, et al. Result of endoscopic biliary drainage in hilar cholangiocarcinoma. J Clin Gastroenterol. 2004;38(6):518–23.
33. Takahashi Y, Nagino M, Nishio H, et al. Percutaneous transhepatic biliary drainage catheter tract recurrence in cholangiocarcinoma. Br J Surg. 2010;97(12):1860–6.
34. Gerhards MF, Gonzalez DG, ten Hoopen-Neumann H, et al. Prevention of implantation metastases after resection of proximal bile duct tumours with pre-operative low dose radiation therapy. Eur J Surg Oncol. 2000;26(5):480–5.
35. Kaskarelis IS, Papadaki MG, Papageorgiou GN, et al. Long-term follow-up in patients with malignant biliary obstruction after percutaneous placement of uncovered wallstent endoprostheses. Acta Radiol. 1999;40(5):528–33.
36. Oikarinen H, Leinonen S, Karttunen A, et al. Patency and complications of percutaneously inserted metallic stents in malignant biliary obstruction. J Vasc Interv Radiol. 1999;10(10):1387–93.
37. Hamy A, d'Alincourt A, Paineau J, et al. Percutaneous self-expandable metallic stents and malignant biliary strictures. Eur J Surg Oncol. 1997;23(5):403–8.
38. Roeren T, Tonn W, Richter GM, et al. Percutaneous therapy of malignant obstructive jaundice using expandable metal stents: a prospective study of 92 patients. Rofo. 1996;165(2):181–7.
39. Inal M, Akgul E, Aksungur E, et al. Percutaneous placement of biliary metallic stents in patients with malignant hilar obstruction: unilobar versus bilobar drainage. J Vasc Interv Radiol. 2003;14(11):1409–16.
40. Cotton PB. Endoscopic methods for relief of malignant obstructive jaundice. World J Surg. 1984;8(6):854–61.
41. Maguchi H, Takahashi K, Katanuma A, et al. Preoperative biliary drainage for hilar cholangiocarcinoma. J Hepato-Biliary-Pancreat Surg. 2007;14(5):441–6.
42. van der Gaag NA, Kloek JJ, de Castro SM, et al. Preoperative biliary drainage in patients with obstructive jaundice: history and current status. J Gastrointest Surg. 2009;13(4):814–20.
43. Nagino M, Takada T, Miyazaki M, et al. Preoperative biliary drainage for biliary tract and ampullary carcinomas. J Hepato-Biliary-Pancreat Surg. 2008;15(1):25–30.
44. Cotton PB, Lehman G, Vennes J, et al. Endoscopic sphincterotomy complications and their management: an attempt at consensus. Gastrointest Endosc. 1991;37(3):383–93.
45. dos Santos JS, Junior WS, Modena JL, et al. Effect of preoperative endoscopic decompression on malignant biliary obstruction and postoperative infection. Hepatogastroenterology. 2005;52(61):45–7.
46. Pinol V, Castells A, Bordas JM, et al. Percutaneous self-expanding metal stents versus endoscopic polyethylene endoprostheses for treating malignant biliary obstruction: randomized clinical trial. Radiology. 2002;225(1):27–34.
47. Saluja SS, Gulati M, Garg PK, et al. Endoscopic or percutaneous biliary drainage for gallbladder cancer: a randomized trial and quality of life assessment. Clin Gastroenterol Hepatol. 2008;6(8):944–50.
48. Speer AG, Cotton PB, Russell RC, et al. Randomised trial of endoscopic versus percutaneous stent insertion in malignant obstructive jaundice. Lancet. 1987;2(8550):57–62.
49. Nimura Y. Preoperative biliary drainage before resection for cholangiocarcinoma (Pro). HPB (Oxford). 2008;10(2):130–3.

Portal Vein Embolization

14

T. Hashimoto and M. Makuuchi

Abstract

Preoperative portal vein embolization (PVE) is performed to increase the safety of major hepatic resection which reduces the volume of the liver and raises the portal pressure immediately after operation. PVE induces atrophy of the embolized portion of the liver to be resected, with compensatory hypertrophy of the contralateral portion of the future preserved liver remnant. Today, PVE is widely accepted as a standard preoperative procedure for patients with hilar cholangiocarcinoma.

14.1 Introduction

In patients with hilar cholangiocarcinoma, radical surgery out performs any other therapeutic modalities in survival rate and quality of life [1]. To improve survival for hilar cholangiocarcinoma, curative resection after good preoperative management is an important approach [2]. Minimal resection of the involved segments, such as en-bloc caudate lobectomy, paramedian sectorectomy with caudate lobectomy, and central hepatectomy have been selected on the basis of the extent of cancer invasion to minimize the risk of postoperative hepatic failure [3, 4]. However, in many patients with hilar cholangiocarcinoma, limited hepatectomy is insufficient, and extended hepatectomy is required to obtain a negative surgical margin for cancer. Extended hemihepatectomy has recently been recognized as the standard curative treatment for hilar bile duct cancer and has an acceptable mortality [5–9]. Major hepatectomy, concomitant with pancreaticoduodenectomy has been applied to selected patients with advanced tumors [7, 8, 10–12]. However, these extensive radical procedures are not always safe, because there are risks of postoperative liver failure, especially after extended right hepatectomy. The greater the volume of liver resected, the greater the risk for patients to develop postoperative hepatic failure due to insufficient remnant liver volume.

In 1982, to overcome this problem, Makkuchi et al. carried out the first preoperative portal vein embolization (PVE) on a patient with hilar bile duct carcinoma scheduled to undergo a major hepatic resection [13, 14]. This approach was based on the concept of hepatic "atrophy-hypertrophy complex". The concept dates back to 1920 when Rous and Larimore ligated a major branch of the portal vein in a rabbit, and successfully acquired atrophy of the ipsilateral hepatic lobe and hypertrophy of the contralateral lobe [15]. Later, in 1975, in an effort to suppress tumor growth, Honjo et al. ligated the ipsilateral portal venous branch in patients with hepatocellular carcinoma (HCC) [16]. Although the approach did not succeed in preventing tumor growth, it did produce marked atrophy of the occluded part of the liver. Likewise, patients with hilar bile duct carcinoma involving a branch of the portal vein experienced an uneventful postoperative clinical course after extensive hepatectomy as the tumor caused partial liver atrophy and corresponding hypertrophy of the contralateral portion of the liver [17].

Major hepatectomy induces reduction in liver volume and raises portal pressure immediately after operation. If PVE is performed preoperatively, the portal pressure would already have been raised at the time of PVE and a slight increase in size can be observed in the remnant liver. PVE has dramatically increased the safety of hepatic resection, and consequently, the indication for PVE has now been extended to other diseases; such as HCC, intrahepatic cholangiocarcinoma, and metastatic liver tumors [18].

T. Hashimoto, MD, PhD • M. Makuuchi, MD, PhD (✉)
Department of Hepato-Biliary-Pancreatic Surgery,
Japanese Red Cross Medical Center,
Tokyo, Japan
e-mail: makuuchi_masatoshi@med.jrc.or.jp

W.Y. Lau (ed.), *Hilar Cholangiocarcinoma*,
DOI 10.1007/978-94-007-6473-6_14, © Springer Science+Business Media Dordrecht and People's Medical Publishing House 2013

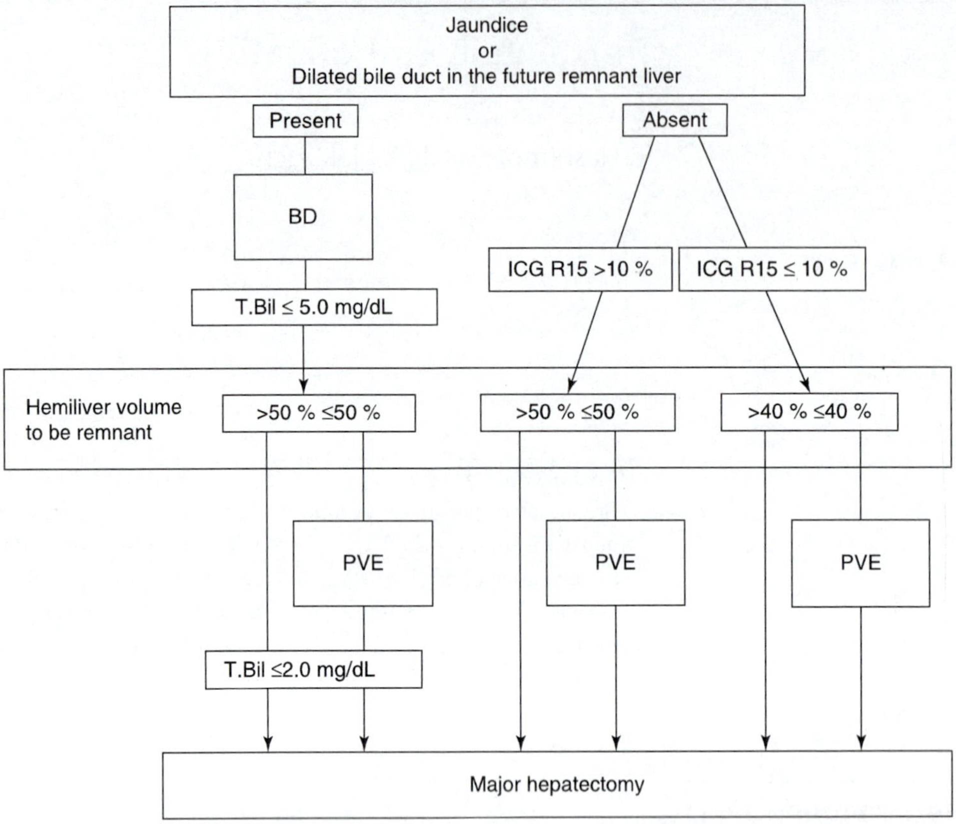

Fig. 14.1 Flowchart for preoperative treatments. When jaundice or dilated bile ducts in the FRL is observed, biliary drainage (*BD*) is performed. Surgical interventions are scheduled after sufficient recovery of the hepatic function. Portal vein embolization (*PVE*) is carried out to avoid postoperative liver failure, which is dependent on the liver function and the liver volume to be resected

14.2 Indications for PVE

Seyama et al. described a safe strategy for hilar bile duct cancer which included biliary drainage and PVE [8]. A flow chart for preoperative treatment is shown in Fig. 14.1. If the patient showed evidence of jaundice, or dilated bile ducts in the future remnant liver (FRL) was detected, biliary drainage was performed, but in principle only to the FRL. Whether PVE was indicated depended on the liver function and the volume of the FRL as calculated by CT volumetry. In patients with normal liver function, i.e. patients with ICG R15 value under 10 %, PVE was indicated when the remnant hemiliver volume was less than 40 %. In patients with jaundice or with ICG R15 value over 10 %, PVE was indicated if the remnant hemiliver volume was less than 50 % [19]. Since the standard operative procedure for hilar bile duct cancer is an extended hemihepatectomy including the whole segment 1, the remaining hemiliver volume should have a margin above the safety zone. After PVE, hepatectomy was performed after re-evaluation of the liver volume, and only when the patient had fulfilled the criteria. Figure 14.2 shows the intraoperative findings after biliary drainage of the FRL followed by PVE of the right portal vein. The right liver was markedly atrophic, and a biliary drainage tube was inserted into the bile duct in segment 3, which drained only the future remnant left liver. Extended right hemihepatectomy was carried out for this patient.

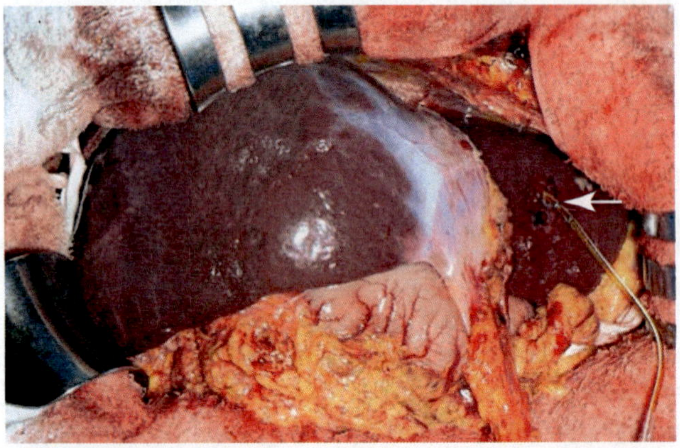

Fig. 14.2 Intraoperative view at laparotomy after biliary drainage and PVE. A percutaneous transhepatic biliary drainage tube (*white arrow*) is inserted into the bile duct of segment 3. The right liver is markedly atrophic, and there is a clear line of demarcation between the right and left liver

Sometimes we experience patients to whom hemihepatic biliary drainage has been carried out but the serum total bilirubin decreases slowly and does not reach the target level of under 5.0 mg/dl, which is the indication criteria for PVE. For such patients, we aggressively perform PVE to the undrained hemiliver before the serum total bilirubin can finally reaches the target level of within the criteria. After PVE, the rate of decrease of the serum total bilirubin rapidly improves. One point never to be forgotten is that during prolonged biliary drainage, cholangiography must not be carried out because it induces cholangitis and increases the risk of postoperative infectious complications. Do not perform cholangiography especially when the right and left bile ducts are not communicating. If a need for cholangiography arises during the prolonged waiting period from the time of the drainage to the operation because of unsatisfactory serum bilirubin or to show regeneration of the FRL, cholangiography should be carried out in the afternoon on the day prior to the radical operation.

14.3 Types of PVE

Basically, the portal branches in the liver to be resected are embolized according to the criteria previously described. In most cases of extended right hemihepatectomy, portal vein embolization of the right hemiliver (right PVE) is required. When the tumor is located predominantly in the left hepatic duct, and left trisectorectomy is scheduled, embolization of the left portal vein and the portal vein of the right paramedian sector is performed. When the FRL volume is smaller than expected for an extended left hemihepatectomy, the left portal vein is embolized. In some cases in which the serum total bilirubin is still high even after adequate biliary drainage, portal vein embolization of the liver to be resected is carried out in order to decrease the serum bilirubin and improve the liver function.

It is still controversial whether the portal branches to segment 4 should be embolized when an extended right hemihepatectomy or a right hemihepatectomy with segment 4 resection is scheduled. Because the portal branches to segments 2, 3, and 4 usually originate from the umbilical portion, insufficient hypertrophy of segments 2 and 3, and unwanted hypertrophy of segment 4 is expected after right portal branch embolization alone. The right plus segment 4 embolizations through an ipsilateral approach have been reported [20, 21]. Right liver plus segment 4 PVE has been proven to be more effective than the standard right PVE as preparation for right hemihepatectomy plus segment 4 resection, and it also has the potential in increasing the safety of high-risk surgery for patients with hilar cholangiocarcinoma. Madoff et al. [22] also reported on the effectiveness of segment 4 embolization. On the other hand, Capussotti et al. [23] reported that extension of embolization to segment 4 portal branches should not be routinely carried out because a similar volume increase of segments 2–3 could simply be achieved by right PVE. In general, the portal branching pattern of segment 4 is not simple. Several small branches run to the segment 4 from the umbilical portion, in addition to the major branches which run to the superior and inferior parts of the segment 4. The liver volume supplied by these small branches cannot be neglected.

The standard procedure for hilar cholangiocarcinoma is extended right hemihepatectomy. The inferior part of segment 4 is resected with the right hemiliver and the caudate lobe, in order to resect the left hepatic duct as much as possible. Before this procedure, right PVE had been performed for anatomical reasons as described before. The postoperative courses of our patients were uneventful.

14.4 Technique of PVE

There are three standard approaches which may be chosen for PVE: the intraoperative transileocolic venous approach; the transhepatic contralateral approach (i.e., portal access via the FRL); and the transhepatic ipsilateral approach (i.e., portal access via the liver to be resected). In general, an approach is chosen based on the type of hepatic resection planned, location of tumor, extent of embolization, and availability of the surgical and radiological facilities. For most patients with hilar cholangiocarcinoma, the first choice is the transhepatic ipsilateral approach. This procedure is ideal because the FRL would not be injured by the puncture. However, when the bile ducts in the future resected liver are dilated and are not drained, this procedure may carry the risk of bile leakage from the needle tract. Intraoperative transileocolic venous approach is generally the second choice.

In every step of the procedures, portal vein anomalies should be investigated by ultrasound (US) or computed tomography (CT) prior to PVE (Fig. 14.3), and by direct portography at the commencement of embolization (Fig. 14.4), paying particular attention to whether or not second-order branches originate close to, or independently of, the main portal trunk. Right anterolateral fluoroscopy is recommended during embolization of the branches to segments 6 and 7. Rare but indismissible technical failures are usually associated with difficulty in catheterization due to severe angulations between the portal branches and the migration of embolization materials. To overcome the narrow angulations, several preshaped catheters should be prepared. Use of a balloon-tipped catheter is advocated to avoid the complication of migration of embolization materials.

14.4.1 Transileocolic Venous Approach

Transileocolic venous approach is performed during laparotomy under general anesthesia by direct cannulation of a catheter into the ileocolic vein inserted and advanced under the guidance of a wire, which is then replaced by a balloon catheter at the portal vein for subsequent embolization under fluoroscopic guidance [13, 14]. This approach is often performed when an interventional radiology suite is not available, percutaneous approach is not feasible, or when an

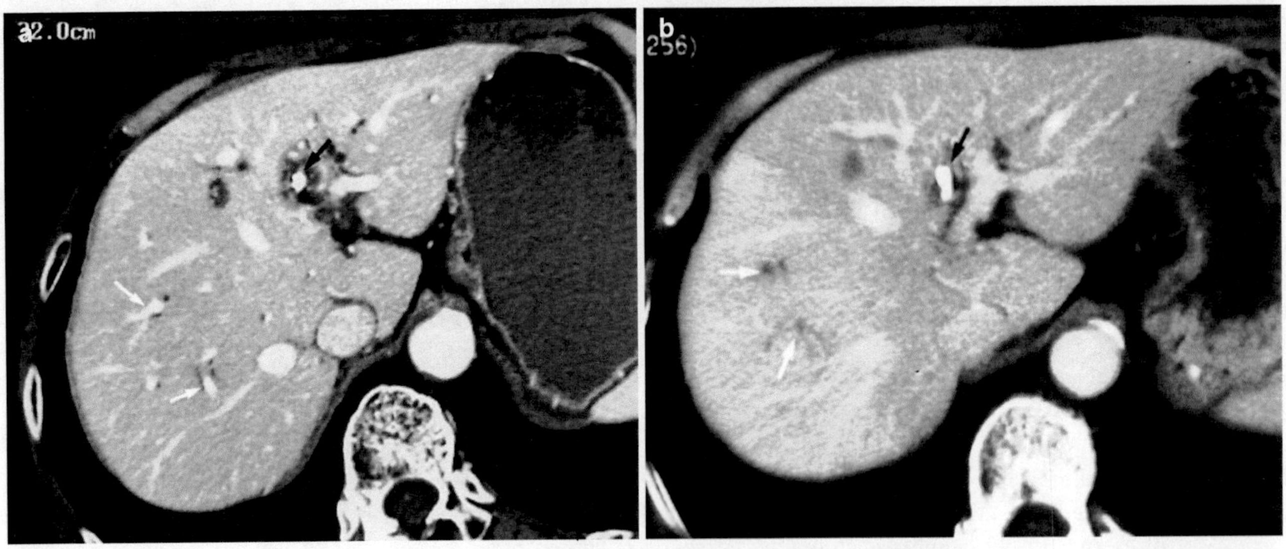

Fig. 14.3 CT scan images of a 70-year-old woman with hilar bile duct carcinoma (**a**) before and (**b**) 2 weeks after PVE carried out to the right liver with gelatin sponge particles and thrombin. Coil was not used for this patient. The *black arrow* indicates a percutaneous transhepatic biliary drainage catheter. The *white arrows* indicate portal tributaries to segment 8. Note the cessation of portal flow and the attenuation difference by HABR in the right liver after PVE

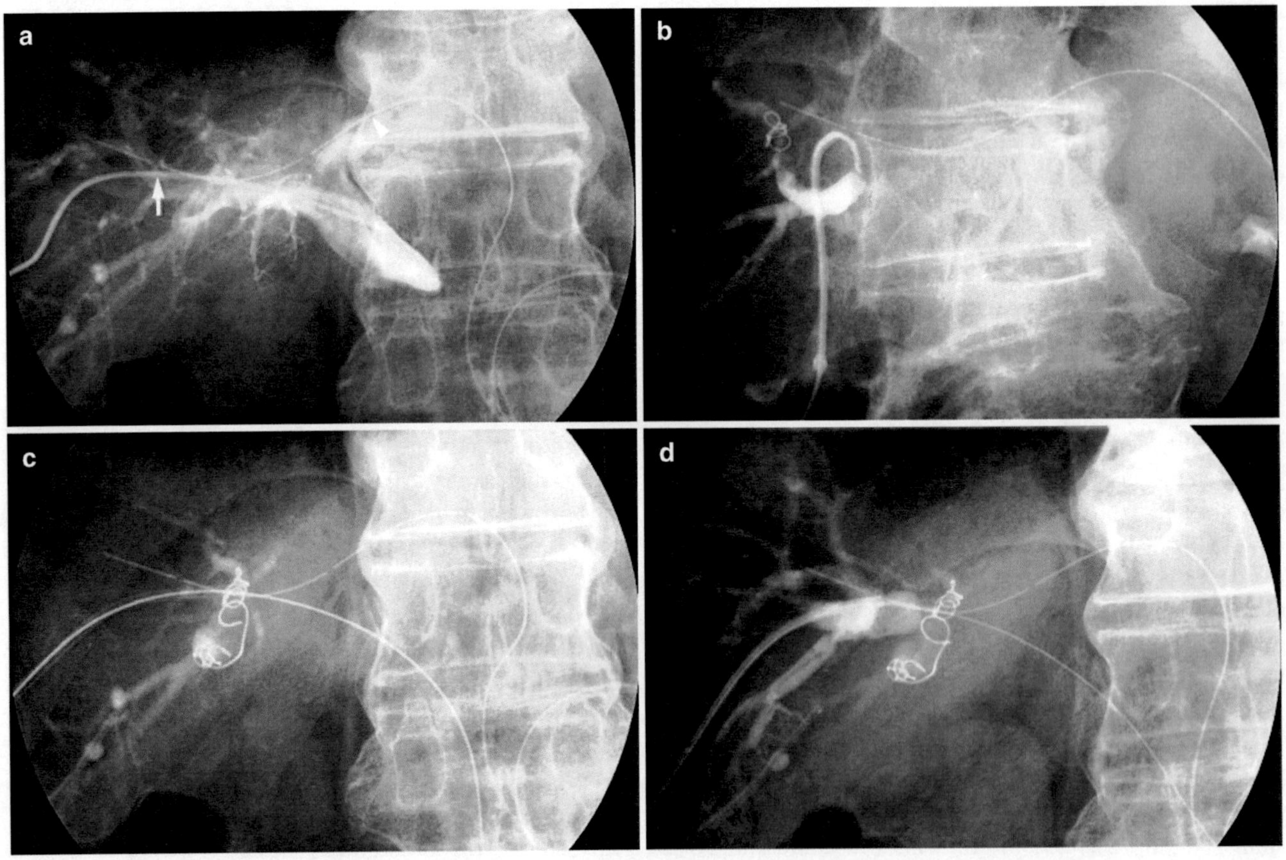

Fig. 14.4 Transhepatic ipsilateral right PVE with gelatin sponge particles, thrombin, and coils carried out on a 72-year-old man with hilar bile duct carcinoma. (**a**) Anteroposterior flush portogram obtained before right PVE with the use of a 6-F vascular sheath in segment 5 portal branch, and a 5-F flush catheter in the main portal vein (*arrow*). The *arrowhead* indicates the percutaneous transhepatic biliary drainage catheter (anteroposterior fluoroscopy view). (**b**) Embolization was commenced from the portal branch to segment 7 with a reverse-curve catheter with distal end-hole under right anterolateral fluoroscopy (anterolateral fluoroscopy view). (**c**) Completion of the embolization carried out to portal branches to segments 6 and 7. Tip of the catheter was placed in the main portal vein (anteroposterior fluoroscopy view). (**d**) Embolization of portal branches to segments 5 and 8 with proximal side-hole type catheter (anterolateral fluoroscopy view). (**e**) Completion of PVE. Coils were placed at the root of the portal branches to segments 5, 6, 7 and 8 (anterolateral fluoroscopy view)

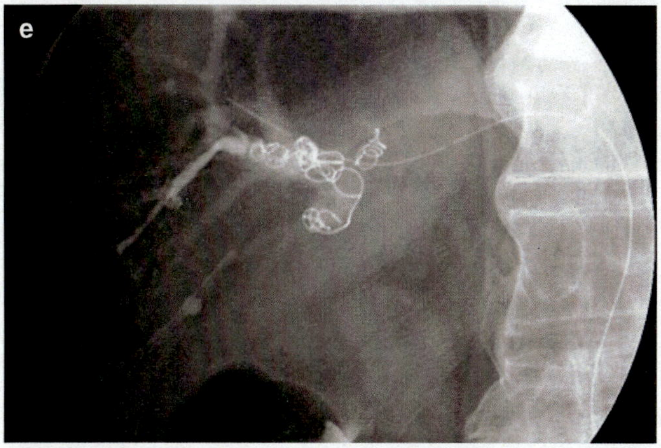

Fig. 14.4 (continued)

additional treatment which may be carried out during the procedure has become necessary [24]. One of the advantages of this approach is that it is possible to evaluate the extent of the tumor at the time of PVE including peritoneal dissemination and hilar lymph node metastases [25]. Catheterization of all portal tributaries is simple even in cases with anatomical variations. However, open laparotomy under general anesthesia is required and this technique is not suitable for patients with a history of prior lower abdominal surgery. Intestinal ileus has been reported to occur [25].

14.4.2 Transhepatic Approach

Transhepatic procedure may be performed under local anesthesia, and intravenous sedatives may or may not be administered. US examination of the liver is carried out to determine the most favorable access route into the portal venous system. Under sterile condition, access into the portal venous system is gained under ultrasonic and fluoroscopic guidance. The contralateral approach (access through the FRL) is technically easier than the ipsilateral approach (access through the portion of the liver to be resected), especially in the presence of anatomical variations [26].

The transhepatic contralateral approach was the most commonly used technique in the early periods [27]. For embolization of the right portal branches, a branch of the left portal system is chosen for access, and a balloon occlusion catheter is advanced through an introducer into the branches of the right portal tree. The major advantage of this approach is the operative simplicity. Catheterization of the desired right PV branches is easily accomplished from the left side. The drawback of this method on the other hand, is that the portal vein in the FRL is punctured. Iatrogenic lesions of the FRL lobe, including hematoma, portal vein wall dissection, and portal vein thrombosis, have been reported in a multicenter review [28].

Transhepatic ipsilateral approach was first described by Nagino et al. [29]. The peripheral portal vein branch in the liver to be resected is secured, and a sheath is inserted through. One apparent advantage of the ipsilateral approach is that the FRL is not injured. Embolization materials or coils are placed along the puncture line upon completion of the procedure to prevent post-PVE hemorrhage. However, this approach is technically more demanding than the contralateral approach. A balloon occlusion catheter with a side lumen opening just proximal to the balloon is occasionally required to avoid unintended embolization of the FRL. When the angle of the right portal branches is severe, the use of reverse-curved catheters becomes necessary. Furthermore, it is usually difficult to perform post-PVE portography or portal pressure measurement to confirm the efficacy of embolization with this procedure.

14.5 Embolization Materials

There is no clear general consensus on the choice of embolization material for PVE. Biomaterials including gelatin sponge particles or powder with thrombin [25] and fibrin glue (combination of fibrinogen and thrombin) [29, 30], synthetic glue (n-butyl-2-cyanoacrylate) [26], synthetic embolization particles (polyvinyl alcohol) [31, 32], coils, iodized oil, and absolute ethanol [33] are used. These materials have yielded different rates or degrees of hypertrophy of the unembolized segments, and the choice of embolization material usually depends on each surgeon's or institute's preference [34]. While absorbability of biomaterials allow unwanted recanalization, the same characteristic also keeps the damage caused by unintended migration of embolization materials during the procedure into the portal branches of the FRL to a minimum or is completely absent [25]. N-butyl-2-cyanoacrylate immediately polymerizes upon contact with blood (water) and has a permanent embolizing effect. However, massive peribiliary fibrosis and portal vein casting [26] it induces may lead to difficulty in dissecting the hilar region or in evaluating tumor invasion [33]. Polyvinyl alcohol particles have a smaller diameter (150–100 μm) than gelatin sponge (500–100 μm). This material is selected for its safety in use, minimal periportal reaction, and sustainable embolization effect when used in combination with coils [32]. Coils and iodized oil are usually used in combination with these materials. Iodized oil in particular is used because of its long-lasting "portal cast" effect which may be viewed on follow up plain X-ray film and CT scans. PVE with absolute ethanol had been proposed because of its strong coagulation effect [33], and hypertrophy appeared to be more significant than with other materials. However, PVE with absolute ethanol has been associated with a marked increase in serum aspartate aminotransferase

(AST) and alanine aminotransferase (ALT) levels, which in turn, may lead to necrosis of the embolized region [33]. We have to be careful when selecting absolute ethanol, especially for patients undergoing hemiliver biliary drainage. Damage inflicted to liver parenchyma by ethanol injection would be more severe on the hemiliver without biliary drainage than on the hemiliver with adequate biliary drainage. If the whole right hemiliver is necrotized by using absolute ethanol, critical hepatic failure would occur and postoperative course after PVE would be miserable. The basic concept of PVE is that it induces increment of portal pressure, and progression of apotosis of the embolized liver, which in turn gradually produces atrophic and hypertrophic changes of the liver. However, if increment of portal pressure and necrosis occur at the same time from using ethanol, the clinical course is the same as that of extended hepatectomy without preoperative PVE.

We routinely use gelatin sponge powder with thrombin. This material is less harmful than others and the effect is enough for sequential hepatic resection. When recanalization of the embolized portal branches is detected during the follow up period, the recanalized portal branches are selectively punctured to inject absolute ethanol. The use of absolute ethanol for embolization in a small part of the liver is considered acceptable.

14.6 Portal Pressure After PVE

Total portal venous flow (ml/min) is unaffected by PVE because the liver does not have an intrinsic ability to modulate portal flow, and that it is a function of extrahepatic and systemic factors. In a PVE study on human, this was confirmed using Doppler US [35]. Because the same volume of portal flow prior to PVE enters the non-embolized lobe after PVE, portal pressure in the non-embolized liver is elevated immediately after PVE by 4.9±2.7 cm H_2O [36]. A similar increase was observed in cirrhotic patients with a higher baseline portal pressure [37]. The elevation of portal pressure is transient, with pressure gradually returning to the baseline value in 2–3 weeks, as indicated by the portal flow velocity (cm/s) changes measured by Doppler ultrasound [38].

14.7 Clinical Course After PVE

Signs and symptoms of postembolization syndrome due to PVE itself, such as pain, fever, nausea, and vomiting, are milder and less than transcatheter arterial embolization (TAE). Most patients experience a mild fever following PVE, which subsides within 2–3 days. Changes in liver function as reflected by an increased total bilirubin and prolonged prothrombin time are mild and transient, returning to their baseline values 2–3 days after PVE. Serum levels of AST and ALT are stable in about 50 % of patients. They are mildly elevated on day 1, then returning to the baseline values in 4–7 days after PVE. These findings suggest that inflammatory and/or necrotic reactions after PVE are minimal, if at all, present [25]. The exceptions are when absolute ethanol is used [33] for embolization. When absolute ethanol is used for PVE, it is followed by a marked rise in serum AST and ALT, though both tend to return to their baseline values by 2 weeks before the scheduled hepatectomy.

In western countries, an evaluation of liver volume is carried out 4–6 weeks after PVE. The waiting period between PVE and operation is reported to be shorter in Japan (2–3 weeks), but this has been proven to be quite adequate in performing hepatic resection safely.

14.8 Volumetric Changes After PVE

In order to determine whether PVE is necessary before hepatic resection, and to assess the degree of FRL hypertrophy, the ratio of "FRL volume/Total liver volume-Tumor volume" (the FRLV/TLV ratio) is widely used as a parameter. CT scan with contrast material is the most commonly used method for calculating noncancerous total liver volume and FRL volume. Examination using CT scan should be performed before and after PVE. Multi-slice helical CT scan or multidetector CT scan with contrast material allows accurate volumetric measurement by subtracting the small tumor volumes and vasculo-biliary structures at the Couinaud's segment level.

PVE leads to an increase in the segmental volume of a non-embolized liver, and a decrease in an embolized liver, homogeneously maintaining a constant total liver volume. The regeneration rate of the non-cirrhotic liver has been reported to be 12 cm^3/day 2 weeks after PVE [30, 39], then falling to 11 cm^3/day at 4 weeks [30], and 6 cm^3/day at 32 days [26]. In general, a 30 % increase in the non-embolized liver volume being an absolute value, and a 10 % increase as expressed by the FRLV/TLV ratio, are attained 2 weeks after right liver PVE.

Various factors have been reported to affect the regeneration rate after PVE. The greater the FRL volume before PVE, the smaller the volume increase after PVE [25, 40, 41]. The magnitude of hypertrophy differs with the materials used for PVE. Hypertrophy appears to be moderate when biological materials such as gelfoam and fibrin glue are used, most probably because of their progressive recanalization effect. Absolute alcohol has been reported to achieve the highest degree of regeneration. However, it is accompanied by marked increases in serum AST and ALT, and an increased risk of liver necrosis. Thus, absolute alcohol is not a good choice as an embolic material for PVE. Diabetes, obstructive jaundice, and active hepatitis have been reported to hamper the regeneration process [25, 30]. In cirrhotic patients, the regeneration rate is smaller than in non-cirrhotic patients. Their reported regeneration rate is 9 cm^3/day at 2 weeks [26, 39].

14.9 Histological Changes After PVE

In a human study, liver tissues obtained 3 weeks after PVE have shown almost normal microscopic structures in both the embolized and the non-embolized lobes. However, in the embolized lobe, dilatation of sinusoids with decreased hepatocyte density and hepatocyte apoptosis, especially in the pericentral area, were observed [42]. There were no signs of necrosis or inflammation in the embolized lobe, except for the liver tissues of the embolized lobe which had undergone PVE using absolute ethanol [33], with clear evidence of necrosis. When cyanoacrylate is used for PVE, peribiliary fibrosis is induced [26]. Microscopic findings of the non-embolized liver on the other hand, have shown hepatocyte replication as evidenced by increased mitotic figures and other parameters of cell proliferation such as the levels of proliferative cell nuclear antigen and Ki-67 [42, 43]. Hepatocytes in this liver were histologically characterized by basophilic cytoplasm, abundant binuclear cells, and they were small. The observation provides indirect evidence of hepatocyte proliferation [42].

14.10 Functional Changes After PVE

Considering proliferating isolated hepatocytes lose their differentiated hepatocyte-specific functions, cellular hyperplasia and the resulting partial hypertrophy do not necessarily signify functional gain in the corresponding part of the liver. Most reports investigating liver function after PVE had assessed the whole liver function, including both the embolized and the non-embolized lobe. The overall functional hepatocyte number, as estimated by the clearance of antipyrine, a prototype low-extractable drug, has shown similar values before and 2 weeks after PVE [44]. When ATP concentrations and hepatic energy reserves per *g* of liver tissue were assessed in the non-embolized lobe 3 weeks after PVE, the values were similar to those of the control tissue [45]. Likewise, the non-embolized lobe uptake of technetium-99 m-galactosyl human serum albumin (^{99m}Tc-GSA), a ligand bound to asialoglycoprotein receptors on the hepatocyte cell membrane, showed a rapid increase 1–2 weeks after PVE [46, 47]. These findings demonstrate that the volume increase in the non-embolized liver is accompanied by a parallel increment of liver function in the corresponding part.

Conclusion

PVE is indispensable for extensive liver resection for hilar cholangiocarcinoma. Although randomized controlled study has not been conducted, its effectiveness is widely accepted. However, one should not forget that PVE is only a "preoperative procedure" whose aim is to assist in the safety of liver resection. Complications arising from PVE therefore are preposterous. PVE should be performed promptly and without any complications.

References

1. Khan SA, Thomas HC, Davidson BR, et al. Cholangiocarcinoma. Lancet. 2005;366:1303–14.
2. Nimura Y, Kamiya J, Kondo S, et al. Aggressive preoperative management and extended surgery for hilar cholangiocarcinoma: nagoya experience. J Hepatobiliary Pancreat Surg. 2000;7:155–62.
3. Nagino M, Nimura Y, Kamiya J, et al. Segmental liver resections for hilar cholangiocarcinoma. Hepatogastroenterology. 1998;45:7–13.
4. Shimada H, Izumi T, Note M, et al. Anterior segmentectomy with caudate lobectomy for hilar cholangiocarcinoma. Hepatogastroenterology. 1993;40:61–4.
5. Kawasaki S, Makuuchi M, Miyagawa S, et al. Radical operation after portal embolization for tumor of hilar bile duct. J Am Coll Surg. 1994;178:480–6.
6. Miyagawa S, Makuuchi M, Kawasaki S. Outcome of extended right hepatectomy after biliary drainage in hilar bile duct cancer. Arch Surg. 1995;130:759–63.
7. Kawasaki S, Imamura H, Kobayashi A, et al. Results of surgical resection for patients with hilar bile duct cancer: application of extended hepatectomy after biliary drainage and hemihepatic portal vein embolization. Ann Surg. 2003;238:84–92.
8. Seyama Y, Kubota K, Sano K, et al. Long-term outcome of extended hemihepatectomy for hilar bile duct cancer with no mortality and high survival rate. Ann Surg. 2003;238:73–83.
9. Hemming AW, Reed AI, Fujita S, et al. Surgical management of hilar cholangiocarcinoma. Ann Surg. 2005;241:693–9; discussion 699–702.
10. Mimura H, Kim H, Ochiai Y, et al. Radical block resection of hepatoduodenal ligament for carcinoma of the bile duct with double catheter bypass for portal circulation. Surg Gynecol Obstet. 1988;167:527–9.
11. Nimura Y, Hayakawa N, Kamiya J, et al. Hepatopancreatoduodenectomy for advanced carcinoma of the biliary tract. Hepatogastroenterology. 1991;38:170–5.
12. Miyagawa S, Makuuchi M, Kawasaki S, et al. Outcome of major hepatectomy with pancreatoduodenectomy for advanced biliary malignancies. World J Surg. 1996;20:77–80.
13. Makuuchi M, Takayasu K, Takuma T, et al. Preoperative transcatheter embolization of the portal venous branch for patients receiving extended lobectomy due to the bile duct carcinoma. J Jpn Surg Assoc. 1984;45:1558–64.
14. Makuuchi M, Thai BL, Takayasu K, et al. Preoperative portal embolization to increase safety of major hepatectomy for hilar bile duct carcinoma: a preliminary report. Surgery. 1990;107:521–7.
15. Rous P, Larimore LD. Relation of the portal blood to liver maintenance: a demonstration of liver atrophy conditional on compensation. J Exp Med. 1920;31:609–32.
16. Honjo I, Suzuki T, Ozawa K, et al. Ligation of a branch of the portal vein for carcinoma of the liver. Am J Surg. 1975;130:296–302.
17. Takayasu K, Muramastu Y, Shima Y, et al. Hepatic lobar atrophy following obstruction of the ipsilateral portal vein from cholangiocarcinoma. Radiology. 1986;160:389–93.
18. Kawasaki S, Makuuchi M, Kakazu T, et al. Resection for multiple metastatic liver tumors after portal embolization. Surgery. 1994;115:674–7.
19. Kubota K, Makuuchi M, Kusaka K, et al. Measurement of liver volume and hepatic functional reserve as a guide to decision-making in resectional surgery for hepatic tumors. Hepatology. 1997;26:1176–81.
20. Nagino M, Nimura Y, Kamiya J, et al. Right or left trisegment portal vein embolization before hepatic trisegmentectomy for hilar bile duct carcinoma. Surgery. 1995;117:677–81.
21. Nagino M, Kamiya J, Kanai M, et al. Right trisegment portal vein embolization for biliary tract carcinoma: technique and clinical utility. Surgery. 2000;127:155–60.
22. Madoff DC, Abdalla EK, Gupta S, et al. Transhepatic ipsilateral right portal vein embolization extended to segment IV: improving

hypertrophy and resection outcomes with spherical particles and coils. J Vasc Interv Radiol. 2005;16:215–25.
23. Capussotti L, Muratore A, Ferrero A, et al. Extension of right portal vein embolization to segment IV portal branches. Arch Surg. 2005;140:1100–3.
24. Azoulay D, Raccuia JS, Castaing D, et al. Right portal vein embolization in preparation for major hepatic resection. J Am Coll Surg. 1995;181:266–9.
25. Imamura H, Shimada R, Kubota M, et al. Preoperative portal vein embolization: an audit of 84 patients. Hepatology. 1999;29: 1099–105.
26. De Baere T, Roche A, Elias D, et al. Preoperative portal vein embolization for extension of hepatectomy indications. Hepatology. 1996;24:1386–91.
27. Kinoshita H, Sakai K, Hirohashi K, et al. Preoperative portal vein embolization for hepatocellular carcinoma. World J Surg. 1986; 10:803–8.
28. Di Stefano DR, de Baere T, Denys A, et al. Preoperative percutaneous portal vein embolization: evaluation of adverse events in 188 patients. Radiology. 2005;234:625–30.
29. Nagino M, Nimura Y, Kamiya J, et al. Selective percutaneous transhepatic embolization of the portal vein in preparation for extensive liver resection: the ipsilateral approach. Radiology. 1996;200:559–63.
30. Nagino M, Nimura Y, Kamiya J, et al. Changes in hepatic lobe volume in biliary tract cancer patients after right portal vein embolizaiton. Hepatology. 1995;21:434–9.
31. Abdalla EK, Barnett CC, Doherty D. Extended hepatectomy in patients with hepatobiliary malignancies with and without preoperative portal vein embolization. Arch Surg. 2002;137: 675–81.
32. Madoff DC, Hicks ME, Abdalla EK, et al. Portal vein embolization with polyvinyl alcohol particles and coils in preparation for major liver resection for hepatobiliary malignancy: safety and effectiveness- study in 26 patients. Radiology. 2003;227:251–60.
33. Shimamura T, Nakajima Y, Une Y, et al. Efficacy and safety of preoperative percutaneous transhepatic portal embolization with absolute ethanol: a clinical study. Surgery. 1997;121:135–41.
34. Elias D, Ouellet JF, De Baere T, et al. Preoperative selective portal vein embolization before hepatectomy for liver metastases: long-term results and impact on survival. Surgery. 2002;131:294–9.
35. Denys AL, Abehsera M, Leloutre B, et al. Intrahepatic hemodynamic changes following portal vein embolization: a prospective Doppler study. Eur Radiol. 2000;10:1703–7.
36. Takayama T, Makuuchi M, Kosuge T, et al. Preoperative portal embolization. Ann Ital Chir. 1997;68:745–50.
37. Aoki T, Imamura H, Hasegawa K, et al. Sequential preoperative arterial and portal venous embolizations in patients with hepatocellular carcinoma. Arch Surg. 2004;139:766–74.
38. Goto Y, Nagino M, Nimura Y. Doppler estimation of portal blood flow after percutaneous transhepatic portal vein embolization. Ann Surg. 1998;228:209–13.
39. Lee KC, Kinoshita H, Hirohashi K, et al. Extension of surgical indications for hepatocellular carcinoma by portal vein embolization. World J Surg. 1993;17:109–15.
40. Yamakado K, Takeda K, Matsumura K, et al. Regeneration of the un-embolized liver parenchyma following portal vein embolization. J Hepatol. 1997;27:871–80.
41. Kokudo N, Tada K, Seki M, et al. Proliferative activity of intrahepatic colorectal metastases after preoperative hemihepatic portal vein embolization. Hepatology. 2001;34:267–72.
42. Harada H, Imamura H, Miyagawa S, et al. Fate of the human liver after hemihepatic portal vein embolization: cell kinetic and morphometric study. Hepatology. 1997;26:1162–70.
43. Kusaka K, Imamura H, Tomiya T, et al. Expression of transforming growth factor-alpha and -beta in hepatic lobes after hemihepatic portal vein embolization. Dig Dis Sci. 2006;51:1404–12.
44. Shimada R, Imamura H, Nakayama, et al. Changes in blood flow and function of the liver after right portal vein embolization. Arch Surg. 2002;137:1384–8.
45. Chijiiwa K, Saiki S, Noshiro H, et al. Effect of preoperative portal vein embolization on liver volume and hepatic energy status of the nonembolized liver lobe in humans. Eur Surg Res. 2000;32:94–9.
46. Nishiguchi S, Shiomi S, Sasaki N, et al. Course before and after percutaneous transhepatic portal vein embolization of a patient with cholangiocarcinoma monitored by schintigraphy with Tc-99m galactosyl human serum albumin. Ann Nucl Med. 2000;14:231–4.
47. Hirai I, Kimura W, Fuse A, et al. Evaluation of preoperative portal vein embolization for safe hepatectomy, with special reference to assessment of nonembolized lobe function with 99mTc-GSA SPECT scintigraphy. Surgery. 2003;133:495–506.

15 Anesthesia for Patients with Hilar Chlolangiocarcinoma

S.S. Ho and M.T.V. Chan

Patients with hilar cholangiocarcinoma require anesthesia for a number of surgical procedures. This ranges from minimally invasive surgery, such as diagnostic laparoscopy, to major procedures including liver transplantation. Anesthetic management in these patients is not only dependent on the magnitude of surgery, but also on any concurrent illnesses. In this chapter, we outlined the principles of anesthesia and perioperative management for patients with hilar cholangiocarcinoma undergoing a variety of surgery.

15.1 Preoperative Considerations

Patients with hilar cholangiocarcinoma are usually asymptomatic until late in the development of their disease [1–6]. Therefore, when patients are presented for surgery, there are often serious complications and will require careful evaluation.

15.1.1 Obstructive Jaundice

Post-hepatic obstructive jaundice is the commonest presenting feature of hilar cholangiocarcinoma [1–7]. However, secondary biliary cirrhosis with intrahepatic cholestasis should be considered if plasma bilirubin concentration remains elevated (>68 μmol/L) after biliary drainage [1, 3]. The anesthetic implication of obstructive jaundice is however, related to fat malabsorption, particularly for fat-soluble vitamin K. This is because chronic vitamin K deficiency will lead to a decrease in the production of clotting factors (II, VII, IX and X), and bleeding tendency.

S.S. Ho, MBBS, MRCP, FANZCA, FHKCA, FHKAM
M.T.V. Chan, MBBS, FANZCA, FHKCA, FHKAM (✉)
Department of Anesthesia and Intensive Care,
The Chinese University of Hong Kong,
Shatin, New Territories, Hong Kong
e-mail: mtvchan@cuhk.edu.hk

15.1.2 Cholangitis

More importantly, obstructive jaundice may predispose patients to acute suppurative cholangitis [1–7]. Other contributing factors include an elevated intraluminal pressure, and bacterial colonization in the bile [8]. It is commonly believed that bacteria access the biliary system from the duodenum. As the pressure within the biliary lumen builds up, bacteria are pushed into the biliary canaliculi, hepatic veins, and perihepatic lymphatics, leading to bacteremia and systemic sepsis in about 25–40 % of patients [8]. It is important that empirical antibiotics are given early. Antibiotics against gram-negative enteric organisms (e.g. *Escherichia coli, Klebsiella* and *Enterobacter* species), gram-positive organisms (e.g. *Enterococcus* and *Streptococcus* species), and anaerobes (e.g. *Bacteroides fragilis, Clostridium perfringens*), such as a combination of extended-spectrum cephalosporin, metronidazole, and ampicillin would be appropriate [8, 9]. In addition, decompression of the biliary system with endoscopic retrograde cholangiopancreatography (ERCP) or percutaneous drainage should be performed, whenever feasible, prior to major definitive surgery [4, 7].

15.1.3 Infection

Immunosuppression is common among patients with hilar cholangiocarcinoma, and may be related to malignancy, malnutrition and cholestasis. It is important to look for respiratory and urinary tract infections. In a systematic review, it was reported that 9 % of patients had fever at presentation [5]. Infections should be treated promptly with appropriate antibiotics before elective surgery is scheduled.

15.1.4 Bleeding Tendency

This is related to liver failure and hypersplenism, and is characterized by prolonged international normalized ratio of

W.Y. Lau (ed.), *Hilar Cholangiocarcinoma*,
DOI 10.1007/978-94-007-6473-6_15, © Springer Science+Business Media Dordrecht and People's Medical Publishing House 2013

(INR) the prothrombin time (PT) and thrombocytopenia. In addition, patients may receive drugs that could induce bleeding tendency. Typically, this includes non-steroidal anti-inflammatory drugs (NSAIDs). These agents are known to impair platelet function and are best avoided during the week prior to surgery. Patients with concurrent coronary artery disease and stroke are often taking antiplatelet agents, such as aspirin and clopidogrel, either alone or in combination. Although it is clear that these agents prevent major cardiac event in the non-operative setting, there are uncertainty whether the risk of perioperative bleeding will outweigh the benefits [10–12]. Stopping aspirin for 72 h will ensure substantial (if not complete) recovery of platelet function [13, 14]. Clopidogrel should be discontinued for 7 days prior to surgery [12]. Similarly, the risk of starting prophylactic anticoagulation (e.g. low molecular weight heparin) for the prevention of deep venous thrombosis has to be carefully considered, because significant bleeding may occur during major hepatobiliary surgery [12]. Furthermore, over-the-counter herbal products and traditional Chinese medicine, such as ginkgo and ginseng, are known to affect coagulation and should be discontinued long before surgery [15]. Finally, it is important to ensure patients with known clotting defects are actually receiving their treatment before the scheduled procedure (e.g. desmopressin for von Willebrand disease).

15.1.5 Renal Impairment

The causes of renal failure are often multifactorial and are related to sepsis and pre-existing renal failure. The contribution of nephrotoxic drugs, such as antibiotics and NSAIDs should not be overlooked. Perioperative renal replacement therapy and optimization of drug treatment should be considered. Renal impairment before surgery is a predictor of post-operative hepatorenal syndrome.

15.1.6 Underlying Liver Disease

Hypoperfusion during surgery and anesthetic drugs per se may exacerbate underlying liver dysfunction, leading to postoperative liver failure. In this regard, preoperative coagulopathy, hypoglycemia and encephalopathy are clear indicators of end-stage liver failure. They are strong predictors for postoperative complications and death. However, clinical features for significant liver dysfunction can be subtle. Therefore, it is important to look for an objective measure to quantify the severity of underlying liver disease.

The Child-Turcotte-Pugh score assesses plasma concentrations of bilirubin and albumin, the presence of ascites and encephalopathy (Table 15.1). It was originally derived to predict mortality after emergency ligation of esophageal varices in the 1960s–1970s, and is still commonly used to assess the severity of underlying liver dysfunction [16, 17]. Patients who scored between 5 and 6 points (class A), 7–9 (class B) and 10–15 (class C) had a perioperative risk of ≤5 %, 10 and 50 %, respectively.

Table 15.1 Child-Turcotte-Pugh score [16, 17]

Clinical and biochemical measurements	Points scored for worsening abnormality		
	1	2	3
Encephalopathy[a]	None	Stages 1–2	Stages 3–4
Ascites	None	Slight	Moderate
Plasma total bilirubin concentration (μmol/L)[b]	<2	2–3	>3
Plasma albumin (g/L)	>35	28–35	<28
International normalized ratio of prothrombin time	<1.7	1.7–2.3	>2.3

[a]The severity of hepatic encephalopathy is graded according to the West Haven Criteria: Grade 0—Subclinical; normal mental status, but minimal changes in memory, concentration, intellectual function, coordination; Grade 1—Mild confusion, depression, inattention, showiness, irritable, inverted sleep cycle; Grade 2—Drowsiness, lethargy, unable to perform mental tasks, personality changes, inappropriate behavior, intermittent disorientation (usually with time); Grade 3—Somnolent but rousable, confusion, amnesia, incomprehensible speech; Grade 4—Coma

[b]In patients with primary biliary cirrhosis or primary sclerosing cholangitis, the upper limit for 1 point is 68 μmol/L and that for 2 points is 170 μmol/L

Alternatively, the (Mayo) Model for End-Stage Liver Disease (MELD) could be used to assess liver reserve [18]. MELD is an objective measure that calculates the relative contributions of INR, plasma concentrations of creatinine and total bilirubin to predict mortality in patients with liver failure. Its variations also include plasma concentration of sodium to reflect the severity of ascites and hepatorenal syndrome (Table 15.2) [19–21]. In a patient undergoing liver resection, a MELD score ≤ 8 seems to carry minimal risk. Although both Child-Turcotte-Pugh and MELD scoring systems correlate with postoperative outcomes, their prediction accuracy in subclinical liver disease remains unclear [19].

With the development of technology, dynamic assessment of liver function can be performed as a bedside test [22–24]. The use of indocynaine green (ICG) retention test is one of the common techniques that is commercially available [25–28]. ICG is a tricarbocyanine dye that is rapidly extracted by the liver. By measuring plasma ICG concentration using noninvasive pulse spectrophotometry [26], hepatic clearance of ICG can be calculated. This is usually expressed as the proportion of ICG remained in the plasma, 15 min after injection (ICG R_{15}) or the elimination rate constant of ICG [ICG(K) or ICG-PDR, Fig. 15.1]. Although it has not been fully validated, ICG R_{15} > 15 % [27], or ICG(K) (or ICG-PDR) < 7.5 %/min usually indicate limited liver reserve [22–28]. As hilar cholangiocarcinoma commonly presents with obstructive jaundice and obstruction to the biliary system affects the ICG test, the results of ICG R15 in patients

Table 15.2 Models for end-stage liver disease

$$\text{MELD score} = 9.57 \cdot ln[\text{creatinine}] + 3.78 \cdot ln[\text{bilirubin}] + 11.2 \cdot ln[\text{international normalized ratio of prothrombin}] + 6.43$$

where [creatinine] = plasma concentration of creatinine (mg/dl)when patient received dialysis twice in the prior week or continuous hemodialysis within the past 24 h, plasma creatinine concentration should be set as 4 mg/dl

[bilirubin] = plasma concentration of bilirubin (mg/dl)

$$\text{MELD-}Na = \text{MELD} + 1.59 \cdot (135 - [\text{sodium}])$$

$$\text{iMELD} = \text{MELD} + [0.3 * \text{age}(\text{year})] - (0.7 + [\text{sodium}]) + 100$$

$$\text{MESO} = \{\text{MELD} / [\text{sodium}]\} * 10$$

where [sodium] = plasma concentration of sodium (mmol/L), the maximum and minimum plasma sodium concentrations are 135 and 120, respectively

MELD Models for End-Stage Liver Disease [18], *MELD-Na* MELD with the incorporation of serum sodium [19], *iMELD* integrated MELD [20], *MESO* MELD to sodium index [21]

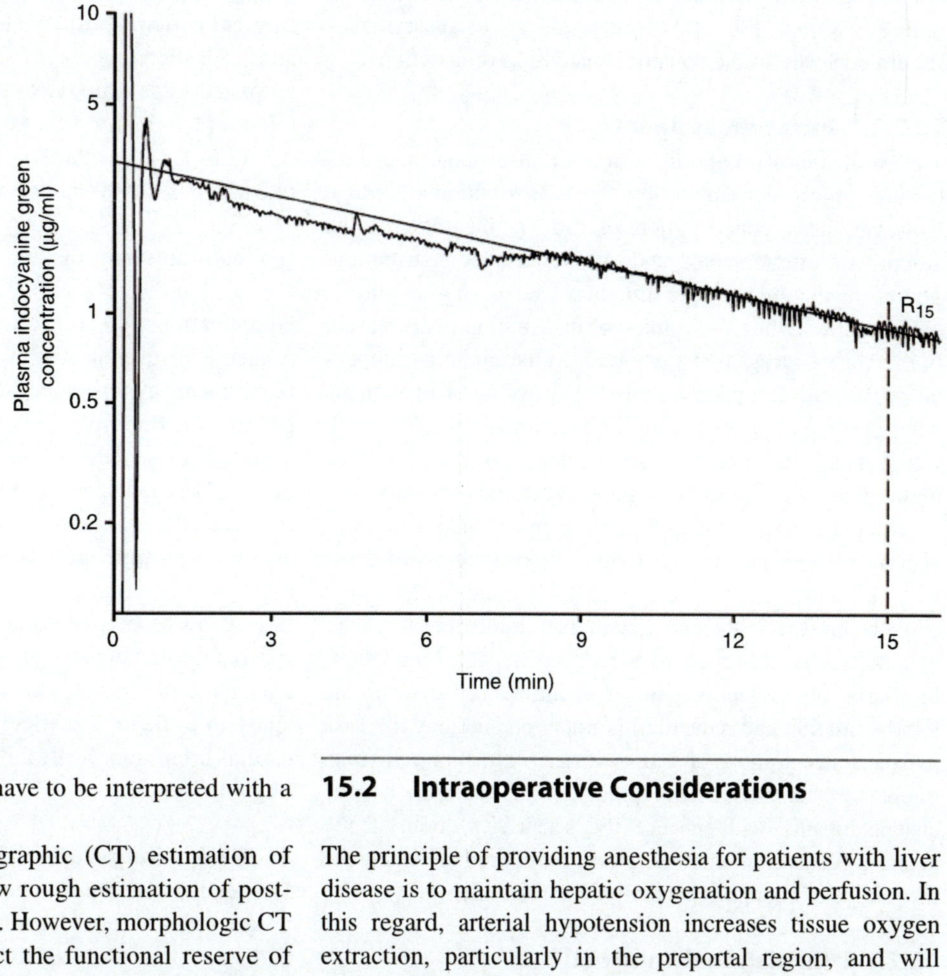

Fig. 15.1 Typical elimination curve of indocyanine green (*ICG*). A bolus of ICG dye 20 mg was injected intravenously. Plasma ICG concentration was measured by pulse dye-densitometry (DDG–2001A/K, Nihon Kohden, Shinjuku-ku, Toyoko, Japan) using an optical probe attached to the patient's finger. The terminal elimination rate of ICG(K) was calculated using linear regression (6.9 %/min). The proportion of ICG remained in plasma at 15 min (ICG R_{15}) was 28.5 %. Both values indicate poor liver reserve

with hilar cholangiocarcinoma have to be interpreted with a lot of caution.

Finally, computerized tomographic (CT) estimation of remnant liver volume may allow rough estimation of postoperative liver function [23, 28]. However, morphologic CT assessment alone cannot predict the functional reserve of the remaining liver. Therefore, further imaging studies may be required. Examples of functional imaging of the liver include 31-phosphorus magnetic resonance spectroscopy and 99mTc-galactosyl-human serum albumin scintigraphy [29, 30].

Intuitively, an integrated assessment system combining clinical features, biochemical changes and imaging modalities would produce the best prediction model for postoperative outcome. However, data confirming the usefulness of such integrated system remain preliminary [31].

15.2 Intraoperative Considerations

The principle of providing anesthesia for patients with liver disease is to maintain hepatic oxygenation and perfusion. In this regard, arterial hypotension increases tissue oxygen extraction, particularly in the preportal region, and will decrease venous oxygen content in portal venous system. Under physiologic condition, vasodilation in the hepatic artery provides compensatory perfusion. However, in patients with limited liver reserve and autoregulatory failure, the hepatic artery is already maximally dilated. Therefore a decrease in portal perfusion will lead to frank ischemia [32, 33]. In this regard, arterial hypotension with deep anesthesia and positive pressure ventilation should be avoided. Systemic hypovolemia must be treated aggressively. There is also portosystemic shunting, so that despite an increase in cardiac output by as much as 50–100 %, there is inadequate liver perfusion [32–34].

Maintaining systemic oxygenation could also be a challenge. At least 50 % of patients have significant intrapulmonary shunting and ventilation-perfusion mismatch [33, 35]. This is made worse with pleural effusion, and diaphragmatic splinting with ascites. Diuretic therapy, such as spironolactone, and paracentesis may improve oxygenation, and should be considered before induction of anesthesia.

15.2.1 Pharmacological Changes

The liver has a large functional reserve. Therefore altered drug metabolism may not be obvious until fulminant liver failure develops [36, 37]. Nevertheless, anesthesiologists should be aware of the potential changes in drug actions.

15.2.1.1 Intravenous Agents

The onset and offset of drug action for intravenous anesthetics are largely determined by the redistribution of drugs. However, peak concentration of drug is the ratio of the amount of drug injected and the volume of distribution. Therefore, the same dose of drug may lead to a higher plasma concentration when the volume of distribution is decreased. In this regard, drugs that are bound to albumin (e.g. thiopental) will have a smaller volume of distribution in patients who are malnourished with hypoalbuminemia [38, 39]. Consequently, a standard dose of thiopental might produce higher plasma concentration and exaggerated hypotension.

There are other changes in the pharmacokinetics of intravenous anesthetics with liver failure. Bioavailability of drugs with high extraction ratio (e.g. propofol, etomidate, ketamine) could be unexpectedly increased in liver failure, because liver metabolism is decreased with reduced hepatic blood flow. Similarly, phase I elimination (predominantly cytochrome P450 oxidation and reduction) is impaired and may increase plasma concentrations of drugs with low extraction ratio (e.g. thiopental, benzodiazepine) [36, 39]. In addition, hepatic encephalopathy will enhance the sensitivity of anesthetic agents [40]. Overall, there is an increase in drug effect, but the magnitude of change is generally unpredictable.

15.2.1.2 Inhalational Anesthetics

All commonly used inhalational anesthetics including isoflurane, sevoflurane and desflurane, can be safely administered to patients with liver disease [39, 41]. Minor changes in liver enzymes have been reported after surgery and may be the results of perioperative hypotension and surgical trauma. There are however, anecdotal reports of massive liver necrosis after inhalational agents [42–44]. This is thought to be related to the formation of fluroacylated proteins in the liver, leading to autoimmune hepatitis. Nevertheless, billions of patients have received these agents in the past, and the fact that only a handful of patients had proven anesthesia-induced hepatitis would suggested that the disease entity is extremely rare. Currently, no risk factor has been identified.

15.2.1.3 Nitrous Oxide

The use of nitrous oxide (N_2O), as an inhalational anesthetic, deserves further discussion. Although it was the first anesthetic since 1844, N_2O is still widely used today as part of the anesthetic regimen. N_2O is usually given at ≥50 % in oxygen, it is inexpensive and is widely available. It provides substantial analgesia and reduces exposure of other anesthetic agents [45].

However, recent data have challenged the use of N_2O. In a large multicenter randomized controlled trial of 2,050 surgical patients [46]. We have recently reported that N_2O administration increased the risk of wound infection [adjusted odds ratio, OR (95 % confidence intervals, CI): OR 1.4 (1.1–1.9), $P=0.04$], severe vomiting [OR(95 %CI): 2.5 (2.0–3.2), $P<0.001$], atelectasis [OR(95 %CI): 1.8 (1.3–2.5), $P<0.001$], and pneumonia [OR(95 %CI): 2.0 (1.1–3.7), $P=0.04$]. N_2O patients also had a longer intensive care unit stay [hazard ratio (95 %CI): 1.4 (1.1–1.7); $P=0.02$], indicating an increased incidence of more serious complications [46, 47]. Many of these adverse events were related to irreversible inhibition of methionine synthetase, resulting in hyperhomocysteinemia, folate deficiency and genomic instability [48]. Other adverse effects include enlarged air spaces, bowel distension after prolonged surgery [45]. The use of N_2O also limits oxygen delivery and increases the likelihood of hypoxia (e.g. diffusion hypoxia and crossed pipelines). Current evidence would suggest that administration of N_2O in major surgery increases the rate of postoperative complications. Interestingly, replacing N_2O with medical air and other expensive anesthetic agents did not increase cost of hospital stay [49]. A further study to evaluate the effect of N_2O on postoperative myocardial infarction, heart failure and arrhythmia is currently ongoing [50–52].

15.2.1.4 Analgesics

Despite the concerns of respiratory depression and sedation, potent opioids can be administered safely in patients with end-stage liver disease [53]. In moderate doses, fentanyl (3–5 μg/kg) does not decrease hepatic oxygenation or perfusion. Remifentanil, an ultra-short acting opioid, can be given in large doses, even during anhepatic phase of liver transplantation. The time required for plasma concentration of remifentanil to decrease by 50 % after cessation of drug administration (context sensitive half time) is 3.5 min regardless the duration of infusion [54, 55]. Therefore, respiratory depression in the postoperative period after remifentanil is not a concern.

Tramadol is a popular analgesic given for postoperative pain. It blocks the μ-opioid, serotonin ($5HT_{2C}$) and NMDA receptors. Reuptake of norepinephrine is also inhibited [56]. Tramadol is primarily metabolized in the liver. Both tramadol and its active metabolite *O*-desmethyltramadol contribute to analgesia. Although there is no evidence that pharmacology of tramadol is altered in advanced liver disease, it is advisable to reduce dosage because of concerns about serotonergic syndrome [57].

Large doses of paracetamol may induce liver failure, owing to the formation of *N*-acetyl-*p*-benzoquinoneimine. This binds to hepatocytes and causes tissue necrosis. The reaction is normally protected by glutathione in the liver but this may be depleted in pre-existing liver disease. Dosage of paracetamol should be reduced in patients with mild liver dysfunction and probably should be avoided in those with significant liver disease [53, 58].

The pharmacology of morphine and pethidine is not significantly altered with liver disease. However, concomitant renal failure may lead to accumulation of active and potent metabolites, such as morphine-6-glucuronide and norpethidine, respectively [57].

15.2.1.5 Neuromuscular Blocking Agents [59]

The pharmacology of neuromuscular blocking agents is not affected by liver disease. Clinically, any neuromuscular blocking agent can be used, however, atracurium and cis-atracurium have theoretical advantage because their metabolisms are independent to liver function. In end-stage liver disease, there is a decrease in cholinesterase activity which may prolong the effect of succinylcholine. Titration of neuromuscular blocking effect using transcutaneous nerve stimulator is recommended.

15.2.2 Regional Anesthesia and Analgesia

Regional blockade (nerve block, epidural or spinal block) in combination of general anesthesia is thought to be beneficial because it prevents nociceptive transmission during surgery and provides postoperative pain relief [60–62]. In this regard, regional block reduces neuroendocrine stress response and tampers perioperative sympathetic activity. Despite the initial enthusiasm, clinical trials have failed to prove any outcome benefit with regional block. The Veterans Affairs Cooperative Studies Program (VACS) compared postoperative outcomes in 489 patients receiving combined general/epidural anesthesia with 495 patients having general anesthesia alone after abdominal surgery [63]. Although postoperative pain score was lower in the combined general/epidural anesthesia group, there was no difference in the death rate and other complications (cardiac events, myocardial infarction, respiratory failure and pneumonia) within 30 days after randomization. In a subgroup of patients undergoing aortic surgery ($n=374$), myocardial infarction in the epidural group, 2.7 %, was lower than that of the control (i.e. general anesthesia alone), 7.9 % [OR(95 %CI): 0.3 (0.1–0.9), $P=0.02$]. However, the number of events were few ($n=20$) and the confidence intervals were wide. The single positive finding in the VACS trial should not be considered as conclusive evidence.

Similarly, the Multicentre Australian Study of Epidural Anesthesia (MASTER) trial found that adverse postoperative outcomes in high-risk patients undergoing major abdominal surgery were not reduced by use of combined epidural and general anesthesia. There was a modest decrease in respiratory failure (needing prolonged ventilation or re-intubation) after epidural block (23.3 %) compared with control (30.2 %, $P=0.02$), but the number needed to treat (95 %CI) was large, 15 (7.9–91.9) [64, 65].

Using a population-based administrative database, Wijeysundera and co-workers evaluated 259,037 anesthetics (epidural 56,556; general anesthetics 202,481) performed in Ontario, Canada between 1994 and 2004 [66]. Although there was a small reduction in 30-day mortality (1.7 % vs. 2.0 %; $P=0.02$), the result was biased with the lower death rate in patients undergoing orthopedic surgery and the number needed to treat was 477. In a subgroup analysis of 73,635 patients undergoing abdominal surgery (epidural 21,988; general anesthetics 51,647), mortality at 30 days after indexed surgery was not significantly reduced between groups, relative risk (95 %CI): 0.93 (0.82–1.06).

There are other perceived advantages of providing perioperative epidural. In animal studies it was shown that inhalational anesthetics and opioid inhibited cellular and humoral immunity [67]. It has been therefore proposed that epidural block with local anesthetics, by reducing exposure of anesthetics and postoperative opioids, might decrease metastatic burden, and tumor recurrence. Despite encouraging data from breast and prostatic cancer, MASTER trial showed no difference in 5-years cancer-free survival between groups in patients undergoing hepatobiliary, gastric and colonic surgery (epidural 40 % vs. general anesthetics 38 %, $P=0.58$) [67–69].

Taken together, it would appear that epidural block provides better analgesia during surgery and in the early postoperative period. However, there is no convincing evidence that this advantage will translate into outcome benefit. On the contrary, placement of epidural block is associated with procedural complications [70]. These include epidural hematoma, abscess, nerve injury and hemodynamic instability (with sympathetic block). The risk is substantially higher in patients with bleeding tendency [71]. Thus, it is considered unsafe to place an epidural catheter if INR > 1.5, platelet count < 75×10^9/L and particularly if both parameters are rapidly deteriorating. The same criteria should be adopted

Table 15.3 Hemostatic agents: clinical uses and mechanisms of action

Drug	Dosage	Mechanism of action	Side effects
Tranexamic acid	Loading dose 10 mg/kg during induction of anesthesia Maintenance dose 1–2 mg/kg/h	Lysine analogue that inhibits the binding of plasmin to fibrin	Thromboembolism
ε-aminocaproic acid (EACA)	Loading dose 150 mg/kg during induction of anesthesia Maintenance dose 10–15 mg/kg/h	As above	As above
Desmopressin (Deamino-8-d-arginine-vasopressin, DDAVP)	Slow infusion 0.3 μg/kg over 30 min	Release of von Willebrand factor	Possible increase in myocardial infarction
Recombinant activated factor VII (rFVIIa)	30–120 μg/kg every 2 h for three doses	Binds with subendothelial tissue factor that in the exposed vessel wall. The binding complexes subsequently generate thrombin that in turn facilitate conversion of fibrinogen to fibrin	Thromboembolism

when removing a catheter. Currently the risk of placing epidural catheter on causing localized infection, epidural abscess and meningitis has not been defined [72]. Nevertheless, vigilance and frequent neurologic monitoring are required to ensure early recognition of injury, so that timely treatment can be provided.

There are other regional blocks that may incur less risk. Thoracic paraverteberal (T5/6) block [73], transversus abdominis plane (TAP) block and continuous wound instillation with local anesthetics are getting popular [74, 75]. These blocks are less demanding on technical skills and may be safer in patients with mild coagulopathy. However the risk of local anesthetic toxicity remains [39].

15.2.3 Bleeding: Prevention and Management

Despite recent advances in surgery and technology, bleeding remains a major problem during hepatobiliary surgery [2, 4], especially in patients with pre-existing coagulopathy and sepsis.

Minimizing blood loss during surgery will require effective communication and close collaboration among the team [12]. Nevertheless, the anesthesiologists should be concerned with the following roles:

1. Preoperative autologous donation program asks patients to donate several units of blood before surgery [76]. During and after surgery, patients received their own stored blood when clinically indicated. The major drawback of this technique is that it only applies to elective surgery when procedures are planned weeks ahead. It should also be clear that the risk of clerical error, bacterial contamination and complications associated with stored blood are not modified. The program is also useless in malnourished patients who are already anemic prior to surgery.
2. Acute normovolemic hemodilution (ANH) may decrease loss of hemoglobin during surgery [77]. In this technique, blood is removed (down to a hematocrit value of 20–30 %) and circulating volume is restored with crystalloids or colloids prior to an anticipated episode of bleeding. The blood collected is then returned to the patient after hemostasis is achieved. Therefore, only diluted blood with lower hematocrit is being lost during surgery. Additional advantages of ANH are that it uses patient's own blood and that the clotting factors and platelets in it will improve hemostasis. However, the volume of blood that can be collected is limited.
3. Perioperative red cell salvage involves collection of bloodshed during surgery and reinfused to the patients following appropriate filtering and treatment [78, 79]. The technique may reduce allogenic transfusion, but the effect is often small and costly. It remains controversial whether perioperative red cell salvage can be used in surgery for infective or malignant disease.
4. Apart from local control of bleeding, hemostasis may also be enhanced with administration of hemostatic drugs [80]. Table 15.3 summarizes the clinical uses, mechanisms of action and potential side effects of these agents. In the literature, prophylactic use of tranexamic acid or recombinant activated factor VII (rFVIIa) significantly decreases blood loss and the need for allogenic blood transfusion. However, they also increase the risk of thromboembolism, especially in patients with proven history or at risk of atherosclerosis or thrombosis. Currently, tranexamic acid and rFVIIa should only be given to patients when massive hemorrhage is anticipated.

15.3 Postoperative Considerations

The extent of postoperative monitoring will depend on the likelihood of complications after surgery. In a large survey ($n = 363{,}897$) from the American College of Surgeons National Surgical Quality Improvement Program in 2005–2007 [81], it was noted that between 13.6 and 19.3 % of patients undergoing major abdominal surgery had at least one major complication (e.g. pneumonia, wound infection,

Table 15.4 International Study Group of Liver Surgery (ISGLS) grading of post-hepatectomy liver failure [85]

	Grades of post-hepatectomy liver failure		
	Grade A	Grade B	Grade C
Hepatic function			
INR	<1.5	1.5–1.9	≥2.0
Consciousness	No neurologic symptoms	Confusion, somnolence	Hepatic encephalopathy
Renal function			
Urine output	>0.5 ml/kg/h	≤0.5 ml/kg/h	≤0.5 ml/kg/h, despite diuretics
Plasma urea concentration	<54 μmol/L	<54 μmol/L	≥54 μmol/L
Pulmonary function			
PaO_2	>90 %	<90 % despite supplemental O_2	≤85 %
Treatment options	None required	1. Correction of coagulopathy 2. Diuretics 3. ± Mechanical ventilation	1. Correct hypoglycemia 2. Renal replacement therapy 3. Mechanical ventilation 4. Extracorporeal liver support 5. Liver transplantation

INR International normalized ratio of prothrombin time, *PaO_2* arterial oxygen tension

postoperative bleeding) during their hospital stay. These complications are serious, because on average 11.4–26.3 % of patients died after the events. Interestingly, 6.3–8.1 % of patients required mechanical ventilation > 48 h after surgery, 3.6–4.6 % had unplanned tracheal intubation and 1.4–2.5 % had septic shock. These data strongly suggested patients undergoing major abdominal surgery should be carefully monitored, preferably in a high dependency or intensive care unit.

Three groups of postoperative complications deserve further discussion:

1. Postoperative vascular complications
   Patients undergoing abdominal surgery are at risk of perioperative vascular events, such as vascular death, myocardial infarction (MI), arrhythmias, heart failure and stroke. Currently, based on the revised cardiac risk index, 1.3–9.0 % of patients, at risk of atherosclerosis, had a major vascular event after surgery [82]. Unfortunately, only a fraction of these patients are symptomatic for MI, therefore we believe the incidence of postoperative vascular events is almost certainly an underestimate [83, 84]. In this regard, the data from the Peri-Operative ISchemic Evaluation (POISE) trial were alarming. In this trial, plasma cardiac troponin concentrations were measured daily in 8,351 patients during the first 3 days after surgery. 415 (5.0 %) patients had a rise in troponin concentrations (>99th centile of adult population) and were adjudicated to have MI within 30 days of randomization [84, 85]. Only 34.7 % of these patients had ischemic symptoms. Interestingly, patients with asymptomatic MI had a higher risk of dying at 30 days, OR(95 %CI) 4.0 (2.7–6.1) [84, 85]. These findings would indicate that routine surveillance, after major abdominal surgery, with regular electrocardiograms and cardiac enzymes measurements are justified to facilitate early detection of problems and may improve patient outcome.
2. Postoperative acute liver failure
   Postoperative liver failure is one of the most feared complications after hepatobiliary surgery especially associated with portal vein resection. It is characterized by progressive deterioration in synthetic (hypoalbuminemia and coagulopathy), excretory (hyperbilirubinemia) and detoxifying functions (encephalopathy) of the liver on or after postoperative day 5 (Table 15.4). The clinical effects are variable and can range from simple changes in biochemistry to multiple organ dysfunction [86]. In a recent report, the mortality of postoperative liver failure was up to 14 % [4, 7]. Current treatment strategy is largely supportive.
3. Postoperative acute renal failure [87]
   Acute renal failure following major hepatobiliary surgery can be due to a number of reasons. However, hepatorenal syndrome should be considered in patients with concomitant liver failure. Hepatorenal syndrome is a diagnosis of exclusion, so that common causes of renal failure such as hypovolemina, sepsis, obstructive uropathy, nephrotoxicity (e.g. aminoglycoside related) and parenchymal injury should be carefully discarded. Established hepatorenal syndrome carries a high mortality, 80 % at 30 days and 90 % in 6 months [87]. The pathophysiology is probably related to severe vasospasm of the renal circulation in the setting of splanchnic vasodilation. The end result is shunting of blood to the splanchnic vasculature, leading to renal ischemia [87]. In the non-operative setting, normovolemia and replacement with albumin appear to prevent hepatorenal syndrome, however their use after surgery remains inconclusive. Recommended treatments also include splanchnic vasoconstriction with vasopressin and albumin infusion.

Table 15.5 Continuum of depth of sedation

	Anxiolysis	Conscious sedation	Deep sedation/analgesia	General anesthesia
Responsiveness	Normal to verbal command	Purposeful response to touch	Purposeful response to touch	Unarousable
Airway	Unaffected, no intervention required	Unaffected, no intervention required	Intervention may be required	Intervention often required
Spontaneous ventilation	Unaffected	Adequate	May be inadequate	Frequently inadequate
Cardiovascular function	Unaffected	Usually maintained	Usually maintained	May be impaired

Modified from American Society of Anesthesiologists [89]

15.4 Anesthetic Management for Specific Procedures

15.4.1 Biliary Decompression

As previously mentioned, patients with hilar cholangiocarcinoma often presented with biliary obstruction and will require external and internal drainage either as part of their preoperative workup or for palliative treatment. Common procedures include percutaneous transhepatic biliary drainage (PTBD) and therapeutic ERCP [1–7].

PTBD is generally performed without anesthesia or sedation. The puncture wound is infiltrated with local anesthetics and the entire procedure is usually well tolerated. Occasionally, anesthesiologists are involved for airway support and cardiorespiratory monitoring in patients with ongoing sepsis.

ERCP is usually performed with sedation [88]. Combinations of benzodiazepine and opioid are widely used to produce amnesia and analgesia, respectively. However, there are substantial variations in dosing regimens. For instance, in a survey of 76 endoscopy units in UK, the average dose of midazolam given for ERCP was 5.7 mg, but the dose range is large (95 %CI: 1–12.1 mg). Similarly, there was a huge differences in the dose of pethidine administered (mean: 50.8 mg; 95 %CI: 10–110 mg) [89]. Alternatively, infusions of propofol and fentanyl can be used to provide sedation [88]. These drugs have distinct advantages, in that the onset of drug effect is rapid and the duration of action is short [39, 88]. It is therefore suitable to match the changes in stimulation (e.g. sphincterotomy and stent deployment) with varying rates of infusion. It should be clear that the therapeutic windows of these drugs are narrow [39]. Therefore, although we intend to provide "conscious" sedation (Table 15.5) during ERCP, drug effect could be unpredictable, and may result in deep sedation or even general anesthesia [90]. Anesthesiologists must be prepared for emergency management of airway and ventilation. Several techniques have been proposed to improve patient safety during propofol/fentanyl infusion.

1. Patient controlled sedation (PCS) uses the ordinary patient controlled analgesia (PCA) device and delivers drug boluses [propofol (10 mg/ml) and fentanyl (5 μg/ml); bolus of 1 ml at 200 ml/h; effective lockout time 18 s] upon patient demand to match with sedation requirement [91]. Theoretically, PCS should prevent drug overdose, because a sedated patient will not trigger another demand for drug delivery.
2. Patient maintained computer assisted target controlled infusion, uses similar principle as with PCS, but specific pharmacokinetic model is incorporated to the PCA system in order to avoid overshoot of drug effect [92].
3. There are also measures of electroencephalogram (e.g. bispectral index, BIS) that will assist anesthesiologists to titrate drug infusions. In a preliminary report, BIS was incorporated into a closed-loop control infusion system for sedation during endoscopy [93].

15.4.2 Laparoscopic Assisted Surgery

Laparoscopy has become widely accepted for the diagnosis and staging of the hilar cholangiocarcinoma. With technological advances and accumulation of surgical experience, major complex hepatobiliary resection can also be performed using laparoscopic approach. The documented benefits of laparoscopic assisted surgery over laparotomy include early mobilization, less postoperative ileus, smaller wound and shorter hospital stay. Postoperative respiratory function and cosmetic results are also improved [94]. The anesthetic implications of laparoscopic surgery are related to the changes of intra-abdominal pressure (IAP) after carbon dioxide (CO_2) pneumoperitoneum [93–96].

1. When IAP ≤ 15 mmHg, venous return from splanchnic circulation is increased. However, when IAP is above 15 mmHg, the inferior vena cava becomes compressed, and venous return is reduced. Other hemodynamic changes include vagal bradycardia when the peritoneum is stretched with trocar insertion. However, delayed tachycardia may occur as increasing amount of CO_2 is being absorbed. These changes are well tolerated in healthy adults, however, heart rate responses and hypotension could be exaggerated in patients with pre-existing anemia, hypovolemia and those with limited cardiac reserve.
2. Similarly, an increase in IAP > 15 mmHg produces splinting of the diaphragm and results in a decrease in lung volumes. There is preferential ventilation of the

non-dependent parts of the lung as the diaphragm is pushed up to compress the lung bases. The end result is lung atelectasis, intrapulmonary shunting and pulmonary vasoconstriction [94].

The choice of anesthetic technique is therefore largely limited to general anesthesia for cardiorespiratory management and patient comfort after pneumoperitoneum [94]. Controlled ventilation of the lungs, tracheal intubation and adequate muscle relaxation are required to prevent pulmonary aspiration, removal of CO_2 and to facilitate surgical exposure. The extent of intraoperative monitoring will depend on the magnitude of surgery. Postoperative analgesia with local anesthetic infiltration to the port sites and oral paracetamol may be all that is required after diagnostic laparoscopy [96]. Shoulder tip pain is common after surgery and is probably due to diaphragmatic stretching and distension during pneumoperitonium. It is usually self-limiting and is effectively treated with NSAIDs. Analgesia for more extensive surgery is provided by PCA morphine. Regional block, such as T4/5 epidural, paravertebral block are rarely used. Laparoscopic procedure is associated with postoperative nausea and vomiting [94–96], routine prophylactic antiemetic drug (e.g. ondansetron 4 mg at the end of surgery) is recommended.

15.4.3 Major Curative Resection

Curative surgery for hilar cholangiocarcinoma involves extensive hepatic resection, lymphadenectomy, bile duct and portal vein resection [4, 7]. This is a technically demanding surgery and in the hands of the most experienced surgeon, the procedure is likely to be prolonged and is associated with substantial blood loss. Therefore, surgery required general anesthesia with tracheal intubation and controlled ventilation. Warming devices and rapid infusion system should be prepared. Arterial and central venous cannulae are inserted for blood sampling, and invasive hemodynamic monitoring. The merit of combined regional and general anesthesia and other perioperative considerations have been discussed in previous sections.

In order to decrease blood loss during surgery, hemodynamic manipulation to maintain central venous pressure (CVP) ≤5 mmHg has been suggested [97, 98]. A low CVP reduces congestion in the hepatic vein and the venous sinusoids and should limit bleeding during parenchymal transection. This is achieved by fluid restriction, administration of diuretics, vasodilators and deepening of anesthesia. There are however a number of problems with this technique. A low CVP may induce systemic tissue hypoxia, and air embolism. There is also risk of rebleeding in the early postoperative period [99]. In this regard, small venous branches may be overlooked during hemostasis when the CVP is low, these vessels may then be opened up when CVP rises with patient awakening [100]. There is no randomized controlled trial to evaluate the relative risks and benefits of maintaining a low

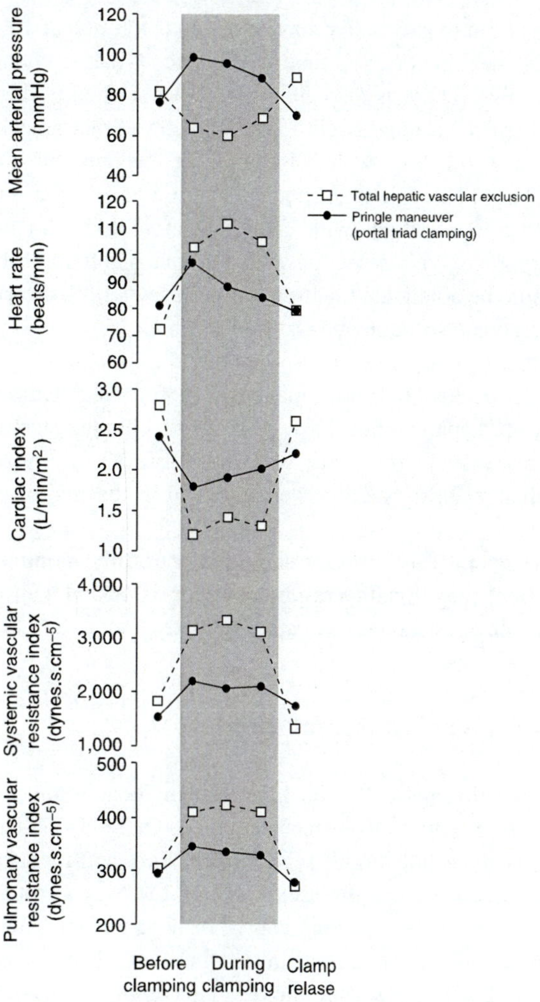

Fig. 15.2 Hemodynamic changes after total hepatic vascular (inflow and outflow) exclusion (□) and Pringle maneuver with portal triad (inflow) clamping (●). *Shaded area* clamping period

CVP during major liver resection. However, it would be logical to avoid high CVP during surgery.

Temporary vascular occlusion may also be required during radical liver resection [101]. In the extreme situation, hepatic vascular inflow is occluded with vascular clamps or tourniquet (Pringle maneuver). This is followed by cross-clamping of the infrahepatic inferior vena cava and then the suprahepatic vena cava, distal to the openings of hepatic veins. These maneuvers effectively exclude the liver from the systemic circulation. Following liver resection and vascular reconstruction, the clamps are removed sequentially. Total hepatic vascular (inflow and outflow) exclusion however presents specific challenges to the anesthesiologist. Cross clamping of inferior vena cava reduces venous return by>50 %, this is compensated by an increase in afterload. The end result is a precipitous decrease (>50 %) in cardiac output and the arterial pressure is reduced by about 20 % (Fig. 15.2). These changes may precipitate heart failure in patients with underlying coronary artery disease. Preloading with colloid (e.g. 6 % hydroxyethyl starch solution at 10 ml/kg) has been reported to modify the hemodynamic changes [101, 102]. There is also concern of liver ischemia during total hepatic vascular occlusion. It is believed that a healthy adult may tolerate "warm" ischemia of the liver for up to 60–90 min. Nevertheless, anhepatic period of 5.5 h has been reported in a patient with cholangiocarcinoma who have undergone ex-vivo resection with autotransplantation [103]. It should be noted that the liver was perfused with University of Wisconsin solution and was cooled on ice.

Other techniques have also been used to produce hepatic vascular occlusion. Pringle maneuver (portal triad clamping) interrupts hepatic inflow [101, 104]. This technique increases systemic vascular resistance by 30–60 % (Fig. 15.2). However the changes are generally well tolerated in the majority of patients.

Postoperatively, patients should be carefully monitored. Infection, coagulopathy, respiratory depression and hemodynamic changes should be treated promptly.

15.4.4 Liver Transplantation

Occasionally, patients with hilar cholangiocarcinoma may undergo orthotopic liver transplantation (OLT) [1–7]. These patients are usually highly selected, who have non-metastatic but locally advanced disease. Based on the Mayo protocol, patients will receive a long course of neoadjuvant external beam radiotherapy and concomitant fluorouracil and capecitabine [105, 106]. Patients who develop complications or fail to respond to the neoadjuvant therapy are usually excluded for OLT. Specific anesthetic challenges occur during the following stages of the procedure [107].

Preanhepatic stage: Bleeding during mobilization and dissection of the liver is related to pre-existing coagulopathy, portal hypertension, and complexity of surgery.

Anhepatic stage: Hemodynamic changes may be associated with total hepatic vascular occlusion (Fig. 15.2) [101, 108]. Venovenous bypass is sometimes used to divert venous return from the femoral vein to the superior vena cava. This should reduce hemodynamic changes, avoid splanchnic congestion and improve renal perfusion. However, bypass related thromboembolism and inadvertent decannulation could result in fatal complications [107]. Plasma glucose concentration should be regularly monitored and hypoglycemia should be treated promptly.

Neohepatic stage: The reperfusion syndrome is characterized by arterial hypotension and pulmonary hypertension within 5 min after graft reperfusion. This is due to the release of vasoactive substances (including hydrogen and potassium ions) from the graft liver. Constituents in the preservation solution, such as adenosine, may also produce clinically significant bradycardia [107, 108]. Fibrinolysis is another major problem and should be treated with fresh frozen plasma, cryoprecipitate and other hemostatic agents listed in Table 15.3.

15.5 Summary

This chapter summarizes the anesthetic issues during surgery for hilar cholangiocarcinoma. Anesthetic requirement varies with different surgical procedures. There are also important changes in physiology and pharmacology associated with liver disease. Anesthesiologists should understand these possible changes in order to facilitate surgery for achieving the best possible outcome.

References

1. Zografos GN, Farfaras A, Zagouri F, et al. Cholangiocarcinoma: principles and current trends. Hepatobiliary Pancreat Dis Int. 2011;10:10–20.
2. Regimbeau JM, Fuks D, Le Treut YP, et al. Surgery for hilar cholangiocarcinoma: a multi-institutional update on practice and outcome by the AFC-HC study group. J Gastrointest Surg. 2011;15:480–8.
3. Cai WK, Sima H, Chen BD, et al. Risk factors for hilar cholangiocarcinoma: a case-control study in China. World J Gastroenterol. 2011;17:249–53.
4. Ito F, Cho CS, Rikkers LF, et al. Hilar cholangiocarcinoma: current management. Ann Surg. 2009;250:210–8.
5. Chamberlain RS, Blumgart LH. Hilar cholangiocarcinoma: a review and commentary. Ann Surg Oncol. 2000;7:55–66.
6. de Martel C, Plummer M, Franceschi S. Cholangiocarcinoma: descriptive epidemiology and risk factors. Gastroenterol Clin Biol. 2010;34:173–80.
7. Jonas S, Benckert C, Thelen A, et al. Radical surgery for hilar cholangiocarcinoma. Eur J Surg Oncol. 2008;34:263–71.
8. Hanau LH, Steigbigel NH. Acute (ascending) cholangitis. Infect Dis Clin North Am. 2000;14:521–46.
9. Lee JG. Diagnosis and management of acute cholangitis. Nat Rev Gastroenterol Hepatol. 2009;6:533–41.
10. Squizzato A, Keller T, Romualdi E, et al. Clopidogrel plus aspirin versus aspirin alone for preventing cardiovascular disease. Cochrane Database Syst Rev. 2011;19(1):CD005158.
11. Pulmonary Embolism Prevention (PEP) trial Collaborative Group. Prevention of pulmonary embolism and deep vein thrombosis with low dose aspirin: Pulmonary Embolism Prevention (PEP) trial. Lancet. 2000;355:1295–302.
12. Levy JH, Azran M. Anesthetic concerns for patients with coagulopathy. Curr Opin Anaesthesiol. 2010;23:400–5.
13. Bradlow BA, Chetty N. Dosage frequency for suppression of platelet function by low dose aspirin therapy. Thromb Res. 1982;27:99–110.
14. Patrono C, Ciabattoni G, Patrignani P, et al. Clinical pharmacology of platelet cyclooxygenase inhibition. Circulation. 1985;72:1177–84.
15. Cheng B, Hung CT, Chiu W. Herbal medicine and anaesthesia. Hong Kong Med J. 2002;8:123–30.
16. Child CG. The liver and portal hypertension. Philadelphia: Saunders; 1964.
17. Pugh RN, Murray-Lyon IM, Dawson JL, et al. Transection of the oesophagus for bleeding oesophageal varices. Br J Surg. 1973; 60:646–9.

18. Kamath PS, Wiesner RH, Malinchoc M, et al. A model to predict survival in patients with end-stage liver disease. Hepatology. 2001;33:464–70.
19. Biggins SW, Kim WR, Terrault NA, et al. Evidence-based incorporation of serum sodium concentration into MELD. Gastroenterology. 2006;130:1652–60.
20. Luca A, Angermayr B, Bertolini G, et al. An integrated MELD model including serum sodium and age improves the prediction of early mortality in patients with cirrhosis. Liver Transpl. 2007;13:1174–80.
21. Huo TI, Wang YW, Yang YY, et al. Model for end-stage liver disease score to serum sodium ratio index as a prognostic predictor and its correlation with portal pressure in patients with liver cirrhosis. Liver Int. 2007;27:498–506.
22. Sakka SG. Assessing liver function. Curr Opin Crit Care. 2007;13:207–14.
23. Fazakas J, Mándli T, Ther G, et al. Evaluation of liver function for hepatic resection. Transplant Proc. 2006;38:798–800.
24. Morris-Stiff G, Gomez D, Prasad R. Quantitative assessment of hepatic function and its relevance to the liver surgeon. J Gastrointest Surg. 2009;13:374–85.
25. Seibel A, Müller A, Sakka SG. Indocyanine green plasma disappearance rate for monitoring hepatosplanchnic blood flow. Intensive Care Med. 2011;37:357–9.
26. Reekers M, Simon MJ, Boer F, et al. Pulse dye densitometry and indocyanine green plasma disappearance in ASA physical statusI-II patients. Anesth Analg. 2010;110:466–72.
27. Fan ST. Liver functional reserve estimation: state of the art and relevance for local treatments: the eastern perspective. J Hepatobiliary Pancreat Sci. 2010;17:380–4.
28. Schneider PD. Preoperative assessment of liver function. Surg Clin North Am. 2004;84:355–73.
29. Mann DV, Lam WW, Hjelm NM, et al. Metabolic control patterns in acute phase and regenerating human liver determined in vivo by 31-phosphorus magnetic resonance spectroscopy. Ann Surg. 2002;235:408–16.
30. Wakamatsu H, Nagamachi S, Kiyohara S, et al. Predictive value of Tc-99m galactosyl human serum albumin liver SPECT on the assessment of functional recovery after partial hepatectomy: a comparison with CT volumetry. Ann Nucl Med. 2010;24:729–34.
31. Manizate F, Hiotis SP, Labow D, et al. Liver functional reserve estimation: state of the art and relevance to local treatments. Oncology. 2010;78 Suppl 1Suppl 1:131–4.
32. Jakob SM. Splanchnic blood flow in low-flow states. Anesth Analg. 2003;96:1129–38.
33. Groszmann RJ, Abraldes JG. Portal hypertension: from bedside to bench. J Clin Gastroenterol. 2005;39(4 Suppl 2):S125–30.
34. Asfar P, De Backer D, Meier-Hellmann A, et al. Clinical review: influence of vasoactive and other therapies on intestinal and hepatic circulations in patients with septic shock. Crit Care. 2004;8:170–9.
35. Vedrinne JM, Duperret S, Bizollon T, et al. Comparison of transesophageal and transthoracic contrast echocardiography for detection of an intrapulmonary shunt in liver disease. Chest. 1997;111:1236–40.
36. Williams RL. Drug administration in hepatic disease. N Engl J Med. 1983;309:1616–22.
37. Rodighiero V. Effects of liver disease on pharmacokinetics. An update. Clin Pharmacokinet. 1999;37:399–431.
38. Wood M. Plasma drug binding: implications for anesthesiologists. Anesth Analg. 1986;65:786–804.
39. Stoelting RK, Hiller AC. Pharmacology and physiology in anesthetic practice. Philadelphia: Lippincott Williams and Wilkins; 2006.
40. Merritt WT. Perioperative concerns in acute liver failure. Int Anesthesiol Clin. 2006;44:37–57.
41. Reichle FM, Conzen PF. Halogenated inhalational anaesthetics. Best Pract Res Clin Anaesthesiol. 2003;17:29–46.
42. Sinha A, Clatch RJ, Stuck G, et al. Isoflurane hepatotoxicity: a case report and review of the literature. Am J Gastroenterol. 1996; 91:2406–9.
43. Singhal S, Gray T, Guzman G, et al. Sevoflurane hepatotoxicity: a case report of sevoflurane hepatic necrosis and review of the literature. Am J Ther. 2010;17:219–22.
44. Berghaus TM, Baron A, Geier A, et al. Hepatotoxicity following desflurane anesthesia. Hepatology. 1999;29:613–4.
45. Myles PS, Leslie K, Silbert B, et al. A review of the risks and benefits of nitrous oxide in current anaesthetic practice. Anaesth Intensive Care. 2004;32:165–72.
46. Myles PS, Leslie K, Chan MTV, ENIGMA Trial Group, et al. Avoidance of nitrous oxide for patients undergoing major surgery: a randomized controlled trial. Anesthesiology. 2007;107: 221–31.
47. Leslie K, Myles PS, Chan MTV, et al. Risk factors for severe postoperative nausea and vomiting in a randomised trial of nitrous oxide-based versus nitrous oxide-free anaesthesia. Br J Anaesth. 2008;101:498–505.
48. Myles PS, Chan MTV, Leslie K, et al. Effect of nitrous oxide on plasma homocysteine and folate in patients undergoing major surgery. Br J Anaesth. 2008;100:780–6.
49. Graham AM, Myles PS, Leslie K, et al. A cost-benefit analysis of the ENIGMA trial. Anesthesiology. 2011;115:265–72.
50. Myles PS, Chan MTV, Kaye DM, et al. Effect of nitrous oxide anesthesia on plasma homocyst(e)ine and endothelial dysfunction. Anesthesiology. 2008;109:657–63.
51. Myles PS, Leslie K, Peyton P, ANZCA Trials Group, et al. Nitrous oxide and perioperative cardiac morbidity (ENIGMA-II) trial: rationale and design. Am Heart J. 2009;157:488–94.
52. Leslie K, Myles PS, Chan MTV, et al. Nitrous oxide and long-term morbidity and mortality in the ENIGMA trial. Anesth Analg. 2011;112:387–93.
53. Delcò F, Tchambaz L, Schlienger R, et al. Dose adjustment in patients with liver disease. Drug Saf. 2005;28:529–45.
54. Glass PS, Hardman D, Kamiyama Y, et al. Preliminary pharmacokinetics and pharmacodynamics of an ultra-short-acting opioid: remifentanil (GI87084B). Anesth Analg. 1993;77:1031–40.
55. Richardson SP, Egan TD. The safety of remifentanil by bolus injection. Expert Opin Drug Saf. 2005;4:643–51.
56. Grond S, Sablotzki A. Clinical pharmacology of tramadol. Clin Pharmacokinet. 2004;43:879–923.
57. Murphy EJ. Acute pain management pharmacology for the patient with concurrent renal or hepatic disease. Anaesth Intensive Care. 2005;33:311–22.
58. Prescott LF. Paracetamol: past, present, and future. Am J Ther. 2000;7:143–7.
59. Craig RG, Hunter JM. Neuromuscular blocking drugs and their antagonists in patients with organ disease. Anaesthesia. 2009;64 Suppl 1Suppl 1:55–65.
60. Curatolo M. Adding regional analgesia to general anaesthesia: increase of risk or improved outcome? Eur J Anaesthesiol. 2010;27:586–91.
61. Fischer B. Benefits, risks, and best practice in regional anesthesia: do we have the evidence we need? Reg Anesth Pain Med. 2010;35:545–8.
62. Marret E, Remy C, Bonnet F, Postoperative Pain Forum Group. Meta-analysis of epidural analgesia versus parenteral opioid analgesia after colorectal surgery. Br J Surg. 2007;94:665–73.
63. Park WY, Thompson JS, Lee KK. Effect of epidural anesthesia and analgesia on perioperative outcome: a randomized, controlled veterans affairs cooperative study. Ann Surg. 2001;234:560–9.
64. Rigg JR, Jamrozik K, Myles PS, MASTER Anaethesia Trial Study Group, et al. Epidural anaesthesia and analgesia and outcome of major surgery: a randomised trial. Lancet. 2002;359: 1276–82.

65. Peyton PJ, Myles PS, Silbert BS, et al. Perioperative epidural analgesia and outcome after major abdominal surgery in high-risk patients. Anesth Analg. 2003;96:548–51.
66. Wijeysundera DN, Beattie WS, Austin PC, et al. Epidural anaesthesia and survival after intermediate-to-high risk non-cardiac surgery: a population-based cohort study. Lancet. 2008;372:562–9.
67. Exadaktylos AK, Buggy DJ, Moriarty DC, et al. Can anesthetic technique for primary breast cancer surgery affect recurrence or metastasis? Anesthesiology. 2006;4:660–4.
68. Biki B, Mascha E, Moriarty DC, et al. Anesthetic technique for radical prostatectomy surgery affects cancer recurrence: a retrospective analysis. Anesthesiology. 2008;109:180–7.
69. Myles PS, Peyton P, Silbert B, for the ANZCA Trials Group Investigators, et al. Perioperative epidural analgesia for major abdominal surgery for cancer and recurrence-free survival: a randomised trial. BMJ. 2011;342:d1491.
70. Neal JM, Bernards CM, Hadzic A, et al. ASRA practice advisory on neurologic complications in regional anesthesia and pain medicine. Reg Anesth Pain Med. 2008;33:404–15.
71. Horlocker TT, Wedel DJ, Rowlingson JC, et al. Regional anesthesia in the patient receiving antithrombotic or thrombolytic therapy: American Society of Regional Anesthesia and Pain Medicine Evidence-Based Guidelines (third edition). Reg Anesth Pain Med. 2010;35:64–101.
72. Horlocker TT, Wedel DJ. Infectious complications of regional anesthesia. Best Pract Res Clin Anaesthesiol. 2008;22:451–75.
73. Richardson J, Lönnqvist PA, Naja Z. Bilateral thoracic paravertebral block: potential and practice. Br J Anaesth. 2011;106:164–71.
74. Siddiqui MR, Sajid MS, Uncles DR, et al. A meta-analysis on the clinical effectiveness of transversus abdominis plane block. J Clin Anesth. 2011;23:7–14.
75. Forastiere E, Sofra M, Giannarelli D, et al. Effectiveness of continuous wound infusion of 0.5 % ropivacaine by On-Q pain relief system for postoperative pain management after open nephrectomy. Br J Anaesth. 2008;101:841–7.
76. Goodnough LT. Autologous blood donation. Anesthesiol Clin North America. 2005;23:263–70.
77. Maithel SK, Jarnagin WR. Adjuncts to liver surgery: is acute normovolemic hemodilution useful for major hepatic resections? Adv Surg. 2009;43:259–68.
78. Pape A, Habler O. Alternatives to allogeneic blood transfusions. Best Pract Res Clin Anaesthesiol. 2007;2:221–39.
79. Carless PA, Henry DA, Moxey AJ, et al. Cell salvage for minimizing perioperative allogeneic blood transfusion. Cochrane Database Syst Rev. 2010(4):CD001888.
80. Gurusamy KS, Li J, Sharma D, et al. Pharmacological interventions to decrease blood loss and blood transfusion requirements for liver resection. Cochrane Database Syst Rev. 2009(4):CD008085.
81. Ghaferi AA, Birkmeyer JD, Dimick JB. Variation in hospital mortality associated with inpatient surgery. N Engl J Med. 2009;361:1368–75.
82. Lee TH, Marcantonio ER, Mangione CM, et al. Derivation and prospective validation of a simple index for prediction of cardiac risk of major noncardiac surgery. Circulation. 1999;100:1043–9.
83. Devereaux PJ, Chan MTV, Eikelboom J. Major vascular complications in patients undergoing non-cardiac surgery: magnitude of the problem, risk prediction, surveillance, and prevention. In: Yusuf S, Cairns JA, Camm AJ, et al., editors. Evidence based cardiology. 3rd ed. West Sussex: Wiley-Blackwell; 2010. p. 47–62.
84. Devereaux PJ, Pogue J, Guyatt G, et al. Characteristics and short-term prognosis of perioperative myocardial infarction in patients undergoing noncardiac surgery: a cohort study. Ann Intern Med. 2011;154(8):523–8.
85. Devereaux PJ, Yang H, Yusuf S, on behalf of POISE Investigators, et al. Effects of metoprolol succinate extended-release in patients undergoing noncardiac surgery: a randomised controlled trial. Lancet. 2008;371:1839–47.
86. Rahbari NN, Garden OJ, Padbury R, et al. Posthepatectomy liver failure: a definition and grading by the International Study Group of Liver Surgery (ISGLS). Surgery. 2011;149:713–24.
87. Ginès P, Guevara M, Arroyo V, et al. Hepatorenal syndrome. Lancet. 2003;362:1819–27.
88. Bamji N, Cohen LB. Endoscopic sedation of patients with chronic liver disease. Clin Liver Dis. 2010;14:185–94.
89. Williams EJ, Taylor S, Fairclough P, BSG Audit of ERCP, et al. Are we meeting the standards set for endoscopy? Results of a large-scale prospective survey of endoscopic retrograde cholangio-pancreatograph practice. Gut. 2007;56:821–9.
90. American Society of Anesthesiologists Task Force on Sedation and Analgesia by Non-Anesthesiologists. Practice guidelines for sedation and analgesia by non-anesthesiologists. Anesthesiology. 2002;96:1004–17.
91. Heuss LT, Drewe J, Schnieper P, et al. Patient-controlled versus nurse-administered sedation with propofol during colonoscopy. A prospective randomized trial. Am J Gastroenterol. 2004;99: 511–8.
92. Campbell L, Imrie G, Doherty P, et al. Patient maintained sedation for colonoscopy using a target controlled infusion of propofol. Anaesthesia. 2004;59:127–32.
93. Chen SC, Rex DK. An initial investigation of bispectral monitoring as an adjunct to nurse-administered propofol sedation for colonoscopy. Am J Gastroenterol. 2004;99:1081–6.
94. Chui PT, Gin T, Oh TE. Anaesthesia for laparoscopic general surgery. Anaesth Intensive Care. 1993;21:163–71.
95. Cunningham AJ. Anesthetic implications of laparoscopic surgery. Yale J Biol Med. 1998;71:551–78.
96. Gerges FJ, Kanazi GE, Jabbour-Khoury SI. Anesthesia for laparoscopy: a review. J Clin Anesth. 2006;18:67–78.
97. Alkozai EM, Lisman T, Porte RJ. Bleeding in liver surgery: prevention and treatment. Clin Liver Dis. 2009;13:145–54.
98. Schroeder RA, Kuo PC. Pro: low central venous pressure during liver transplantation—not too low. J Cardiothorac Vasc Anesth. 2008;22:311–4.
99. Massicotte L, Beaulieu D, Thibeault L. Con: low central venous pressure during liver transplantation. J Cardiothorac Vasc Anesth. 2008;22:315–7.
100. Kim YK, Chin JH, Kang SJ, et al. Association between central venous pressure and blood loss during hepatic resection in 984 living donors. Acta Anaesthesiol Scand. 2009;53:601–6.
101. Lau WY, Lai EC, Lau SH. Methods of vascular control technique during liver resection: a comprehensive review. Hepatobiliary Pancreat Dis Int. 2010;9:473–81.
102. Fu SY, Lau WY, Li AJ, et al. Liver resection under total vascular exclusion with or without preceding Pringle manoeuvre. Br J Surg. 2010;97:50–5.
103. Chui AK, Island ER, Rao AR, et al. The longest survivor and first potential cure of an advanced cholangiocarcinoma by ex vivo resection and autotransplantation: a case report and review of the literature. Am Surg. 2003;69:441–4.
104. Fu SY, Lai EC, Li AJ, et al. Liver resection with selective hepatic vascular exclusion: a cohort study. Ann Surg. 2009;249:624–7.
105. De Vreede I, Steers JL, Burch PA, et al. Prolonged disease-free survival after orthotopic liver transplantation plus adjuvant chemoirradiation for cholangiocarcinoma. Liver Transpl. 2000;6:309–16.
106. Rea DJ, Heimbach JK, Rosen CB, et al. Liver transplantation with neoadjuvant chemoradiation is more effective than resection for hilar cholangiocarcinoma. Ann Surg. 2005;242:451–8.
107. Ozier Y, Klinck JR. Anesthetic management of hepatic transplantation. Curr Opin Anaesthesiol. 2008;21:391–400.
108. Della Rocca G, Brondani A, Costa MG. Intraoperative hemodynamic monitoring during organ transplantation: what is new? Curr Opin Organ Transplant. 2009;14:291–6.

Selection of Patients for Liver Resection and Liver Transplantation

16

J.J. Schwartz, J. Sorensen, and R. Kim

16.1 Introduction

Complete excision of viable tumor offers the only chance for cure for hilar cholangiocarcinoma. Resection and liver transplantation have each evolved to offer significant survival advantages over non-surgical treatments. Although the two options beg comparison, currently the indications for each are different.

Although early attempts at liver transplantation for hilar cholangiocarcinoma were associated with poor cancer-related survival [1–12], more recent results with neoadjuvant chemoradiation followed by liver transplantation have shown significant improvements [13–15]. Despite the renewed interest in liver transplantation, the global limitation of organ availability and the lack of Level I data tempers its widespread use.

Resection for hilar cholangiocarcinoma, or Klatskin tumor, has also evolved. The initial poor survival rates, associated with limited duct resection [16] (see Chap. 23) have increased with bile duct and extended liver resections [17–21] performed in high-volume centers (see Chap. 18). The resection rates, documented in various series containing over 50 patients from 1990 to 2006, have ranged from 45 to 94 % (Table 16.1). In these same series, the mortality and 5-year survival rates have ranged from 0 to 15 %, and 11 to 41 %, respectively [22–24]. In this chapter, we discuss the considerations when selecting a patient for resection or liver transplantation in the setting of hilar cholangiocarcinoma.

J.J. Schwartz, MD (✉)
Department of Gastroenterological Surgery, Graduate School of Medicine, Yokohama City University, Yokohama, Japan
e-mail: jason.schwartz@hsc.utah.edu

J. Sorensen, MD • R. Kim, MD
Department of Surgery, University of Utah, Salt Lake City, UT, USA

16.2 Populations at Risk

As development of cholangiocarcinoma is predicated on the existence of chronic inflammation, it may theoretically be possible to identify patients at increased risk of harboring the disease. While numerous conditions have been found to predispose to its development, protocol-based methods for surveillance and detection are currently employed with the intent of unearthing localized, resectable hilar disease. Other candidates include those with disease confined to the extrahepatic bile duct in which underlying biliary inflammation and impaired hepatic function would otherwise obviate extended surgical resection.

With a cancer incidence ranging from 7 to 42 % [25–29] and a cumulative neoplasia risk of 11 % within the first 10 years of diagnosis [26], patients with primary sclerosing cholangitis (PSC) can be regarded as a population specifically at risk [22, 29, 30]. There are, unfortunately, no existing features to identify those with PSC who will go on to develop cholangiocarcinoma, making PSC patients obvious candidates for surveillance protocols. It is noteworthy that a majority of patients with PSC (80 %) will also harbor a concomitant diagnosis of inflammatory bowel disease (IBD), either ulcerative colitis or Crohn's disease [31]. It is currently unknown whether patients with a non-cholestatic pattern of blood chemistries and normal radiographic findings who harbor a diagnosis of IBD are at increased risk for developing PSC and subsequent cholangiocarcinoma, but they are widely assumed to be at low risk for these disorders [32]. Certainly, the sudden manifestation of right upper quadrant pain, cholangitis, or signs of biliary obstruction in an individual with stable IBD should prompt an evaluation of the biliary tree. Similarly, the appearance of abnormal liver function tests or elevated tumor markers in a patient with Crohn's disease or ulcerative colitis merits similar investigation.

W.Y. Lau (ed.), *Hilar Cholangiocarcinoma*,
DOI 10.1007/978-94-007-6473-6_16,

Table 16.1 Series of over 50 patients resected for hilar cholangiocarcinoma

Authors	Liver resection (%)	Negative margin (%)	Resection (n)	Year published	5-year survival (%)
Nakeeb*	14	26	56	1996	11
Gerhards*	29	14	112	2000	NA
Launois*	32	NA	151	2000	NA
Dinant*	38	31	99	2006	27
Todoroki*	58	14	101	2000	28
Seyama*	67	64	87	2003	40
Kawarada*	75	64	65	2002	26
Klempnauer [131]	77	77	151	1997	28
Jarnagin [75]	78	78	80	2001	26
Kosuge*	50	52	65	1999	40
Jarnagin*	82	77	106	2005	NA
Neuhaus [84]	85	61	80	1999	22
Miyazaki [85]	86	71	76	1998	26
Kawasaki [133]	54	68	79	2003	30
Nimura [97]	70	100	46	1990	41
Hemming*	66	80	53	2005	35

*References found in Suggested Reading List

16.3 Diagnostics

16.3.1 Serological Testing and Imaging

Except in cases where palliation is the chief consideration, a tissue diagnosis of cholangiocarcinoma informs all subsequent decision making. Early detection of cholangiocarcinoma, however, is a formidable obstacle. Current diagnostic approaches offer suboptimal yield and must rely on a combination of serologic testing, imaging modalities, pathologic analyses, and a high index of clinical suspicion. Often times, an elevation in tumor associated markers, particularly CA 19-9, initiates further workup by clinicians to establish the presence of biliary pathology. The diagnosis of cholangiocarcinoma on the basis of this test alone is problematic, however. For example, in patents without PSC, a sensitivity of 53 % is reported at a value of 100 U/ml. This decreases to 33 % for patients with early-stage cholangiocarcinoma [33]. In these individuals, the negative predictive value ranged from 76 to 92 %. In the PSC population, sensitivity and specificity for cholangiocarcinoma detection were improved at 89 and 86 %, respectively. Increasing the threshold of concern to 129 U/ml for PSC patients improved the specificity to 98.5 %, but lowered the sensitivity to 78.6 %. In these patients, the positive predictive value was 57 % [34–36]. An elevation in CA 19-9 is also observed in the setting of cholangitis and hepatolithiasis [34], but is missing entirely in patients lacking the blood type Lewis antigen [36, 37]. For these reasons, in the absence of known risk factors or virtually diagnostic imaging studies, a diagnosis of cholangiocarcinoma should not be entertained on the basis of this tumor marker alone [34]. Conversely, additional testing should be sought if warranted by clinical suspicion despite near normal CA 19-9 levels.

An elevated CA 19-9 ordinarily precipitates further imaging of the liver and biliary tree, which should be employed with the intent of assessing tumor extent, the level of biliary obstruction, the technical feasibility of resection, and the calculation of a future liver remnant when resection is entertained [36]. While abdominal ultrasound can sometimes reveal the presence of biliary ductal dilatation, establish a diagnosis of hepatolithiasis, and provide evidence of biliary mass lesions, it can also be used in duplex mode to assess the degree to which central tumors impinge on vascular structures [22, 38, 39]. However, ultrasonographic findings have largely been supplanted by the use of cross-sectional imaging. Computed tomography (CT) is helpful in this regard and is often the first modality employed in a patient with an elevated CA 19-9 or obstructive jaundice. A typical finding is the presence of biliary ductal dilatation proximal to a blocked choledochus. Not infrequently, lobar atrophy is present from long-standing biliary obstruction or portal vein involvement on the side of tumor. However, an obvious mass is sometimes lacking on CT despite findings that would otherwise suggest neoplasia. For this reason, magnetic resonance imaging (MRI) coupled with magnetic resonance cholangiopancreatography (MRCP) is emerging as the imaging modality of choice given its ability to provide superior anatomic resolution of the intra- and extrahepatic bile ducts and adjacent vascular structures. Cholangiocarcinomas, appearing hypointense on T1-weighted images, and hyperintense on T2, can be further delineated using gadolinium contrast enhancement, which can help further define vascular encasement. Additional information can be gained with respect to invasion of adjacent liver parenchyma as well as the presence of distant and nodal metastases [22, 34, 36, 40–44]. While sensitivity and positive predictive value are roughly equivalent

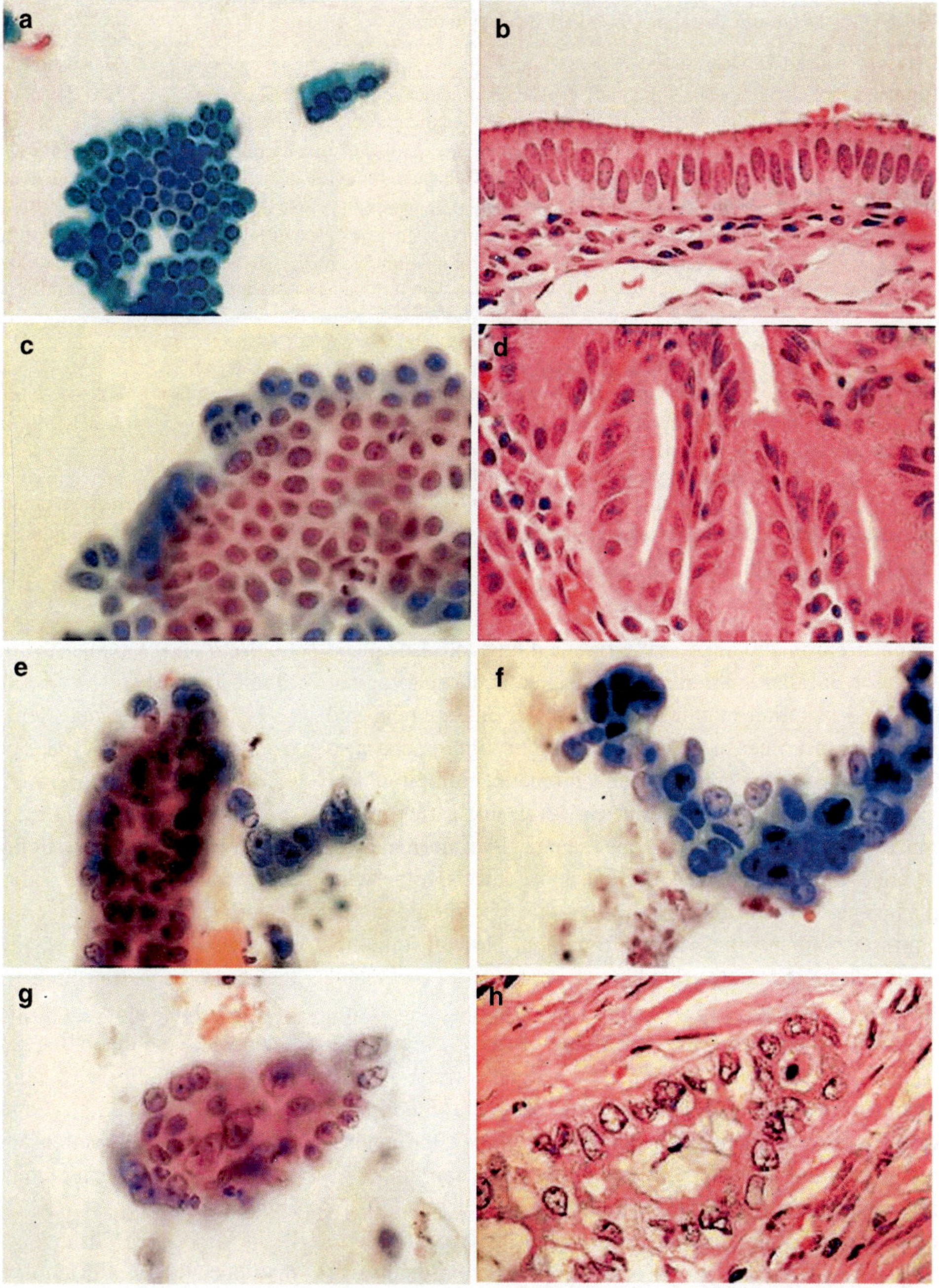

Fig. 16.1 Cytology. (**a**) Cytology of benign bile duct epithelium with sheets and strips of cells with bland round to oval nuclei (Papanicolaou). (**b**) Histology of benign bile duct epithelium with a single layer of columnar cells (H&E). (**c**) Cytology of reactive bile duct epithelium with mildly enlarged nuclei, prominent nuclei, and overlying inflammation. (**d**) Histology of reactive bile duct epithelium. (**e–g**) Cytology of adenocarcinoma with irregularly arranged groups of cells with increased nuclear: cytoplasmic ratio and nuclear molding, as well as increased nuclear size, anisonucleosis, and marked nuclear irregularity. (**h**) Histology of adenocarcinoma (cholangiocarcinoma) (Figure and legend reproduced with permission from Advances in Anatomic Pathology [47])

between the two modalities, comparisons in the literature have noted superior diagnostic accuracy for MRI/MRCP (92 % versus 56–84 % for CT), an improved specificity (79 % versus 33–57 %), and a higher negative predictive value (73 % versus 7–50 %) [36, 45, 46].

16.3.2 Cytologic Evaluation

Whereas imaging remains a vital component in the multimodality approach to diagnosis, pathologic evaluation is considered the gold standard. In these cases, a tissue diagnosis often hinges on cytology, which is not always confirmatory, and sometimes difficult to acquire. Diagnostic attempts via percutaneous fine needle aspiration (FNA) should be discouraged due to the theoretical risk of tumor seeding. Preferably, tissue sampling is obtained by endoscopic retrograde cholangiopancreatography (ERCP) in conjunction with over-the-wire brush sampling of a malignant-appearing stricture. Accessing the biliary tree in this manner allows for characterization of benign, atypical, suspicious, and overtly malignant-appearing epithelia (Fig. 16.1) [47]. After processing, Papanicolaou-stained slides of benign-appearing cells appear as sheet-like monolayers and orderly palisades with

Table 16.2 Diagnostic categories for biliary brush cytology

Diagnostic category	Definition	Management
Unsatisfactory	Specimen is nondiagnostic: insufficient cellular material for diagnosis, extensive artifact or specimen obscured by acellular debris	Additional attempts at biliary access required
Negative for malignancy	Benign-appearing cells in cohesive monolayers (honeycombing) and / or orderly palisades. Material is adequate for cytologic interpretation.	Additional testing unwarranted unless inconsistent with abnormal clinical or radiologic findings
Atypical indeterminate	Cells demonstrate benign, reactive changes which may manifest as nuclear enlargement, mild variation in nuclear size, and 1–2 prominent nucleoli. Occasional mitotic figures and degenerative changes may be present. Cells maintain normal tissue architecture with little crowding or overlap. Normal N/C ratio and nuclear contours are observed. Although malignancy cannot be excluded, changes are likely a function of associated ductal inflammation. This category may encompass what was previously regarded as low-grade dysplasia	Must be correlated with available clinical and radiologic data which. Timing of follow-up and repeat cytology predicated on suspicion for neoplasia
Suspicious for malignancy	Highly-dysplastic cells that display some, but not all of the features of malignancy. This may include clumping of cells with prominent nuclear crowding; irregular nuclear membranes; high N/C ratio; coarse chromatin and distinct; prominent nucleoli	Timely follow-up required. Repeat biliary access recommended in 1–3 months. May be interpreted in context of additional clinical and radiographic studies
Adenocarcinoma	Cells with unquestionable features of malignancy	No additional confirmation required

Modified from deBellis et al. [49], Henke et al. [47] and Lograno and Waxman [53]

granular chromatin and basally-oriented nucleoli. Localized infection or biliary inflammation can alter the morphology of collected material, manifesting as nuclear enlargement and increased prominence of nucleoli. Mitotic figures can also appear, as can hyperchromasia, chromatin clumping, and vacuolization of the cytoplasm. However, nuclear/cytoplasmic ratio remains unaltered, cells maintain their normal level of cohesiveness, and their nuclear appearance is otherwise unchanged [47]. Reactive changes of this type should not be confused with neoplastic transformation. Notwithstanding, some cytologic features should raise awareness of the potential for malignant progression. These include clustering of cells and crowding or overlapping of nuclei; increasing irregularity of nuclear membranes; a trend toward a more abundant nuclear: cytoplasmic ratio; coarse chromatin; and distinct, prominent nucleoli [48, 49]. Although the natural history of these lesions is currently unknown, they should be regarded with suspicion, particularly in patients with PSC or other chronic inflammatory lesions of the bile duct, where they may represent a point on a neoplastic continuum. In this setting, the theoretical risk of malignant transformation should stimulate more rigorous follow-up and encourage more frequent biliary sampling.

Although the ability to discriminate between dysplasia and overt malignancy can be difficult with cytology, features used to distinguish benign from malignant strictures include the presence of nuclear molding, chromatin clumping, and a substantially increased nuclear-cytoplasmic ratio [50]. Adenocarcinoma of the biliary tract can also harbor anisonucleosis, irregular nuclear contours/grooves, enlarged nuclei/nucleoli, and altered cell polarity, amongst other features [47]. Because of the subjective nature of cytologic interpretation and the potential for interobserver variation [49, 51, 52], we endorse the system proposed by Logrono and Waxman for the reporting of biliary cytology (Table 16.2) [53].

In reality, little may separate higher grades of dysplasia from what is clearly malignant. This, coupled with a lack of uniform interpretation of diagnostic criteria, has caused reported sensitivities for brush cytology to vary widely. With sensitivities typically ranging from 20 to 60 % [36, 54, 55], the inability to secure a diagnosis with this technique can be influenced by a variety of additional factors. As cholangiocarcinomas are tumors of the bile duct epithelium, those that fail to penetrate into the lumen (submuscosal spread) will not be sampled appropriately. Sampling error can also be encountered due to the paucicellular, desmoplastic nature of the surrounding environment in which these tumors frequently arise. The chronic inflammatory milieu common to the biliary tree in patients with PSC can introduce further ambiguity. Well-differentiated tumors such as mucinous and papillary types may also generate false negatives as these tumors are difficult to interpret on cytology. Tumors may occur at sites difficult to access, their location obviating the use of various biopsy techniques. Finally, collected material may be insufficient for analysis [36, 54]. In contrast, the diagnostic specificity of this technique has seldom been questioned, consistently approaching 100 % in most studies [54].

To improve the diagnostic yield of cytology, the use of repeat over-the wire brushings during separate procedures has been advocated in the setting of dysplasia or when cholangiocarcinoma is suspected [56–61]. Two advanced cytologic techniques have also emerged recently as important aids to diagnosis. Both techniques, fluorescent in situ hybridization (FISH) and digital image analysis (DIA), capitalize on the near-universal propensity for biliary cancer to exhibit chromosomal instability. Fluorescently-labeled DNA

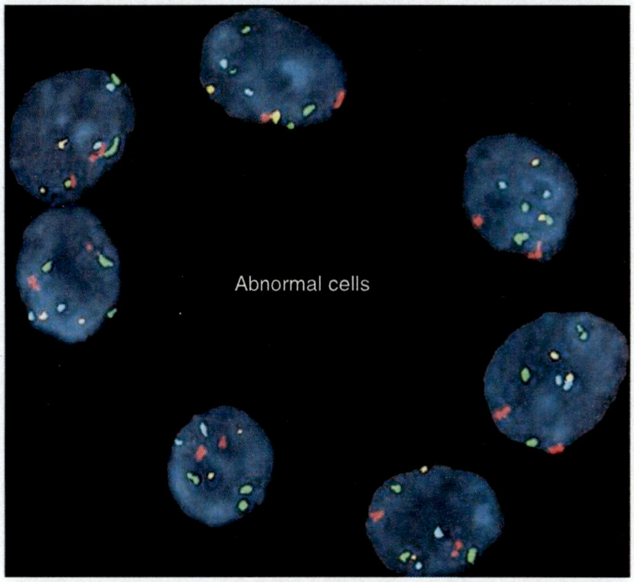

Fig. 16.2 Fluorescence in situ hybridization of biliary brushing. A representative fluorescence micrograph of biliary brushings from a patient with cholangiocarcinoma is shown here. Each colored spot represents one chromosome; therefore, two spots per color are indicative of the normal diploid state. In this example, >2 spots are seen for more than one color (indicating more than one chromosome pair is abnormal), leading to a diagnosis of polysomy (Figure reproduced with permission from the *Journal of Hepatology* [34])

probes are used in the case of FISH to detect aneuploidy or abnormalities of particular loci (gain or deletion), while DIA utilizes the stoichiometric binding properties of a cytochemical stain to quantitate nuclear DNA as a ratio of normal ploidy. Chromosomes specifically affected include 3, 7, and the 9p21 band. In this context, a finding of FISH polysomy can be equated with cytologic malignancy (Fig. 16.2). In like manner, DNA tetraploidy (DNA index >1.89) in non-PSC patients can be viewed similarly. Investigators who have examined the use of these techniques in conjunction with conventional cytology have noted an overall improvement in sensitivity without compromising specificity in patients with malignant-appearing strictures. In this population, results demonstrate that FISH has the highest sensitivity amongst those without PSC, while retaining appropriate levels of specificity. In patients with PSC, FISH retains the highest sensitivity of the three techniques. Specificity is lower, however. DIA results demonstrating aneuploidy (DNA index from 1.12 to 1.89) appear to have intermediate sensitivity and specificity compared to cytology and FISH, but its addition to PSC and non-PSC groups increases the malignant detection rate by twofold relative to cytology alone when clinical decision-making is predicated strictly on unequivocally positive cytologic results (Tables 16.3 and 16.4) [62]. As such, the inclusion of such diagnostic methodologies should be viewed as a requirement for institutions contemplating the implementation of transplant-based protocols.

16.3.3 Adjunctive Measures

Newer techniques of endoscopic retrograde cholangioscopy may facilitate direct examination of suspicious lesions and subsequent biopsy [63–67]. This method has been used extensively in the therapeutic approach to benign biliary disease. However, in the setting of cholangiocarcinoma, its utility as a screening or diagnostic tool has yet to be confirmed in a sizable cohort. With advancements in fiberoptics, it is expected that this technology will continue to evolve. The newly developed-SpyGlass Direct Visualization System™ is one such example. Cholangioscopy using this system allows for intraductal biliary imaging in all four quadrants, thereby permitting tissue sampling under direct visualization. Experience gained with its use may eventually increase the ability to discriminate benign from malignant biliary lesions.

On many occasions, a combination of methods is required when evaluating a suspicious biliary lesion. If an initial ERCP and/or cytologic diagnosis is evasive, then endoscopic ultrasound (EUS) may prove useful when examining this region. In this regard, EUS can offer greater resolution when compared to conventional cholangiography, thereby allowing the detection of a tumor mass or an infiltrating process. Vascular invasion can also be identified as can the presence of malignant-appearing lymph nodes [54]. Moreover, EUS-guided FNA of strictures, masses, and suspicious lymph nodes can supplement conventional techniques when cholangiography and/or cytology proves unremarkable. The technique frequently requires sphincterotomy and is procedurally difficult. A compilation of studies has revealed its overall cancer detection rate to be 33 % [49]. However, with some reports indicating a sensitivity closer to 100 % [61, 68, 69], the skill of the endoscopist, the experience of the cytopathologist, and the stringency of the cytologic criteria used likely inform results.

Historically, a variety of endoluminal sampling techniques have been applied to cytodiagnosis. Duodenal aspirates used in 1960's and 70's carried a high false positive rate. This technique was largely supplanted by intraductal bile aspiration cytology, the sensitivity of which ranged from 6 to 32 % across multiple studies. Despite their simplicity and low cost, these techniques should be considered inferior to contemporary cytologic methodologies [49, 54]. Neither approach should be employed routinely in surveillance protocols.

Occasionally, cytopathologic evaluation can be conducted on the material retrieved from occluded biliary stents. With diagnosis being deferred until after stent removal, the clinical utility of this sampling technique is questionable in most settings. However, in situations where frequent stent exchanges are required to maintain biliary patency, the examination of stent-adherent material may complement other sampling

Table 16.3 Sensitivity, specificity, positive predictive value, and negative predictive value of cytology, DIA, and FISH for the detection of malignancy by stricture classification

	Sensitivity (95 % CI)	Specificity (95 % CI)	PPV (95 % CI)	NPV (95 % CI)
Non-PSC patients				
Proximal				
Cytology (positive or suspicious)	9 % (0.01–0.30)	100 % (0.71–1)	100 % (0.16–1)	37 % (0.20–0.56)
Positive	4 % (0.001–0.24)	100 % (0.71–1)	100 % (–)	35 % (0.19–0.55)
Suspicious	4 % (0.001–0.24)	100 % (0.71–1)	100 % (–)	35 % (0.19–0.55)
DIA (aneuploid or tetraploid)	30 % (0.12–0.54)	90 % (0.55–1)	86 % (0.42–1)	39 % (0.20–0.61)
Tetraploid	5 % (0.001–0.25)	100 % (0.69–1)	100 % (–)	34 % (0.18–0.54)
Aneuploid	25 % (0.09–0.49)	90 % (0.55–1)	83 % (0.36–0.99)	37 % (0.19–0.59)
FISH (polysomy or trisomy)	63 % (0.38–0.84)	100 % (0.66–1)	100 % (0.73–1)	56 % (0.30–0.80)
FISH polysomy	31 % (0.12–0.56)	100 % (0.66–1)	100 % (0.54–1)	41 % (0.21–0.64)
FISH trisomy	31 % (0.12–0.56)	100 % (0.66–1)	100 % (0.54–1)	41 % (0.21–0.64)
Distal				
Cytology (positive or suspicious)	41 % (0.29–0.54)	96 % (0.86–0.99)	93 % (0.77–0.99)	54 % (0.43–0.65)
Positive	20 % (0.11–0.31)	100 % (0.93–1)	100 % (0.75–1)	47 % (0.37–0.58)
Suspicious	21 % (0.12–0.33)	96 % (0.86–0.99)	87 % (0.62–0.98)	47 % (0.37–0.57)
DIA (aneuploid or tetraploid)	49 % (0.36–0.62)	98 % (0.88–1)	97 % (0.84–1)	57 % (0.45–0.69)
Tetraploid	16 % (0.08–0.27)	100 % (0.92–1)	100 % (0.69–1)	45 % (0.35–0.56)
Aneuploid	33 % (0.22–0.46)	98 % (0.88–1)	95 % (0.77–1)	50 % (0.39–0.62)
FISH (polysomy or trisomy)	59 % (0.46–0.71)	92 % (0.80–0.98)	90 % (0.77–0.97)	63 % (0.50–0.74)
FISH polysomy	48 % (0.35–0.60)	100 % (0.93–1)	100 % (0.88–1)	59 % (0.48–0.70)
FISH trisomy	11 % (0.04–0.21)	92 % (0.80–0.98)	64 % (0.31–0.89)	44 % (0.34–0.54)
PSC patients				
Cytology (positive or suspicious)	41 % (0.18–0.67)	97 % (0.90–1)	78 % (0.40–0.97)	87 % (0.77–0.93)
Positive	18 % (0.04–0.43)	100 % (0.95–1)	100 % (0.29–1)	83 % (0.73–0.90)
Suspicious	23 % (0.07–0.50)	97 % (0.90–1)	67 % (0.22–0.96)	83 % (0.73–0.91)
DIA (aneuploid or tetraploid)	43 % (0.18–0.71)	87 % (0.76–0.94)	43 % (0.18–0.71)	87 % (0.76–0.94)
Tetraploid	14 % (0.02–0.43)	95 % (0.86–0.99)	40 % (0.05–0.85)	83 % (0.72–0.91)
Aneuploid	28 % (0.08–0.58)	92 % (0.82–0.97)	44 % (0.14–0.79)	85 % (0.74–0.92)
FISH (polysomy or trisomy 7 or 3)	70 % (0.44–0.90)	86 % (0.75–0.93)	57 % (0.34–0.78)	92 % (0.82–0.97)
FISH polysomy	47 % (0.23–0.72)	100 % (0.94–1)	100 % (0.63–1)	88 % (0.78–0.94)
FISH trisomy	23 % (0.07–0.50)	86 % (0.75–0.93)	31 % (0.09–0.61)	81 % (0.69–0.89)

Reprinted with permission from *Gastroenterology* [62]
PPV positive predictive value, *NPV* negative predictive value, *CI* confidence interval, (–) insufficient number of patients to calculate 95 % CI

methods when a lesion appears suspicious for malignancy. Pooled data indicates the overall sensitivity of stent examination to be 32 % [49].

Finally, techniques which can obtain more substantial tissue samples offer the prospect of improving diagnostic yield through the maintenance of tissue architecture, an essential component in pathologic diagnosis. The use of endoscopic forceps biopsy appears to corroborate this assertion, especially when combined with biliary brushings where in some cases it has contributed to a two-fold increase in diagnostic sensitivity [54]. Similar to EUS, the technique requires advanced endoscopic proficiency and may not be suitable for some lesions. Theoretically, an increased risk of bile duct injury is also incurred. This approach may be considered when a diagnosis is in question. Likewise, the introduction of various cutting and scraping devices, through pre-existing percutaneous transhepatic biliary drainage (PTBD) tubes, may also contribute to enhanced diagnostic yield. Two studies examining the use of the 9- French Simpson atherectomy catheter, which can obtain tissue samples 0.5–2.0 cm in length, noted sensitivities of 79 and 97 %, respectively. Specificity was retrospectively reported to be 100 %, positive predictive value 100 %, and negative predictive value 93 % [54, 70]. At the University of Utah, we have used the modern-day Silverhawk™ atherectomy catheter to similar effect.

Access to the biliary tree through pre-existing PTBD tubes can also facilitate a rendezvous approach when selective bile duct cannulation fails or a tight stricture interferes with conventional endoscopic techniques [70–73]. The rendezvous procedure combines an endoscopic technique with PTBD access to allow the antegrade passage of a guidewire through the native papilla for the purpose of establishing ERCP access. This technique can be combined with variety of biopsy and visualization techniques including EUS,

Table 16.4 Sensitivity, specificity, positive predictive value, and negative predictive value of cytology, DIA, and FISH for the detection of malignancy by stricture classification when cytology is *neither positive nor suspicious*

	Sensitivity (95 % CI)	Specificity (95 % CI)	PPV (95 % CI)	NPV (95 % CI)
Non-PSC patients				
Proximal				
DIA (tetraploid or aneuploid)	28 % (0.1–0.53)	90 % (0.55–1)	83 % (0.36–0.99)	41 % (0.21–0.64)
Tetraploid	5 % (0.001–0.27)	100 % (0.69–1)	100 % (–)	37 % (0.19–0.58)
Aneuploid	22 % (0.06–0.48)	90 % (0.55–1)	80 % (0.28–0.99)	39 % (0.20–0.61)
FISH (polysomy or trisomy 7 or 3)	59 % (0.33–0.81)	100 % (0.66–1)	100 % (0.69–1)	56 % (0.30–0.80)
FISH polysomy	23 % (0.07–0.50)	100 % (0.66–1)	100 % (0.40–1)	41 % (0.21–0.64)
FISH trisomy (7 or 3)	35 % (0.14–0.62)	100 % (0.66–1)	100 % (0.54–1)	45 % (0.23–0.68)
FISH (polysomy or trisomy) and DIA (aneuploid or tetraploid)	23 % (0.07–0.50)	100 % (0.66–1)	100 % (0.40–1)	41 % (0.21–0.64)
FISH (polysomy or trisomy) or DIA (aneuploid or tetraploid)	65 % (0.38–0.86)	89 % (0.52–1)	92 % (0.61–1)	57 % (0.29–0.82)
Distal				
DIA (aneuploid or tetraploid)	25 % (0.12–0.42)	98 % (0.87–0.99)	90 % (0.55–1)	60 % (0.48–0.72)
Tetraploid	5 % (0.007–0.19)	100 % (0.91–1)	100 % (0.16–1)	55 % (0.43–0.67)
Aneuploid	19 % (0.08–0.36)	98 % (0.87–0.99)	87 % (0.47–1)	58 % (0.46–0.70)
FISH (polysomy or trisomy 7 or 3)	35 % (0.20–0.52)	93 % (0.82–0.99)	81 % (0.54–0.96)	64 % (0.51–0.75)
FISH polysomy	22 % (0.10–0.38)	100 % (0.92–1)	100 % (0.63–1)	61 % (0.49–0.72)
FISH trisomy (7 or 3)	13 % (0.04–0.29)	93 % (0.82–0.99)	62 % (0.24–0.91)	57 % (0.45–0.69)
FISH (polysomy or trisomy) and DIA (aneuploid or tetraploid)	15 % (0.05–0.31)	98 % (0.87–1)	83 % (0.36–0.99)	58 % (0.46–0.70)
FISH (polysomy or trisomy) or DIA (aneuploid or tetraploid)	48 % (0.31–0.66)	93 % (0.80–0.98)	85 % (0.62–0.97)	68 % (0.55–0.80)
PSC patients				
DIA (aneuploid or tetraploid)	14 % (0.004–0.58)	88 % (0.77–0.95)	12 % (0.003–0.53)	90 % (0.79–0.96)
Tetraploid	0 (0–0.41)	97 % (0.88–0.99)	0 (0–0.84)	89 % (0.79–0.95)
Aneuploid	14 % (0.004–0.58)	91 % (0.81–0.97)	17 % (0.004–0.64)	90 % (0.79–0.96)
FISH (polysomy or trisomy 7 or 3)	60 % (0.26–0.88)	87 % (0.76–0.94)	43 % (0.18–0.71)	93 % (0.83–0.98)
FISH polysomy	20 % (0.02–0.56)	100 % (0.94–1)	100 % (0.16–1)	88 % (0.79–0.95)
FISH trisomy (7 or 3)	40 % (0.12–0.74)	87 % (0.76–0.94)	33 % (0.10–0.65)	90 % (0.79–0.96)
FISH (polysomy or trisomy) and DIA (aneuploid or tetraploid)	14 % (0.004–0.58)	98 % (0.91–1)	50 % (0.01–0.99)	90 % (0.80–0.96)
FISH (polysomy or trisomy) or DIA (aneuploid or tetraploid)	67 % (0.30–0.92)	75 % (0.62–0.86)	30 % (0.12–0.54)	93 % (0.82–0.99)

Reprinted with permission from *Gastroenterology* [62]
PPV positive predictive value, *CI* confidence interval, *NPV* negative predictive value, (–) insufficient number of patients to calculate 95 % CI

cholangioscopy, forceps biopsy, and endoscopic brushings to improve diagnostic yield.

16.4 Liver Resection

16.4.1 Assessing Resectability

The surgeon must determine two things for resectability: (1) whether an R0 resection can be achieved and (2) the minimum amount of remnant liver volume needed to survive. Distant metastatic disease (including liver lesions not contiguous with the primary biliary tumor) and involvement of Level (L) three lymph nodes (those along the celiac artery, the superior mesenteric artery or the aortocaval groove) preclude curative resection. Otherwise, it is the extent of local disease that determines whether the cancer is resectable.

16.4.1.1 Assessing the Possibility of an R0 Resection

Hilar cholangiocarcinoma lesions are often not visible as discrete masses on imaging as the majority are of the sclerosing macroscopic subtype [74]. Obtaining tissue confirmation is therefore difficult and diagnosis is often made through a combination of factors including patient age and risk factors, signs and symptoms, CA19-9, and pattern of ductal dilatation (see Diagnostics, above) [26, 33].

The ability to resect for cure has been redefined by reports of significantly improved survival from high-volume centers describing aggressive resections of not

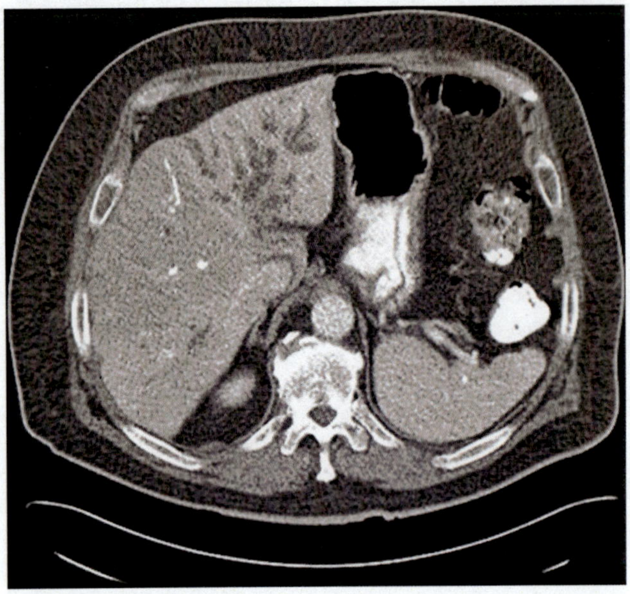

Fig. 16.3 CT scan demonstrating in a patient with hilar cholangiocarcinoma showing left-dominant biliary ductal dilatation without a common confluence suggesting involvement of the second-order biliary radicals

Table 16.5 Proposed clinical T stage criteria for hilar cholangiocarcinoma from MSKCC [131]

Clinical Stage	Criteria
T1	Tumor involving biliary confluence ± unilateral extension to second order biliary radicals
T2	Tumor involving biliary confluence ± unilateral extension to second order biliary radicals and ipsilateral portal vein involvement ± ipsilateral hepatic lobar atrophy
T3	Tumor involving biliary confluence + bilateral extension to second order biliary radicals, unilateral extension to second order biliary radicals with contralateral portal vein involvement, unilateral extension to second order biliary radicals with contralateral hepatic lobar atrophy, or main portal vein involvement

only the bile duct lesion, but also the ipsilateral liver and draining nodes [17–21]. Surgery is avoided if the disease in the potential remnant liver involves the second order biliary radicals, as the risk of complications from multiple biliary anastomoses (bile leaks, anastomotic strictures, residual intrahepatic disease) is greater [75, 76]. If the retropancreatic bile duct is involved, an added pancreaticoduodenectomy can offer a survival advantage [24]. In cases where a discrete mass is not visible, the longitudinal extent of disease is determined by the pattern of intrahepatic bile duct dilatation proximal to the lesion (Fig. 16.3). Circumferential involvement of portal structures [right, left, or proper hepatic artery(ies); right, left, or main portal vein(s)] may preclude resection as these vessels must be preserved to guarantee perfusion I the remnant liver. Other factors important in determining resectability include bilateral involvement in any combination of: (1) lobar atrophy, (2) tumor at second order biliary radicals, and (3) tumor at the hepatic artery or portal vein that precludes attempts at reconstruction.

The value of a given imaging modality (US, CT scan, MRI/MRCP, ERCP, EUS and PTC) [22, 34, 36, 38–44, 47, 49, 71–73] rests on its ability to demonstrate the local and regional extent of disease (see Diagnostics: Serological Testing and Imaging). Although the pattern of disease and extent may be classified by the modified Bismuth-Corlette system [17] (see Chap. 4), this system only partly answers the question of resectability as it describes only the side of the disease in relation to the bifurcation. This system is further limited by not providing information on the radial extent, vascular involvement, and longitudinal extent of the disease (i.e., involvement beyond second order biliary radicals).

The more useful classification system from Memorial Sloan Kettering Cancer Center (MSKCC) was created based on their experience treating 225 patients with hilar cholangiocarcinoma (Table 16.5) [75]. Unresectable local disease was defined as tumors involving (1) bilateral second order biliary radicals, (2) ipsilateral second order biliary with contralateral portal vein involvement, (3) ipsilateral second order biliary with contralateral hepatic lobar atrophy, or (4) main or bilateral portal vein involvement. Using this system, patients with stage T3 disease are considered unresectable given the inability to obtain an R0 resection while preserving a viable sector of remnant liver. MSKCC used this system to achieve resectability rates for T1, T2 and T3 tumors of 59, 31 and 0 %, respectively. Median survival after resection was similarly documented at 20, 13 and 8 months. Currently, the MSKCC classification system with pre-operative imaging is employed by most hepatobiliary surgeons to determine whether a patient is a candidate for resection.

As of this writing American Joint Committee on Cancer staging manual (AJCC 2010, Seventh Edition) [77] has incorporated the MSKCC System into the Primary Tumor (T) category to define resectable local disease (Table 16.6). Thus AJCC T4 is equivalent to the MSKCC T3 disease, both of which are unresectable. This system will likely supplant the MSKCC system as not only does it surgically stage the local disease, but it incorporates information on nodal disease, metastases, and tumor grade to predict both resectability and survival.

In planning a resection, the surgeon must decide if the lesion is left or right dominant as this initial designation will determine whether the resection will be left or right-sided. Central lesions are approached as right-dominant lesions as the right bile duct is shorter than the left and the right hepatic

Table 16.6 TNM classification of hilar cholangiocarcinomas [132]

Primary tumor (T)			
TX	Primary tumor cannot be assessed		
T0	No evidence of primary tumor		
Tis	Carcinoma in situ		
T1	Tumor confined to the bile duct, with extension up to the muscle layer or fibrous tissue		
T2a	Tumor invades beyond the wall of the bile duct to surrounding adipose tissue		
T2b	Tumor invades adjacent hepatic parenchyma		
T3	Tumor invades unilateral branches of the portal vein or hepatic artery		
T4	Tumor invades main portal vein or its branches bilaterally; or the common hepatic artery; or the second order biliary radicals bilaterally; or unilateral second order biliary radicals with contralateral portal vein or hepatic artery involvement		
Regional lymph nodes (N)			
NX	Regional lymph nodes cannot be assessed		
N0	No regional lymph node metastasis		
N1	Regional lymph node metastasis (including nodes along the cystic duct, common bile duct, hepatic artery, and portal vein)		
N2	Metastasis to periaortic, pericaval, super mesenteric artery, and/or celiac artery lymph nodes		
Distant metastasis (M)			
M0	No distant metastasis		
M1	Distant metastasis		
Anatomic stage/prognostic groups			
Stage 0	Tis	N0	M0
Stage I	T1	N0	M0
Stage II	T2a–b	N0	M0
Stage IIIA	T3	N0	M0
Stage IIIB	T1–3	N1	M0
Stage IVA	T4	N0–1	M0
Stage IVB	Any T	N2	M0
	Any T	Any N	M1

artery is more often involved with tumor than the left. Therefore, a resection of the right liver and reconstruction to the left hepatic duct will more likely achieve a negative margin. In general, the standard operation to achieve an R0 resection for hilar cholangiocarcinoma is an extended liver resection with caudate lobectomy, extrahepatic bile duct resection to the remnant intrahepatic bile duct, portal lymphadenectomy, and hepaticojejunostomy [18, 19, 23, 78–82].

16.4.1.2 Assessing the Future Remnant Liver

The major challenge of hilar cholangiocarcinoma is its central location and proximity to the hepatic artery and portal vein. In this setting, minimal radial extension can compromise the inflow to the liver. In various series of resected Klatskin tumors, portal vein involvement has been found in 16–22 % of patients [76, 83]. In addition, its propensity to spread along the length of the bile duct and nerves that accompany the hepatic and celiac arteries, as well as its direct spread to lymph nodes (53 %) and adjacent liver parenchyma has made it difficult to achieve an R0 resection with removal of the duct alone [16]. Over the past 20 years, extended liver and bile duct resection has become the standard of care for hilar cholangiocarcinoma. This strategy facilitates negative margins despite multiple modes of spread by sacrificing the ipsilateral pedicle rather than "scraping" tumor from these pedicles, or aborting altogether. Extended liver/bile duct resections have thus increased the frequency of R0 resections, while at the same time improving recurrence-free survival [21, 75, 80, 84, 85]. In this context, studies have demonstrated improved survival in groups undergoing extended liver resection over bile duct resection alone, even when both groups had R0 duct resections [75, 84, 85]. The improvement in survival in patients undergoing extended liver resection suggests that pathologic assessment may be inaccurate when a limited specimen is submitted, and supports the concept of multiple modes of spread.

As the resection required to achieve negative tumor margins for hilar cholangiocarcinoma requires an extended hepatic lobectomy, the surgeon must confirm that the future liver remnant will be functionally adequate. A work-up for possible underlying liver disease is also needed to make this assessment. Accordingly, risk factors for intrinsic liver disease should be elicited. This could include a history of inflammatory bowel disease (PSC), intravenous drug use (hepatitis C), and either alcohol abuse or obesity (non-alcoholic steatohepatitis). Patients should be examined for signs and symptoms of cirrhosis and portal hypertension (i.e. ascites, caput medusa, splenomegaly, hepatomegaly, and jaundice), while liver function tests, serum albumin, coagulation studies, and platelet count are used for additional screening. In general, a remnant consisting of 20–30 % of the total liver mass is sufficient to prevent liver failure following resection as long as this remaining portion is not compromised to accomplish these aims, [36, 86]. To accomplish these aims, we employ volumetric studies performed by radiologists of the total and future remnant liver volumes.

The purpose of preoperative percutaneous transhepatic cholangiocatheterization (PTC) in patients with jaundice is to: (1) delineate the extent of biliary disease, (2) drain biliary sepsis and, (3) minimize hepatocellular damage in the future remnant for maximal post-operative liver function. Because of the potential risks (tumor seeding, bleeding, and bile leaks), and the lack of benefit found by some [87], drainage has not been universally accepted. In one series of 57 patients randomized to preoperative drainage or no drainage, the peri-operative mortality was not improved with drainage (14 % versus 15 %, respectively) [88]. Still, many groups advocate pre-operative PTC for the listed reasons, citing no increase in complications, with increased resection rates [89, 90]. Our center supports the use of preoperative PTC drainage in order to improve liver function and prevent biliary sepsis and renal insufficiency. Although some centers perform a single PTC to the future liver remnant alone [91], we have found that bilateral PTCs improve anorexia while more efficiently decreasing bilirubin and rates of biliary sepsis.

As resection of 80 % or more of uninjured liver parenchyma (or 65 % of an injured liver as in case of biliary obstruction) is associated with significant morbidity including infection and hepatic insufficiency [36, 86], the ability to offer extended liver resection may be limited by liver anatomy (i.e. the size of the remnant in relation to total size). Portal vein embolization (PVE) to the side of the future specimen takes advantage of the atrophy-hypertrophy complex to induce growth of the future remnant sector over 6 weeks [92]. In addition, the absence of liver growth may suggest chronic injury that may preclude resection altogether. A number of studies document the safety and efficacy of portal vein embolization [86, 90, 92]. Nagino et al. found that in 132 patients with cholangiocarcinoma who underwent extended hepatectomy after PVE, the 5-year survival was similar to that of 136 patients with cholangiocarcinoma who underwent a less than 50 % resection of the liver without PVE (26.8 % versus 27.6 %, respectively). These authors concluded that the PVE facilitated extended liver resections with similar outcomes to patients requiring lesser resections [93]. Others have validated PVE as means of screening potential resection candidates, as they found that patients with <5 % liver growth after PVE had a higher surgical mortality as compared to patients who had >10 % liver growth (mortality 50 % versus 0, respectively) [94].

16.4.2 Intraoperative Techniques and Decision-Making

As 40–50 % of patients with Klatskin tumors undergoing surgery are found to be unresectable despite thorough pre-operative staging [21, 75], staging laparoscopy has been advocated in an attempt to decrease the morbidity of open exploration. Using this approach, the accuracy of laparoscopy (number of unresectable patients detected by laparoscopy divided by the total number of unresectable cases) for hilar cholangiocarcinoma was found to be between 42 and 53 % in some reports [95]. The addition of laparoscopic ultrasound improved the detection of unresectable tumor. In a study of 84 patients undergoing laparoscopic staging for hilar cholangiocarcinoma, the yield (number of unresectable patients detected divided by the number of patients undergoing laparoscopy) with laparoscopy alone was 24.3 % (20 of 82), but 41.5 % (35 of 82) when intraoperative ultrasound was added, for an overall accuracy of 53.1 % (35 of 66). From this, the authors concluded that staging laparoscopy could be justified in the sense that it prevented unnecessary laparotomies in 42.2 % of patients [96]. With small foci of metastatic disease not readily discernible by conventional pre-operative imaging techniques, laparoscopy is mainly useful for detecting occult, superficial liver or peritoneal metastases under 1 cm. These patients are candidates for neither resection nor transplantation. In patients without these lesions, even if unresectable due to locally advanced disease, laparoscopy only adds time and cost to the procedure as these patients will require laparotomy in order to understand the local stage. In an effort to minimize unneeded laparoscopy, Weber et al. used the MSKCC system to predict patients with occult metastases and found evidence o such for 36 % of patients with T2/T3 disease had occult metastases versus 9 % of patients with T1 disease ($P=0.02$) [95]. They concluded that staging laparoscopy should be reserved for patients with MSKCC T2/T3 disease—a criterion which our group uses.

Patients deemed resectable by pre-operative staging (up to AJCC 2010 T1–3/N0–1/M0 or Stage IIIB) undergo open exploration and possible resection (of the liver, bile duct, and lymph nodes) for hilar cholangiocarcinoma (for details see Chap. 20). In the majority of patients classifies as T1 (91 %) and T2/T3 (64 %), it is local extent of disease rather than metastases that will preclude curative resection. Thus the initial challenge at open exploration is to determine whether an R0 resection can be achieved based on visualization and palpation of (1) the nodal disease, (2) the proximal extent and laterality of the primary hilar tumor, (3) the degree of cholestasis and possible fibrosis of the liver, and (4) the freedom of remnant vascular structures from tumor. The operation is then performed in a deliberate sequence to determine these four characteristics before reaching a "point of no return" in the resection (i.e. devascularizing the ipsilateral liver). Despite these attempts, a proportion of cases will reach this point only to learn (as the surgery progress, at the time of frozen section pathology report, or days later at final pathology) that an R0 resection was not possible.

A caudate resection is routinely added because its drainage enters near the bile duct confluence (primarily the left duct) and may be involved with tumor in 40–98 % of the time [97–100]. A number of centers have shown that in selected cases, a caudate resection may be associated with decreased local recurrence and increased 5-year survival [101]. In one series of 75 patients undergoing resection, the 5-year survival for those undergoing combined caudate lobectomy (n = 17) was significantly better than for patients who did not have a caudate lobectomy (25 % versus 5 %, respectively) [102].

Controversy remains over whether the survival advantage and prognostic information offered by nodal dissection justifies the potential morbidity incurred by the procedure. Along these lines, Kitagawa et al. found that in 110 resections for Klatskin tumors with routine L1 and L2 nodal dissections, the 5-year survival was lower for node-positive patients (30 % for node-negative, 15 % for L1 and 12 % for L2). However, these authors pointed out that when compared to patients who were not resected, patient resected with L1 nodal disease may still receive improved long term survival [103]. Other groups do not routinely dissect lymph nodes beyond the hepatoduodenal ligament as they are fatalistic about the decreased survival noted in patients with nodal disease [21, 22]. Based on these reports, and our own experience, we advocate aggressive surgical management (including lymph node dissection) for L2 disease as it may offer improved survival, particularly when there are no other curative options available.

16.5 Liver Transplantation

While surgical outcomes continue to improve, radical bile duct resection and partial hepatectomy must be capable of eliminating all gross and microscopic disease in order to achieve a disease-free resection margin (R0 resection). Leading to improved 3- and 5-year survival rates, this objective has been more readily attainable in contemporary series. However, most patients remain ineligible for resection based on well-defined oncologic principles [75]. As such, total hepatectomy and orthotopic liver transplantation (OLT) have evolved to therapeutically encompass a subset of patients with localized disease who may theoretically benefit from surgical extirpation, but who nevertheless fall outside of standard resection criteria. Despite two decades of experience in which results were less than encouraging [1–12], improved patient selection and the addition of neoadjuvant chemoradiation have re-vitalized interest in the curative potential of this approach. Recent successes in this area have been grounded in a protocol-based methodology which focuses on at-risk populations, incorporates emerging screening and surveillance techniques, retains stringent selection criteria, and makes appropriate use of scarce donor resources.

16.5.1 Screening and Surveillance Protocols

The success of current neoadjuvant protocols has been predicated on patient selection and well-defined treatment algorithms (Fig. 16.4) [11, 13–15, 104, 105]. As eligibility for transplant is restricted to stage I and II disease, early stage detection is mandatory. Unfortunately, many small tumors are asymptomatic. The goal of screening protocols should therefore be one of targeted surveillance in patients with known risk factors or high degrees of clinical suspicion. At our institution, this includes all patients with PSC or IBD who develop the sudden onset of pruritis, jaundice, rapid weight loss, or abnormalities in serum biochemistries. Patients without a mass on imaging or history of a dominant stricture undergo ERCP with brushing of the right and left hepatic ducts, main hepatic duct, and common bile duct. In those with normal cytology, patients are followed at 6-month intervals and re-brushed if they fail to improve, or if otherwise indicated. If cytology harbors evidence of cellular atypia, FISH and DIA are performed. Positive results are referred for transplant. Patients with cellular atypia or indeterminate results otherwise undergo repeat ERCP and follow-up cytology at 6–12 month intervals. The continued presence of cytologic atypia on these exams or its return after an intervening normal cytologic result should prompt the use of adjunctive diagnostic measures (forceps biopsy, cholangioscopy, EUS, etc). Resolution of atypia mandates clinical follow-up only. A patient whose cytological results are viewed as suspicious or dysplastic, in whom FISH/DIA are otherwise negative or equivocal, undergo repeat brushings within 1–3 months of their reference ERCP. Patients with overt evidence of malignancy (adenocarcinoma) are referred for additional staging to determine eligibility for transplant. Like many authors, we do not endorse routine screening of otherwise asymptomatic PSC patients due to the potential for ERCP-induced pancreatitis [34].

Using a similar approach, Wu et al. examined 119 patients with PSC over a 13 year period. In these individuals, 273 ERCPs were performed (2.3 ERCPs per patient). None of the patients with normal cytology went on to develop cholangiocarcinoma. Forty-two (35 %) were found to have abnormal reference cytologies. Of these, three tumors were found at initial evaluation. In five additional patients who originally showed evidence of atypical cells or dysplasia, cholangiocarcinoma was eventually discovered on cytology during

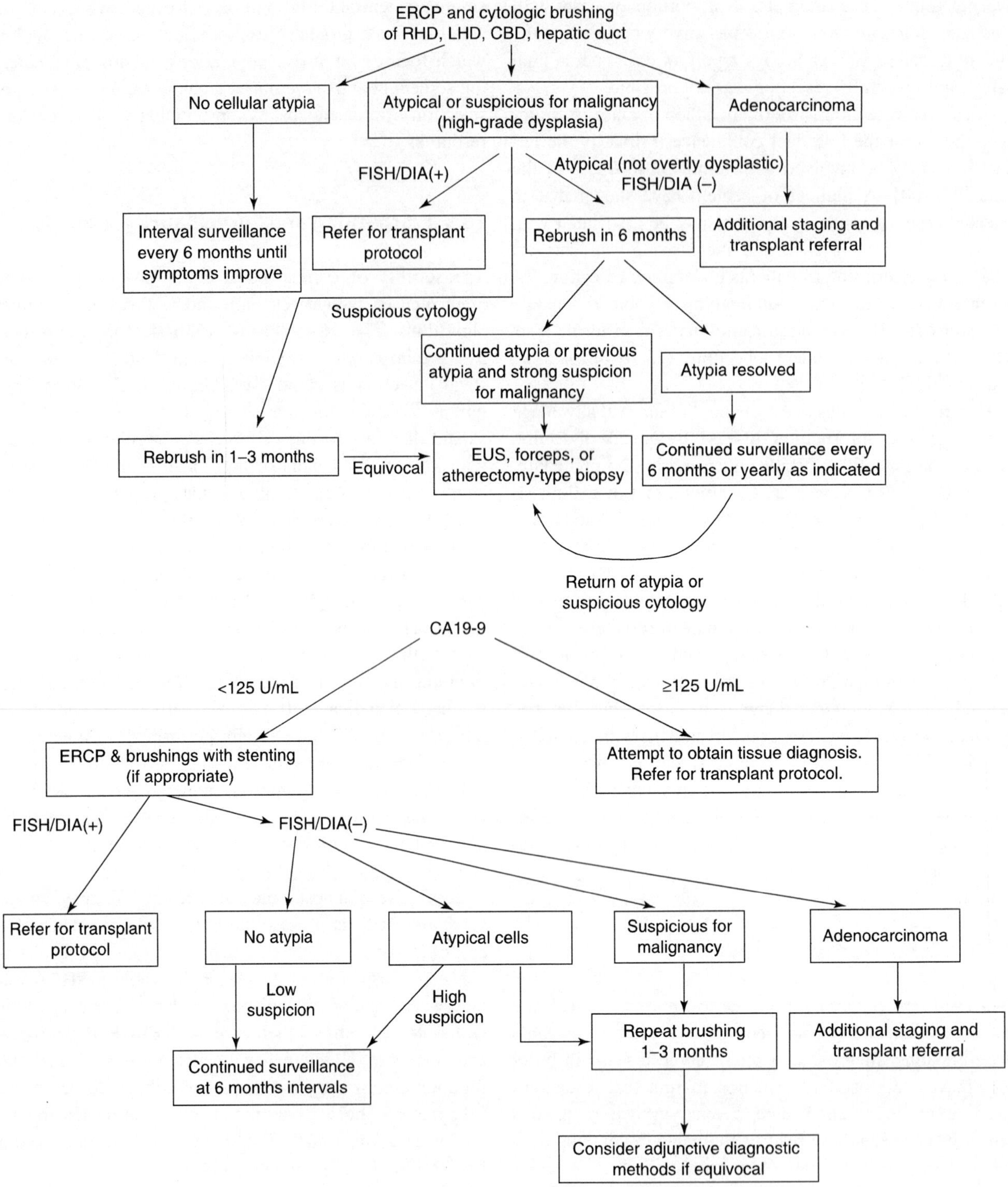

Fig. 16.4 Screening algorithm for cholangiocarcinoma. (**a**) Using ERCP and cytologic brushing as the first screening test. (**b**) Using CA 19-9 as the first screening test. *CA 19-9* Carbohydrate antigen 19-9, *ERCP* endoscopic retrograde cholangiopancreatography, *FISH* fluorescence in situ hybridization, *DIA* digital image analysis, *RHD* right hepatic duct, *LHD* left hepatic duct, *CBD* common bile duct, *EUS* endoscopic ultrasound

subsequent exams. Despite multiple ERCPs, no episodes of pancreatitis or cholangitis were reported to occur [61].

In the setting of a known dominant stricture or mass lesion, CA 19-9 levels should be examined at least semiannually. In this scenario, PSC or IBD patients with elevated CA 19-9 levels are candidates for additional staging and transplant referral [34, 106, 107]. Under these conditions, a confirmatory tissue diagnosis should be sought, but an equivocal result, particularly in the presence of a suspicious mass, does not automatically preclude transplant eligibility. Sudden clinical deterioration in a PSC patient with a high-grade stricture and equivocal CA 19-9 levels is ominous and should trigger an aggressive search for malignancy. Initial maneuvers should include conventional brush cytology, FISH/DIA, forceps biopsy, EUS, EUS-guided FNA, and an atherectomy approach and/or rendezvous procedure if first-line attempts fail. Urgent follow-up is warranted in 1–3 months if a tissue diagnosis cannot be established by a combination of these techniques.

16.5.2 Staging and Selection of Patients for Transplant

All in all, diagnosis and staging should be undertaken using a multimodality approach that includes clinical appraisal, laboratory analysis, as well as radiologic and pathologic assessment [36]. In this context, it is important to remember that an indisputable tissue diagnosis is not always possible. In these cases, diagnosis can be corroborated by a combination of radiographic and serological testing in patients deemed to be at high risk. Our selection criteria for protocol enrollment mirrors that employed by the Mayo Clinic and are demonstrated in Table 16.7. Once a diagnosis of cholangiocarcinoma has been entertained, cross-sectional imaging of the liver and hilar region should be performed, if not done already, preferably with MRI/MRCP. Those with hilar lesions should be evaluated by an experienced hepatobiliary surgeon for the purpose of determining resectability, which should take precedence over transplant referral if technically feasible. Cross-sectional imaging is also performed to establish tumor size and relationship to adjacent structures. Mass lesions below the cystic duct should negatively impact the decision to proceed with transplant. An exception to these guidelines ensues in the case of PSC patients with disease confined to the extrahepatic bile duct who otherwise do not exceed staging criteria. In these individuals, the entire biliary tree should be viewed as tissue at risk for malignant transformation. As well, many will not tolerate extensive hepatic resection as a result of intrinsic liver disease. Because of the difficulty in determining submucosal spread of tumor, its longitudinal extent along a duct does not influence suitability for transplant [108]. However, due to the negative prognostic influence of larger primary tumors, their propensity for lymphatic invasion, and their predilection to grow along neighboring bile duct walls, eligibility for protocol enrollment is predicated on a radial tumor diameter which does not exceed 3 cm on cross-sectional imaging [109–111]. Vascular encasement, per se, does not necessarily disqualify a patient. Alternatively, the failure to visualize a major branch of the portal vein on contrast-enhanced MR venography or comparable imaging study raises the specter of vascular invasion and should obviate further consideration of transplantation.

Table 16.7 Inclusion criteria for transplant protocol

Diagnosis of cholangiocarcinoma by brush cytology, endoscopic forceps biopsy, EUS-guided FNA, or atherectomy-type biopsy
Above cystic duct and unresectable by conventional surgical techniques (unless arising in setting of PSC)
CA 19-9 ≥125 U/ml with dominant stricture and/or mass on cross-sectional imaging
Stricture and FISH polysomy or FISH trisomy (7 or 3)
DIA greater than 1.89 in isolation (FISH negative, routine cytology negative)
FISH polysomy in absence of malignant stricture
Tumor unresectable by conventional techniques
Radial tumor diameter ≤3 cm
No medical contraindications to liver transplantation

Abbreviations: *CA 19-9* carbohydrate antigen 19-9, *DIA* digital image analysis, *FISH* fluorescence in-situ hybridization, *PSC* primary sclerosing cholangitis

Transplantation is not contemplated in patients with prior attempts at resection or in situations where transperitoneal biopsy has been pursued because in most cases, these practices favor peritoneal dissemination of tumor. Prior administration of chemotherapy, external beam radiation therapy, or brachytherapy is also discouraged in the absence of appropriate staging and diagnostic work-up. Patients with gallbladder cancer are excluded due to a tumor predilection to recur at distant sites [13] and due the lack of proven efficacy of chemoradiation. Transplant is similarly avoided in those harboring peripheral (non-hilar) or intra-hepatic cholangiocarcinomas (ICC) owing to rapid recurrence in these individuals [10, 108]. The largest series examining outcomes in this group was reported by the European Transplant Registry, which reported only a 29 % 5-year survival [33, 112]. Patients with combined features of ICC and hepatocellular carcinoma deserve special mention. These tumors have a propensity to infiltrate the portal venous system and share features of cholangiocarcinoma due to their predilection for regional lymph node metastasis [113, 114]. Limited data exists on the outcome after transplant. Existing series of 1–3 patients do not paint an optimistic picture despite patients remaining within Milan criteria [114–116]. As such, surgical resection with hilar lymph node dissection should be considered the most appropriate treatment for the combined variant in the absence of overt cirrhosis, with transplant being reserved for small lesions only, or in cases of hepatic decompensation [114, 117, 118].

Extrahepatic disease is an absolute contraindication to transplantation and should merit consideration for palliative treatment. Resultantly, an aggressive search for metastatic cholangiocarcinoma is required. This can take the form of cross-sectional imaging of the chest, abdomen, or pelvis (CT or MRI) in conjunction with bone scan. More recently, the authors have incorporated ^{18}F-fluorodeoxyglucose positron emission tomography (^{18}F-FDG-PET) scanning into their staging algorithm based on reports which suggest they may offer an additional degree of sensitivity in depicting extrahepatic disease [119–123]. We have introduced this prior to neoadjuvant treatment to help exclude patients with metastatic disease who may progress while on treatment.

16.5.2.1 Role of Staging Laparotomy

A major consideration is the presence of metastatic disease in regional hepatic lymph nodes, which are found in 30–50 % of patients undergoing resection [21, 22, 75, 103]. It is expected that regional lymph node involvement contributes to local as well as distant treatment failures. All in all, patients with regional lymph node positivity do poorly in the context of transplantation [13]. As such, transplant protocols have evolved to include formal operative staging. Once neoadjuvant therapy is complete, patients undergo thorough operative staging to ascertain the presence of N2 nodal disease (celiac, periduodenal, superior mesenteric nodal basins). A formal sampling of the nodes along the common hepatic artery and hepatoduodenal ligament is thus undertaken. Evidence of gross or microscopic disease at the N2 level is a harbinger of distant recurrence and is considered a contraindication to transplant. In most cases, N1 disease (cystic and pericholedochal nodes) can be extirpated during transplant hepatectomy, but their presence portends a high risk of localized recurrence following transplant. A thorough abdominal exploration should also ensue. Specific attention is afforded to periduodenal and superior mesenteric nodal basins to rule out gross disease. The liver is inspected for the presence of intrahepatic metastases and caudate involvement. Examination of peritoneal surfaces is conducted to rule out the presence of tumoral dissemination within the coelomic cavity, a task well-suited to the laparoscope.

In regions where the interval from completion of neoadjuvant therapy to transplant is protracted (>100 days), the ideal timing for staging is a matter of debate. In these instances, it may be advantageous to delay the staging procedure until the time when transplant is imminent or during the actual transplant procedure itself (prior to hepatectomy). In the setting of nodal or extrahepatic disease, the procedure should be aborted and the donor liver re-allocated. Where living donors have been identified, the staging operation is conducted 1–3 days prior to transplant.

Table 16.8 Exclusion criteria for cholangiocarcinomas

Tumor resectable by conventional approaches
Medically unfit for transplant
Prior surgical resection or transperitoneal biopsy
Extrahepatic disease on metastatic work up
Regional lymph nodes positive for metastases on EUS or staging laparotomy
Evidence of intrahepatic spread
Prior administration of chemotherapy and /or radiation
Gallbladder cancer
Combined cholangiocarcinoma/hepatocellular carcinoma variants
Tumor size ≥3 cm on cross-sectional imaging or growth while on neoadjuvant protocol

On the whole, 20–25 % of patients are excluded due to findings wrought by the staging operation [13]. With the advent of EUS-guided FNA, regional lymph nodes can be sampled and a formal staging laparotomy avoided if nodes are positive. In a report by Gleeson et al., 70 lymph nodes in 47 patients with unresectable cholangiocarcinoma were sampled. Nine malignant nodes were detected in eight patients. In these individuals, no morphologic features predicted metastases [124]. Performed prior to neoadjuvant therapy, patients discovered using this approach are likely to have progressed during neoadjuvant treatment [108]. It is estimated that its introduction into transplant protocols prior to neoadjuvant therapy can decrease the likelihood of positive staging laparotomies by 50 % [11]. A full list of exclusion criteria can be found in Table 16.8.

16.5.2.2 Role of Positron Emission Tomography

Aside from regional lymph node infiltration, factors associated with adverse tumor biology include perineural invasion and high-grade differentiation, amongst others [104]. Unfortunately, these characteristics are not appreciated using conventional staging methodologies and are only discovered on explant. It is reasonable to assume that patient selection can further be enhanced in cases where negative prognostic indicators are known prior to transplant. In addition to its ability to foretell the existence of extrahepatic disease, PET scanning has recently been used as a tool to predict biological tumor behavior and outcome after transplantation. In a study by Kornberg et al., 13 patients with Type IV Klatskin tumors (unresectable, bilobar involvement) were examined using PET and findings correlated with histopathologic tumor characteristics and patient outcome after transplantation. Eight patients were PET-avid prior to transplant. Allograft dysfunction resulted in one patient death. All seven of the remaining PET-avid patients developed tumor recurrence. In these cases, PET-avidity was positively correlated with perineural invasion and had a positive predictive value of 89 % [125]. Conversely, all PET (−) patients were tumor-free and alive at a median of 76 months following transplant. The authors concluded that patients with non-PET-avid cholangiocarcinoma are more likely to achieve recurrence-free long-term survival [125]. It seems defensible, as the authors suggest, that a switch from PET (−) status to one of PET-avidity during the course of neoadjuvant therapy may represent a shift in biological tumor behavior from a less aggressive to more aggressive phenotype, thereby disqualifying a patient from subsequent transplant [125]. This notion awaits prospective confirmation, however.

16.5.2.3 A Therapeutic Dilemma

Due to the difficulty in evaluating longitudinal extent of disease, evidence of malignancy below the cystic duct in a PSC patient represents a therapeutic dilemma. This is compounded by evidence which suggests that cholangiocarcinoma in PSC may be distributed widely, surfacing in multiple areas of dysplasia simultaneously [34, 61, 126]. As a consequence, up to 15 % of PSC patients have been found to have a positive distal bile duct margin at hepatectomy [11]. Surgeons must therefore be prepared for this contingency. Accordingly, it is our practice to perform pancreaticoduodenectomy in conjunction with liver transplantation in a stable recipient if the distal bile duct margin is positive by frozen section. Often times, definite confirmation will await permanent tissue fixation. In such cases, completion pancreaticoduodenectomy can be performed during the index hospitalization to effect an R0 resection. In patients with early stage disease undergoing surveillance and neoadjuvant therapy, this approach has been validated with respect to safety and efficacy. In a recent update of the Mayo series, ten concomitant pancreaticoduodenectomies have been performed since 1993. In seven cases, microscopic disease was noted at the time of hepatectomy. Five patients remained alive 1–9 years after transplantation. Two died secondary to arterial complications [11]. These results have been authenticated in a similar group of PSC patients undergoing regular surveillance. Wu and colleagues performed combined Whipple-transplant, which entailed *en bloc* total hepatectomy-pancreaticoduodenectomy in six patients [61]. All patients received combined external beam and brachytherapy. Operative time ranged from 6 to 7 h. Mean intraoperative blood loss was 3.5 units (range 0–13 units). Median post-operative length of stay was 21 days (range 16–138 days). Morbidity included two intra-abdominal infections and a pancreatic leak requiring revision. One patient developed a pancreatic duct stricture proximal to the pancreaticojejunostomy 22 months following Whipple secondary to chronic pancreatitis. There was one episode of chronic renal failure secondary to transplant immunosuppression requiring kidney transplantation 44 months following the combined procedure [61]. One patient died 55 months post-transplant from a non-tumor, unrelated cause. Upon publication, five were well at 5.7, 7.0, 8.7, 8.8, and 10.1 years following transplant. All had returned to full-time employment without evidence of tumor recurrence [61]. For patients enrolled in suitable staging and neoadjuvant protocols, these results support the concept of combining hepatectomy and pancreaticoduodenectomy, followed by orthotopic liver transplantation, in patients with early stage hilar disease. Extirpation of the entire biliary system appears to be well-tolerated and offers long-term tumor-free survival with acceptable rates of morbidity and mortality.

16.6 Resection or Transplantation for Cholangiocarcinoma?

While cholangiocarcinoma remains a surgical disease, treatment and diagnosis must be integrated using a multimodality approach to care. Along these lines, it is clear that favorable outcomes after resection or transplant are dependent on a combination of early detection, appropriate staging, and in the case of transplant, neoadjuvant chemoradiation. In arriving at a diagnosis and treatment plan, it is oftentimes necessary to assimilate information from a wide array of sources. From an institutional perspective, this mandates a full complement of interested pathologists, diagnostic radiologists, medical oncologist, interventional radiologists, endoscopists, radiation oncologists, and hepatologists. Impacting this disease at a treatable stage requires the adherence to targeted surveillance protocols. These algorithms should be developed using multidisciplinary input and may be institution-dependent. However, they should reflect the current state of knowledge regarding screening in at-risk populations. In cases where disease is resectable, recent improvements in outcomes following extended bile duct resection and partial hepatectomy have relied on strict adherence to resection criteria. Similarly, the improvement in transplant outcomes for unresectable hilar disease has been predicated on patient selection and stringent observance of staging and neoadjuvant protocols.

The decision of whether to resect or transplant should be guided by a surgeon or team experienced in performing both complex hepatobiliary resections and liver transplantation, so that bias in choosing between the two curative options is minimized. Identifying patients who should undergo liver transplantation should be the first priority. These include those with end stage liver disease (ESLD), or any one of the following: Childs-Pugh B or C functional status, cirrhosis, or portal hypertension. These individuals are not candidates for liver resection and should be considered for transplantation [75]. Patients with underlying liver disease approaching end stage or with risk factors for the development of cholangiocarcinoma (i.e., primary sclerosing cholangitis) should also be considered for transplantation due to the risk of hepatic decompensation or recurrence in the remnant liver [14].

Patients with MSKCC T3 or AJCC 2010 T4N0 lesions representing unresectable local disease should also be considered for transplantation. However, these patients must be carefully evaluated for nodal disease, a contraindication to transplantation. It is estimated that 13 % of transplant, and 25 % of resection candidates harbor such disease [14]. The remaining group of patients with hilar cholangiocarcinoma represents the majority of individuals, all of which should be considered for curative resection [127–129]. It is rarely possible to switch strategies mid-course as the reasons that preclude resection also preclude transplantation. These reasons include: (1) discovery of nodal, liver, or distant metastases, (2) involvement of neighboring structures, or (3) failed attempt at resection which, in many cases, upstages tumor due to disruption of lymphatic drainage patterns and intraperitoneal tumor dissemination [14].

The largest study to date comparing liver transplantation to resection from the Mayo Clinic did so in a retrospective, case-controlled fashion. With the intention of preventing local recurrence and intraoperative tumor dissemination, patients in this series underwent neoadjuvant chemoradiation prior to liver transplantation. One, 3- and 5-year survival rates for transplant were 92 %, 82 %, and 82 %, versus 82 %, 48 %, and 21 % for resection. In this fashion, liver transplantation with neoadjuvant chemoradiation offered improved survival over resection ($P=0.022$). In this study however, contrasts between the two groups are problematic and confounded by the lack of neoadjuvant therapy in the resection group, the younger age of transplant recipients, and the fact that all transplant patients R0 resection in the setting of node negative disease. With a higher rate of PSC in the transplant group, a potential selection bias can be entertained [14, 15]. However, transplantation in the setting of *de novo* cholangiocarcinoma improved survival as well. The meticulous selection process has also been implicated in the promising results observed in the Mayo series, where 38 of 71 patients entering the neoadjuvant protocol eventually underwent transplant. However, nine patients died before staging due to complications of therapy and ten additional patients were awaiting transplant at the time of the report, making this position difficult to endorse. In transplanted cases, the hepatectomy specimen failed to identify residual disease in 16 of 38 explants, perhaps inferring favorable outcomes were merely a reflection of strict inclusion criteria favoring less aggressive disease [14, 15].

These concerns are justified, but other reports tend to corroborate the Mayo data [3, 12, 15, 130–132]. Currently reported 1-, 3, and 5- year patient survival rates are 84 %, 67 %, 56 % after the start of therapy (n = 167) and 96, 83, and 72 % (n = 111) in patients undergoing transplant [11]. In examining the characteristics which predict recurrence, the Mayo group identified the following: (1) a discreet mass seen on pre-transplant imaging, (2) residual tumor >2 cm at explantation, (3) tumor grade and perineural invasion in the explanted tumor, (4) increased patient age, (5) CA 19-9 > 100 at the time of transplant (but not at enrollment), and prior cholecystectomy. Additionally, an increasing interval from enrollment to transplant (>100 days) was suggestive of a higher recurrence rate [104]. A thorough accounting of these factors is recommended when an individual's transplant candidacy is under consideration.

Despite the limitations of the Mayo series, these data are persuasive. It is not yet clear, however, whether this approach is warranted in patients with resectable disease. Lacking evidence, a transplant-based approach in this setting is difficult to defend. In the future, this may change with improvements in chemoradiotherapeutics. At the present time, however, resection should remain the primary consideration for patients presenting with hilar cholangiocarcinoma, and transplantation reserved for patients with ESLD, PSC, or locally unresectable disease.

References

1. Abu-Elmagd KM, Malinchoc M, Dickson ER, et al. Efficacy of hepatic transplantation in patients with primary sclerosing cholangitis. Surg Gynecol Obstet. 1993;177:335–44.
2. Ahrendt SA, Pitt HA, Nakeeb A, et al. Diagnosis and management of cholangiocarcinoma in primary sclerosing cholangitis. J Gastrointest Surg. 1999;3:357–67; discussion 67–8.
3. Becker NS, Rodriguez JA, Barshes NR, et al. Outcomes analysis for 280 patients with cholangiocarcinoma treated with liver transplantation over an 18-year period. J Gastrointest Surg. 2008;12:117–22.
4. Brandsaeter B, Isoniemi H, Broome U, et al. Liver transplantation for primary sclerosing cholangitis; predictors and consequences of hepatobiliary malignancy. J Hepatol. 2004;40:815–22.
5. Ghali P, Marotta PJ, Yoshida EM, et al. Liver transplantation for incidental cholangiocarcinoma: analysis of the Canadian experience. Liver Transpl. 2005;11:1412–6.
6. Goldstein RM, Stone M, Tillery GW, et al. Is liver transplantation indicated for cholangiocarcinoma? Am J Surg. 1993;166:768–71; discussion 71–2.
7. Goss JA, Shackleton CR, Farmer DG, et al. Orthotopic liver transplantation for primary sclerosing cholangitis. A 12-year single center experience. Ann Surg. 1997;225:472–81; discussion 81–3.
8. Iwatsuki S, Todo S, Marsh JW, et al. Treatment of hilar cholangiocarcinoma (Klatskin tumors) with hepatic resection or transplantation. J Am Coll Surg. 1998;187:358–64.
9. Lindner P, Norrby J, Olausson M, et al. Survival after liver transplantation for cholangiocarcinoma has increased during the last decade. Transplant Proc. 2003;35:811–2.
10. Meyer CG, Penn I, James L. Liver transplantation for cholangiocarcinoma: results in 207 patients. Transplantation. 2000;69:1633–7.
11. Rea DJ, Rosen CB, Nagorney DM, et al. Transplantation for cholangiocarcinoma: when and for whom? Surg Oncol Clin N Am. 2009;18:325–37, ix.
12. Robles R, Figueras J, Turrion VS, et al. Spanish experience in liver transplantation for hilar and peripheral cholangiocarcinoma. Ann Surg. 2004;239:265–71.
13. Heimbach JK, Gores GJ, Nagorney DM, et al. Liver transplantation for perihilar cholangiocarcinoma after aggressive neoadjuvant therapy: a new paradigm for liver and biliary malignancies? Surgery. 2006;140:331–4.

14. Rea DJ, Heimbach JK, Rosen CB, et al. Liver transplantation with neoadjuvant chemoradiation is more effective than resection for hilar cholangiocarcinoma. Ann Surg. 2005;242:451–8.
15. Schwartz JJ, Hutson WR, Gayowski TJ, et al. Liver transplantation for cholangiocarcinoma. Transplantation. 2009;88:295–8.
16. Bismuth H, Corlette MB. Intrahepatic cholangioenteric anastomosis in carcinoma of the hilus of the liver. Surg Gynecol Obstet. 1975;140:170–8.
17. Bismuth H, Nakache R, Diamond T. Management strategies in resection for hilar cholangiocarcinoma. Ann Surg. 1992;215:31–8.
18. Chen XP, Lau WY, Huang ZY, et al. Extent of liver resection for hilar cholangiocarcinoma. Br J Surg. 2009;96:1167–75.
19. Dinant S, Gerhards MF, Busch OR, et al. The importance of complete excision of the caudate lobe in resection of hilar cholangiocarcinoma. HPB (Oxford). 2005;7:263–7.
20. Hirano S, Kondo S, Tanaka E, et al. No-touch resection of hilar malignancies with right hepatectomy and routine portal reconstruction. J Hepatobiliary Pancreat Surg. 2009;16:502–7.
21. Ito F, Agni R, Rettammel RJ, et al. Resection of hilar cholangiocarcinoma: concomitant liver resection decreases hepatic recurrence. Ann Surg. 2008;248:273–9.
22. Ito F, Cho CS, Rikkers LF, et al. Hilar cholangiocarcinoma: current management. Ann Surg. 2009;250:210–8.
23. Jarnagin WR, Shoup M. Surgical management of cholangiocarcinoma. Semin Liver Dis. 2004;24:189–99.
24. Hemming AW, Magliocca JF, Fujita S, et al. Combined resection of the liver and pancreas for malignancy. J Am Coll Surg. 2010; 210:808–16.
25. Bergquist A, Glaumann H, Persson B, et al. Risk factors and clinical presentation of hepatobiliary carcinoma in patients with primary sclerosing cholangitis: a case-control study. Hepatology. 1998;27:311–6.
26. Broome U, Olsson R, Loof L, et al. Natural history and prognostic factors in 305 Swedish patients with primary sclerosing cholangitis. Gut. 1996;38:610–5.
27. Farges O, Malassagne B, Sebagh M, et al. Primary sclerosing cholangitis: liver transplantation or biliary surgery. Surgery. 1995;117:146–55.
28. Ramage JK, Donaghy A, Farrant JM, et al. Serum tumor markers for the diagnosis of cholangiocarcinoma in primary sclerosing cholangitis. Gastroenterology. 1995;108:865–9.
29. Rosen CB, Nagorney DM, Wiesner RH, et al. Cholangiocarcinoma complicating primary sclerosing cholangitis. Ann Surg. 1991; 213:21–5.
30. Marsh Jr JW, Iwatsuki S, Makowka L, et al. Orthotopic liver transplantation for primary sclerosing cholangitis. Ann Surg. 1988;207:21–5.
31. Mahadevan U, Bass N. Sclerosing cholangitis and recurrent pyogenic cholangitis. In: Feldman M, Friedman LS, Scleisenger MH, editors. Gastrointestinal and liver disease: pathophysiology diagnosis management. Philadelphia: Saunders; 2003. p. 1131.
32. Erichsen R, Jepsen P, Vilstrup H, et al. Incidence and prognosis of cholangiocarcinoma in Danish patients with and without inflammatory bowel disease: a national cohort study, 1978—2003. Eur J Epidemiol. 2009;24:513–20.
33. Singal A, Welling TH, Marrero JA. Role of liver transplantation in the treatment of cholangiocarcinoma. Expert Rev Anticancer Ther. 2009;9:491–502.
34. Malhi H, Gores GJ. Cholangiocarcinoma: modern advances in understanding a deadly old disease. J Hepatol. 2006;45:856–67.
35. Patel AH, Harnois DM, Klee GG, et al. The utility of CA 19-9 in the diagnoses of cholangiocarcinoma in patients without primary sclerosing cholangitis. Am J Gastroenterol. 2000;95:204–7.
36. Petrowsky H, Hong JC. Current surgical management of hilar and intrahepatic cholangiocarcinoma: the role of resection and orthotopic liver transplantation. Transplant Proc. 2009;41:4023–35.
37. Vestergaard EM, Hein HO, Meyer H, et al. Reference values and biological variation for tumor marker CA 19-9 in serum for different Lewis and secretor genotypes and evaluation of secretor and Lewis genotyping in a Caucasian population. Clin Chem. 1999;45:54–61.
38. Hann LE, Greatrex KV, Bach AM, et al. Cholangiocarcinoma at the hepatic hilus: sonographic findings. AJR Am J Roentgenol. 1997;168:985–9.
39. Okuda K, Ohto M, Tsuchiya Y. The role of ultrasound, percutaneous transhepatic cholangiography, computed tomographic scanning, and magnetic resonance imaging in the preoperative assessment of bile duct cancer. World J Surg. 1988;12:18–26.
40. Manfredi R, Barbaro B, Masselli G, et al. Magnetic resonance imaging of cholangiocarcinoma. Semin Liver Dis. 2004;24:155–64.
41. Yeh TS, Jan YY, Tseng JH, et al. Malignant perihilar biliary obstruction: magnetic resonance cholangiopancreatographic findings. Am J Gastroenterol. 2000;95:432–40.
42. Zhang Y, Uchida M, Abe T, et al. Intrahepatic peripheral cholangiocarcinoma: comparison of dynamic CT and dynamic MRI. J Comput Assist Tomogr. 1999;23:670–7.
43. Peterson MS, Murakami T, Baron RL. MR imaging patterns of gadolinium retention within liver neoplasms. Abdom Imaging. 1998;23:592–9.
44. Lee MG, Park KB, Shin YM, et al. Preoperative evaluation of hilar cholangiocarcinoma with contrast-enhanced three-dimensional fast imaging with steady-state precession magnetic resonance angiography: comparison with intraarterial digital subtraction angiography. World J Surg. 2003;27:278–83.
45. Kim JY, Kim MH, Lee TY, et al. Clinical role of 18F-FDG PET-CT in suspected and potentially operable cholangiocarcinoma: a prospective study compared with conventional imaging. Am J Gastroenterol. 2008;103:1145–51.
46. Petrowsky H, Wildbrett P, Husarik DB, et al. Impact of integrated positron emission tomography and computed tomography on staging and management of gallbladder cancer and cholangiocarcinoma. J Hepatol. 2006;45:43–50.
47. Henke AC, Jensen CS, Cohen MB. Cytologic diagnosis of adenocarcinoma in biliary and pancreatic duct brushings. Adv Anat Pathol. 2002;9:301–8.
48. Layfield LJ, Wax TD, Lee JG, et al. Accuracy and morphologic aspects of pancreatic and biliary duct brushings. Acta Cytol. 1995;39:11–8.
49. de Bellis M, Sherman S, Fogel EL, et al. Tissue sampling at ERCP in suspected malignant biliary strictures (part 2). Gastrointest Endosc. 2002;56:720–30.
50. Cohen MB, Wittchow RJ, Johlin FC, et al. Brush cytology of the extrahepatic biliary tract: comparison of cytologic features of adenocarcinoma and benign biliary strictures. Mod Pathol. 1995;8:498–502.
51. Gupta DK, Komaromy-Hiller G, Raab SS, et al. Interobserver and intraobserver variability in the cytologic diagnosis of normal and abnormal metaplastic squamous cells in pap smears. Acta Cytol. 2001;45:697–703.
52. Hahm GK, Niemann TH, Lucas JG, et al. The value of second opinion in gastrointestinal and liver pathology. Arch Pathol Lab Med. 2001;125:736–9.
53. Logrono R, Waxman I. Interactive role of the cytopathologist in EUS-guided fine needle aspiration: an efficient approach. Gastrointest Endosc. 2001;54:485–90.
54. Lin A, Jonnalagadda S, Edmundowicz S. Diagnosis of malignant biliary strictures. Tech Gastrointest Endosc. 2002;4:102–12.
55. Harewood GC, Baron TH, Stadheim LM, et al. Prospective, blinded assessment of factors influencing the accuracy of biliary cytology interpretation. Am J Gastroenterol. 2004;99:1464–9.
56. Rabinovitz M, Zajko AB, Hassanein T, et al. Diagnostic value of brush cytology in the diagnosis of bile duct carcinoma: a study in 65 patients with bile duct strictures. Hepatology. 1990;12:747–52.
57. Glasbrenner B, Ardan M, Boeck W, et al. Prospective evaluation of brush cytology of biliary strictures during endoscopic retrograde cholangiopancreatography. Endoscopy. 1999;31:712–7.

58. Ailwala J, Fogel EL, Sherman S, et al. Triple-tissue sampling at ERCP in malignant biliary obstruction. Gastrointest Endosc. 2000;51:383–90.
59. Lindberg B, Arnelo U, Bergquist A, et al. Diagnosis of biliary strictures in conjunction with endoscopic retrograde cholangiopancreaticography, with special reference to patients with primary sclerosing cholangitis. Endoscopy. 2002;34:909–16.
60. Lal A, Okonkwo A, Schindler S, et al. Role of biliary brush cytology in primary sclerosing cholangitis. Acta Cytol. 2004;48:9–12.
61. Wu Y, Johlin FC, Rayhill SC, et al. Long-term, tumor-free survival after radiotherapy combining hepatectomy-Whipple en bloc and orthotopic liver transplantation for early-stage hilar cholangiocarcinoma. Liver Transpl. 2008;14:279–86.
62. Moreno Luna LE, Kipp B, Halling KC, et al. Advanced cytologic techniques for the detection of malignant pancreatobiliary strictures. Gastroenterology. 2006;131:1064–72.
63. Muralikrishna P, Madhu K, Aditya A, et al. Peroral cholangioscopy: new approach with a balloon enteroscope. Endoscopy. 2008;40 Suppl 2Suppl 2:E234.
64. Choi HJ, Moon JH, Ko BM, et al. Overtube-balloon-assisted direct peroral cholangioscopy by using an ultra-slim upper endoscope (with videos). Gastrointest Endosc. 2009;69:935–40.
65. El Fouly A, Dechene A, Gerken G. Surveillance and screening of primary sclerosing cholangitis. Dig Dis. 2009;27:526–35.
66. Igarashi Y, Okano N, Ito K, et al. Effectiveness of peroral cholangioscopy and narrow band imaging for endoscopically diagnosing the bile duct cancer. Dig Endosc. 2009;21 Suppl 1Suppl 1:S101–2.
67. Petersen BT. Cholangioscopy for special applications: primary sclerosing cholangitis, liver transplant, and selective duct access. Gastrointest Endosc Clin N Am. 2009;19:579–86.
68. Chang KJ. State of the art lecture: endoscopic ultrasound (EUS) and FNA in pancreatico-biliary tumors. Endoscopy. 2006;38 Suppl 1Suppl 1:S56–60.
69. DeWitt J, Misra VL, Leblanc JK, et al. EUS-guided FNA of proximal biliary strictures after negative ERCP brush cytology results. Gastrointest Endosc. 2006;64:325–33.
70. Kaufman D, Widlus D, Lazinger M, et al. Diagnostic accuracy of Simpson atherectomy catheter biopsy in detecting pancreaticobiliary malignancy. Am J Gastroenterol. 2001;96:1054–8.
71. Tsukui D, Yano T, Nakazawa K, et al. Rendezvous technique combining double-balloon endoscopy with percutaneous cholangioscopy is useful for the treatment of biliary anastomotic obstruction after liver transplantation (with video). Gastrointest Endosc. 2008;68:1013–5.
72. Kim YS, Gupta K, Mallery S, et al. Endoscopic ultrasound rendezvous for bile duct access using a transduodenal approach: cumulative experience at a single center. A case series. Endoscopy. 2010;42:496–502.
73. Lee TH, Park SH, Lee SH, et al. Modified rendezvous intrahepatic bile duct cannulation technique to pass a PTBD catheter in ERCP. World J Gastroenterol. 2010;16:5388–90.
74. Weinbren K, Mutum SS. Pathological aspects of cholangiocarcinoma. J Pathol. 1983;139:217–38.
75. Jarnagin WR, Fong Y, DeMatteo RP, et al. Staging, resectability, and outcome in 225 patients with hilar cholangiocarcinoma. Ann Surg. 2001;234:507–17.
76. Parikh AA, Abdalla EK, Vauthey JN. Operative considerations in resection of hilar cholangiocarcinoma. HPB (Oxford). 2005;7:254–8.
77. Edge S, Byrd DR, Compton CC, et al. Perihilar bile ducts. In: Edge S, Byrd DR, Compton CC, editors. AJCC cancer staging handbook. New York: Springer; 2010. p. 263–9.
78. Paik KY, Choi DW, Chung JC, et al. Improved survival following right trisectionectomy with caudate lobectomy without operative mortality: surgical treatment for hilar cholangiocarcinoma. J Gastrointest Surg. 2008;12:1268–74.
79. Miyazaki M, Kimura F, Shimizu H, et al. One hundred seven consecutive surgical resections for hilar cholangiocarcinoma of Bismuth types II, III, IV between 2001 and 2008. J Hepatobiliary Pancreat Sci. 2010;17:470–5.
80. Shi Z, Yang MZ, He QL, et al. Addition of hepatectomy decreases liver recurrence and leads to long survival in hilar cholangiocarcinoma. World J Gastroenterol. 2009;15:1892–6.
81. Sotiropoulos GC, Lang H, Molmenti EP, et al. Partial or complete mesohepatectomy combined with resection of the hilar bifurcation in cases of Klatskin tumors: a reasonable strategy? Am J Surg. 2009;198:297–8.
82. Unno M, Katayose Y, Rikiyama T, et al. Major hepatectomy for perihilar cholangiocarcinoma. J Hepatobiliary Pancreat Sci. 2010; 17:463–9.
83. Nguyen KT, Steel J, Vanounou T, et al. Initial presentation and management of hilar and peripheral cholangiocarcinoma: is a node-positive status or potential margin-positive result a contraindication to resection? Ann Surg Oncol. 2009;16:3308–15.
84. Neuhaus P, Jonas S, Bechstein WO, et al. Extended resections for hilar cholangiocarcinoma. Ann Surg. 1999;230:808–18.
85. Miyazaki M, Ito H, Nakagawa K, et al. Aggressive surgical approaches to hilar cholangiocarcinoma: hepatic or local resection? Surgery. 1998;123:131–6.
86. Hemming AW, Reed AI, Howard RJ, et al. Preoperative portal vein embolization for extended hepatectomy. Ann Surg. 2003;237:686–91.
87. McPherson GA, Benjamin IS, Hodgson HJ, et al. Pre-operative percutaneous transhepatic biliary drainage: the results of a controlled trial. Br J Surg. 1984;71:371–5.
88. Hatfield AR, Tobias R, Terblanche J, et al. Preoperative external biliary drainage in obstructive jaundice. A prospective controlled clinical trial. Lancet. 1982;2:896–9.
89. Ebata T, Nagino M, Kamiya J, et al. Hepatectomy with portal vein resection for hilar cholangiocarcinoma: audit of 52 consecutive cases. Ann Surg. 2003;238:720–7.
90. Seyama Y, Kubota K, Sano K, et al. Long-term outcome of extended hemihepatectomy for hilar bile duct cancer with no mortality and high survival rate. Ann Surg. 2003;238:73–83.
91. Belghiti J, Ogata S. Preoperative optimization of the liver for resection in patients with hilar cholangiocarcinoma. HPB (Oxford). 2005;7:252–3.
92. Kim RD, Kim JS, Watanabe G, et al. Liver regeneration and the atrophy-hypertrophy complex. Semin Intervent Radiol. 2008;25: 92–103.
93. Nagino M, Kamiya J, Nishio H, et al. Two hundred forty consecutive portal vein embolizations before extended hepatectomy for biliary cancer: surgical outcome and long-term follow-up. Ann Surg. 2006;243:364–72.
94. Ogata S, Belghiti J, Farges O, et al. Sequential arterial and portal vein embolizations before right hepatectomy in patients with cirrhosis and hepatocellular carcinoma. Br J Surg. 2006:93: 1091–8.
95. Weber SM, DeMatteo RP, Fong Y, et al. Staging laparoscopy in patients with extrahepatic biliary carcinoma. Analysis of 100 patients. Ann Surg. 2002;235:392–9.
96. Connor S, Barron E, Wigmore SJ, et al. The utility of laparoscopic assessment in the preoperative staging of suspected hilar cholangiocarcinoma. J Gastrointest Surg. 2005;9:476–80.
97. Nimura Y, Hayakawa N, Kamiya J, et al. Hepatic segmentectomy with caudate lobe resection for bile duct carcinoma of the hepatic hilus. World J Surg. 1990;14:535–44.
98. Mizumoto R, Kawarada Y, Suzuki H. Surgical treatment of hilar carcinoma of the bile duct. Surg Gynecol Obstet. 1986;162: 153–8.
99. Ogura Y, Mizumoto R, Tabata M, et al. Surgical treatment of carcinoma of the hepatic duct confluence: analysis of 55 resected carcinomas. World J Surg. 1993;17:85–92.
100. Sugiura Y, Nakamura S, Iida S, et al. Extensive resection of the bile ducts combined with liver resection for cancer of the main hepatic duct junction: a cooperative study of the Keio Bile Duct Cancer Study Group. Surgery. 1994;115:445–51.

101. Rea DJ, Munoz-Juarez M, Farnell MB, et al. Major hepatic resection for hilar cholangiocarcinoma: analysis of 46 patients. Arch Surg. 2004;139:514–23.
102. Gazzaniga GM, Filauro M, Bagarolo C, et al. Surgery for hilar cholangiocarcinoma: an Italian experience. J Hepatobiliary Pancreat Surg. 2000;7:122–7.
103. Kitagawa Y, Nagino M, Kamiya J, et al. Lymph node metastasis from hilar cholangiocarcinoma: audit of 110 patients who underwent regional and paraaortic node dissection. Ann Surg. 2001;233:385–92.
104. Heimbach JK, Gores GJ, Haddock MG, et al. Predictors of disease recurrence following neoadjuvant chemoradiotherapy and liver transplantation for unresectable perihilar cholangiocarcinoma. Transplantation. 2006;82:1703–7.
105. Heimbach JK. Successful liver transplantation for hilar cholangiocarcinoma. Curr Opin Gastroenterol. 2008;24:384–8.
106. Nichols JC, Gores GJ, LaRusso NF, et al. Diagnostic role of serum CA 19-9 for cholangiocarcinoma in patients with primary sclerosing cholangitis. Mayo Clin Proc. 1993;68:874–9.
107. Levy C, Lymp J, Angulo P, et al. The value of serum CA 19-9 in predicting cholangiocarcinomas in patients with primary sclerosing cholangitis. Dig Dis Sci. 2005;50:1734–40.
108. Rosen CB, Heimbach JK, Gores GJ. Liver transplantation for cholangiocarcinoma. Transpl Int. 2010;23:692–7.
109. Sasaki A, Aramaki M, Kawano K, et al. Intrahepatic peripheral cholangiocarcinoma: mode of spread and choice of surgical treatment. Br J Surg. 1998;85:1206–9.
110. Sasaki A, Kawano K, Aramaki M, et al. Correlation between tumor size and mode of spread in mass-forming intrahepatic cholangiocarcinoma. Hepatogastroenterology. 2004;51:224–8.
111. Kaseb A, Thomas M, Curley S. Gallbladder and bile duct cancer. In: Hong W, Bast R, Hait W, et al., editors. Holland frei cancer medicine. 8th ed. Beijing: People's Medical Publishing House; 2006.
112. Pascher A, Jonas S, Neuhaus P. Intrahepatic cholangiocarcinoma: indication for transplantation. J Hepatobiliary Pancreat Surg. 2003;10:282–7.
113. Yano Y, Yamamoto J, Kosuge T, et al. Combined hepatocellular and cholangiocarcinoma: a clinicopathologic study of 26 resected cases. Jpn J Clin Oncol. 2003;33:283–7.
114. Maganty K, Levi D, Moon J, et al. Combined hepatocellular carcinoma and intrahepatic cholangiocarcinoma: outcome after liver transplantation. Dig Dis Sci. 2010;55:3597–601.
115. Chan AC, Lo CM, Ng IO, et al. Liver transplantation for combined hepatocellular cholangiocarcinoma. Asian J Surg. 2007;30: 143–6.
116. Kim KH, Lee SG, Park EH, et al. Surgical treatments and prognoses of patients with combined hepatocellular carcinoma and cholangiocarcinoma. Ann Surg Oncol. 2009;16:623–9.
117. Liver Cancer Study Group of Japan. Primary liver cancer in Japan. Clinicopathologic features and results of surgical treatment. Ann Surg. 1990;211:277–87.
118. Maeda T, Adachi E, Kajiyama K, et al. Combined hepatocellular and cholangiocarcinoma: proposed criteria according to cytokeratin expression and analysis of clinicopathologic features. Hum Pathol. 1995;26:956–64.
119. Kato T, Tsukamoto E, Kuge Y, et al. Clinical role of (18)F-FDG PET for initial staging of patients with extrahepatic bile duct cancer. Eur J Nucl Med Mol Imaging. 2002;29:1047–54.
120. Anderson CD, Rice MH, Pinson CW, et al. Fluorodeoxyglucose PET imaging in the evaluation of gallbladder carcinoma and cholangiocarcinoma. J Gastrointest Surg. 2004;8:90–7.
121. Breitenstein S, Apestegui C, Clavien PA. Positron emission tomography (PET) for cholangiocarcinoma. HPB (Oxford). 2008;10:120–1.
122. CorveraCU, BlumgartLH, AkhurstT, etal. 18F-fluorodeoxyglucose positron emission tomography influences management decisions in patients with biliary cancer. J Am Coll Surg. 2008;206:57–65.
123. Seo S, Hatano E, Higashi T, et al. P-glycoprotein expression affects 18F-fluorodeoxyglucose accumulation in hepatocellular carcinoma in vivo and in vitro. Int J Oncol. 2009;34:1303–12.
124. Gleeson FC, Rajan E, Levy MJ, et al. EUS-guided FNA of regional lymph nodes in patients with unresectable hilar cholangiocarcinoma. Gastrointest Endosc. 2008;67:438–43.
125. Kornberg A, Kupper B, Thrum K, et al. Recurrence-free long-term survival after liver transplantation in patients with 18F-FDG non-avid hilar cholangiocarcinoma on PET. Am J Transplant. 2009;9:2631–6.
126. Johlin F, Voight M, Wu Y. Surveillance Cytology (SC) in the detection of asymptomatic progression to cholangiocarcinoma (CCC) in patients with primary sclerosing cholangitis (PSC). Hepatology. 1998;28:393A.
127. De Vreede I, Steers JL, Burch PA, et al. Prolonged disease-free survival after orthotopic liver transplantation plus adjuvant chemoirradiation for cholangiocarcinoma. Liver Transpl. 2000;6:309–16.
128. Heimbach JK, Gores GJ, Haddock MG, et al. Liver transplantation for unresectable perihilar cholangiocarcinoma. Semin Liver Dis. 2004;24:201–7.
129. Hassoun Z, Gores GJ, Rosen CB. Preliminary experience with liver transplantation in selected patients with unresectable hilar cholangiocarcinoma. Surg Oncol Clin N Am. 2002;11:909–21.
130. Sudan D, DeRoover A, Chinnakotla S, et al. Radiochemotherapy and transplantation allow long-term survival for nonresectable hilar cholangiocarcinoma. Am J Transplant. 2002;2:774–9.
131. Klempnauer J, Ridder GJ, von Wasielewski R, et al. Resectional surgery of hilar cholangiocarcinoma: a multivariate analysis of prognostic factors. J Clin Oncol. 1997;15:947–54.
132. American Joint Committee on Cancer. The AJCC Cancer Staging Manual and Handbook. 7th ed. New York: Springer; 2010.
133. Kawasaki S, Imanura H, Kobayaski A, et al. Results of surgical resection for patients with hilar bile duct cancer. Application of extended hepatectomy after biliary drainage and hemihepatic portal vein embolization. Ann Surg. 2003;338:84–92.

Suggested Reading

Dinant S, Gerhards MF, Rauws EA. Improved outcome of resection of hilar cholangiocarcinoma (Klatskin tumor). Ann Surg Oncol. 2006;13:872–80.

Gerhards MF, van Gulik TM, de Wit LT, et al. Evaluation of morbidity and mortality after resection for hilar cholangiocarcinoma—a single center experience. Surgery. 2000;127:395–404.

Hemming AW, Reed AI, Fujita S, et al. Surgical management of hilar cholangiocarcinoma. Ann Surg. 2005;241:693–9.

Jarnagin WR, Bowne W, Klimsgtra DS, et al. Papillary phenotype confers improved survival after resection for hilar cholangiocarcinoma. Ann Surg. 2005;241:703–14.

Kawarada Y, Das BS, Naganuma T, et al. Surgical treatment of hilar bile duct carcinoma: experience with 25 consecutive hepatectomies. J Gastrointest Surg. 2002;6:617–24.

Kosuge T, Yamamot J, Shimada K, et al. Improved surgical results for hilar cholangiocarcinoma with procedures including major hepatic resection. Ann Surg. 1999;230:663–71.

Launois B, Reding R, Lebeau G, et al. Surgery for hilar cholangiocarcinoma: French experience in a collective survey of 552 extrahepatic bile duct cancers. J Hepatobiliary Pancreat Surg. 2000;7:128–34.

Nakeeb A, Pitt HA, Sohn TA, et al. Cholangiocarcinoma. A spectrum of intrahepatic, perihilar, and distal tumors. Ann Surg. 1996;224:463–73.

Seyama Y, Kubota K, Sano K, et al. Long-term outcome of extended hemihepatectomy for hilar bile duct cancer with no mortality and high survival rate. Ann Surg. 2003;238:720–7.

Todoroki T, Kawamoto T, Koike N, et al. Radical resection of hilar bile duct carcinoma and predictors of survival. Br J Surg. 2000;87: 306–13.

History of Surgery in Hilar Cholangiocarcinoma

17

S.H.Y. Lau and W.Y. Lau

17.1 Introduction

In 1965, Dr. Gerald Klatskin reported in the American Journal of Medicine an article "*Adenocarcinoma of the Hepatic Duct at Its Bifurcation Within the Porta Hepatis*" [1]. The purpose of this report by Dr. Klatskin on 13 patients was "to draw attention to the unusual features of adenocarcinomas that arise in the hepatic duct at its bifurcation within the porta hepatis". Thereafter, this tumor is named after him as Klatskin tumor. Actually, tumors of this type have been reported before him [2–7], but the distinctive manifestations of this tumor have not received sufficient emphasis. Dr. Klatskin stated in his paper that "tumors of this type are frequently overlooked during laparotomy …, death in this disease is usually attributable to hepatocellular failure and/or hepatobiliary infection secondary to unrelieved biliary obstruction rather than to massive invasion of the liver by tumor or to extrahepatic metastases, palliative surgery aimed at relieving biliary obstruction may restore the patient to a good state of health for a remarkable long period of time, and such palliation may be achieved by internal drainage of only one of the major intrahepatic bile ducts". Some of these observations are still true even today on these tumors which for one reason or another cannot be resected!

The development of biliary enteric anastomoses has been extensively reviewed and reported by Ahrendt and Pitt [8] and by Braasch [9]. At the time when Dr. Klatskin published this landmark paper, biliary surgery and imaging were both at their embryonic stages. The first cholecystectomy was carried out by Carl Langenbuch in 1882 [10]. The first use of contrast to show the gallbladder in humans as quoted by Braasch [9], was carried out in 1924. The bile ducts were first visualized by injection of contrast into a biliary fistula in 1918 by Reich [11], Mirizzi first reported the use of operative cholangiogram [12]. Frommhold in 1953 introduced intravenous cholangiography which is now rarely used [13] and cannot be used in patients with obstructive jaundice. After the study by Carter and Saypol in 1952, percutaneous transhepatic cholangiography (PTBD) started to become available clinically [14]. PTBD was, however sparingly used because of its serious complications until the introduction of the Chiba or "skinny needle" technique by Okuda et al. in 1975 [15]. The first cannulation of the ampulla of Vater was in 1968 by McCune et al. [16] Oi in 1970 [17] and other Japanese groups, working with instrument manufacturers developed endoscopic retrograde cholangiopancreatogram [9]. Ultrasonography gradually established its foot-hold in the investigation of biliary tract disease in the twentieth century [18].

17.2 Early Attempts of Surgical Treatment

Surgical treatment of hilar cholangiocarcinoma is technically challenging because of the central location of the tumor in the liver hilum and its intimate relationships with adjacent liver parenchyma, the portal vein and its branches, and the hepatic arteries. Furthermore, the diagnosis and the assessment of the extent of local tumor infiltration of hilar cholangiocarcinoma has been a constant challenge to surgeons since the first description of this tumor by Durand-Fardel in 1840 (as quoted by Rershaw in 1922) [2] and its detailed pathological and clinical description by Klatskin in 1965 [1].

The early attempts of surgical treatment of hilar cholangiocarcinoma aimed primarily at palliation, with generally poor long-term survival outcomes. However, the short-term outcomes were rewarding, with relieve of jaundice and its associated pruritus, and prolongation in survival. Moreover, laparotomy was also used to provide an opportunity to diagnose hilar cholangiocarcinoma in patients with obstructive

S.H.Y. Lau, MBChB(CUHK), MRCS(Ed)
Department of Surgery, Queen Elizabeth Hospital, Kowloon, Hong Kong

W.Y. Lau, MD(CUHK), DSc(CUHK), FRCS, FACS, FRACS(Hon) (✉)
Faculty of Medicine, The Chinese University of Hong Kong, Shatin, New Territories, Hong Kong
e-mail: josephlau@cuhk.edu.hk

W.Y. Lau (ed.), *Hilar Cholangiocarcinoma*,
DOI 10.1007/978-94-007-6473-6_17, © Springer Science+Business Media Dordrecht and People's Medical Publishing House 2013

jaundice "by retrograde probing and cholangiography through the common hepatic duct …. and transhepatic cholangiography at the time of surgery" (to avoid the serious complications of bile peritonitis and cholangitis of preoperative percutaneous transhepatic cholangiography) [1].

Klatskin [1], and the surgeons before his time [6, 7] usually drained "only one of the two major hepatic ducts within the liver … by internal drainage via a T tube or vitallium tube threaded through the constricted bifurcation from below, or external drainage via a catheter inserted proximal to the stricture". Surgical stenting of malignant biliary stricture was soon replaced by other less-invasive and safer alternatives. The period of 15 or 20 years from the mid-1970s saw the technical development and maturation of endoscopic biliary procedures [19]. Endoscopic papillotomy, bile duct exploration, biliary stenting and other biliary tract procedures were established. At around the same time, percutaneous transhepatic external/externo-internal/internal biliary drainage procedures were developed. Unfortunately, these stents/tubes often become obstructed by tumor or cause cholangitis as a consequence of the presence of foreign bodies. Although these stents/tubes can be changed, patients often require repeated admissions into hospitals to treat complications and to change the stents/tubes. The alterative to stenting is internal biliary-enteric bypass, which is more invasive than endoscopic/percutaneous stenting but it results in less requirements for subsequent readmission into hospital to deal with complications arising from stenting. The methods and the choice of internal biliary-enteric bypass procedures have been extensively reviewed [8, 9].

17.3 Local Resection of Hilar Cholangiocarcinoma

In the 1910s, surgical management of hilar cholangiocarcinoma gradually evolved from primarily palliative with stenting or internal biliary-enteric bypass to curative resection [20, 21]. Early reports of resection of hilar cholangiocarcinoma typically involved local resections of the bile duct with hepaticojejunostomy [22, 23]. This operation resulted in low R0 resection rates at the expense of significant perioperative morbidity and mortality [24]. In a recent article by Ito et al. [25], the authors concluded after reviewing the medical literatures that R0 resection remains the most effective and only potentially curative therapy for hilar cholangiocarcinoma, and negative resection margins are associated with improved outcomes.

Local excision of the bile duct is not an adequate curative operation for hilar cholangiocarcinoma [26], except perhaps for small papillary Klatskin tumors without bile duct confluence involvement (type 1, Bismuth-Corlette classification) [22] confined to the bile duct wall (Tis and T1, AJCC staging for extrahepatic cholangiocarcinoma [27]). This can be explained by the patterns of spread of cholangiocarcinoma. The mean length of longitudinal spread along the bile duct is 6–10 mm for invasive filtration and 10–20 mm of superficial spread [28]. Therefore, a gross surgical margin of more than 1 cm in the infiltration type and more than 2 cm in the papillary and nodular types is required to achieve a R0 resection [29]. Furthermore, about 75 % of hilar cholangiocarcinoma is associated with perineural invasion (a prognostic factor for poor survival) [30, 31], 80 % has extended into the liver parenchyma [32, 33], 30 % involves the portal vein [32, 33] and around 45 % has metastases to the lymph nodes [29].

A more aggressive surgical approach is required to achieve better long-term survivals for patients with hilar cholangiocarcinoma.

17.4 Local Resection Versus Hepatic Resection for Hilar Cholangiocarcinoma: Operative Safety and Effectiveness

As the pathologic characteristics and the local invasive patterns of hilar cholangiocarcinoma are better understood, it becomes obvious that local excision is inadequate for radical resection of this tumor. Over the past two decades, there has been an increase in the use of hepatic resection to treat hilar cholangiocarcinoma, aiming at a wider resection to cure the disease.

There is little doubt that local resection is safer than liver resection in patients with hilar cholangiocarcinoma [34–36]. In a review article published by Boerema in 1990, perioperative mortality was significantly lower after bile duct resection than after hepatectomy (8 % vs. 15 %) [37]. In 1992, the group from Memorial Sloan-Kettering reported no mortality and 25 % morbidity after local excision compared with 8 and 36 %, respectively, after extended procedures [38]. In 1996, Pichlmayr et al. reported mortality rates of 12.7 % after liver surgery associated with bile duct resection versus 3.3 % after local resection [35]. In the 1990s, surgeons argued that the higher mortality after liver resection was a clear indication that local resection was the operation of choice, even though associated liver resection could improve radicality because long-term benefits were lost in the high operative mortality rates in liver resection [26, 34]. With better patient selection and improvement in perioperative management, postoperative mortalities and morbidities have significantly improved in the past few years [39–43]. In 2000, Launois published a study on the French experience, operative mortality rates were high but similar in patients with and without liver resection (17 % vs. 14 %) [44]. In 2000, Tsao et al. compared the results of surgical treatment in a Japanese center (Nagoya) where liver resection was performed routinely, with those of an American Center (Lahey Clinic) where isolated bile duct resection was

Table 17.1 Association between hepatectomy rate and R0 resection rate for hilar cholangiocarcinomas

Series	Year	Hepatectomy rate (%)	R0 resection rate (%)
Tsao et al. [45] (Lahey)	2000	16	28
Cameron et al. [24]	1990	20	15
Hadjis et al. [48]	1990	60	56
Burke et al. [47]	1998	73	83
Lai and Lau [51]	2005	89	72
Tsao et al. [45] (Nagoya)	2000	89	79
Capussotti et al. [43]	2002	89	89
Nimura et al. [49]	1990	98	89

preferred. The short term outcomes were good and similar between the two groups: mortality rate 4 % vs. 8 % and morbidity 44 % vs. 51 %, respectively [45]. Some Japanese groups have reported no mortality after bile duct resection associated with hepatectomy [39, 41, 42].

There are enough evidence to support that the rate of R0 resection increases with the rate of associated liver resections for hilar cholangiocarcinoma [26, 46–51], although R0 resection can still be achieved in some patients with isolated bile duct resection (Table 17.1).

The caudate lobe ducts join the left and right hepatic ducts near to their conference, explaining why the lobe is involved by hilar cholangiocarcinoma in 40–98 % of patients [49, 52– 54]. Retrospective studies have shown a decrease in local recurrence [55] and improvement in 5-year survival [25, 56, 57] when concomitant caudate lobe resection is performed. Tsao et al. stated that combining hilar resection and partial hepatectomy with complete caudate lobe resection can be performed safely in the hands of experienced surgeons who are familiar with caudate lobe anatomy [45]. This operation is now adopted by most Japanese and some Western surgeons [58–60].

17.5 Combined Liver Resection for Hilar Cholangiocarcinoma

In the past two decades, there has been an increased use of hepatic resection in patients with hilar cholangiocarcinoma. Major hepatic resection with caudate lobectomy addresses both direct hepatic invasion and intraductal extension of hilar cholangiocarcinoma to achieve a wider and, therefore, a higher chance of negative radial and longitudinal resection margins. Incorporating a major hepatic resection as a fundamental surgical strategy for hilar cholangiocarcinoma has increased the R0 resection rate [32, 36, 60–62], improved recurrence-free survivals, and decreased the incidence of hepatic recurrence [62].

In the review article by Ito et al. [25], the published 5-year survival rates after surgical resection for hilar cholangiocarcinoma vary from 25 to 40 %. Clinicopathological factors which have been shown to have a positive impact on long-term survivals include negative histologic margin status, concomitant hepatic resection, lack of nodal involvement, lower AJCC T stage, well-differentiated tumor grade, papillary tumor morphology and lack of perineural invasion. Of these, complete resection with histologically negative margins is the only modifiable factor and should therefore be the primary goal of surgical therapy. If the histological margin is involved by tumor (R1 resection), it is still controversial in the surgical literature as to whether R1 resection provides any survival benefits to patients when compared with patients with unresectable disease [41, 45, 62–68].

Long-term survival data coming from a single institution comparing local bile duct resection with combined hepatectomy should be interpreted with caution as these data concern hilar cholangiocarcinoma with different extension into the bile ducts. Patients undergoing local excision probably had tumors without (or at the most with minimal) involvement of the bile duct confluence. This is not clearly defined in most of the published articles, and the treatment was most likely planned according to tumor location, and that liver resection was scheduled for patients with more extensive diseases. It is, therefore, not surprising to find reports showing no evidence of any statistical difference in long-term survival after local resection when compared with extended surgery with liver resection [34, 35, 37, 38, 44, 69–73]. On the other hand, studies from single institution reported significantly increased survival after associated liver resection [26, 32, 37, 42, 58]. The evidence supporting associated liver resection to treat hilar cholangiocarcinoma came from the study by Tsao on comparing oriental and US experiences, reporting on significantly better long-term survival in Japanese patients undergoing more aggressive surgical strategy (5- and 10-year survival rates were 16 % and 12 % vs. 7 % and 2 %, respectively) [45]. Additional supporting evidence came from the report in 2005 by Dinant et al. from the Netherlands. With a change in policy to treat hilar cholangiocarcinoma with aggressive surgery, there was a higher R0 resection rate and an improvement in long-term survival, with no increase in operative morbidity or mortality [58].

To clarify whether local resection may have a role in patients with hilar cholangiocarcinoma, Capussotti et al. reviewed the medical literature and focused their analysis on the reported results in Bismuth-Corletter (BC) types I to II hilar cholangiocarcinoma [26]. In selected cases, long term survival without recurrence was achievable with local resection [59, 71, 74]. However, the results of local resection have been reported to be poorer than with associated liver resection [26, 41–43, 75–77]. In the Neuhaus series, local resection achieved a R0 resection in two of six patients in BC type I, and one of four in BC type II tumors. However, no patient survived 5 years [75].

The Nagoya group reviewed 54 patients with BC types I, II tumors. Local resection was carried out in 14 patients.

Based on their experience, the authors suggested a surgical approach based on cholangiographic tumor type: extended hepatectomy was always necessary in the nodular or infiltrative tumor, while bile duct resection with or without limited hepatectomy could be performed in papillary tumor without superficial cancer spreading [78]. Capussotti et al., after reviewing the medical literature on local surgical resection of hilar cholangiocarcinoma, concluded that local resection should be scheduled only for small papillary Klatskin tumors without bile duct confluence involvement (type I) confined to the bile duct wall (Tis and T1). These tumours form a small minority of hilar cholangiocarcinoma. Extension of treatment should always be determined in accordance with the patient's condition [26]. To confirm histologically-negative resection margins, intraoperative frozen section examinations of the bile ducts have been advocated [29, 79, 80], especially in local resection, to plan the extent of surgical resection.

17.6 Developments in the Advances in Preoperative Management

Three major advances in the preoperative management of hilar cholangiocarcinoma need to be discussed in slightly more detail:

1. Preoperative Biliary Drainage
   The preoperative relief of obstructive jaundice and the reversal of its hepatic and systemic effects by biliary drainage have been proposed as a method to decrease the risk of surgery in patients with obstruction to the biliary system. In several prospective randomized studies, the routine use of preoperative biliary drainage, either in the form of percutaneous transhepatic or endoscopic, failed to show any benefit [81–84]. A meta-analysis concluded that preoperative biliary drainage increased rather than decreased overall complications and provided no benefit in terms of reduced mortality or decreased hospital stay [85] because postoperative septic complications were common after biliary drainage. A major criticism of these prospective studies is that the duration of preoperative drainage (10–18 days) were not long enough to reverse the metabolic and immunologic abnormalities associated with obstructive jaundice. However, for malignant obstructive jaundice, the wait for surgery cannot be too long or the tumor might have progressed and become unresectable. Another criticism is that the results of these studies may not be applicable to hilar cholangiocarcinoma as most of the patients in these studies received no liver resection, and liver resection is commonly used in hilar cholangiocarcinoma.

   A recently published systematic review on preoperative biliary drainage for resection of hilar cholangiocarcinoma concluded that there was no clinical benefit of using preoperative biliary drainage, and preoperative drainage resulted in significant increase in postoperative complication rates and postoperative infectious complication rates [86].

   Although all these data suggest that preoperative biliary drainage is not beneficial in the routine management of patients, preoperative biliary drainage may have some value in selected patients with advanced malnutrition, biliary sepsis, prolonged delay in surgery to wait for the effects of portal vein embolization or chemotherapy/radiotherapy.
2. Portal Vein Embolization (PVE)
   Most patients with hilar cholangiocarcinoma present with jaundice and are considered to have cholestasis-induced compromised liver function. Portal vein embolization should be considered for patients with potentially resectable tumors with compromised liver function when the anticipated future liver remnant is below 40 % of the total liver volume [25]. The potential benefits of PVE are its ability to induce hypertrophy in the future liver remnant (FLR), thereby reducing the risk of postoperative liver failure, and its ability to permit curative resection for patients who otherwise would be considered unresectable due to insufficient FLR. This strategy has been used prior to major hepatic resection for hilar cholangiocarcinoma [28, 63, 87–89]. Currently, there is no evidence to support the routine use of PVE for hilar cholangiocarcinoma. The major disadvantages of PVE in hilar cholangiocarcinoma are the waiting time for the FLR to hypertrophy, and the occasional difficulty in deciding preoperatively whether a right or a left hemihepatectomy will be required if the tumor is placed centrally at the hilus [25].
3. Staging Laparoscopy and Laparoscopic Ultrasound
   Despite exhaustive preoperative investigations, a significant proportion of patients are found to have unresectable disease at the time of laparotomy [32, 62]. Of the patients who are explored with curative intent, only 40–50 % are ultimately resectable [25]. The yield and accuracy of laparoscopy to determine resectability is between 25–42 % and 42–53 %, respectively [89–93]. Laparoscopy is more likely to detect occult metastases from T2/T3 extrahepatic bile duct cancer than T1 tumors (36 % vs. 9 %, respectively) [89]. Laparoscopic ultrasonography increased the yield of laparoscopy by up to 17 % [91].

17.7 Curative Surgery Beyond Liver Resection

Metastasis to regional lymph nodes is common and is an important prognostic factor for long-term survival after resection for hilar cholangiocarcinoma [25, 62, 64, 72, 94]. Studies showed poor survival for patients who had nodal involvement beyond the hepatoduodenal ligament with

5-year survival of 0–6 % [64, 72, 94]. Routine lymph node dissection beyond the hepatoduodenal ligament is not recommended. Patients with grossly involved lymph nodes beyond the hepatoduodenal ligament are considered to have unresectable disease [25].

Combined portal vein resection and reconstruction for hilar cholangiocarcinoma produce conflicting results [75, 95–97]. Several retrospective studies have shown combined portal vein resection does not add to the operative mortality [75, 96, 97]. The impact of combined resection of the portal vein on long-term survival is less clear [25]. Neuhaus proposed routine portal vein resection as part of "no touch" resection of tumor and adjacent tissue [75]. However, the 60-day mortality after portal vein resection was 17 % as compared with 5 % for patients without portal vein resection. When the 60-day mortalities were excluded, portal vein resections were identified as an independent positive prognostic factor in their multivariate analysis of patients undergoing R0 resection. Other authors show equivalent or worse survival in patients undergoing *en bloc* resection of the portal vein [96–99]. We need a properly conducted randomized clinical trial to find out whether routine resection of the portal vein as advocated by Neuhaus is beneficial or not.

17.8 Palliative Surgery

Patients with hilar cholangiocarcinoma who are not candidates for resection on investigation because of locally extensive disease, distant metastases or serious associated medical illness are usually treated non-surgically by percutaneous or endoscopic biliary stenting. Patients who receive chemotherapy or radiotherapy also require optimal hepatic function prior to these treatments, and thus require biliary drainage as well. An operative biliary decompression procedure is usually only performed for patients with locally advanced tumors who are found to be unresectable at laparotomy, and have therefore already encountered the potential morbidity of laparotomy [25]. In the absence of cholangitis, a unilateral biliary drainage is generally sufficient to relieve jaundice.

17.9 Ex Situ Ex Vivo Liver Resection and Autotransplantation

Ex situ ex vivo liver resection and subsequent autotransplantation was first carried out by Pichlmayr et al. in 1988 for a patient with bilateral liver metastases of a leiomyosarcoma [100]. This procedure was subsequently carried out five times up to the year 2003 for cholangiocarcinoma, and our group carried out the six cases with the longest survival [101, 102]. This procedure is technically difficult and few centers are experienced with this technique. Results with ex situ ex vivo liver surgery with hilar cholangiocarcinoma have generally been poor, and these patients often die of postoperative hepatic insufficiency [103]. This is believed to be due to the longstanding cholestasis associated with this disease which reduces the liver tolerance to ischaemia. Ex situ ex vivo surgery for hilar cholangiocarcinoma is an aggressive surgical treatment which should only be attempted in experienced centers on carefully selected patients.

17.10 Liver Transplantation

Orthotopic liver transplantation (OLT) offers the advantages of resection of all structures that may be involved by hilar cholangiocarcinoma including portal vein, bilateral hepatic ducts, atrophic liver lobes and hepatic artery. Total hepatectomy may therefore permit R0 resection for locally advanced tumors which are beyond the ordinary criteria for resection using partial hepatectomy. The early experience of OLT for hilar cholangiocarcinoma unfortunately was disappointing with early tumor recurrence and poor 5 year survival of 28–30 % [104–107]. As a consequence of these early results and the limited availability of cadaveric livers, hilar cholangiocarcinoma was considered to be a relative contraindication to OLT.

Recently a "Mayo protocol" has been developed to treat a highly selected group of patients with unresectable hilar cholangiocarcinoma or hilar cholangiocarcinoma arising from a setting of primary sclerosing cholangitis. There are very strict inclusion and exclusion criteria [103]. Patient received neoadjuvant chemoradiation and then a staging laparotomy to rule out metastatic nodal disease. Patients without disease progression undergo OLT. This highly rigorous selection process may result in a selection bias in favor of patients with biological favourable disease. Very encouraging results have been reported [108, 109]. At present OLT cannot be recommended for patients with resectable hilar cholangiocarcinoma. Further studies are required to fully define the role of OLT. As primary sclerosing cholangitis commonly develops into cholangiocarcinoma, OLT carried out for primary sclerosing cholangitis often has an associated high rate of unsuspected cholangiocarcinoma [110–112].

17.11 Conservative Combined Liver Resection

Surgical resection of hilar cholangiocarcinoma with adequate resection margins is the only form of treatment that offers the potential of cure. In an attempt to achieve a high rate of R0 resection, major hepatic resections such as left hepatectomy, right hepatectomy, left trisectionectomy and right trisectionectomy have been advocated [56, 73, 113–117]. However, major liver resection in patients with obstructive jaundice results in high surgical mortality and morbidity [98]. High operative mortality rate of 17 % for major liver resection [50] and 23 % for left trisectionectomy have been reported.

As an alterative to using preoperative biliary drainage and portal vein embolization to reduce the perioperative risk of liver resection for hilar cholangiocarcinoma, we have been using a strategy of minor liver resection (defined as resection of less than three Couinaud liver segments) in selected patients with hilar cholangiocarcinoma, so that a sufficient hepatic mass is preserved after surgery [118]. As the hilar bifurcation of the bile ducts is near to liver segments 4, 5 and 1, adequate resection of these liver segments together with their bile ducts can result in cure in selected patients. For obvious reasons, for hilar cholangiocarcinoma that involves the right and left hepatic arteries, or portal vein, or for Bismuth-Corletter type IV tumors, the surgical option is to carry out a right/extended right or left/extended left hepatectomy. With a predetermined selection criteria to choose patients with hilar cholangiocarcinoma for minor or major hepatectomy, we were able to achieve a 0 mortality rate, and a 29.7 % morbidity rate. There was no significant difference in the 5-year survival rates of 34 % in the minor liver resection group compared with the major liver resection group. Although resecting Couinaud's liver segments 1, 4, 5 is called a minor liver resection in this study, this operation is technically more difficult than most of the major liver resections because it involved: (1) a mesohepatectomy with two liver transection planes and the need to preserve the blood supply to the left outer section (segments 2, 3) and the right posterior section (segment 6, 7) [119]; (2) many intrahepatic ductal openings are left in the remnant liver after liver resection and these ducts need to be anastomosed to a roux-en-y loop of jejunum. We have devised a special technique in hepaticojejunostomy to solve this problem [118, 120].

Central lobe resection (or mesohepatectomy) in selected patients with hilar cholangiocarcinoma requires good technical skills. The initial good results need to be confirmed by more studies.

Conclusion

The surgical treatment of hilar cholangiocarcinoma has evolved through many stages. The changes involved improve the immediate and long-term results of this tumour. Hilar cholangiocarcinoma is still a disease which is difficult to cure. Further studies are needed to further improve on the management of this disease.

References

1. Klatskin G. Adenocarcinoma of the hepatic duct at its bifurcation within the porta hepatis. Am J Med. 1965;38:241–56.
2. Renshaw K. Malignant neoplasms of the extrahepatic biliary ducts. Ann Surg. 1922;76:205–21.
3. Altemeier WA, Gall EA, Sinninger MM, et al. Sclerosing carcinoma of the major intrahepatic bile ducts. Arch Surg. 1957;75:450–60.
4. Edmundson HA. Tumors of the liver and intrahepatic bile ducts. Atlas of tumor pathology. Washington, DC: Armed Forces Institute of Pathology; 1958. p. 86. Fascicle 25, Section VII.
5. Alvarez AF. Carcinoma of the main hepatic ducts within the liver: a report of two cases treated by intrahepatic cholangiojejunostomy. Ann Surg. 1958;148:733–82.
6. Thorbjarnarson B. Carcinoma of the intrahepatic bile ducts. Arch Surg. 1958;77:908–17.
7. Meyerowitz RB, Aird I. Carcinoma of the hepatic ducts within the liver. Br J Surg. 1962;50:178–84.
8. Ahrendt SA, Pitt HA. A history of the bilioenteric anastomosis. Arch Surg. 1990;125:1493–500.
9. Braasch JW. History of biliary surgery. In: Braasch JW, Tompkins RK, editors. Surgical diseases of the biliary tract and pancreas—multidisciplinary management. St Louis: Mosby; 1994. p. 3–12, section 1, chapter 1.
10. Langenbuch CJA. Ein fall von exstirpation der gallenblase wegen chronischer cholelithiasis: heilung. Berlin Klin Wochenschr. 1882;19:725–7.
11. Reich A. Accidental injection of bile ducts with petrolatum and bismuth paste. JAMA. 1918;71:1555–6.
12. Mirizzi PL. La colangiografia durante las operaciones de las vias biliares. Bol Trab Soc Cir B Aires. 1932;16:1133–61.
13. Frommhold W. Ein neuartiges kontrastmittel für die intravenose cholezystographie. Fortschr Geb Rontgenstr. 1953;79:283–91.
14. Carter RF, Saypol GM. Transabdominal cholangiography. JAMA. 1952;148:253–5.
15. Okuda K, Tanikawa K, Emura T, et al. Non-surgical, percutaneous transhepatic cholangiography: diagnostic significance in medical problems of the liver. Am J Dig Dis. 1974;19:21–36.
16. McCune WS, Shorb PE, Moscovitz H. Endoscopic cannulation of the ampulla of Vater: a preliminary report. Ann Surg. 1968;167:752–6.
17. Oi I. Fiberduodenoscopy and endoscopic pancreatocholangiography. Gastrointest Endosc. 1970;17:59–62.
18. Cooperberg PL, Durhenne HJ. Real-time ultrasonography: diagnostic technique of choice in calculous gallbladder disease. N Engl J Med. 1980;302:1277–9.
19. Cotton PB. ERCP overview—a 30-year perspective. In: Cotton PB, Leng J, editors. Advanced digestive endoscopy: ERCP. Massachusetts: Blackwell; 2006. p. 1–8, chapter I.
20. Bismuth H, Malt RA. Current concepts in cancer: carcinoma of the biliary tract. N Eng J Med. 1979;301:704–6.
21. Bismuth H, Castaing D, Traynor O. Resection or palliation priority of surgery in the treatment of hilar cancer. World J Surg. 1988;12:39–47.
22. Bismuth H, Corlette MB. Intrahepatic cholangioenteric anastomosis in carcinoma of the hilus of the liver. Surg Gynecol Obstet. 1975;140:170–8.
23. Tompkins PK, Thomas D, Wile A, et al. Prognostic factors in bile duct carcinoma: analysis of 96 cases. Ann Surg. 1981;194:447–57.
24. Cameron JL, Pitt HA, Zinner MJ, et al. Management of proximal cholangiocarcinomas by surgical resection and radiotherapy. Am J Surg. 1990;159:91–7.
25. Ito F, Cho CS, Rikkers LF, et al. Hilar cholangiocarcinoma: current management. Ann Surg. 2009;250:210–8.
26. Capussotti L, Vigano L, Ferrero A, et al. Local surgical resection of hilar cholangiocarcinoma: is there still a place? HPB. 2008;10:174–8.
27. Greene FL, Page DL, Fleming ID. AJCC (American Joint Committee on Cancer) cancer staging manual. 6th ed. New York: Springer; 2002.
28. Ebata T, Watanabe H, Ajioka Y, et al. Pathological appraisal of lines of resection for bile duct carcinoma. Br J Surg. 2002;89:1260–7.

29. Aljiffy M, Walsh MJ, Molinari M. Advances in diagnosis, treatment and palliation of cholangiocarcinoma: 1990–2009. World J Gastroenterol. 2009;15:4240–62.
30. Yamaguchi K, Chijiiwa K, Saiki S, et al. Carcinoma of extrahepatic bile duct: mode of spread and its prognostic implications. Hepatogastroenterology. 1997;44:1256–61.
31. He P, Shi JS, Chen WK, et al. Multivariate statistical analysis of clinicopathologic factors influencing survival of patients with bile duct carcinoma. World J Gastroenterol. 2002;8:943–6.
32. Jarnagin WR, Fong Y, DeMatteo RP, et al. Staging resectability, and outcome in 225 patients with hilar cholangiocarcinoma. Ann Surg. 2001;234:507–17.
33. Nagorney DM, Kendrick ML. Hepatic resection in the treatment of hilar cholangiocarcinoma. Adv Surg. 2006;40:157–71.
34. Nakeeb A, Pitt HA, Sohn TA, et al. Cholangiocarcinoma. A spectrum of intrahepatic, perihilar and distal tumors. Ann Surg. 1996; 224:463–73.
35. Pichlmayr R, Weimann A, Klempnauer J, et al. Surgical treatment in proximal bile duct cancer. A single-center experience. Ann Surg. 1996;224:628–38.
36. Miyazaki M, Ito H, Nakagawa K, et al. Aggressive surgical approaches to hilar cholangiocarcinoma: hepatic or local resection? Surgery. 1998;123:131–6.
37. Boerma EJ. Research into the results of resection of hilar bile duct cancer. Surgery. 1990;108:572–80.
38. Baer HU, Stain SC, Dennison AR, et al. Improvements in survival by aggressive resection of hilar cholangiocarcinoma. Ann Surg. 1993;217:20–7.
39. Sano T, Shimada K, Sakamoto Y, et al. One hundred and two consecutive hepatobiliary resections for perihilar cholangiocarcinoma with zero mortality. Ann Surg. 2006;244:240–7.
40. Kawasaki S, Imamura H, Kobayashi A, et al. Results of surgical resection for patients with hilar bile duct cancer: application of extended hepatectomy after bilary drainage and hemihepatic portal vein embolization. Ann Surg. 2003;238:84–92.
41. Seyama Y, Kubota K, Sano K, et al. Long-term outcome of extended hemihepatectomy for hilar bile duct cancer with no mortality and high survival rate. Ann Surg. 2003;238:73–83.
42. Kondo S, Hirano S, Ambo Y, et al. Forty consecutive resections of hilar cholangiocarcinoma with no postoperative mortality and no positive ductal margins: results of a prospective study. Ann Surg. 2004;240:95–101.
43. Capussotti L, Muratore A, Polastri R, et al. Liver resection for hilar cholangiocarcinoma: in hospital mortality and long-term survival. J Am Coll Surg. 2002;195:641–7.
44. Launois B, Reding R, Lebeau G, et al. Surgery for hilar cholangiocarcinoma: French experience in a collective survey of 552 extrahepatic bile duct cnacers. J Hepatobiliary Pancreat Surg. 2000;7:128–34.
45. Tsao JI, Nimura Y, Kamiya J, et al. Management of hilar cholangiocarcinoma: comparison of an American and a Japanese experience. Ann Surg. 2000;232:166–74.
46. Saldinger PF, Blumgart LH. Resection of hilar cholangiocarcinoma—a European and United States experience. J Hepatobiliary Pancreat Surg. 2000;7:111–4.
47. Burke EC, Jarnagin WR, Hockwald SN, et al. Hilar cholangiocarcinoma: patterns of spread, the importance of hepatic resection for curative operation, and a presurgical clinical staging system. Ann Surg. 1998;228:385–94.
48. Hadjis NS, Blenkharn JI, Alexander N, et al. Outcome of radical surgery for hilar cholangiocarcinoma. Surgery. 1990;101:597–604.
49. Nimura Y, Hayakawa N, Kamiya J, et al. Hepatic segmentectomy with caudate lobe resection fo bile duct carcinoma of the hepatic hilus. World J Surg. 1990;14:535–44.
50. Klempnauer J, Ridder GJ, Werner M, et al. What constitutes long-term survival after surgery for hilar cholangiocarcinoma? Cancer. 1997;79:26–34.
51. Lai ECH, Lau WY. Aggressive surgical resection for hilar cholangiocarcinoma. ANZ J Surg. 2005;75:981–5.
52. Mizumoto R, Kawarada Y, Suzuki H, et al. Surgical treatment of hilar carcinoma of the bile duct. Surg Gynecol Obstet. 1986;162: 153–8.
53. Ogura Y, Mizumoto R, Tabata M, et al. Surgical treatment of carcinoma of the hepatic duct confluence: analysis of 55 resected carcinomas. World J Surg. 1993;17:85–92.
54. Sugiura Y, Nakamura S, Iida S, et al. Extensive resection of the bile ducts combined with liver resection for cancer of the main hepatic duct junction: a cooperative study of the Keio Bile Duct Cancer Study Group. Surgery. 1994;115:445–51.
55. Gazzaniga GM, Ciferri E, Bagarolo C, et al. Primitive hepatic hilum neoplasm. J Surg Oncol Suppl. 1993;3:140–6.
56. Rea DJ, Munoz-Juarez M, Farnell MB, et al. Major hepatic resection for hilar cholangiocarcinoma: analysis of 46 patients. Arch Surg. 2004;139:514–23.
57. Gazzaniga GM, Filauro M, Bagarolo C, et al. Surgery for hilar cholangiocarcinoma: an Italian experience. J Hepatobiliary Pancreat Surg. 2000;7:122–7.
58. Dinant S, Gerhards MF, Busch OR, et al. The importance of complete excision of the caudate lobe in resection of hilar cholangiocarcinoma. HPB. 2005;7:263–7.
59. Bismuth H, Nakache R, Diamond T. Management strategies in resection for hilar cholangiocarcinoma. Ann Surg. 1992;215:31–8.
60. Neuhaus P, Jonas S, Settmacher U, et al. Surgical management of proximal bile duct cancer: extended right lobe resection increases resectability and radicality. Langenbecks Arch Surg. 2003;388:194–200.
61. Lee SG, Lee YJ, Park KM, et al. One hundred and eleven liver resections for hilar bile duct cancer. J Hepatobiliary Pancreat Surg. 2000;7:135–41.
62. Ito F, Agni R, Rettammel RJ, et al. Resection of hilar cholangiocarcinoma: concomitant liver resection decreases hepatic recurrence. Ann Surg. 2008;248:273–9.
63. Hemming AW, Reed AI, Howard RJ, et al. Preoperative portal vein embolization for extended hepatectomy. Ann Surg. 2003;237: 686–91.
64. Klempnauer J, Ridder GJ, von Wasielewski R, et al. Resectional surgery of hilar cholangiocarcinoma: a multivariate analysis of prognostic factors. J Clin Oncol. 1997;15:947–54.
65. Baton O, Azoulay D, Adam DV, et al. Major hepatectomy for hilar cholangiocarcinoma type 3 and 4: prognostic factors and long-term outcomes. J Am Coll Surg. 2007;204:250–60.
66. Jarnagin WR, Shoup M. Surgical management of cholangiocarcinoma. Semin Liver Dis. 2004;242:189–99.
67. Hemming AW, Reed AI, Fujita S, et al. Surgical management of hilar cholangiocarcinoma. Ann Surg. 2005;241:693–9.
68. IJitsma AJ, Appeltans BM, de Jong KP, et al. Extrahepatic bile duct resection in combination with liver resection for hilar cholangiocarcinoma: a report of 42 cases. J Gastrointest Surg. 2004;8:686–94.
69. Tabata M, Kawarada Y, Yokoi H, et al. Surgical treatment for hilar cholangiocarcinoma. J Hepatobiliary Pancreat Surg. 2000;7: 148–54.
70. DeOliveira ML, Cunningham SC, Cameron JL, et al. Cholangiocarcinoma: thirty-one-year experience with 564 patients at a single institution. Ann Surg. 2007;245:755–62.
71. Jang JY, Kim SW, Park DJ, et al. Actual long-term outcome of extrahepatic bile duct cancer after surgical resection. Ann Surg. 2005;241:77–84.
72. Kosuge T, Yamamoto J, Shimada K, et al. Improved surgical results for hilar cholangiocarcinoma with procedures including major hepatic resection. Ann Surg. 1999;230:663–71.
73. Witzigmann H, Berr F, Ringel U, et al. Surgical and palliative management and outcome in 184 patients with hilar cholangiocarcinoma: palliative photodynamic therapy plus stenting is comparable to R1/R2 resection. Ann Surg. 2006;244:230–9.

74. Launois B, Terblanche J, Lakehal M, et al. Proximal bile duct cancer; high resectability rate and 5-year survival. Ann Surg. 1999; 230:266–75.
75. Neuhaus P, Jonas S, Bechstein WO, et al. Extended resection for hilar cholangiocarcinoma. Ann Surg. 1999;230:808–18.
76. Su CH, Tsay SH, Wu CC, et al. Factor influencing post-operative morbidity, mortality, and survival after resection for hilar cholangiocarcinoma. Ann Surg. 1996;223:284–94.
77. van Gulik TM, Gerhards M, de Vries J, et al. Local resection of biliopancreatic cancer. Ann Oncol. 1990;10 Suppl 4Suppl 4:243–6.
78. Ikeyama T, Nagino M, Oda K, et al. Surgical approach to Bismuth type I and II hilar cholangiocarcinomas: audit of 54 consecutive cases. Ann Surg. 2007;246:1052–7.
79. Nathan H, Aloia TA, Vauthey JN, et al. A proposal staging system from intrahepatic cholangiocarcinoma. Ann Surg Oncol. 2009;16:14–22.
80. Endo I, House MG, Klimstra DS, et al. Clinical significance of intraoperative bile duct margin assessment for hilar cholangiocarcinoma. Ann Surg Oncol. 2008;15(8):2104–12.
81. Hatfield AR, Tobias AR, Terblanche J, et al. Preoperative external biliary drainage in obstructive jaundice: a prospective controlled clinical trial. Lancet. 1982;2:886–9.
82. McPherson GA, Benjamin IS, Hodgson HJ, et al. Pre-operative percutaneous transhepatic biliary drainage: the results of a controlled trial. Br J Surg. 1984;71:371–5.
83. Pitt HA, Gomes AS, Lois JF, et al. Does preoperative procedures biliary drainage reduce operative risk or increase hospital cost? Ann Surg. 1985;201:545–53.
84. Lai ECS, Mok KP, Fan ST, et al. Preoperative endoscopic drainage for malignant obstructive jaundice. Br J Surg. 1994;81:1195–8.
85. Sewnath ME, Karsten TM, Prins MH, et al. A meta-analysis on the efficacy of preoperative biliary drainage for tumors causing obstructive jaundice. Ann Surg. 2002;236:17–27.
86. Liu F, Li Y, Wei YG, et al. Preoperative biliary drainage before resection for hilar cholangiocarcinoma: whether or not? A systematic review. Dig Dis Sci. 2011;56:663–72.
87. Imamura H, Shimada R, Kubota M, et al. Preoperative portal vein embolization: an audit of 84 patients. Hepatology. 1999;29:1099–105.
88. Makuuchi M, Thai BL, Takayasu K, et al. Preoperative portal embolization to increase safety of major hepatectomy for hilar hile duct carcinoma: a preliminary report. Surgery. 1990;107:521–7.
89. Weber SM, DeMatteo RP, Fong Y, et al. Staging laparoscopy in patients with extrahepatic biliary carcinoma. Analysis of 100 patients. Ann Surg. 2002;235:392–9.
90. Palavecino M, Abdalla EK, Madoff DC, et al. Portal vein embolization in hilar cholangiocarcinoma. Surg Oncol Clin N Am. 2009;18: 257–67.
91. Connor S, Barron E, Wigmore SJ, et al. The utility of laparoscopic assessment in the preoperative staging of suspected hilar cholangiocarcinoma. J Gastrointest Surg. 2005;9:476–80.
92. Goere D, Wagholikar GD, Pessaux P, et al. Utility of staging laparoscopy in subsets of biliary cancers: laparoscopy is a powerful diagnostic tool in patients with intrahepatic and gallbladder carcinoma. Surg Endosc. 2006;20(5):721–5.
93. Corvera CU, Weber SM, Jarnagin WR. Role of laparoscopy in the evaluation of biliary tract cancer. Surg Oncol Clin N Am. 2002; 11(4):877–91.
94. Kitagawa Y, Nagino M, Kamiya J, et al. Lymph node metastasis from hilar cholangiocarcinoma: audit of 110 patients who underwent regional and paraaortic node dissection. Ann Surg. 2001; 233:385–92.
95. Todoroki T, Kawanmoto T, Kioke N, et al. Radical resection of hilar bile duct carcinoma and predictors of survival. Br J Surg. 2000; 87:306–13.
96. Ebata T, Nagino M, Kamiya J, et al. Hepatectomy with portal vein resection for hilar cholangiocarcinoma: audit of 52 consecutive cases. Ann Surg. 2003;238:720–7.
97. Hemming AW, Kim RD, Mekeel KL, et al. Portal vein resection of hilar bile duct carcinoma. Am Surg. 2006;72:599–604.
98. Miyazaki M, Kato A, Mto H, et al. Combined vascular resection in operative resection for hilar cholangiocarcinoma: does it work or not? Surgery. 2007;141:581–8.
99. Muñoz L, Roayaie S, Maman D, et al. Hilar cholangiocarcinoma involving the portal vein bifurcation: long-term results after resection. J Hepatobiliary Pancreat Surg. 2002;9(2):237–41.
100. Pichlmayr R, Bretschneider HJ, Kichner E, et al. Ex situ operation of the liver: a new possibility in liver surgery. Langenbecks Arch Chir. 1988;27:44–8.
101. Chui AK, Rao AR, Wang J, et al. Ex situ ex vivo liver resection, partial liver autotransplantation for advanced hilar cholangiocarcinoma: a case report. Transplant Proc. 2003;35:402–3.
102. Chui AK, Island ER, Rao AR, et al. The longest survivor and first potential cure of an advanced cholangiocarcinoma by ex vivo resection and autotransplantation: a case report and review of the literature. Am Surg. 2003;69:441–4.
103. Oldhafer KJ, Lang H, Schlitt HJ, et al. Long term experience after ex situ liver surgery. Surgery. 2000;127:520–7.
104. Goldstein RM, Stone M, Tilley GW, et al. Is liver transplantation indicated for cholangiocarcinoma? Am J Surg. 1993;166:768–71.
105. Meyer CG, Penn I, James L. Liver transplantation for cholangiocarcinoma: results in 207 patients. Transplantation. 2000;69:1633–7.
106. Robles R, Figueras J, Turiòn VS, et al. Spanish experience in liver transplantation for hilar and peripheral cholangiocarcinoma. Ann Surg. 2004;239:265–71.
107. Shimoda M, Farmer DG, Colquhoun SD, et al. Liver transplantation for cholangiocellular carcinoma: analysis of a single-center experience and review of the literature. Liver Transpl. 2001;7: 1023–33.
108. Rea DJ, Heimbach JK, Rosen CB, et al. Liver transplantation with neoadjuvant chemoradiation is more effective resection for hilar cholangiocarcinoma. Ann Surg. 2005;242:451–8.
109. Heimbach JK, Gores GJ, Haddock MG, et al. Predictors of disease recurrence following neoadjuvant chemoradiotherapy and liver transplantation for unresectable perihilar cholangiocarcinoma. Transplantation. 2006;82:1703–7.
110. Rosen CB, Nagorney DM, Wiesner RH, et al. Cholangiocarcinoma complicating primary sclerosing cholangitis. Ann Surg. 1991;213:21–5.
111. Marsh Jr JW, Iwatsuki S, Makowka L, et al. Orthotopic liver transplantation for primary sclerosing cholangitis. Ann Surg. 1988;207:21–5.
112. Goss JA, Shackleton CR, Farmer DG, et al. Orthotopic liver transplantation for primary sclerosing cholangitis. A 12-year single center experience. Ann Surg. 1997;225:472–81.
113. Belghiti J, Ogata S. Preoperative optimization of the liver for resection in patients with hilar cholangiocarcinoma. HPB. 2005;7:252–3.
114. Parikh AA, Abdalla EK, Vauthey JN. Operative considerations in resection of hilar cholangiocarcinoma. HPB. 2005;7:254–8.
115. Pinson CW, Rossi RC. Extended right liver lobectomy, left hepatic lobectomy and skeletonization resection for proximal bile duct cancer. World J Surg. 1988;12:52–9.
116. Jonas S, Benchert C, Thelen A, et al. Radical surgery for hilar cholangiocarcinoma. Eur J Surg Oncol. 2008;34:263–71.
117. Nishio H, Nagino M, Nimura Y. Surgical management of hilar cholangiocarcinoma: the Nagoya experience. HPB. 2005;7:259–62.
118. Chen XP, Lau WY, Huang ZY, et al. Extent of liver resection for hilar cholangiocarcinoma. Br J Surg. 2009;96:1167–75.
119. Chen XP, Qiu FZ, Lau WY, et al. Mesohepatectomy for hepatocellular carcinoma: a study of 256 patients. Int J Colorectal Dis. 2008;23:543–6.
120. Chen XP, Zhang ZW, Huang ZY, et al. The technique modified biliary tract reconstruction after resection of hilar cholangiocarcinoma. Chin J Surg. 2006;46:634–5.

Radical Resection and Its Limits

18

T. Sano and Y. Nimura

18.1 Introduction

It has been difficult to make an accurate diagnosis of tumor extent and strategy for curative resection of hilar cholangiocarcinoma (HCCa) [1] even in this era of sophisticated imaging diagnostic modalities such as multidetector row computed tomography (MDCT) [2]. An increasing resection rate of HCCa has been achieved and the surgical procedures for HCCa are changing from hilar local resection or limited hepatectomy [3] to major or extensive hepatobiliary resection including caudate lobectomy [1], which remains technically demanding and calls for a high level of skill in biliary and hepatic surgeries. Although the histological curative resection with negative surgical margins (R0) offers the only chance for cure in patients with HCCa, the gold standard for the treatment strategy for HCCa has not yet been determined. To achieve a R0 resection, an extensive hepatectomy (hepatic trisectionectomy) with vascular resection and reconstruction [4, 5], or pancreatoduodenectomy (HPD) [6, 7] is essential in some patients with advanced or extensive disease. Since the majority of patients with HCCa have cholestatic liver damage due to bile duct obstruction, major hepatobiliary resection carries a considerable risk of serious postoperative morbidity and mortality [8]. The limitations for radical resection for HCCa are mainly determined in terms of two factors: whether R0 resection is possible or not against the local tumor extension and whether the functional reserve of the future remnant liver is adequate or not to tolerate the surgical stress. We have a dilemma as to whether extensive hepatobiliary resection is advisable to achieve a R0 resection, or whether less extensive resection is a prerequisite for patients with impaired functional reserve of the liver. Currently, we have adopted a management strategy for patients with HCCa, including preoperative biliary drainage, portal vein embolization (PVE) [9–12] and major hepatobiliary resection [13, 14].

In this chapter, we introduced our current standard approach and surgical techniques in radical resection of HCCa referring to the limits.

18.1.1 Fundamental Principles of HCCa Surgery in Terms of Limits

Glisson's capsule includes hepatic artery, portal vein, and segmental bile duct, and their detachment from each other is impossible in the liver parenchyma. Detachment of the hepatic artery and portal vein from the segmental bile duct prior to cutting the segmental bile duct at the expected line is essential to preserve the affected liver parenchyma. Hence, if it is impossible to dissociate from the feeding vasculatures and the segmental bile duct upstream of the expected resection line, the affected liver segment must be included in the resected liver segments to achieve a R0 resection (Fig. 18.1). The limitation of the detachment of the segmental bile duct and vasculature is usually determined by the individual anatomical relationship between the vasculature and bile duct system. On the other hand, not only the cancer-free proximal and distal bile duct margins but also the cancer-free dissection margin around the hepatoduodenal ligament is also an important issue in accomplishing a R0 resection [15].

18.1.2 Proximal Limit of Bile Duct Resection Line During HCCa Surgery

The proximal limit of resection of intrahepatic segmental and/or segmental bile ducts is differentially dependent upon

T. Sano, MD
Hepato-Biliary and Pancreatic Surgery Division,
Aichi Cancer Center Hospital,
Nagoya, Japan

Y. Nimura, MD (✉)
Division of Gastroenterological Surgery,
Aichi Cancer Center Hospital,
Nagoya, Japan
e-mail: ynimura@aichi-cc.jp

W.Y. Lau (ed.), *Hilar Cholangiocarcinoma*,
DOI 10.1007/978-94-007-6473-6_18, © Springer Science+Business Media Dordrecht and People's Medical Publishing House 2013

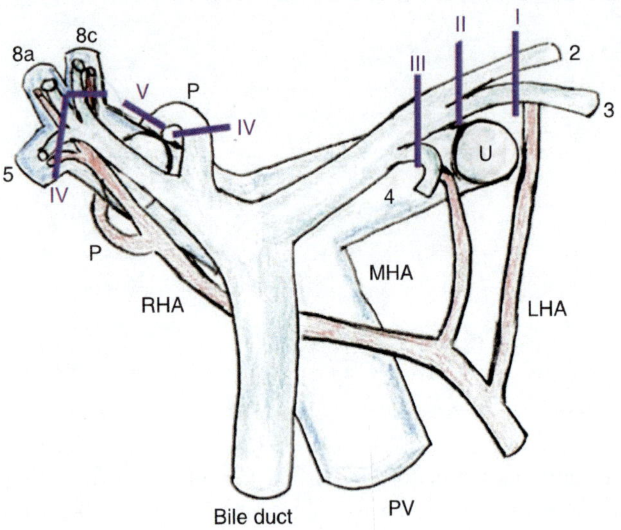

Fig. 18.1 The proximal limit of the resection intrahepatic segmental ducts is schematically illustrated in terms of type of hepatectomy. Numerals indicate Couinauld's segment of the liver. *U* umbilical portion of the left portal vein, *P* right posterior section, *8a* a ventral branch of the right anterosuperior segmental glisson, *8c* a dorsal branch of the right anterosuperior segmental glisson, *PV* portal vein, *LHA* left hepatic artery, *MHA* middle hepatic artery, *RHA* right hepatic artery, *I* right trisectionectomy (anatomical), *II* right trisectionectomy (classical), *III* right hemihepatectomy, *IV* left hemihepatectomy, *V* left trisectionectomy

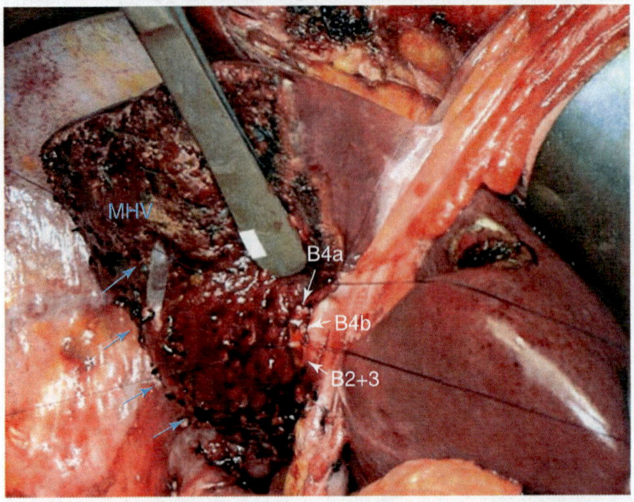

Fig. 18.2 Intraoperative photograph after right hepatectomy with caudate lobectomy shows openings of the left intrahepatic segmental ducts, and completed hepaticoplasty. Middle hepatic vein (*MHV*) indicated with *blue arrows* is clearly exposed on the raw surface of the liver. *B2* left lateral inferior segmental duct, *B3* left lateral superior segmental duct, *B4a* left medial inferior subsegmental duct, *B4b* left medial superior subsegmental duct. The *white arrows* point to B2+3, B4b and B4a

the type of hepatectomy (Fig. 18.1). In a right-sided hepatobiliary resection, the positive cancer involvement of the left medial segmental duct usually does not indicate a right hemihepatectomy but a right trisectionectomy to obtain the proximal tumor-free resection margin. The tumor involvement extends around the confluence of the left lateral anterior and posterior segmental ducts, in which case the limitation of the resecting line of the bile duct must correspond to the left side border of the umbilical portion of the left portal vein. Anatomic right trisectionectomy [16] is a potential option for such patients with right-side predominant extensive disease. This procedure is the ultimate for patients with the right-side predominant HCCa to obtain the proximal tumor-free resection margin. In a right hemihepatectomy, the left hepatic duct should be finally divided in the ventral to dorsal direction. Usually, the orifices of the left medial sectional (B4), the left lateral superior segmental (B3), and the left lateral inferior segmental (B2) bile ducts can be identified in order (Fig. 18.2). The limit of the resection line is the right-side border of the umbilical portion of the left portal vein. This line is somewhat oblique from the point at which the middle hepatic artery runs into the liver parenchyma.

In a left-sided hepatobiliary resection, the cancer involvement extends over the confluence of the right posterosuperior (B7) and posteroinferior segmental ducts (B6). It is usually difficult to secure the cancer-free resection margin even though a left trisectionectomy is performed. With a left hemihepatectomy, three to four proximal bile duct stumps appearing on the raw surface of the right liver is the limit. The orifices of the anteroinferior segmental duct (B5) and/or ventral branch of the anterosuperior segmental duct (B8a), dorsal branch of the anterosuperior segmental duct (B8c), and the posterior sectional duct are arranged in order from the ventral to dorsal direction. The orifice of the transected posterior sectional duct is located cranially to the right portal vein and at the right side border of the inferior vena cava (IVC) (Fig. 18.3).

18.1.3 Distal Limit of Bile Duct Resection Line During HCCa Surgery

As for distal tumor extension along the bile duct, it is theoretically possible to secure a cancer-free margin through concomitant pancreatoduodenectomy (HPD) [6, 7]. HPD usually involves concomitant pancreatoduodenectomy in a hemihepatectomy or more extended hepatobiliary resection in surgery for HCCa (Fig. 18.4). Right-sided hepatectomy is more often involved in HPD than left-sided hepatectomy according to the tumor extent; there is a risk of potential invasion of the right hepatic artery. This procedure is one of the most delicate operations in terms of the degree of invasiveness, and often carries high morbidity and mortality rates. With improved perioperative management and surgical techniques, the short-term outcome for patients undergoing HPD has improved, but the current results are still unsatisfactory [7, 17]. Thus, the selection criteria for HPD should be strict in selected patients with extensive disease.

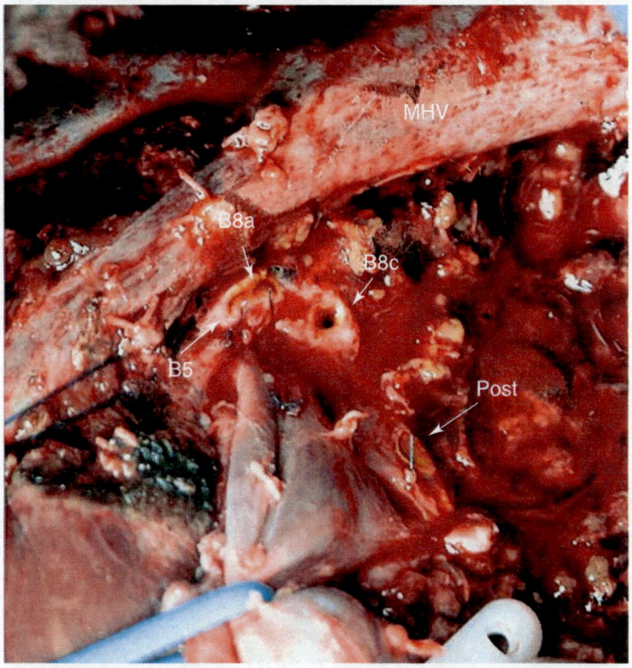

Fig. 18.3 The representative case of left hemihepatectomy with caudate lobectomy depicts bile duct stumps around the right portal vein and the right hepatic arterial branches on the raw surface of the liver. *MHV* middle hepatic vein, *B5* right anteroinferior segmental duct, *B8a* ventral branch of the right anterosuperior segmental duct, *B8c* dorsal branch of the right anterosuperior segmental duct, *Post* right posterior sectional duct

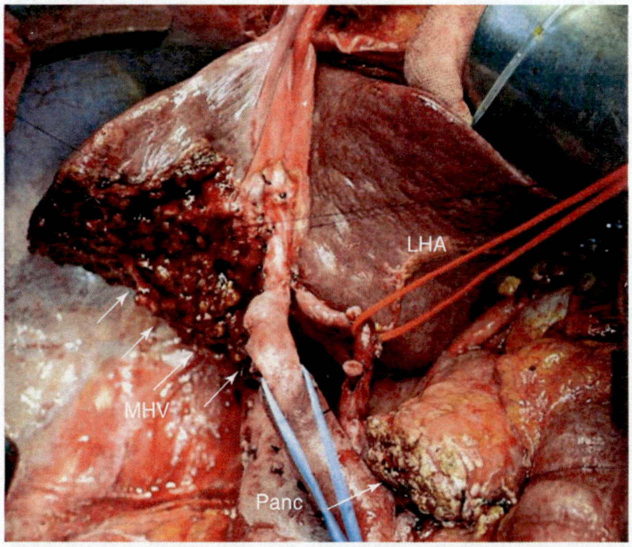

Fig.18.4 This is an intraoperative photograph after the right hepatopancreatoduodenectomy (right hemihepatectomy with pancreatoduodenectomy) with caudate lobectomy. *LHA* left hepatic artery, *MHV* middle hepatic vein, *Panc* stump of the pancreas

Several predictive factors affecting postoperative survival after surgery for HCCa are reported in the literature. Although in situ cancer at the proximal bile duct margin does not have a strong impact on survival compared with a positive bile duct margin with invasive cancer [18, 19], needless to say, a R0 resection is the ideal option for cure. Resected cases of biliary malignancies by HPD still remain few, so the future accumulation and analyses of HPD cases will delineate the patient profile with large benefit from this invasive operation [3, 19, 20].

18.1.4 Preoperative Staging of HCCa

Preoperative staging is an important issue to estimate the possibility of radical surgery. The first step for staging of HCCa is now ultrasonography (US) followed by multidetector row computed tomography (MDCT) [2, 21] and it should be undertaken prior to biliary drainage for preventing modifications of the bile duct wall by a drainage catheter. The side of the liver resection can be determined by MDCT, and endoscopic naso-biliary drainage (ENBD) for the future remnant liver is performed to relieve cholestasis of the future remnant liver. Recently, ENBD is the first choice and percutaneous transhepatic biliary drainage (PTBD) is the second. Patients with endoscopic retrograde biliary drainage (ERBD) after developing clogging and/or segmental cholangitis, eventually require PTBD to recover from those serious complications. In an actual case of Bismuth type III and IV [22], multiple biliary drainages are often required. Only an endoscopic approach for biliary drainage using three or more stents is usually difficult, so additional PTBD is eventually indicated. We minimize PTBD sessions or the number of PTBD catheters which potentially causes seeding or implantation metastasis along the sinus tract of the PTBD [23]. PTBD still has a strong therapeutic impact on segmental cholangitis, which is a significant risk factor for postoperative morbidity and mortality [24]. Magnetic resonance cholangiopancreatography (MRCP) is insufficient to diagnose the difficult local anatomy of the separated intrahepatic segmental ducts and to design an appropriate operative procedure in patients with Bismuth type III or IV tumor [22]. Both proximal and distal cancer extension along the bile duct is evaluated by the combined use of percutaneous selective cholangiography and endoscopic retrograde cholangiography (ERC) or MRCP, and the resection lines of the separated intrahepatic segmental ducts in the future remnant liver are determined. Mapping biopsy under fluoroscopic guidance, peroral or percutaneous transhepatic cholangioscopy is also useful, especially in cases suspected of superficially spreading cholangiocarcinoma, to define the expected resection line of the proximal or distal bile duct [25].

Thanks to recent advances in imaging techniques, MDCT and three-dimensional CT angiography have replaced conventional angiography to assess the degree of vascular involvement and to delineate the vascular anatomy in each individual HCCa case [2, 21].

18.1.5 Limit of Liver Resection Volume for HCCa

The limit of the liver resection rate is critical to the strategy or decision regarding a radical resection in patients with HCCa. Currently, there is no definitive answer to the question: how much liver volume should be preserved to assure a feasible, safe resection? We routinely examine the indocyanine green (ICG) 15-min retention rate (R15), and the ICG clearance (K-value) is calculated when the serum total bilirubin level has decreased below 3 mg/dl. CT-volumetry is used to estimate the volume of the entire liver and the future remnant liver. PVE for the liver segment to be resected, has been advocated as a useful option to induce compensatory hypertrophy of the future remnant liver [10, 11]. If the estimated resection volume exceeds 55–60%of the whole liver, one must take into consideration the hepatic functional reserve or invasiveness of the additional procedure with concomitant vascular resection and/or pancreatic head resection. We can calculate ICG-K of the future remnant liver (ICG-Krem) according to CT-volumetric analysis by multiplying the ICG-K value by the ratio of future remnant liver volume. The guiding value of ICG-Krem for a safe operation is 0.06, and a 0.05 is considered as the minimal requirement to tolerate major hepatobiliary resection in our current treatment strategy. The actual future remnant liver volume and resection rate are another prime concern; the present ceiling is considered to be 250 mm [3] and 75 %, respectively. In CT-volumetry 2 weeks after PVE, there is an approximately 10 % volume gain in the future remnant liver, whereas there is a 10 % volume loss in the embolized liver to be resected [10, 11]. Although clinical utility and feasibility have been reported, the indication of preoperative PVE has still not been established. Cherqui et al. [26] reported the surgical results of major hepatobiliary resection without preoperative biliary drainage in 20 biliary cancer patients; the postoperative morbidity was significantly higher in the patients with jaundice, while the postoperative liver failure rate was 5 %, and mortality was documented in the same cases. The limit of the preoperative serum total bilirubin level for performing major hepatobiliary resection is also controversial. We usually perform resectional surgery 2–4 weeks after PVE, and when the serum total bilirubin level decreases below 2 mg/dl.

18.2 Surgery

18.2.1 Extent of Lymph Node and Nerve Plexus Dissection During HCCa Surgery

Although lymph node metastasis is known as one of the poor prognostic factors, there is no golden standard with regard to the extent of lymph node dissection. En-bloc dissection of the regional (cystic duct, pericholedochal, periportal, periduodenal, peripancreatic head, celiac) nodes is routine for radical resection for HCCa (Figs. 18.5, 18.6, 18.7, and 18.8). Inspection and sampling dissection of the paraaortic lymph node followed by intraoperative frozen section examination are often included. In a case with definitive paraaortic lymph node metastasis, the long-term outcome is usually disappointing [27], so the indications for aggressive surgery such as HPD [6] or extended hepatobiliary resection with complex vascular reconstruction [5] may require careful reconsideration.

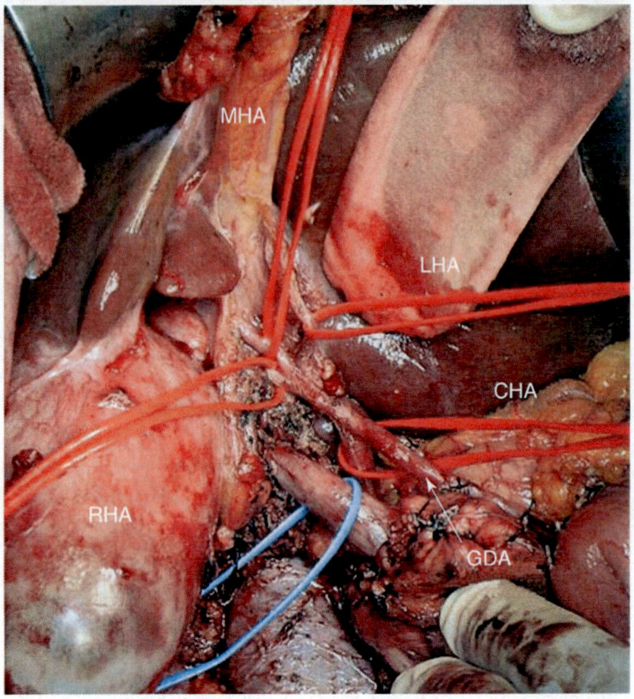

Fig. 18.5 An intraoperative photograph shows skeletonization of the hepatoduodenal ligament prior to right hemihepatectomy with caudate lobectomy. Various arteries and portal vein are isolated with a silicon rubber tape. *CHA* common hepatic artery, *GDA* gastroduodenal artery, *LHA* left hepatic artery, *MHA* middle hepatic artery, *RHA* right hepatic artery

On the other hand, we consider not only lymph nodes but also connective tissue clearance, especially the autonomic nerve plexus around the common hepatic, proper hepatic, and right or left hepatic arteries, is crucial for radical resection. Although the clinical impact or efficacy of nerve plexus dissection has not been established, biliary cancer is often associated with perineural invasion which is identified as a significant prognostic factor in bile duct [28] and gallbladder cancers [29]. Thus, we perform complete skeletonization of the hepatoduodenal ligament to achieve cancer-free dissection margins in radical resection for HCCa (Figs. 18.5, 18.6, 18.7, and 18.8). It is advisable to use topical application of

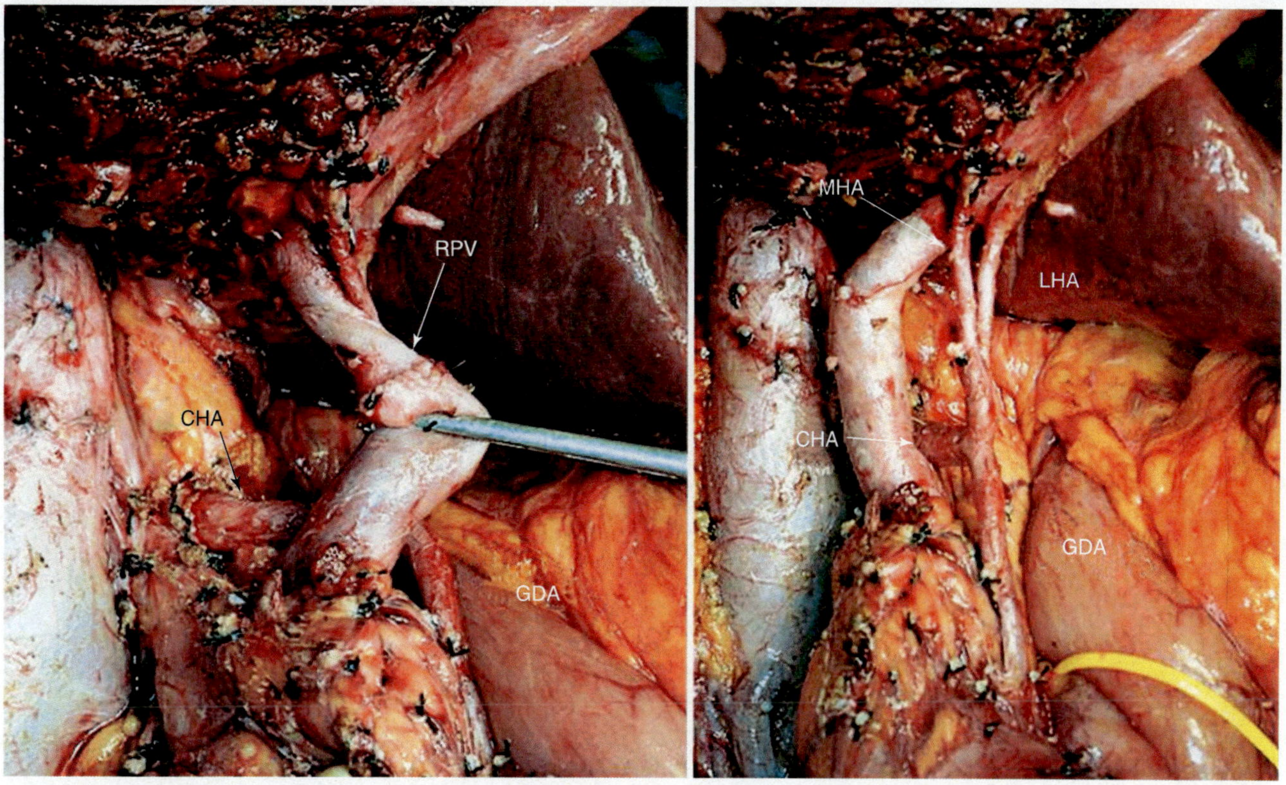

Fig. 18.6 Intraoperative photographs after a right hemihepatectomy with caudate lobectomy show complete skeletonization of the hepatoduodenal ligament and clearance of retropancreatic, celiac, and common hepatic lymph nodes. *CHA* common hepatic artery, *GDA* gastroduodenal artery, *LHA* left hepatic artery, *MHA* middle hepatic artery, *RPV* stump of the right portal vein

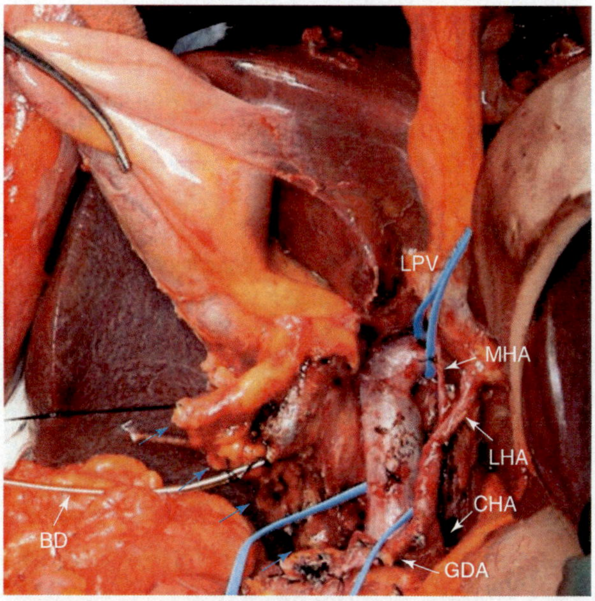

Fig. 18.7 An intraoperative photograph just prior to transecting the right portal vein depicts *en bloc* skeletonized connective tissue and lymph nodes surrounding the bile duct (*blue arrows*). The left portal vein (*LPV*) and portal vein are encircled with a silicon rubber tape. *BD* a tube for intraoperative biliary drainage, *CHA* common hepatic artery, *GDA* gastroduodenal artery, *LHA* left hepatic artery, *MHA* middle hepatic artery, *LPV* left portal vein

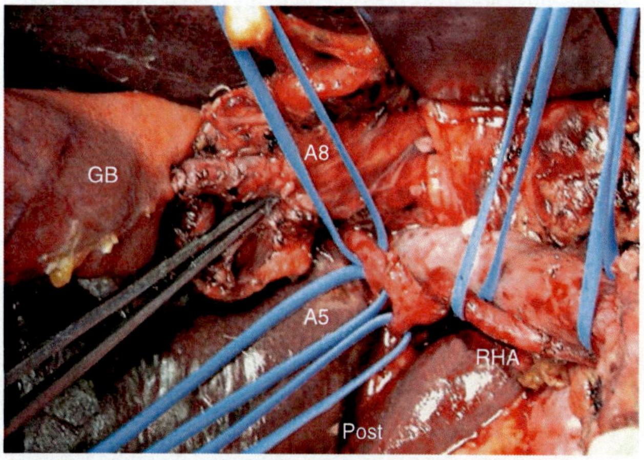

Fig. 18.8 An intraoperative photograph shows skeletonization of the hepatoduodenal ligament during the left hemihepatectomy with caudate lobectomy. Branches of the replaced right hepatic artery are isolated with silicon rubber tape. *GB* gallbladder, *A5* anteroinferior segmental branch of the right hepatic artery, *A8* anterosuperior segmental branch of the right hepatic artery, *Post* posterior sectional branch of the right hepatic artery, *RHA* replaced right hepatic artery from superior mesenteric artery

1 % procaine solution for the skeletonized hepatic artery to prevent spastic reaction of the artery followed by unexpected thrombosis.

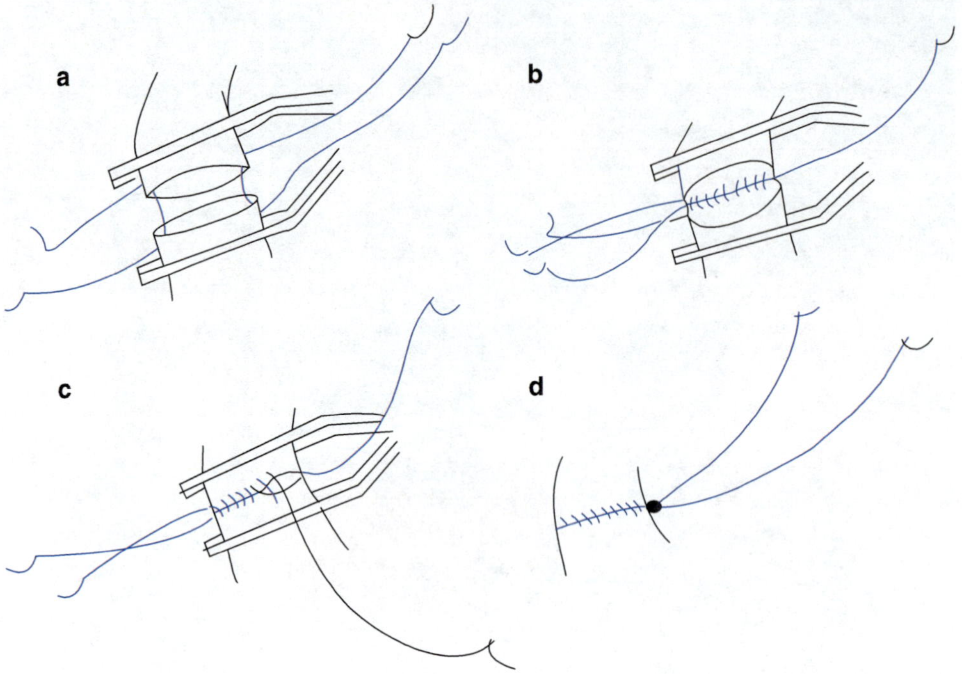

Fig. 18.9 Schematic drawing of the portal vein resection and reconstruction. At first, stay suture is placed bilaterally (**a**), and intraluminal technique is used for the posterior wall suture (**b**). Next, anterior wall anastomosis is performed using the same string (**c**), then single string continuous suture is completed (**d**)

18.2.2 Limit of Portal Vein Resection and Reconstruction

In right-sided hepatectomies, portal vein resection and reconstruction prior to liver parenchymal transection are feasible [30]. The wedge resection or segmental resection with end-to-end anastomosis is possible in many cases (Fig. 18.9), and segmental resection with an autologous vein grafting is uncommon in a right-sided hepatectomy. If the length of the portal vein resection exceeds 5 or 6 cm, an interposition graft must be required (Figs. 18.10 and 18.11). An external iliac vein is usually harvested through an extraperitoneal approach as an autologous graft for portal vein reconstruction, because the diameter of the external iliac vein is similar to that of the portal veins for reconstruction. Roughly one-fourth of the external iliac veins have a valve, so normograde reconstruction of the portal vein using an external iliac vein is essential to prevent portal thrombosis. In portal vein reconstruction using an interposition graft, the proximal anastomosis precedes the distal anastomosis. After releasing of the proximal clamp to expand the anastomotic side, the distal anastomosis is then performed. In left sided-hepatectomies, portal vein resection and reconstruction prior to liver resection are difficult and rare, and segmental autologous vein grafting is often required for reconstruction. Depending upon the defect of the resected portal vein to be reconstructed, a direct transverse suture, patch graft repair, or segmental vein grafting are selected for portal vein reconstruction. The limit of the portal vein resection and reconstruction during right-sided hepatectomies is the feasibility of cross-clamping of the root of the umbilical portion of the left portal vein. There is an exceptional case in which the left lateral inferior and umbilical portion of the left portal vein are isolated and separately clamped for the portal vein reconstruction during right hepatectomy. In left-sided hepatectomies, isolation and clamping of the right posterior sectional and/or the right anterior sectional portal vein are the critical procedure. For the end-to-end portal vein anastomosis, a stay stitch is placed on both sides and an intraluminal technique is usually used for the posterior wall suture, followed by anterior wall anastomosis using the over and over suture technique with 6-0 prolene.

In most cases undergoing portal vein resection and reconstruction, anticoagulant therapy is not employed. Color Doppler ultrasonography is used to examine the perioperative portal blood flow for patients undergoing portal vein resection and reconstruction [31]. We consider that the portal vein resection and reconstruction per se does not increase the operative risk during hepatobiliary resection; moreover, long-term survival is actually expected after this aggressive surgery [32]. Thus, the hepatobiliary surgeon should not hesitate to perform portal vein resection and reconstruction during hepatobiliary resection in case of a promising R0 resection for a locally advanced HCCa.

18.2.3 Hepatic Arterial Resection and Reconstruction During HCCa Surgery

Concomitant left hepatic arterial resection and reconstruction during right-sided hepatobiliary resection is uncommon and an extremely rare. The left hepatic artery usually runs along

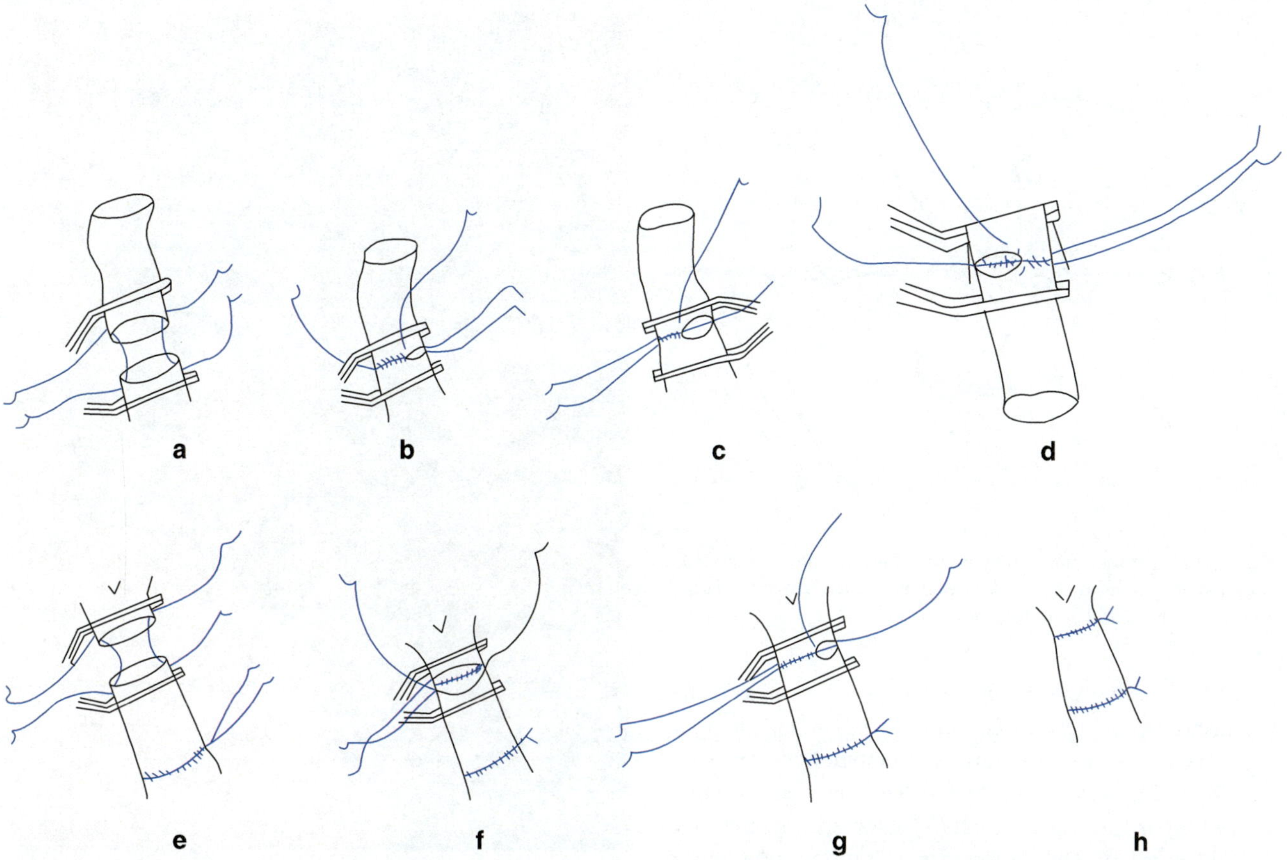

Fig. 18.10 Scheme of the interposition grafting for the portal vein reconstruction is illustrated. The proximal single-string continuous suture is performed (**a–d**), followed by the distal anastomosis (**e–h**). In case of the proximal anastomosis, over and over suture for both anterior and posterior wall is capable in terms of inversion of the graft (d)

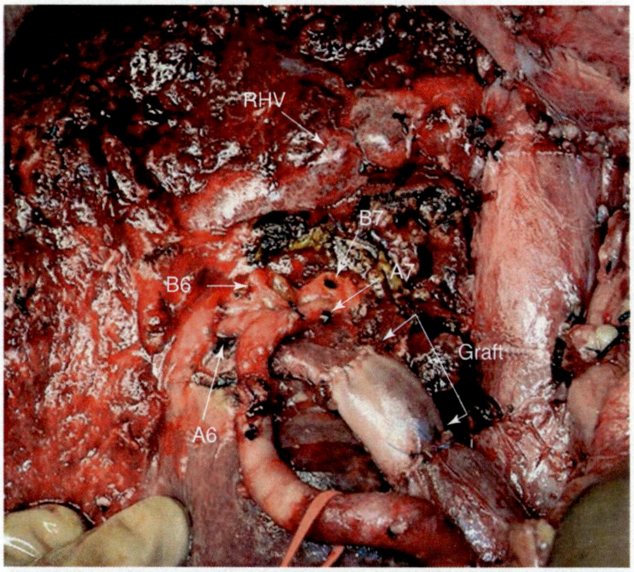

Fig. 18.11 Left trisectionectomy with caudate lobectomy with portal vein resection and reconstruction using an external iliac vein graft. There is no obvious caliber change in the reconstructed portal vein. *RHV* right hepatic vein, *A6* posteroinferior branch of the right hepatic artery, *A7* posterosuperior branch of the right hepatic artery, *B6* right posteroinferior segmental duct, *B7* right posterosuperior segmental duct

the left edge of the hepatoduodenal ligament, so a right-side predominant HCCa involving the left hepatic artery implies almost entire invasion of the hepatoduodenal ligament. In this event, it is virtually impossible to obtain tumor-free resection margins even after hepatoduodenal ligamentectomy, major hepatectomy with *en bloc* resection of the hepatic artery, portal vein, and pancreas head. In patients with a replaced left hepatic artery arising from the left gastric artery, hepatic arterial reconstruction is unnecessary for hepatoduodenal ligamentectomy, and the success of R0 resection might be further assured by preserving the replaced arterial blood supply [20].

In case of Bismuth type I or II [22] with definitive or suspected right hepatic arterial invasion, a right hemihepatectomy is ideal to achieve a R0 resection, but a left hemihepatectomy with right hepatic arterial resection and reconstruction is one of the alternative strategies for patients with poor liver functional reserve. Recently, a more aggressive approach to patients with more advanced left-side predominant HCCa has been applied through a left trisectionectomy using right hepatic arterial resection and reconstruction with or without simultaneous portal vein resection and reconstruction [5]. Most of the right hepatic

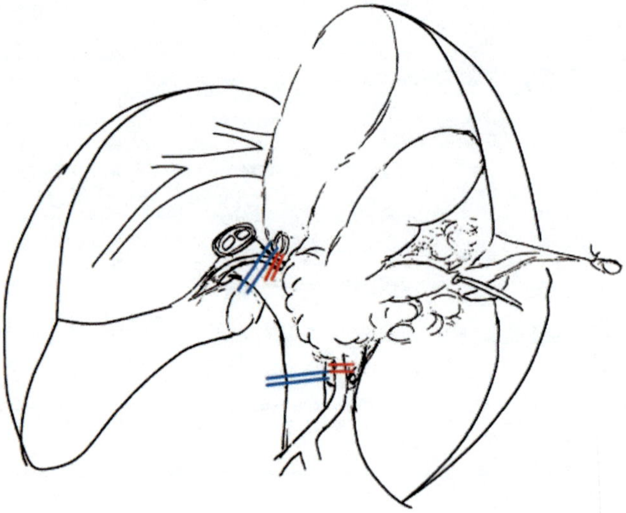

Fig. 18.12 Left trisectionectomy with portal vein and hepatic arterial resection and reconstruction. Portal vein and hepatic arterial resection lines are depicted with *double lines*

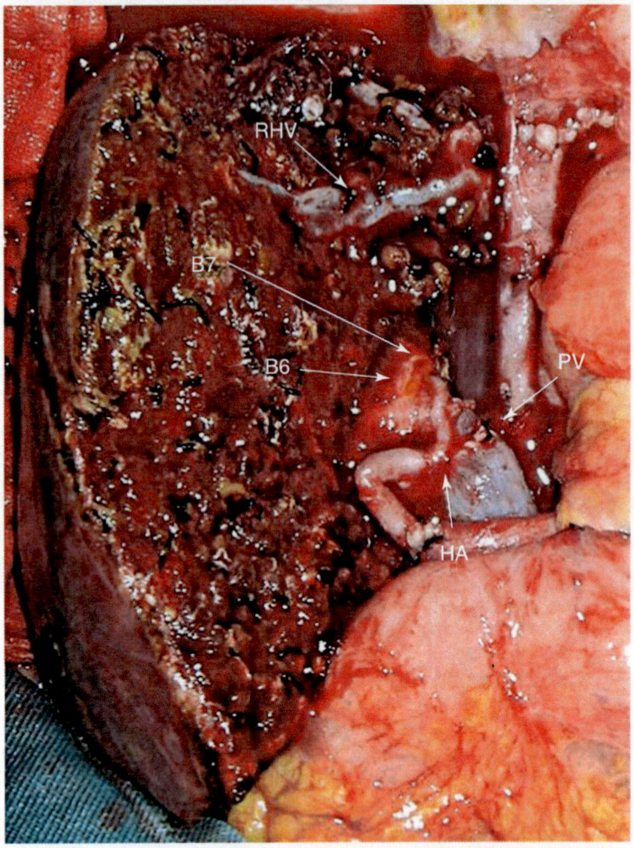

Fig. 18.13 Left trisectionectomy with caudate lobectomy plus portal vein and hepatic arterial resection and reconstruction. Portal vein is reconstructed in end-to-end fashion, and the right hepatic artery is reconstructed by end-to-end anastomosis between the right posterior branch and the proper hepatic artery. There is no obvious caliber change in the reconstructed portal vein. *RHV* right hepatic vein, *B6* right posteroinferior segmental duct, *B7* right posterosuperior segmental duct, *PV* anastomosis of the portal vein, *HA* anastomosis of the hepatic artery

arterial resection and reconstruction is done in left-sided hepatectomy, and reconstruction of the right hepatic artery with an end-to-end anastomosis is a common microsurgical technique (Figs. 18.12 and 18.13). The right gastroepiploic artery [33] or radial artery graft [5] is sometimes selected as a recipient artery. The posterior branch of the right hepatic artery often runs on the caudal side of the posterior branch of the right portal vein in the Rouviere's sulcus, making it easy to assess and ensure the cancer negative dissection of the posterior branch of the right hepatic artery prior to liver parenchymal transaction. On the other hand, the posterior branch of the right hepatic artery occasionally runs on the cranial side of the right portal vein, and it is difficult to assess the capability of securing the distal portion of the posterior branch of the right hepatic artery for reconstructing before proceeding in hepatectomy. This anatomical variation of the posterior branch of the right hepatic artery is a key issue to assess or decide the indication of the right hepatic arterial resection and reconstruction in case of a left-sided hepatectomy.

When arterial reconstruction is impossible, one possible countermeasure is arterialization of the portal vein using arterioportal shunting [34]. Oblique-to-side anastomosis is performed between the common hepatic artery and the main portal vein. Approximately 3 weeks after surgery, transcatheter arterial embolization of the common hepatic artery is carried out to prevent further portal hypertension. This procedure possibly prevents liver infarction or liver abscess in the remnant liver leading to postoperative liver failure. Preoperative left trisectional portal vein embolization is beneficial to enhance not only the compensatory hypertrophy of the future remnant liver, but also easy detection of the right portal fissure as the demarcation line on the liver surface just after clamping of the right hepatic artery in a case of left trisectionactomy.

18.2.4 General Procedures in Resectional Surgery for HCCa

After laparotomy, Kocher's maneuver is performed to mobilize the pancreas head and allow regional lymphadenectomy in the hepatoduodenal ligament and around the retropancreatic, and celiac arteries (Figs. 18.5 and 18.6). Simultaneously, the distal bile duct is isolated and resected at the intrapancreatic portion. The distal margin should be submitted for intraoperative frozen section examination. Once a negative resection margin is confirmed, the bile duct stump is closed with interrupted or continuous sutures of monofilament thread. If the distal bile duct margin is positive for cancer even after additional resection of the intrapancreatic bile

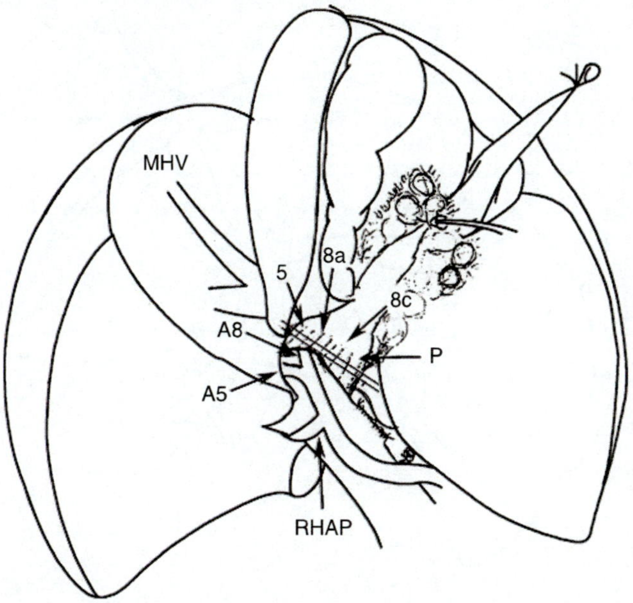

Fig. 18.14 Schematic illustration of left hemihepatectomy just prior to bile duct resection. The resection line is presented with double line. *P* right posterior sectional duct, *8a* ventral branch of the right anterosuperior segmental duct, *8c* dorsal branch of the right anterosuperior segmental duct, *5* right anteroinferior segmental duct, *RHAP* posterior sectional branch of the right hepatic artery, *A5* anteroinferior branch of the right hepatic artery, *A8* anterosuperior branch of the right hepatic artery

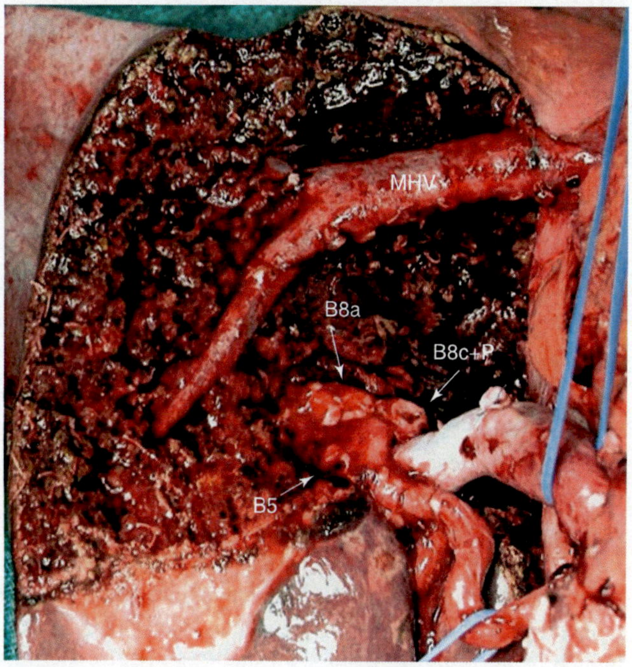

Fig. 18.15 Intraoperative photograph after left hemihepatectomy with caudate lobectomy. Middle hepatic vein (*MHV*) is clearly exposed on the raw surface of the liver and bile duct stumps formed around the right portal vein and the right hepatic arterial branches. *B5* right anteroinferior segmental duct, *B8a* ventral branch of the right anterosuperior segmental duct, *B8c* dorsal branch of the right anterosuperior segmental duct, *P* right posterior sectional duct

duct, indication of concomitant pancreaticoduodenectomy should be decided in terms of the status of the proximal and/or dissected margins. The posterior superior pancreatoduodenal artery should be divided in some cases of more distal intrapancreatic bile duct resection close to the papilla of Vater. Intraoperative biliary drainage through the resected end of the bile duct is advisable for patients with ENBD or ERBD, or without preoperative biliary drainage. Spilled bile contaminated with bacteria or tumor cells may well cause postoperative abdominal sepsis and/or seeding metastasis.

18.2.5 Left Hemihepatectomy with Caudate Lobectomy (Figs. 18.3, 18.8, 18.14, and 18.15)

During skeletonization of the hepatoduodenal ligament, the right gastric artery, then the left hepatic artery is ligated, transfixed, and divided. Next, the middle hepatic artery is divided. The main portal vein is skeletonized and encircled with a vessel loop. Careful division of the several tiny caudate branches around the portal bifurcation makes for easier division of the left portal vein at its origin by ligation with transfixing. Another way to divide the left portal vein is to clamp on the proximal side and the right portal vein, and oversew the venous stump with a transverse running suture of 6-0 prolene. After complete or partial detachment of the gallbladder from the gallbladder bed, the extrahepatic bile duct including lymph nodes and connective tissues is retracted in the cranio-ventral direction and the right hepatic artery is carefully isolated and encircled with a vessel loop; the cystic artery is then ligated and divided at its origin, and the right anterior and posterior branches are isolated. Meticulous manipulation and skeletonization dissection of the nerve plexus around the right hepatic artery is advisable. A demarcation line appearing on the main portal fissure is marked by electrocautery.

For complete mobilization of the left liver, the falciform and coronary ligaments are incised and the triangle ligament is ligated and divided. The root of the left (LHV) and middle hepatic vein (MHV) making a common trunk in many cases should be identified. Next, the distal side of the Arantius canal is ligated and divided, to make it easier to encircle the common trunk of LHV and MHV. The entire caudate lobe is completely mobilized on the right and ventrally and detached from the inferior vena cava (IVC) from the caudal to cranial direction. During this procedure the short hepatic veins (SHV) are carefully ligated and divided step by step. Thick SHV such as the caudate vein [35] often located around one-third of the cranial part of the caudate lobe should be clamped with a vascular forceps, then transected and sutured. Liver parenchymal transection is carried out along the demarcation line using an ultrasonic dissector or the forceps clamp crushing method. Hepatic inflow occlusion is employed for 20 min at 5-min intervals. The MHV appears on the transection plane, the left lateral aspect of the MHV is exposed, and the confluence of the MHV and LHV is identified. The root of the LHV is clamped, divided and closed with running sutures of 4-0 prolene. Then the liver parenchymal transection advances exposing the dorsal wall of the MHV in the direction of the right-side border of the IVC, a critical landmark of the right side margin of the right caudate lobe. Then, the caudate process and posterior section are divided in the cranial direction. Careful dissection of the branches of the right hepatic artery and the right portal vein is critical prior to transection of the right hepatic duct beneath the MHV at the expected point determined preoperatively. Bile duct transection starts from the ventral to the dorsal wall, and usually the orifices of the anteroinferior segmental duct (B5), ventral branch of the anterosuperior segmental duct (B8a), dorsal branch of the anterosuperior segmental duct (B8c), and the posterior sectional duct are observed in that order. These bile duct orifices are noticed around the right portal vein and the right hepatic arterial branches. Frozen sections of the proximal bile duct margins should be submitted to check the negative margins.

After completing hemostasis, hepaticoplasty prior to bilio-enterostomy using a Roux-en-Y jejunal limb is advisable to reduce the number of anastomoses and simplify the procedure. The external biliary stents are usually placed across the bilio-enteric anastomosis. Interrupted or continuous sutures of 5-0 monofilament absorbable thread are used. The enteral feeding tube is sometimes placed through the proximal jejunal limb for replacement of externally drained bile. A retrocolic and retrogastric route [36] is often selected to elevate the jejunal limb.

18.2.6 Right Hemihepatectomy with Caudate Lobectomy (Figs. 18.2, 18.7, 18.16, 18.17, and 18.18)

After retropancreatic lymph node dissection, the distal bile duct is dissected similarly to the *left hemihepatectomy*. Next, skeletonization of the hepatoduodenal ligament is follows, and then the common hepatic, gastroduodenal, and proper hepatic arteries are isolated with the vessel loops. The right gastric artery is ligated and divided, then the middle hepatic and the left hepatic arteries is identified, and the right hepatic artery is ligated, transfixed, and divided at its origin. Next, the portal vein is taped and skeletonized up to the portal bifurcation. After division of the caudate and the quadrate lobe branches, the main, left and right portal veins are encircled with the vessel loops. The right portal vein is transected

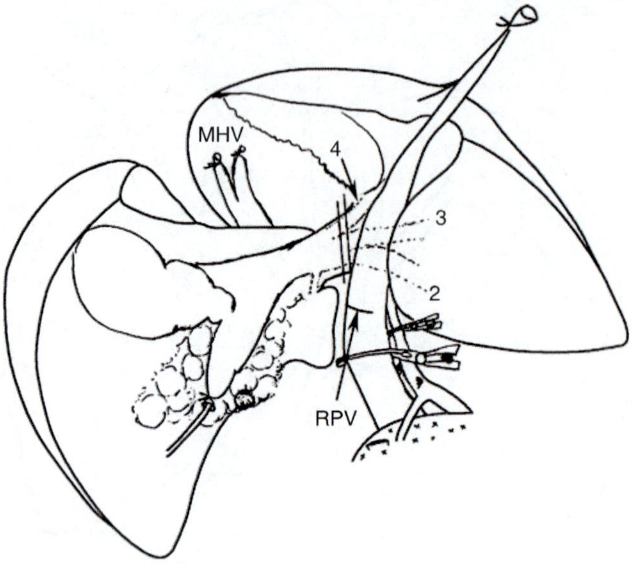

Fig. 18.16 Final step of the right hemihepatectomy. Bile duct resection is indicated by double lines. *2* left lateral inferior segmental duct, *3* left lateral superior segmental duct, *4* left medial sectional duct, *MHV* middle hepatic vein, *RPV* stump of the right portal vein

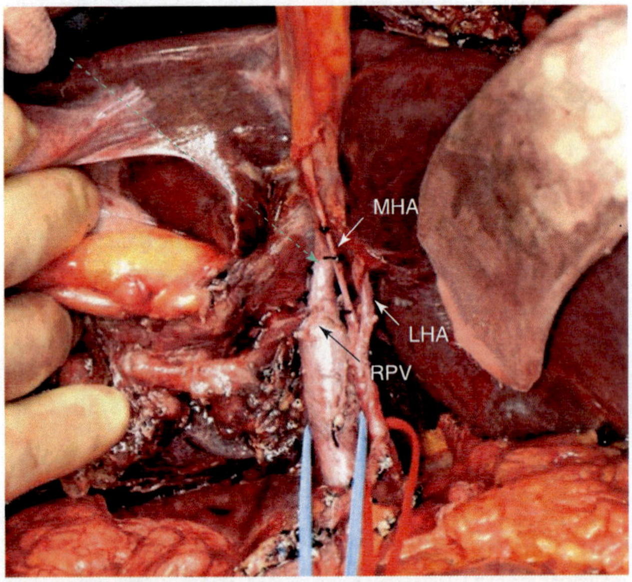

Fig. 18.17 *Dotted line* shows the liver transection line of the ventral part of the left medial section and the solid line depicts expected resection line of the bile duct during right hemihepatectomy with caudate lobectomy. *LHA* left hepatic artery, *MHA* middle hepatic artery, *RPV* stump of the right portal vein

after ligation with a transfixing suture. In patients who have undergone PVE, the main and the left portal vein are clamped with vascular forceps and the origin of the right portal vein is transversely incised to inspect the unexpected embolic material migration in the portal bifurcation. Any embolic materials, if detected, should be removed and washed out from the orifice of the right portal vein with heparinized saline. This

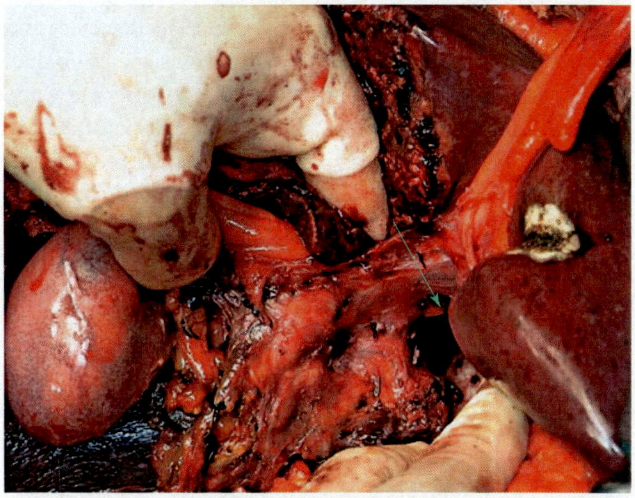

Fig. 18.18 Bile duct transection on the *solid line* is the final step during right hemihepatectomy with caudate lobectomy. The *green line* with an *arrow* indicate the line of bile duct transection as the final step during right hemihepatectomy with caudate lobectomy. The arrow points to the direction of transection from the surgeon's left to right

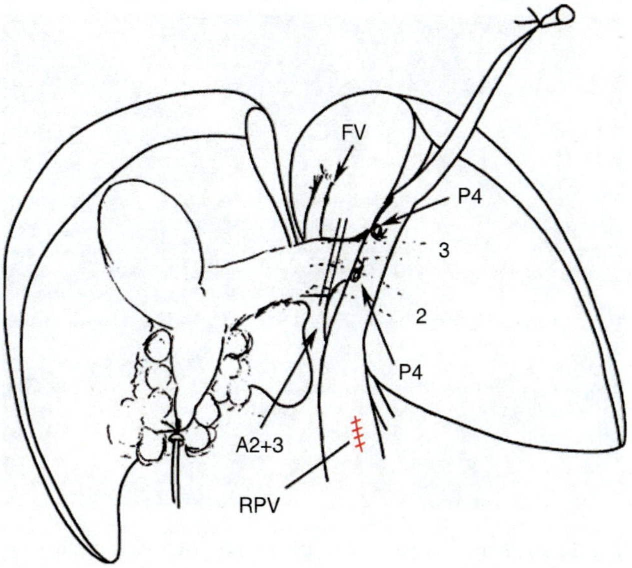

Fig. 18.19 Schematic illustration of anatomical right trisectionectomy just prior to bile duct resection (*double line*) depicts dissection along the cranial aspect of the umbilical portion of the left portal vein and exposure of the umbilical plate. *2* left lateral inferior segmental duct, *3* left lateral superior segmental duct, *FV* fissural vein, *A2+3* left hepatic artery, *RPV* stump of the right portal vein, *P4* stump of the medial sectional portal vein

orifice should be closed with transverse suture to prevent stenosis of the portal vein. On the other hand, in a case with apparent or suspected cancer invasion around the portal bifurcation, combined portal vein resection and reconstruction should be performed to obtain cancer-free dissection margins [4].

Next, the proximal origin of the Arantius canal is ligated and divided, and the Rex's recess is dissected to expose the visceral part of the umbilical portion of the left portal vein. At that time one can identify the left hepatic artery running into the liver from the left side of the umbilical portion of the portal vein. The middle hepatic artery (MHA) usually runs into the liver from the right side of umbilical portion of the left portal vein. Occasionally, the MHA arises from the left hepatic artery in the umbilical plate. On the other hand, MHA sometimes branches from RHA close to the left-side border of the common hepatic duct and may be potentially involved by the tumor. In such cases, combined resection of MHA is advisable to achieve R0 resection. If backflow bleeding from the hepatic-side stump of resected MHA is documented, we consider there is no indication for the reconstruction but simple ligation of MHA is thereby validated [37].

When a demarcation line appears along the main portal fissure, it is marked by electrocautery. On the inferior aspect of the left medial section, the liver transection line should be delimited transversely approximately 1 cm above (ventral to) the hilar plate to secure the negative surgical margin.

During mobilization of the right liver, detachment of the right adrenal gland is carefully carried out because dense adhesion between the right liver and the right adrenal gland is encountered in some patients. The right hepatic vein (RHV) is encircled, divided and closed with manual running sutures or a stapler device. The RHV is usually divided behind the liver before liver transaction which makes complete detachment of the entire caudate lobe from the IVC easier. The managements of SHV are similar to those for the left hemihepatectomy.

Liver parenchymal transection starts along the demarcation line during intermittent inflow occlusion similar to the left hemihepatectomy. The MHV appears on the transection plane, and the tributaries from the right liver should be carefully ligated and divided. From the confluence of the IVC, the dorsal aspect of the MHV is exposed and the operator at the same time pulls and turns the left caudate lobe right dorsally with the left fingers. Finally, the right and the left livers are connected with the left hepatic duct. The right liver with entire caudate lobe is held in the left hand of the operator, and the left hepatic duct is incised in the ventral to dorsal direction. Usually, we can identify orifices of B4, B3, and B2 in order, hepaticoplasty follows, and a bilioenterostomy is created.

18.2.7 Right Trisectionectomy with Caudate Lobectomy (Figs. 18.19, 18.20, and 18.21)

In case of right-sided hepatobiliary resection, especially in the right trisectionectomy, exposure of the umbilical portion of the left portal vein is a fundamental manipulation. We sometimes encounter a bridge in front of the umbilical portion of the left portal vein, so transection of this bridge is the first step to expose the umbilical portion of the left portal

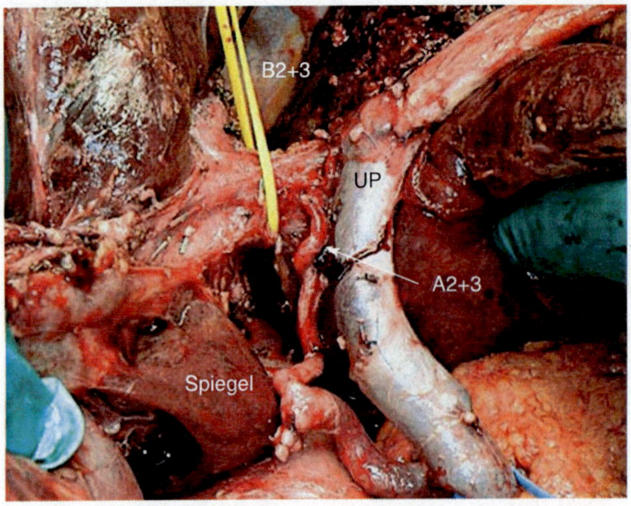

Fig. 18.20 Intraoperative photograph prior to bile duct resection during anatomical right trisectionectomy with caudate lobectomy demonstrates complete mobilization of the umbilical portion of the left portal vein (*UP*) and isolation of the left lateral superior and inferior segmental ducts with silicon rubber tape. The left lateral inferior and superior segmental branches of the hepatic artery is clearly exposed and identified between left lateral segmental ducts and UP. *B2* left lateral inferior segmental duct, *B3* left lateral superior segmental duct, *A2* left lateral inferior segmental branch of the hepatic artery, *A3* left lateral superior segmental branch of the hepatic artery

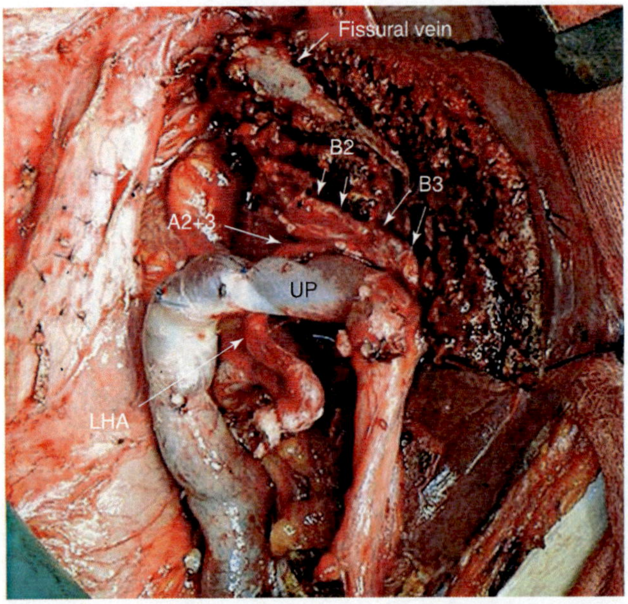

Fig. 18.21 A fissural vein can be identified on the raw surface of the liver after the anatomical right trisectionectomy with caudate lobectomy. Plural left lateral superior and inferior segmental ducts are observed. *B2* left lateral inferior segmental duct, *B3* left lateral superior segmental duct, *A2* left lateral inferior segmental branch of the hepatic artery, *A3* left lateral superior segmental branch of the hepatic artery, *LHA* left hepatic artery, *UP* umbilical portion of the left portal vein

vein. Surgeons must be aware that a thick bridge potentially includes the infra-portal bile duct [38, 39], which should be diagnosed preoperatively by MDCT. If the infra-portal left lateral or left lateral superior bile duct is detected and transected, bilioenteric anastomosis for transected bile duct is mandatory. After division of the middle hepatic artery, the visceral connective tissue of the umbilical portion of the left portal vein is dissected, and portal vein branches for the left medial section are ligated and divided step by step. Simultaneously, the proximal end of the Arantius canal is ligated and divided at the portal elbow.

In case of anatomic (extended) right trisectionectomy, all portal vein branches arising from the dorsal aspect of umbilical portion of the left portal vein should be completely ligated and divided [16]. This procedure provides complete mobilization of the umbilical portion of the left portal vein which can be completely turned out to confirm the root of the left lateral inferior (P2) and the left lateral superior (P3) segmental branches of the portal vein. Also, the left hepatic artery and its branches run through the left side of the umbilical portion of the left portal vein, and can be clearly identified between the bile ducts and the portal veins of the left lateral section. The demarcation line appears not on the right but rather on the left side of the falciform ligament. After complete mobilization of the right liver and caudate lobe similar to the *right hemihepatectomy*, liver parenchymal transection along the demarcation line starts using intermittent inflow occlusion. The fissural vein should be identified by intraoperative ultrasonography and preserved as far as possible. The middle hepatic vein is divided at its root with a stapler or sutured. Finally, the bile ducts are transected in the ventral to dorsal direction, and the left lateral superior segmental duct (B3) and left lateral inferior segmental duct (B2) are identified in order. Separate hepaticojejunostomies for B2 and B3 are required in the case of anatomic right trisectionectomy.

18.2.8 Left Trisectionectomy with Caudate Lobectomy (Figs. 18.11, 18.13, and 18.22)

Similarly to the *left hemihepatectomy*, retropancreatic lymph node dissection, and division of the distal bile duct are the first step. The right gastric, left hepatic, middle hepatic, cystic, and anterior branch of the right hepatic artery are identified, ligated, and divided step by step during the skeletonization of the hepatoduodenal ligament. Tiny branches for the caudate lobe around the portal bifurcation should be carefully ligated and divided, which makes it easier to isolate and encircle the left, right, right anterior, and right posterior portal veins. Preoperative left trisection PVE is indicated for most patients undergoing left trisectionectomy. Therefore, a careful inspection of the embolic material is advisable prior to transecting portal vein branches. If the embolic material migrates to the right or main portal vein, the embolic material must be removed from the right anterior or left portal

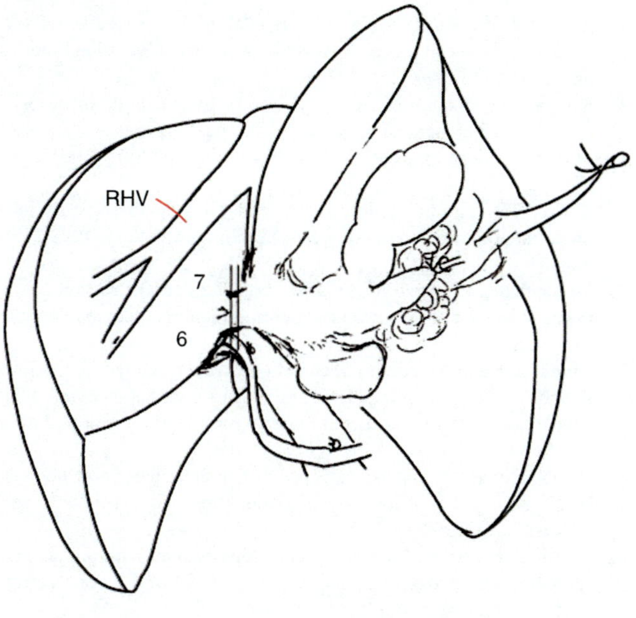

Fig. 18.22 Schematic illustration of the left trisectionectomy just prior to bile duct resection. *6* right posteroinferior segmental duct, *7* right posterosuperior segmental duct, *RHV* right hepatic vein

vein. After division of the left and the right anterior portal vein, both the right posterior branch of the portal and hepatic artery should be dissected further up to the predetermined resection line of the posterior sectional bile duct.

After the above-mentioned manipulations, a demarcation line corresponding to the right portal fissure appears and is marked by electrocautery. The distal portion of the Arantius canal is ligated and divided, which makes it easier to encircle the common trunk of the MHV and LHV. Then mobilization of the left liver and caudate lobe is completed similarly to the *left hemihepatectomy*. We prefer to divide the common trunk of the MHV and LHV with manual suture or a stapler technique prior to liver transection.

Liver transection along the demarcation line starts under intermittent inflow occlusion. The right hepatic vein should be exposed on the raw surface of the liver from the periphery to the confluence of the IVC, and the parenchymal transection between the caudate lobe and right posterior section then starts along the right edge of the IVC. Another critical landmark for transection is the root of the right posterior branch of the portal vein. The transection of the dorsal part of the right portal vein proceeds from the caudal side, and the transection plane is connected to the cranial plane. Finally, the left trisection of the liver and the caudate lobe are simply interconnected with the right posterior section through the posterior sectional bile duct. Adequate isolation of the right posterior portal and hepatic artery is confirmed, then the bile duct is divided for completion of the left hepatic trisectionectomy. Eventually, the bile duct orifices of the right posteroinferior branches (B6) and the right posterosuperior (B7) are sometimes identified separately.

18.2.9 Perioperative Management

Preoperative periodic bile culture, at least once a week, for possible positive bacteria for appropriate use of sensitive antibiotics is routine in patients with biliary drainage. Perioperative septic complications considerably influence surgical outcome [24]. To prevent severe septic complications, appropriate use of antibiotics as well as proper biliary drainage is crucial.

External biliary drainage without bile replacement impairs intestinal barrier function in patients with biliary obstruction, primarily due to physical damage to the integrity of the intestinal mucosa. Therefore, externally drained bile should be replaced as perioperative management for patients with HCCa to prevent bacterial translocation [40, 41]. In this connection, perioperative oral synbiotics administration can enhance immune responses and attenuate systemic postoperative inflammatory responses, as well as improve the intestinal microbial environment [42]. These procedures reduce postoperative infectious complications after major hepatobiliary resection, so perioperative synbiotics treatment deserves consideration as a management of choice for patients with HCCa.

Conclusion

We have various limitations for surgical treatment of HCCa, and the R0 resection still remains a difficult challenge for the surgeon. Coordination of the radicality and the safety of surgery for HCCa is the prime concern, and the many issues remaining to be resolved include precise determination of the tumor extent, liver resection volume, and estimation of the functional reserve of the future remnant liver, when the limitation of surgery for HCCa is discussed. Currently only several large surgical series treating HCCa have been published [14, 43–55]. Forthcoming accumulation of cases and evaluation of the surgical outcome will serve to delineate future problems to be addressed.

References

1. Nimura Y, Hayakawa N, Kamiya J, et al. Hepatic segmentectomy with caudate lobe resection for bile duct carcinoma of the hepatic hilus. World J Surg. 1990;14:535–43.
2. Senda Y, Nishio H, Oda K, et al. Value of multidetector row CT in the assessment of longitudinal extension of cholangiocarcinoma: correlation between MDCT and microscopic findings. World J Surg. 2009;33:1459–67.
3. Miyazaki M, Ito H, Nakagawa K, et al. Parenchyma-preserving hepatectomy in the surgical treatment of hilar cholangiocarcinoma. J Am Coll Surg. 1999;189:575–83.
4. Nimura Y, Hayakawa N, Kamiya J, et al. Combined portal vein and liver resection for carcinoma of the biliary tract. Br J Surg. 1991;78:727–31.

5. Nagino M, Nimura Y, Nishio H, et al. Hepatectomy with simultaneous resection of the portal vein and hepatic artery for advanced perihilar cholangiocarcinoma: an audit of 50 consecutive cases. Ann Surg. 2010;252:115–23.
6. Nimura Y, Hayakawa N, Kamiya J, et al. Hepatopancreatoduodenectomy for advanced carcinoma of the biliary tract. Hepatogastroenterology. 1991;38:170–5.
7. Ebata T, Nagino M, Nishio H, et al. Right hepatopancreatoduodenectomy: improvements over 23 years to attain acceptability. J Hepatobiliary Pancreat Surg. 2007;14:131–5.
8. Nagino M, Nimura Y, Hayakawa N, et al. Logistic regression and discriminant analyses of hepatic failure after liver resection for carcinoma of the biliary tract. World J Surg. 1993;17:250–5.
9. Makuuchi M, Thai BL, Takayasu K, et al. Preoperative portal embolization to increase safety of major hepatectomy for hilar bile duct carcinoma: a preliminary report. Surgery. 1990;107:521–7.
10. Nagino M, Nimura Y, Kamiya J, et al. Changes in hepatic lobe volume in biliary tract cancer patients after right portal vein embolization. Hepatology. 1995;21:434–9.
11. Imamura H, Shimada R, Kubota M, et al. Preoperative portal vein embolization: an audit of 84 patients. Hepatology. 1999;29:1099–105.
12. Nagino M, Kamiya J, Nishio H, et al. Two hundred forty consecutive portal vein embolizations before extended hepatectomy for biliary cancer: surgical outcome and long-term follow-up. Ann Surg. 2006;243:364–72.
13. Nimura Y, Kamiya J, Kondo S, et al. Aggressive preoperative management and extended surgery for hilar cholangiocarcinoma: Nagoya experience. J Hepatobiliary Pancreat Surg. 2000;7:155–62.
14. Sano T, Shimada K, Sakamoto Y, et al. One hundred two consecutive hepatobiliary resections for perihilar cholangiocarcinoma with zero mortality. Ann Surg. 2006;244:240–7.
15. Sakamoto Y, Kosuge T, Shimada K, et al. Prognostic factors of surgical resection in middle and distal bile duct cancer: an analysis of 55 patients concerning the significance of ductal and radial margins. Surgery. 2005;137:396–402.
16. Nagino M, Kamiya J, Arai T, et al. Anatomic right hepatic trisectionectomy (extended right hepatectomy) with caudate lobectomy for hilar cholangiocarcinoma. Ann Surg. 2006;243:28–32.
17. Wakai T, Shirai Y, Tsuchiya Y, et al. Combined major hepatectomy and pancreaticoduodenectomy for locally advanced biliary carcinoma: long-term results. World J Surg. 2008;32:1067–74.
18. Wakai T, Shirai Y, Moroda T, et al. Impact of ductal resection margin status on long-term survival in patients undergoing resection for extrahepatic cholangiocarcinoma. Cancer. 2005;103:1210–6.
19. Ojima H, Kanai Y, Iwasaki M, et al. Intraductal carcinoma component as a favorable prognostic factor in biliary tract carcinoma. Cancer Sci. 2009;100:62–70.
20. Maeba T, Maeta H, Wakabayashi H, et al. Modified hepatoduodenal ligamentectomy for advanced carcinoma of the biliary tract: the importance of preservation of the replaced left hepatic artery. J Hepatobiliary Pancreat Surg. 1998;5:297–302.
21. Sugiura T, Nishio H, Nagino M, et al. Value of multidetector-row computed tomography in diagnosis of portal vein invasion by perihilar cholangiocarcinoma. World J Surg. 2008;32:1478–84.
22. Bismuth H, Corlette MB. Intrahepatic cholangioenteric anastomosis in carcinoma of the hilus of the liver. Surg Gynecol Obstet. 1975;140:170–8.
23. Takahashi Y, Nagino M, Nishio H, et al. Percutaneous transhepatic biliary drainage catheter tract recurrence in cholangiocarcinoma. Br J Surg. 2010;97:1860–6.
24. Kanai M, Nimura Y, Kamiya J, et al. Preoperative intrahepatic segmental cholangitis in patients with advanced carcinoma involving the hepatic hilus. Surgery. 1996;119:498–504.
25. Nimura Y. Staging of biliary carcinoma: cholangiography and cholangioscopy. Endoscopy. 1993;25:76–90.
26. Cherqui D, Benoist S, Malassagne B, et al. Major liver resection for carcinoma in jaundiced patients without preoperative biliary drainage. Arch Surg. 2000;135:302–8.
27. Kitagawa Y, Nagino M, Kamiya J, et al. Lymph node metastasis from hilar cholangiocarcinoma: audit of 110 patients who underwent regional and paraaortic node dissection. Ann Surg. 2001;233:385–92.
28. Bhuiya MR, Nimura Y, Kamiya J, et al. Cinicopathologic studies on perineural invasion of bile duct carcinoma. Ann Surg. 1992;215:344–9.
29. Yamaguchi R, Nagino M, Oda K, et al. Perineural invasion has a negative impact on survival of patients with gallbladder carcinoma. Br J Surg. 2002;89:1130–6.
30. Kondo S, Katoh H, Hirano S, et al. Portal vein resection and reconstruction prior to hepatic dissection during right hepatectomy and caudate lobectomy for hepatobiliary cancer. Br J Surg. 2003;90:694–7.
31. Kin Y, Nimura Y, Hayakawa N, et al. Doppler analysis of hepatic blood flow predicts liver dysfunction after major hepatectomy. World J Surg. 1994;18:143–9.
32. Ebata T, Nagino M, Kamiya J, et al. Hepatectomy with portal vein resection for hilar cholangiocarcinoma: audit of 52 consecutive cases. Ann Surg. 2003;238:720–7.
33. Sakamoto Y, Sano T, Shimada K, et al. Clinical significance of reconstruction of the right hepatic artery for biliary malignancy. Langenbecks Arch Surg. 2006;391:203–8.
34. Kondo S, Hirano S, Ambo Y, et al. Arterioportal shunting as an alternative to microvascular reconstruction after hepatic artery resection. Br J Surg. 2004;91:248–51.
35. Takayama T, Makuuchi M, Kubota K, et al. Living-related transplantation of left liver plus caudate lobe. J Am Coll Surg. 2000;190:635–8.
36. Nagino M, Kamiya J, Kanai M, et al. Hepaticojejunostomy using a roux-en-Y jejunal limb via the retrocolic-retrogastric route. Langenbecks Arch Surg. 2002;387:188–9.
37. Hirano S, Kondo S, Tanaka E, et al. Safety of combined resection of the middle hepatic artery in right hemihepatectomy for hilar biliary malignancy. J Hepatobiliary Pancreat Surg. 2009;16:796–801.
38. Sugiura T, Nagino M, Kamiya J, et al. Infraportal bile duct of the caudate lobe: a troublesome anatomic variation in right-sided hepatectomy for perihilar cholangiocarcinoma. Ann Surg. 2007;246:794–8.
39. Ozden I, Kamiya J, Nagino M, et al. Clinicoanatomical study on the infraportal bile duct of segment 3. World J Surg. 2002;26:1441–5.
40. Kanazawa H, Nagino M, Kamiya S, et al. Synbiotics reduce postoperative infectious complications: a randomized controlled trial in biliary cancer patients undergoing hepatectomy. Langenbecks Arch Surg. 2005;390:104–13.
41. Kamiya S, Nagino M, Kanazawa H, et al. The value of bile replacement during external biliary drainage: an analysis of intestinal permeability, integrity, and microflora. Ann Surg. 2004;239:510–7.
42. Sugawara G, Nagino M, Nishio H, et al. Perioperative synbiotic treatment to prevent postoperative infectious complications in biliary cancer surgery: a randomized controlled trial. Ann Surg. 2006;244:706–14.
43. Seyama Y, Kubota K, Sano K, et al. Long-term outcome of extended hemihepatectomy for hilar bile duct cancer with no mortality and high survival rate. Ann Surg. 2003;238:73–83.
44. Kawasaki S, Imamura H, Kobayashi A, et al. Results of surgical resection for patients with hilar bile duct cancer: application of extended hepatectomy after biliary drainage and hemihepatic portal vein embolization. Ann Surg. 2003;238:84–92.
45. Neuhaus P, Jonas S, Bechstein WO, et al. Extended resections for hilar cholangiocarcinoma. Ann Surg. 1999;230:808–18.
46. Hemming AW, Reed AI, Fujita S, et al. Surgical management of hilar cholangiocarcinoma. Ann Surg. 2005;241:693–702.

47. Klempnauer J, Ridder GJ, von Wasielewski R, et al. Resectional surgery of hilar cholangiocarcinoma: a multivariate analysis of prognostic factors. J Clin Oncol. 1997;15:947–54.
48. Gerhards MF, van Gulik TM, de Wit LT, et al. Evaluation of morbidity and mortality after resection for hilar cholangiocarcinoma – a single center experience. Surgery. 2000;127:395–404.
49. Miyazaki M, Kimura F, Shimizu H, et al. One hundred seven consecutive surgical resections for hilar cholangiocarcinoma of bismuth types II, III, IV between 2001 and 2008. J Hepatobiliary Pancreat Sci. 2010;17:470–5.
50. Unno M, Katayose Y, Rikiyama T, et al. Major hepatectomy for perihilar cholangiocarcinoma. J Hepatobiliary Pancreat Sci. 2010;17:463–9.
51. Young AL, Prasad KR, Toogood GJ, et al. Surgical treatment of hilar cholangiocarcinoma in a new era: comparison among leading Eastern and Western Centers Leeds. J Hepatobiliary Pancreat Sci. 2010;17:497–504.
52. Lee SG, Song GW, Hwang S, et al. Surgical treatment of hilar cholangiocarcinoma in the new era: the Asan experience. J Hepatobiliary Pancreat Sci. 2010;17:476–89.
53. Hirano S, Kondo S, Tanaka E, et al. Outcome of surgical treatment of hilar cholangiocarcinoma: a special reference to postoperative morbidity and mortality. J Hepatobiliary Pancreat Sci. 2010;17: 455–62.
54. Igami T, Nishio H, Ebata T, et al. Surgical treatment of hilar cholangiocarcinoma in the "new era": the Nagoya university experience. J Hepatobiliary Pancreat Sci. 2010;17:449–54.
55. Rocha FG, Matsuo K, Blumgart LH, et al. Hilar cholangiocarcinoma: the memorial Sloan-Kettering cancer center experience. J Hepatobiliary Pancreat Sci. 2010;17:490–6.

Central Lobectomy

19

Z.Y. Huang and X.P. Chen

19.1 Introduction

Hilar cholangiocarcinoma, also known as Klatskin tumor or proximal extrahepatic cholangiocarcinoma, is an uncommon adenocarcinoma which arises from the epithelial cells of the biliary confluence of the right and left hepatic ducts. It accounts for nearly two thirds of cholangiocarcinoma and therefore is the most frequently encountered biliary tumor [1]. The estimated incidence of hilar cholangiocarcinoma is around 1:250,000 population. The cause for hilar cholangiocarcinoma is still unknown, although a variety of chronic inflammatory conditions of the biliary tree, such as sclerosing cholangitis, choledochal cysts, oriental cholangiohepatitis, and biliary parasitic disease, have been reported to increase the risk of bile duct cancers [2].

Unlike intrahepatic or distal cholangiocarcinoma, which can be treated with hepatic resection or pancreaticoduodenectomy, respectively, surgical management of hilar cholangiocarcinoma has evolved since its original description. In earlier decades, surgical management was primarily palliative with generally poor outcomes [3]. Early reports of resection of hilar cholangiocarcinoma typically involved resection of the biliary tree with hepaticojejunostomy [4]. In the last 20 years, surgical management of hilar cholangiocarcinoma has evolved due to improvements in preoperative imaging and an enhanced appreciation of tumor growth characteristics [5]. Unfortunately, despite these surgical advances, a significant proportion of hilar cholangiocarcinoma were deemed unresectable because of the locally aggressive nature of the disease, and survival rates after surgery have not substantially changed over the past 20 years. In a recent review of 25 studies on surgical resection for hilar cholangiocarcinoma published from 1990 to 2008, the resectability for hilar cholangiocarcinoma was 28–95 %, with a median resectability of 70 %. The curative resection rates ranged between 14 and 95 %. The 5-year survival rates varied from 25 to 40 % in recent series (Table 19.1) [5]. As complex biliary and hepatic resections are required to obtain complete resection, the risks of perioperative morbidity and mortality are significant. The median morbidity and mortality rates are 47 % (14–76 %) and 8 % (0–19 %), respectively. Perioperative morbidity includes bleeding, biliary fistula, liver failure, and infectious complications including cholangitis, liver abscess, intra-abdominal abscess, wound infection, and pneumonia. Of these, postoperative hepatic failure was particularly common, and mortality has been associated with the extent of liver resection [5].

Hilar cholangiocarcinoma is a relatively slow growing tumor and is usually tiny at clinical presentation. There is no effective screening for hilar cholangiocarcinoma and most patients with unresectable disease die within 4–8 months of diagnosis [6]. Palliative biliary drainage by stents or prostheses appears to confer a survival benefit of only a few months [7]. Treatment for hilar cholangiocarcinoma has remained challenging because of the lack of effective adjuvant treatment, the close proximity of the tumor to vital biliary and vascular structures as well as to other organs, and a limited ability to achieve complete resection owing to the locally advanced nature of the tumor at presentation [3]. The operative management of hilar cholangiocarcinoma has evolved since its first description by Durand-Fardel in 1840, and surgical resection is the only therapeutic option with a chance of cure. The goals of surgical resection should be complete excision of tumor with negative margins and reconstruction of biliary-enteric continuity. The ability to completely excise the tumor with negative margins is usually limited by its infiltrative and longitudinal spread pattern and its close proximity to the hepatic artery and portal vein. Furthermore, surgical therapy is dictated by the location of the tumor and the presence of underlying liver disease. Surgical therapy for hilar cholangiocarcinoma in the early 1970s was primarily palliative or it involved only bile duct resection and

Z.Y. Huang, MD • X.P. Chen, MD (✉)
Hepatic Surgery Center, Tongji Hospital, Tongji Medical College, Huazhong University of Science and Technology, Wuhan, China
e-mail: chenxp@medmail.com.cn

W.Y. Lau (ed.), *Hilar Cholangiocarcinoma*,
DOI 10.1007/978-94-007-6473-6_19, © Springer Science+Business Media Dordrecht and People's Medical Publishing House 2013

Table 19.1 Results of surgical resection for hilar cholangiocarcinoma

Authors	Published year	Resections (n)	Resectability (%)	Morbidity (%)	Mortality (%)	5-year survival rate (%)
Hadjis et al.	1990	27	NA	NA	7	22
Nimura et al.	1990	55	83	41	6	41[a]
Nakeeb et al.	1996	109	56	47	4	11
Su et al.	1996	49	28	47	10	15
Klempnauer et al.	1997	151	45	NA	10	28
Miyazaki et al.	1998	76	NA	33	13	26
Burke et al.	1998	30	43	NA	6	45
Neuhaus et al.	1999	80	NA	55	8	22
Kosuge et al.	1999	65	73	37	9	33
Launois et al.	2000	131	35	NA	19	NA
Gerhards et al.	2000	112	NA	65	18	NA
Nimura et al.	2000	142	80	49	9	26[b]
Todoroki et al.	2000	101	89	14	4	28
Jarnagin et al.	2001	80	50	64	10	26
Kawarada et al.	2002	65	89	28	2.3	26
Capussotti et al.	2002	36	NA	47	3	27
Kawasaki et al.	2003	79	75	14	1.3	22
Seyama et al.	2003	87	94	43	0	40
Rea et al.	2004	46	NA	52	9	26
Kondo et al.	2004	40	95	48	0	NA
IJitsma et al.	2004	42	NA	76	12	19
Hemming et al.	2005	53	50	40	9	35
Jarnagin et al.	2005	106	70	62	8	NA
Dinant et al.	2006	99	NA	62	15	27
Ito et al.	2008	38	55	32	0	33

NA indicates data not available

[a]Data from the patients who underwent curative resection

[b]Data from the patients who underwent hepatectomy

hepaticojejunostomy. The high rates of disease recurrence and poor survival outcomes after bile duct resection alone had led surgeons to pursue a more radical approach. Early experience using combined liver resection in hilar cholangiocarcinoma resulted in a low R0 resection rate with significantly high perioperative morbidity and mortality [8]. The development and evolution of liver surgery and perioperative care in the past 20 years has significantly improved the surgical management of hilar cholangiocarcinoma. At present, a combined radical bile duct resection and partial hepatectomy is the accepted surgical approach for hilar cholangiocarcinoma. Concomitant liver resection is one of the most important elements of the surgical procedure to achieve negative resection margins. In a report from the Memorial Sloan-Kettering Cancer Center negative margins could be achieved in 84 % of patients who received partial hepatectomy as compared to 56 % of patients who did not have hepatectomy. The 5-year survival in the liver resection group in this series was 39 %, while none of the patients who did not have liver resection survived for 5 years [9]. A recent study demonstrated that the R0 resection rate and patient survival significantly improved over time after the addition of partial hepatectomy to bile duct resection [10]. There was a positive correlation between the rates of R0 resection and partial hepatectomy in surgical therapy for hilar cholangiocarcinoma [11]. Moreover, surgical adjuvant strategies such as portal vein embolization have resulted in increased rates of major liver resections and negative resection margins as well as improved rates in recurrence-free survival [12, 13].

19.2 Major Liver Resection

Surgeons from Japan and the West have performed major liver resection in order to increase the curative resection rate. Neuhaus et al. advocated the inclusion of portal vein resection and showed increased resectability and survival rates [14, 15]. Some centers routinely include hepatic segment 1 resection because of the proximity of the caudate lobe duct to the hilar bifurcation to achieve tumor clearance [16, 17]. Unfortunately, the prognosis of these patients after such extensive surgery has not been significantly improved further and this approach increased the 5-year survival rate to less than 50 % only in one reported series up to the present time [18]. These unsatisfactory results have been attributed largely to the high operative morbidity (40–71.2 %) and mortality

(6.9–17 %) rates after major liver resection in patients with an obstructed biliary system [10, 19–28]. Specifically, in patients with cirrhotic livers or impaired liver function or both, the minimal required amount of functional liver volume in the remnant liver after liver resection increases. Liver failure is one of the main causes of postoperative morbidity and it is directly associated with mortality. In the majority of cases, the liver remnant consists only of 2–3 segments, posing a great risk for postoperative small-for-size syndrome and liver failure. Although a few authors reported that major hepatectomy can be carried out without liver failure or mortality by using preoperative portal vein embolization (PVE) together with preoperative biliary drainage (BD), high mortality rates up to 6.9–17 % after major liver resection have been reported by most authors, with the main causes of death due to insufficient functional liver remnant and liver failure.

19.3 Liver Transplantation

Because of the limitations of surgical resection, orthotopic liver transplantation (OLT) was initially proposed as an optimal solution. Complete hepatectomy followed by transplantation addressed all the problems related to resection margins and the underlying liver disease such as primary sclerosing cholangitis, a primary risk factor for hilar cholangiocarcinoma. Unfortunately, the experience with liver transplantation for hilar cholangiocarcinoma was uniformly disappointing, with a high incidence of disease recurrence and subsequent mortality. In a recent review, Meyer et al. reported the results of liver transplantation for cholangiocarcinoma in 207 patients: the 2- and 5-year survival rates were 48 and 23 %, but >50 % of patients had a recurrence within 2 years, with a median time from transplantation to recurrence of 9 months and a median time between recurrence and death of 2 months [29]. The Spanish liver transplant centers reported a similar result of 30 % 5-year survival and a 53 % tumor recurrence rate for 36 patients with nondisseminated, unresectable hilar cholangiocarcinoma [30]. Recently, the so-called "Mayo protocol" has been developed with the intent of treating a highly selected group of patients with hilar cholangiocarcinoma with a strict regimen of preoperative staging and neoadjuvant treatment followed by OLT [31]. Patients eligible for OLT under this protocol have locally advanced tumors but no pathologic nodal disease. Furthermore, the prolonged course of neoadjuvant therapy, staging laparotomy, and time on the OLT waiting list provide an opportunity to exclude patients demonstrating disease progression. This highly rigorous selection bias in favor of patients with biologically favorable disease is reflected in the early outcomes published from the Mayo group. In 38 patients who received this protocol, a 5-year survival of 82 % was reported (as compared with a 5-year survival of 21 % after resection, which included patients with nodal disease, $P = 0.022$) [32]. The patients who ultimately underwent OLT were generally young (mean age 48 years). Pathologic analysis of the resected specimens confirmed N0 and R0 status in all patients. Later outcomes on 65 patients who received this protocol showed a 1-year survival of 91 % and a 5 year survival of 76 % (mean follow-up 32 months) [33]. Another study by Wu et al. used *en bloc* total hepatectomy-pancreaticoduodenectomy-orthotopic liver transplantation (OLT-Whipple) to achieve a complete eradication of early-stage cholangiocarcinoma (CC) complicating primary sclerosing cholangitis (PSC). Between 1988 and 2001, CC was detected in 8 of 42 PSC patients who were followed-up according to a surveillance protocol, 6 of whom underwent OLT-Whipple. Of these 6 patients, 4 had stage I CC, and 2 had stage II CC. All 6 OLT-Whipple patients received combined external-beam and brachytherapy radiotherapy. One patient died 55 months post-transplant of an unrelated cause, without tumor recurrence. The other 5 were well and without recurrence at 5.7, 7.0, 8.7, 8.8, and 10.1 years. The authors concluded that, for patients with an early-stage hilar CC complicating PSC, broad and lesion-focused radiotherapy combined with OLT-Whipple to remove the biliary epithelium *en bloc* offered promising long-term, tumor-free survival [34]. However, these data originated from a single centre with specialized interest in this disease; the generalizability of this experience remains untested. Thus, OLT in the setting of hilar cholangiocarcinoma is controversial and deserves more studies.

19.4 Central Lobectomy

19.4.1 Anatomic Basis and Rationale

A reduction in morbidity and mortality after liver resection is the key strategy for improving the results of surgical treatment of hilar cholangiocarcinoma. Central lobectomy is a way to resolve this problem. Central lobectomy, a segment-oriented procedure, preserves more functional liver tissue than either extended left or right hepatectomy. More than 30 years ago, McBride and Wallace described central liver resection for a centrally located tumor in a child [35]. This procedure has been referred to by different authors as central hepatectomy, central bi-/trisegmentectomy, middle lobectomy and middle hepatic segments resection. With this form of resection, later named as mesohepatectomy, the central liver segments 4 and/or 5, and 8 ± 1 are removed and the lateral sections remain intact (Fig. 19.1) [36]. This technique requires access to the right anterior portal pedicle and resects the area drained by the middle hepatic vein [37]. Depending on the size of the right and left lateral sections, parenchymal loss with central lobectomy can be up to 35 % less than with

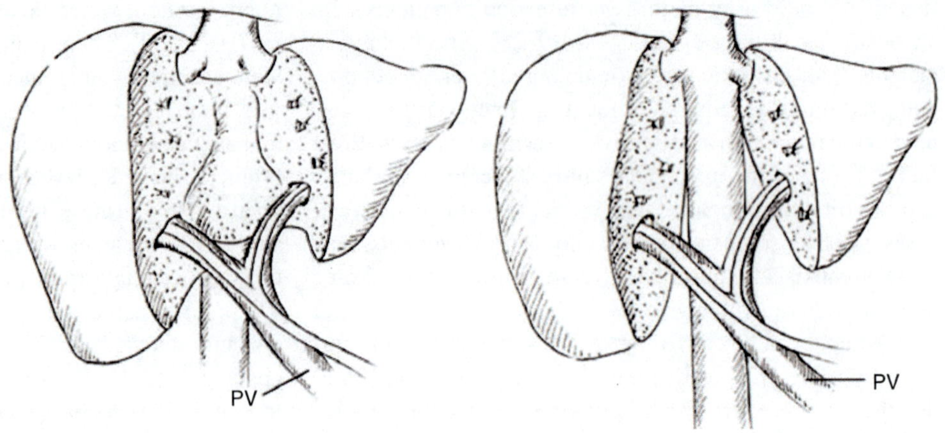

Fig. 19.1 Mesohepatectomy without excision of the caudate lobe (*left*) and with excision of the caudate lobe (*right*). *PV* portal vein

an extended right/left liver resection. Preserving more functional liver tissue is crucial for preventing postoperative liver failure. However, central lobectomy has not been widely applied, perhaps partly because of its complexity and partly because of the difficulties in bile duct reconstruction.

19.4.2 Assessment for Resectability

The American Joint Committee on Cancer (AJCC) TNM staging system is most commonly used to stage hilar cholangiocarcinoma. However, this system is based on pathologic criteria and does not provide information on the potential for resectability. The Bismuth-Corlette classification stratifies patients based on the extent of biliary involvement by tumor, which has been used to predict resectability and to assess the extent of resection [38]. In brief, Type I: tumors below the confluence of the left and right hepatic ducts; Type II: tumors reaching the confluence; Type IIIa and IIIb: tumors occluding the common hepatic duct and either the right or the left hepatic duct, respectively; and Type IV: tumors involving the confluence and both the right and left hepatic ducts [11]. Although it does not incorporate radial tumor extension, it provides a useful preoperative terminology to describe the extent of hepatic resection that will be necessary to encompass the longitudinal intraductal extension of hilar cholangiocarcinoma.

19.4.3 Surgical Principle

We determined the extent of liver resection in central lobectomy based on the Bismuth-Corlette classification of the tumor. Segment IVb resection is performed for type I tumors; segment IVb/extended IVb combined with segment I resection for type II tumors; segment IVb/extended IVb plus V/extended V combined with segment I resection for type IIIa and IIIb tumors without invasion of the right or left branches of the hepatic artery or portal vein; right/extended right hepatectomy combined with segment I resection for type IIIa tumors with invasion of the right branch of the portal vein or type IV tumors; and left/extended left hepatectomy combined with segment I resection for type IIIb tumors with invasion of the left branch of portal vein. On occasions, the extent of liver resection has to be modified during surgery to suit an individual patient. For tumors with invasion of both branches of the portal vein or the main portal vein, resection is not performed. Routine porta hepatis lymph node dissection is carried out with skeletonization of the portal vein and hepatic artery, and nodal clearance up to the celiac origin and around the head of pancreas. Where possible, gross resection margins of 1 cm is achieved for intrahepatic ducts.

19.5 Operative Procedures

19.5.1 Central Lobectomy

An incision is made 2 cm below the right costal margin extending from the midline to the right flank. A thorough exploration followed by intraoperative ultrasonography (IOUS) is performed.

The extent of resection depends on the extent of tumor in the bile duct, and whether the branches of the hepatic artery or portal vein are involved as determined before surgery on medical imaging and during operation by gross examination and IOUS. After porta hepatis lymph node dissection starting from the celiac plexus and the retropancreatic region, and with skeletonization of the hepatic artery and portal vein, the common bile duct is divided at the upper border of the pancreas. The gallbladder is dissected from its bed and the extrahepatic biliary tree dissected up to the hepatic hilum. The tumor is freed from the vessels if they have not been invaded by the tumor. The amount of liver to be resected is determined and the appropriate feeding vessels are ligated and divided. The liver is fully mobilized and the caudate lobe dissected from the inferior vena cava for combined segment

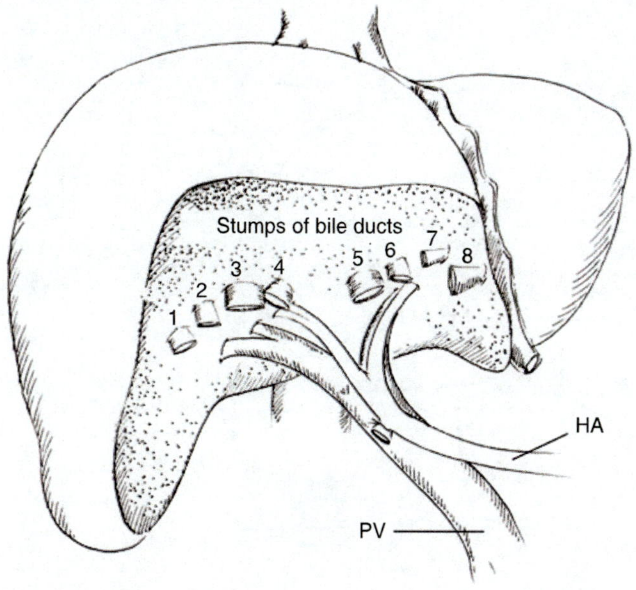

Fig. 19.2 Intrahepatic ductal openings on the remnant liver. *1–8* Stumps of bile duct, *PV* portal vein, *HA* hepatic artery

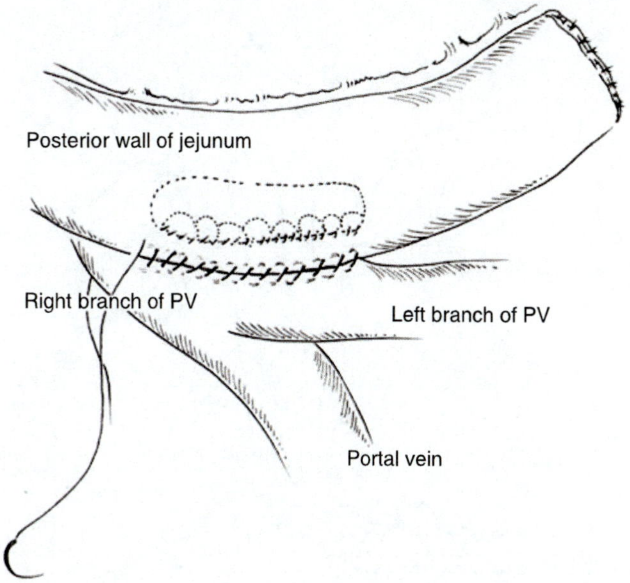

Fig. 19.3 Operative diagram showing anastomosis involving the posterior wall of jejunum: a continuous 4/0 polypropylene suture was used to sew the seromuscular layer of the posterior wall of jejunum to the wall of the right and left branches of the portal vein. *PV* portal vein, *R* right branch of portal vein, *L* left branch of portal vein

I resection. Under IOUS guidance, the line of liver transection is marked on the surface of the liver by diathermy 1 cm away from the margin of the tumor. The liver parenchyma and intrahepatic bile ducts are transected and the specimen is removed *en bloc* with the extrahepatic duct and the gallbladder. There are usually three to five divided openings for right intrahepatic ducts and two to four divided openings for left intrahepatic ducts; the diameter of these openings varied from 0.2 to 1 cm (Fig. 19.2).

19.5.2 Hepaticojejunostomy

Hepaticojejunostomy is made in an end-to-end fashion for patients who have resection of segment IVb with or without segment I, and in an end-to-side fashion in patients who have resection of segments IVb, V and I. First, adjacent hepatic ducts are sutured together to form a single large duct for anastomosis. Mucosal to mucosal anastomosis is then made between a Roux-en-Y loop of jejunum and the bile duct using continuous 4/0 polypropylene. When it is not possible to join the intrahepatic bile ducts because their openings are too far away from one another, the jejunum is sutured to the adjacent liver around the bile duct openings with intermittent 3/0 polypropylene U sutures. When the intrahepatic ducts are small and thin walled, the seromuscular layer of the posterior wall of the jejunum is anastomosed to the adjacent walls of the portal venous branches with continuous 4/0 polypropylene sutures (Fig. 19.3) to ensure stability of the anastomosis. The anterior wall of the anastomosis is made between the jejunum and the liver adjacent to the bile duct openings with intermittent U sutures (Fig. 19.4).

Transhepatic tubes are not used. A drainage tube is placed inside the Roux-en-Y jejunal loop next to the hepatojejunal anastomosis to monitor postoperative bile secretion and to reduce pressure within the loop, thus helping the anastomosis to heal. The tube is brought out from the loop 10 cm away from the anastomosis. Abdominal drainage tubes are placed on either side of the hepatojejunal anastomosis, and brought to the outside through separate stab incisions in the abdominal wall.

19.6 Feasibility and Safety of Central Lobectomy

Mehrabi et al. [36] reviewed and analyzed all reported cases of mesohepatectomy found in the PubMed database between 1972 and April 2008. There were no restrictions on the number of reported patients, although some articles reported on a mixed population of patients who underwent different types of resection. The data of 859 patients (including 48 patients reported by the authors) were analyzed. In 658 patients with available data, the three most common indications for mesohepatectomy were HCC (82.7 %, n=544), liver metastasis (11.1 %, n=73), and hilar cholangiocarcinoma(3.4 %, n=22). The recorded data of 636 patients showed 27.8 % (n=177) had complications after mesohepatectomy. The majority of these complications were pleural effusion or pneumonia (12.6 %, n=80), ascites (4.1 %, n=26), bilioma or bile leakage (3.5 %, n=22), wound infection (1.1 %,

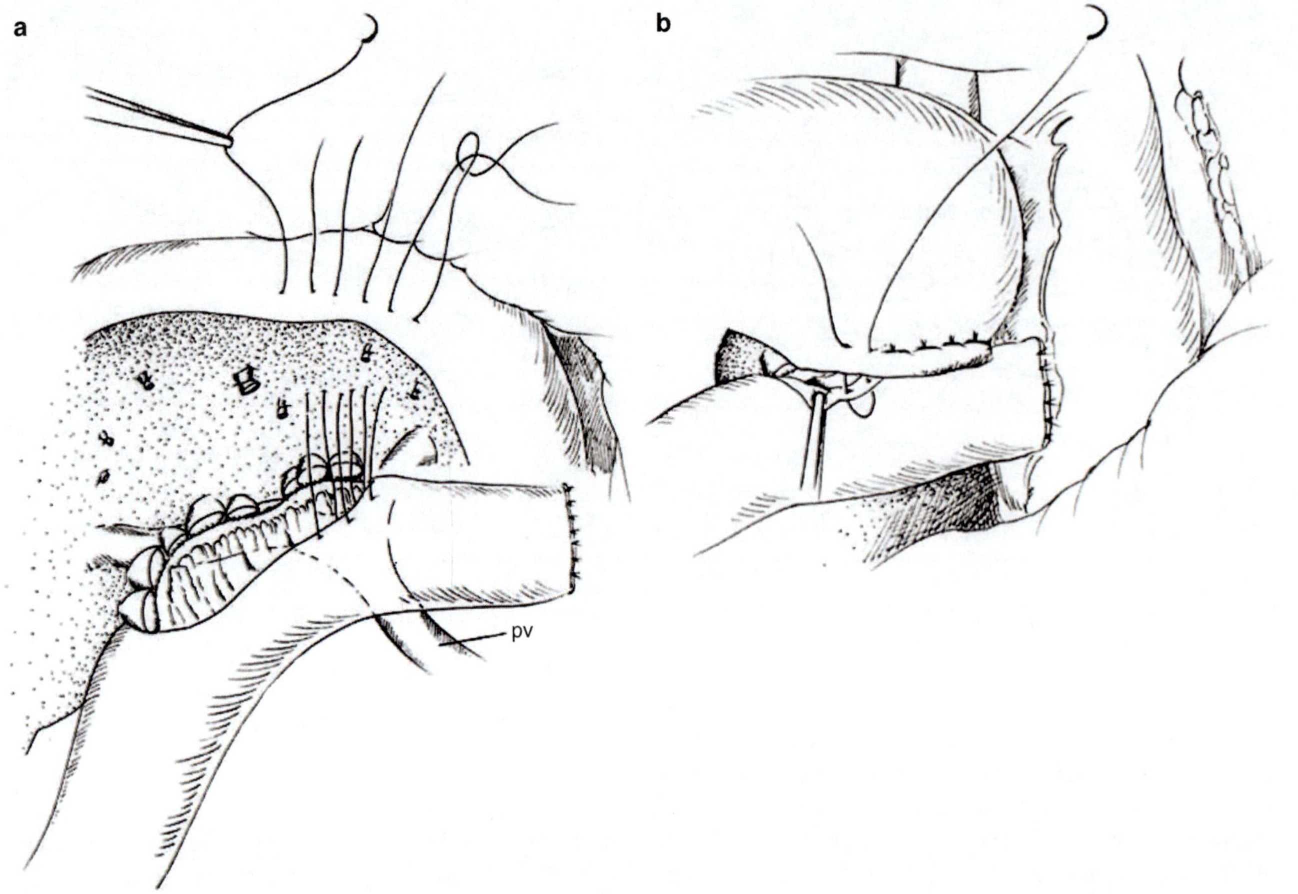

Fig. 19.4 (**a**) Start of the anterior anastomosis: the anterior edge of the jejunal opening was sutured to the edge of the liver adjacent to the bile duct opening. (**b**) Anterior anastomosis almost completed. *PV* portal vein

n=7), intraabdominal/subphrenic abscess (1.1 %, n=7), temporary renal insufficiency (0.6 %, n=4), and hemorrhage/hematoma (0.6 %, n=4). Interestingly, the mortality rate after mesohepatectomy for 756 patients was 1.6 %(n=12) (range 0–6 %), and this was mainly due to liver failure (42 %, 5 of 12) [36]. We previously reported on 256 patients who received mesohepatectomy for hepatocellular carcinoma. The in-hospital mortality rate was 0.4 % and the postoperative morbidity rate was 28.1 % [39]. In another report by us on mesohepatectomy on 93 patients with hilar cholangiocarcinoma, the morbidity and mortality were 22 and 0 %, respectively [40], which were lower than most published reports on extended hepatectomy [5].

19.7 Outcomes of Central Lobectomy for Hilar Cholangiocarcinoma

Between January 2000 and December 2007, 138 (73.8 %) of 187 patients with hilar cholangiocarcinoma who underwent surgical exploration at our centre (the Hepatic Surgery Centre, Tongji Hospital, Wuhan, China) had their tumors resected with an curative intent. There were 86 men and 52 women. The median age was 54 (range 26–72) years. These patients were evaluated before surgery with a baseline history, physical and biochemical examinations. Imaging included ultrasonography, computed tomography (CT) or magnetic resonance cholangiopancreatography, cholangiography through the percutaneous transhepatic or the endoscopic retrograde approach. Preoperative biliary drainage was performed only when jaundice had lasted for more than 4 weeks and the total bilirubin level was 200 μmol/L or higher. Preoperative portal vein embolization was not carried out. The criteria for resectability were absence of peritoneal or liver metastasis, tumor extension beyond the secondary biliary branches bilaterally, or extension to the secondary portal venous branches bilaterally.

With preoperative imaging and intraoperative findings (including IOUS), the Bismuth–Corlette classification of the 138 patients with hilar cholangiocarcinoma was: type I in 11 patients (8.0 %), type II in 34 patients (24.6 %), type IIIa in 43 patients (31.2 %), type IIIb in 35 patients (25.4 %) and type IV in 15 patients (10.9 %). Of the 45 patients who had a major hepatectomy, preoperative biliary drainage was performed in

Table 19.2 Extent of liver resection according to Bismuth–Corlette classification in 138 patients

		Bismuth–Corlette classification				
Extent of liver resection	No. of patients	Type I (n=11)	Type II (n=34)	Type IIIa (n=43)	Type IIIb (n=35)	Type IV (n=15)
Segment IVb/extended IVb resection	24	11	13			
Segment IVb/extended IVb+I resection	30		21	7	2	
Segment IVb/extended IVb+V/extended V + Iresection	39			32	7	
Right/extended right hepatectomy[a]	19			4		15
Left/extended left hepatectomy[a]	26				26	

[a]All left or right hepatectomies combined with segment I resection

11 patients who had jaundice for more than 4 weeks (range 4–7 weeks) and a total bilirubin level of 200 μmol/L or greater (range 200–410 μmol/L). Preoperative biliary drainage was not performed in 34 patients with jaundice for less than 4 weeks (range 4 days to 3 weeks); in five of these patients the total bilirubin level was more than 200 μmol/L (range 210–270 μmol/L). Preoperative biliary drainage was not performed in patients undergoing minor hepatectomy. No patient had preoperative portal vein embolization.

Segment IVb/extended IV resection was carried out in 24 patients with Bismuth–Corlette type I and II tumors that did not involve the cranioposterior wall of the hepatic duct bifurcation and the ducts to segment I. Segment IVb/extended IVb + I resection was performed in 30 patients with type II, IIIa and IIIb tumors with caudate lobe invasion but without vascular invasion. Segment IVb/extended IVb + V/extended V + I resection was carried out in 39 patients with type IIIa and IIIb tumors that had not invaded the right or left branches of the hepatic artery or portal vein. Right/extended right hepatectomy was performed in 19 patients with type IIIa tumors that had invaded the right branch of the hepatic artery or portal vein, or with type IV tumors. Left/extended left hepatectomy was undertaken in 26 patients with type IIIb tumors that had invaded the left branch of the hepatic artery or portal vein (Table 19.2). All left or right hepatectomies/extended hepatectomies were combined with caudate lobectomy, because caudate lobe involvement by tumor was common. Operating time ranged from 166 to 322 (median 195) minutes. Blood loss ranged from 100 to 1,260 (median 470) ml. Twenty-three patients received blood transfusion [median 2 (range 1–4) units].

Portal venous invasion was detected macroscopically in 45 patients (32.6 %) during surgery, and documented microscopically in a further 15 patients (10.9 %) after surgery. Hepatic arterial invasion was detected histopathologically in nine patients (6.5 %). The vascular involvement was ipsilateral to the side of the resected liver in all cases. Bile duct resection margins were negative in 123 patients (89.1 %) and positive in 15 (10.9 %). All patients with caudate lobe resection had negative resection margins, although extension of the tumor into the ducts of the caudate lobe was documented histopathologically in 37 (34.9 %) of 106 patients who had combined caudate lobectomy.

Table 19.3 Relationship between recurrence and extent of hepatectomy in patients with Bismuth–Corlette type IIIa and IIIb tumors

Extent of hepatectomy	No. of patients	IIIa/ IIIb	Tumor recurrence (%)
Minor resection	48	39/9	24 (50 %)
Major resection	30	4/26	16 (53 %)

During follow-up, tumor recurrence was detected in 76 (55.1 %) of 138 patients, at a median of 2.4 years. The longest interval to recurrence was 5.8 years. The relationship between tumor recurrence and surgery in patients with Bismuth–Corlette type IIIa and IIIb tumors is shown in Table 19.3. The liver remnant was the most common site of recurrence (23 patients, 33.8 %), followed by the retroperitoneum (17 patients, 25 %), the biliary tract (14 patients, 21 %), the peritoneum (11 patients, 16 %) and other sites (3 patients, 4 %). Some patients had more than one site of recurrence. Intrahepatic recurrence was usually adjacent to the liver transection plane. The rate of distant metastasis with or without local recurrence was found in 47 patients (69 %). An aggressive treatment was offered to the patients with recurrence, if possible, which included radiofrequency ablation in 22, microwave tissue coagulation in 14 and stereotactic radiotherapy in 11 patients. No patient with tumor recurrence was considered suitable for repeat resection with intent for cure. Systemic chemotherapy was not offered to any patient.

The median overall survival was 3.2 years for patients having a minor resection and 2.5 years for those having a major resection ($P=0.11$). Actuarial 1-, 3- and 5-year survival rates were 87, 54 and 34 % respectively for minor resection and 80, 42 and 27 % for major resection, with no significant difference between the groups ($P=0.300$) . On univariable

Table 19.4 Cox regression analysis of overall survival in 138 patients with hilar cholangiocarcinoma

Variables	Relative risk (95 % confidence interval)	P value
UICC stage	2.43 (0.29, 5.70)	0.001
Histopathological grade	2.50 (0.34, 4.79)	0.003

UICC International Union Against Cancer

Table 19.5 Comparison of outcomes between the extended hepatectomy (EXH) group and the parenchyma-preserving hepatectomy (PPH) group

Extent of hepatectomy	PPH (n=14) (%)	EXH (n=66) (%)	P value
R0 resection rate	93	71	>0.05
5-year survival rate	36	27	>0.05
Morbidity	14	48	<0.05
Hyperbilirubinemia rate	0	29	<0.05
Mortality	7	12	>0.05

Data were extracted from reference Miyazaki et al. [42]

analysis, prognostic factors that impacted significantly on long-term survival were portal vein resection, nodal involvement, vascular invasion, International Union against Cancer (UICC) tumor stage, blood transfusion and histopathological grade. On multivariable analysis, significant factors were UICC tumor stage and histopathological grade (Table 19.4).

Sotiropoulos et al. reported using partial or complete mesohepatectomy combined with resection of the hilar bifurcation to treat three cases of Klatskin tumors [41]. Two men and one woman with a median age of 62 years underwent resection of the hilar bifurcation, cholecystectomy, and lymphadenectomy of the liver hilum for clinically diagnosed Bismuth-Corlette type IV Klatskin adenocarcinoma. The first case entailed complete mesohepatectomy plus caudate lobectomy. Biliary reconstruction comprised 6 hepaticojejunostomies (4 right and 2 left ducts) into a single jejunal Roux-en-Y loop. The second case required resection of the quadrate lobe. To reestablish biliary drainage, 4 bile ducts on the right side and 5 bile ducts on the left side were reconstructed into a right and a left common opening, respectively. Subsequently, each common opening, as well as the caudate lobe duct, was anastomosed onto a single Roux-en-Y jejunal loop. The third case required resection of segment 4a. Biliary reconstruction was achieved with 5 hepaticojejunostomies (3 right and 2 left ducts) onto a single jejunal Roux-en-Y loop. All tumors were moderately differentiated. Histological evaluation of the hilar bifurcation showed Bismuth-Corlette type IV Klatskin carcinomas in the first two cases and type IIIB carcinoma in the third case. There was no lymphatic or hematogenous carcinomatosis, and all resection margins were negative for malignancy (R0 resections). Despite the complexity of the procedures undertaken, all three patients had uneventful post-operative courses. The first patient required reintervention 4 months after the primary surgery to resect a local recurrence on the cut surface of segment 5. No reconstruction of the hepaticojejunostomies was needed. He was alive and well at the time of the reporting, with no evidence of tumor recurrence, 87 months after the initial surgery. The second patient was also alive and tumor free 54 months after surgery. The third patient was diagnosed with tumor recurrence 4 months after the resection and died 8 months later (12 months after surgery).

Miyazaki et al. reported 93 patients with hilar cholangiocarcinoma who underwent surgical treatment (Table 19.5) [42]. The patients were stratified into three groups: the extended hepatectomy (EXH) group (n=66), the parenchyma-preserving hepatectomy (PPH) group (n=14), and the local resection (LR) group (n=13). The EXH group had more extensive hepatectomy than hemihepatectomy, the PPH group had hepatectomy less extensive than hemihepatectomy, and the LR group had extrahepatic bile duct resection without hepatic resection. Surgical curability of the PPH and EXH groups was better than the LR group. Fifty-four percent of patients in the LR group showed positive surgical margins at the hepatic stump of the bile duct, compared with 7 % in the PPH group and 20 % in the EXH group ($P<0.01$ for each comparison). Surgical morbidity was higher in the EXH group (48 %) than in the LR group (8 %) and the PPH group (14 %) ($P<0.01$ and $P<0.05$, respectively). Postoperative hyperbilirubinemia occurred more frequently in the EXH group (29 %) than the LR and PPH groups (0 and 0, respectively, $P<0.05$ for each comparison). Survival rates after resection were significantly higher in patients who underwent hepatectomy, including PPH and EXH, than patients who underwent LR, 29 % versus 8 % at 5 years, respectively ($P<0.05$). However, no significant difference in survival was found between the PPH and EXH groups. The authors concluded that curative resection is possible with PPH which improved the outcomes for patients with hilar cholangiocarcinoma localized at the hepatic duct confluence if vascular resection was not required. PPH provided benefits to highly selected patients chosen because of the local extent of the disease or because of liver dysfunction.

19.8 Further Comments

19.8.1 Local Resection Alone for Bismuth Type I and II Tumors?

Bismuth type I and II hilar cholangiocarcinomas appear less advanced on cholangiography and are easier to resect than Bismuth type III and IV tumors. As a consequence, many surgeons have chosen local or hilar resection (resection of the extrahepatic suprapancreatic biliary tract) as the treatment of choice for Bismuth type I and II tumors. Patients who receive such a limited resection frequently suffer from locoregional recurrence even after a R0 resection, and the prognosis is unexpectedly poor [9, 14, 43]. Neuhaus et al. reported on a dismal outcome after hilar resection in 14 patients with Bismuth type I or II tumors. R0 resection was achieved in only six (42.9 %) patients, and all patients died of recurrence within 5 years [14]. Kondo also reported on a poor prognosis after limited resection. In their series, including 19 patients with Bismuth type I and II tumors, 15 (78.9 %) patients underwent limited resection (bile duct resection in 9, isolated caudate lobectomy in 5, and left hepatectomy in 1). Although R0 resection was achieved in most patients, the 3-year survival rate was approximately 15 % and only one patient survived >3 years [43]. Capussotti et al. analyzed the results of surgery for Bismuth type I and II tumors and found the long-term outcome was markedly worse in the subset of patients who underwent bile duct resection; none survived more than 2 years [44]. These previous reports indicate that local or hilar resection alone is inadequate for Bismuth type I and II tumors.

19.8.2 Major Hepatectomy for Bismuth Type I and II Tumors?

Over the past 20 years, there has been an increase in the use of hepatic resection in patients with hilar cholangiocarcinoma. Major hepatic resection addresses both the problems of direct hepatic invasion and intraductal extension of hilar cholangiocarcinoma to achieve negative radial and longitudinal resection margins. Incorporation of major hepatic resection as a fundamental surgical strategy for this disease has increased the proportion of R0 resections, improved recurrence-free survival outcomes, and decreased the prevalence of hepatic recurrences. There are some authors who recommend right hepatectomy for all Bismuth type I and II tumors. Kawasaki et al. have stressed the importance of performing right hepatectomy with caudate lobectomy in all patients with Bismuth type I, II, IIIa, and IV tumors, and recommended left hepatectomy only in patients with Bismuth type IIIb. They believed that right hepatectomy offers the best chance of cure in Bismuth type I, II, and IV tumors in which the right and left hepatic ducts are involved to a similar extent. Although detailed data were not presented in their report, the mean survival for 17 patients with Bismuth type I and II tumors was reported to be 33.7 months [16]. Seyama et al. also reported on a better prognosis in patients with Bismuth type I and II tumors, who underwent right hepatectomy with caudate lobectomy. In their series, the mean survival for 9 patients with Bismuth type I tumor was 42 months and that for 8 patients with Bismuth type II tumor was 51 months [45]. However, it is still uncertain whether or not major hepatic resection can improve survival for patients with Bismuth and Corlette type I or II hilar cholangiocarcinoma. Ikeyama et al. retrospectively evaluated surgical outcome of 54 patients with Bismuth and Corlette type I and II hilar cholangiocarcinoma, and demonstrated survival benefit from right hepatectomy with caudate lobectomy for nodular and sclerosing tumors, but not for papillary tumors [46]. Others have reported no significant difference in survival between hepatectomy and bile duct resection alone for Bismuth and Corlette type I and II tumors. Besides, major hepatic resection in patients with obstructive jaundice results in high surgical morbidity and mortality [47]. Postoperative hepatic failure and its associated mortality have been associated with the extent of liver resection [5]. In patients with cirrhotic livers or impaired liver function, or both, the minimal required amount of functional liver volume increases. Improving perioperative management of patients with hilar cholangiocarcinoma after extended liver resection does not substantially decrease morbidity and mortality rates associated with this technique. High mortality rates have been reported, with the main cause being liver failure due to insufficient functional liver parenchyma left after liver resection. In the large series reported by Klempnauer et al., an aggressive approach resulted in an operative mortality rate of 17 % [48]. In the study by Nishio and co-workers, the operative mortality rate for left trisectionectomy was 23 % [24].

To reduce the perioperative risk of major liver resection for hilar cholangiocarcinoma, two approaches have been proposed. The first is preoperative biliary drainage of the future hepatic remnant. Reports from the West have shown that preoperative biliary drainage does not reduce perioperative risk, but increases hospital costs as a result of septic complications related to the drainage [49, 50]. The second approach is preoperative portal vein embolization (PVE) of the hepatic segments that are to be resected. Recent reports suggested benefit, but the reduction in postoperative liver failure rate was only 2 % after resection of hilar cholangiocarcinoma [16, 23]. For patients with hilar cholangiocarcinoma, the indications for PVE remain controversial.

19.8.3 Central Lobectomy for Bismuth–Corlette Type I, II and III Tumors Without Vascular Invasion?

Hepatic resection, limited as much as possible to what is necessary for curative resection, might result in fewer postoperative complications, including liver failure, in patients with hilar cholangiocarcinoma. Nimura et al. have also advocated limited hepatic resection according to the tumor extent [42]. Our strategy to reduce perioperative mortality is the use of central lobectomy in selected patients with hilar cholangiocarcinoma, so that a sufficient hepatic mass is preserved.

As the hilar bifurcation of the bile ducts is near to liver segments 4, 5 and 1, adequate liver resection of these segments together with the bile ducts can result in cure. Under intraoperative ultrasonographic guidance, the aim is to resect the liver parenchyma and the bile duct 1 cm away from the tumor. The negative surgical resection margin rate in our hands was 89.1 %, and no serious complications with this operation were encountered. Although there are many arguments for or against central lobectomy for hilar cholangiocarcinoma, our results of 0 mortality, 29.7 % morbidity and 34 % 5-year survival rate are encouraging, and better than the results of other authors. For hilar cholangiocarcinoma that involves the right or left hepatic artery or portal vein, or for Bismuth–Corlette type IV tumors, the only surgical option is to perform a right/extended right or left/extended left hepatectomy.

A negative bile duct resection margin is an important factor, but it is not the only factor that influences prognosis after surgery. Although not all patients with clear surgical resection margins have good prognosis, some of the reported long-term survivors are patients with positive resection margins. Maeno et al. found a 5-year survival rate of 20 % in patients with positive bile duct resection margins (a finding similar to our results of 23 % with R1 resection [40]), and 37 % in patients with clear surgical margins [51]. Kondo et al. reported a 3-year overall survival rate in 40 consecutive patients with hilar cholangiocarcinoma with clear resection margins of only 40 % [43]. Hasegawa and co-workers reported that 60 % of patients with hilar cholangiocarcinoma who had an R0 resection developed tumor metastasis [49]. The 3-year survival rate following liver transplantation for hilar cholangiocarcinoma was 35 % [26]. All of these findings suggest that there are many factors influencing the outcomes of surgical treatment for hilar cholangiocarcinoma [40, 52]. Increasing the extent of liver resection is not necessary. If the tumor can be resected completely, minor liver resection is better in patients with hilar cholangiocarcinoma.

Radical resection of hilar cholangiocarcinoma results in higher morbidity rates (40–71 %) compared with resection of other hepatic tumors; the most common complication is bile leakage, which occurs in about 10 % of patients (range 4–61.9 %) [10, 17, 20, 23, 30, 48, 49, 53]. For this reason, biliary tract reconstruction is the key step in this operation. In minor liver resection for hilar cholangiocarcinoma, the liver has to be transected in two or three planes, leaving behind many intrahepatic bile ductal openings (usually between five and nine). Conventionally, each bile duct opening is anastomosed to the jejunum [54, 55], making the reconstruction very difficult, which is the main disadvantage of this procedure. Using our technique of hepatojejunal anastomosis, the bile leak rate was only 1.4 %.

In conclusion, central lobectomy can be used with good results in selected patients with Bismuth–Corlette type I, II and III tumors without vascular invasion. For type III tumors with vascular invasion and selected type IV lesions, major hepatectomy must be performed.

References

1. Aljiffry M, Walsh MJ, Molinari M. Advances in diagnosis, treatment and palliation of cholangiocarcinoma: 1990–2009. World J Gastroenterol. 2009;15:4240–62.
2. Gatto M, Alvaro D. Cholangiocarcinoma: risk factors and clinical presentation. Eur Rev Med Pharmacol Sci. 2010;14:363–7.
3. Bismuth H, Castaing D, Traynor O. Resection or palliation: priority of surgery in the treatment of hilar cancer. World J Surg. 1988;12:39–47.
4. Tompkins RK, Thomas D, Wile A, et al. Prognostic factors in bile duct carcinoma: analysis of 96 cases. Ann Surg. 1981;194:447–57.
5. Ito F, Cho CS, Rikkers LF, Weber SM. Hilar cholangiocarcinoma: current management. Ann Surg. 2009;250:210–8.
6. Carriaga MT, Henson DE. Liver, gallbladder, extrahepatic bile ducts, and pancreas. Cancer. 1995;75:171–90.
7. Otto G. Diagnostic and surgical approaches in hilar cholangiocarcinoma. Int J Colorectal Dis. 2007;22:101–8.
8. Cameron JL, Pitt HA, Zinner MJ, et al. Management of proximal cholangiocarcinomas by surgical resection and radiotherapy. Am J Surg. 1990;159:91–7; discussion 97–8.
9. Jarnagin WR, Fong Y, DeMatteo RP, et al. Staging, resectability, and outcome in 225 patients with hilar cholangiocarcinoma. Ann Surg. 2001;234:507–17; discussion 517–9.
10. Dinant S, Gerhards MF, Rauws EA, et al. Improved outcome of resection of hilar cholangiocarcinoma (Klatskin tumor). Ann Surg Oncol. 2006;13:872–80.
11. Petrowsky H, Hong JC. Current surgical management of hilar and intrahepatic cholangiocarcinoma: the role of resection and orthotopic liver transplantation. Transplant Proc. 2009;41:4023–35.
12. De Vreede I, Steers JL, Burch PA, et al. Prolonged disease-free survival after orthotopic liver transplantation plus adjuvant chemoirradiation for cholangiocarcinoma. Liver Transpl. 2000;6: 309–16.
13. Hidalgo E, Asthana S, Nishio H, et al. Surgery for hilar cholangiocarcinoma: the leeds experience. Eur J Surg Oncol. 2008;34:787–94.
14. Neuhaus P, Jonas S, Bechstein WO, et al. Extended resections for hilar cholangiocarcinoma. Ann Surg. 1999;230:808–18; discussion 819.
15. Song GW, Lee SG, Hwang S, et al. Does portal vein resection with hepatectomy improve survival in locally advanced hilar cholangiocarcinoma? Hepatogastroenterology. 2009;56:935–42.
16. Kawasaki S, Imamura H, Kobayashi A, et al. Results of surgical resection for patients with hilar bile duct cancer: application of extended hepatectomy after biliary drainage and hemihepatic portal vein embolization. Ann Surg. 2003;238:84–92.
17. Dinant S, Gerhards MF, Busch OR, et al. The importance of complete excision of the caudate lobe in resection of hilar cholangiocarcinoma. HPB (Oxford). 2005;7:263–7.
18. Neuhaus P, Jonas S, Settmacher U, et al. Surgical management of proximal bile duct cancer: extended right lobe resection increases resectability and radicality. Langenbecks Arch Surg. 2003;388: 194–200.
19. Launois B, Reding R, Lebeau G, Buard JL. Surgery for hilar cholangiocarcinoma: French experience in a collective survey of 552 extrahepatic bile duct cancers. J Hepatobiliary Pancreat Surg. 2000; 7:128–34.
20. Witzigmann H, Berr F, Ringel U, et al. Surgical and palliative management and outcome in 184 patients with hilar cholangiocarcinoma: palliative photodynamic therapy plus stenting is comparable to r1/r2 resection. Ann Surg. 2006;244:230–9.

21. Nishio H, Nagino M, Nimura Y. Surgical management of hilar cholangiocarcinoma: the Nagoya experience. HPB (Oxford). 2005;7:259–62.
22. Yokoyama Y, Nagino M, Nishio H, et al. Recent advances in the treatment of hilar cholangiocarcinoma: portal vein embolization. J Hepatobiliary Pancreat Surg. 2007;14:447–54.
23. Rea DJ, Munoz-Juarez M, Farnell MB, et al. Major hepatic resection for hilar cholangiocarcinoma: analysis of 46 patients. Arch Surg. 2004;139:514–23; discussion 523–5.
24. Jonas S, Benckert C, Thelen A, et al. Radical surgery for hilar cholangiocarcinoma. Eur J Surg Oncol. 2008;34:263–71.
25. Hemming AW, Kim RD, Mekeel KL, et al. Portal vein resection for hilar cholangiocarcinoma. Am Surg. 2006;72:599–604; discussion 604–5.
26. Miyazaki M, Kato A, Ito H, et al. Combined vascular resection in operative resection for hilar cholangiocarcinoma: does it work or not? Surgery. 2007;141:581–8.
27. Abdel Wahab M, Fathy O, Elghwalby N, et al. Resectability and prognostic factors after resection of hilar cholangiocarcinoma. Hepatogastroenterology. 2006;53:5–10.
28. Giuliante F, Ardito F, Vellone M, et al. Liver resections for hilar cholangiocarcinoma. Eur Rev Med Pharmacol Sci. 2010;14:368–70.
29. Meyer CG, Penn I, James L. Liver transplantation for cholangiocarcinoma: results in 207 patients. Transplantation. 2000;69:1633–7.
30. Robles R, Figueras J, Turrion VS, et al. Spanish experience in liver transplantation for hilar and peripheral cholangiocarcinoma. Ann Surg. 2004;239:265–71.
31. Shimoda M, Farmer DG, Colquhoun SD, et al. Liver transplantation for cholangiocellular carcinoma: analysis of a single-center experience and review of the literature. Liver Transpl. 2001;7:1023–33.
32. Rea DJ, Heimbach JK, Rosen CB, et al. Liver transplantation with neoadjuvant chemoradiation is more effective than resection for hilar cholangiocarcinoma. Ann Surg. 2005;242:451–8; discussion 458–61.
33. Heimbach JK, Gores GJ, Haddock MG, et al. Predictors of disease recurrence following neoadjuvant chemoradiotherapy and liver transplantation for unresectable perihilar cholangiocarcinoma. Transplantation. 2006;82:1703–7.
34. Wu Y, Johlin FC, Rayhill SC, et al. Long-term, tumor-free survival after radiotherapy combining hepatectomy-Whipple en bloc and orthotopic liver transplantation for early-stage hilar cholangiocarcinoma. Liver Transpl. 2008;14:279–86.
35. McBride CM, Wallace S. Cancer of the right lobe of the liver: a variety of operative procedures. Arch Surg. 1972;105:289–96.
36. Mehrabi A, Mood ZA, Roshanaei N, et al. Mesohepatectomy as an option for the treatment of central liver tumors. J Am Coll Surg. 2008;207:499–509.
37. Chouillard E, Cherqui D, Tayar C, et al. Anatomical bi- and trisegmentectomies as alternatives to extensive liver resections. Ann Surg. 2003;238:29–34.
38. Bismuth H, Corlette MB. Intrahepatic cholangioenteric anastomosis in carcinoma of the hilus of the liver. Surg Gynecol Obstet. 1975;140:170–8.
39. Chen XP, Qiu FZ, Lau WY, et al. Mesohepatectomy for hepatocellular carcinoma: a study of 256 patients. Int J Colorectal Dis. 2008;23:543–6.
40. Chen XP, Lau WY, Huang ZY, et al. Extent of liver resection for hilar cholangiocarcinoma. Br J Surg. 2009;96:1167–75.
41. Sotiropoulos GC, Lang H, Molmenti EP, et al. Partial or complete mesohepatectomy combined with resection of the hilar bifurcation in cases of Klatskin tumors: a reasonable strategy? Am J Surg. 2009;198:297–8.
42. Miyazaki M, Ito H, Nakagawa K, et al. Parenchyma-preserving hepatectomy in the surgical treatment of hilar cholangiocarcinoma. J Am Coll Surg. 1999;189:575–83.
43. Kondo S, Hirano S, Ambo Y, et al. Forty consecutive resections of hilar cholangiocarcinoma with no postoperative mortality and no positive ductal margins: results of a prospective study. Ann Surg. 2004;240:95–101.
44. Capussotti L, Muratore A, Polastri R, et al. Liver resection for hilar cholangiocarcinoma: in-hospital mortality and longterm survival. J Am Coll Surg. 2002;195:641–7.
45. Seyama Y, Kubota K, Sano K, et al. Long-term outcome of extended hemihepatectomy for hilar bile duct cancer with no mortality and high survival rate. Ann Surg. 2003;238:73–83.
46. Ikeyama T, Nagino M, Oda K, et al. Surgical approach to bismuth Type I and II hilar cholangiocarcinomas: audit of 54 consecutive cases. Ann Surg. 2007;246:1052–7.
47. Jang JY, Kim SW, Park DJ, et al. Actual long-term outcome of extrahepatic bile duct cancer after surgical resection. Ann Surg. 2005;241:77–84.
48. Klempnauer J, Ridder GJ, Werner M, et al. What constitutes long-term survival after surgery for hilar cholangiocarcinoma? Cancer. 1997;79:26–34.
49. Hasegawa S, Ikai I, Fujii H, et al. Surgical resection of hilar cholangiocarcinoma: analysis of survival and postoperative complications. World J Surg. 2007;31:1256–63.
50. Pitt HA, Gomes AS, Lois JF, et al. Does preoperative percutaneous biliary drainage reduce operative risk or increase hospital cost? Ann Surg. 1985;201:545–53.
51. Maeno H, Ono T, Yamanoi A, et al. Our experiences in surgical treatment for hilar cholangiocarcinoma. Hepatogastroenterology. 2007;54:669–73.
52. Thelen A, Neuhaus P. Liver transplantation for hilar cholangiocarcinoma. J Hepatobiliary Pancreat Surg. 2007;14:469–75.
53. Pichlmayr R, Ringe B, Lauchart W, et al. Radical resection and liver grafting as the two main components of surgical strategy in the treatment of proximal bile duct cancer. World J Surg. 1988;12:68–77.
54. Miyazaki M, Ito H, Nakagawa K, et al. Segments I and IV resection as a new approach for hepatic hilar cholangiocarcinoma. Am J Surg. 1998;175:229–31.
55. White TT. Skeletization resection and central hepatic resection in the treatment of bile duct cancer. World J Surg. 1988;12:48–51.

Extended Resections

20

D. Seehofer and P. Neuhaus

20.1 Preoperative Considerations

20.1.1 Rational for Extended Hepatectomies

The major goal of oncological surgery is to achieve negative resection margins. Extended hepatectomies are the most radical procedures for resection of hilar cholangiocarcinoma. Due to the longitudinal (bile duct) and vertical (adjacent structures) tumor invasion of hilar cholangiocarcinoma, it is essential to reach tumor free margins at the biliary tree and to resect the liver parenchyma adjacent to the hepatic hilum *en bloc* with the hilar plate. Both is achievable only by extended hemihepatectomies *en bloc* with extrahepatic bile duct resection—if required in combination with pancreatoduodenectomy. Additionally, the growth pattern of hilar cholangiocarcinoma is in the vast majority of cases periductal infiltrating and only very rarely nodular or papillary. This infiltrating growth pattern makes curative tumor resection difficult and requires appropriate safety margins. Moreover, microscopic infiltration of perineural sheaths hinders a clear intraoperative identification of tumor boundaries. This requires a radical surgical strategy with a safety margin as wide as possible. For the reasons that safety margins are naturally small in hilar cholangiocarcinoma, all efforts have to be undertaken to increase the resection margin. Therefore extended hepatectomies have evolved as the standard of curative treatment in hilar cholangiocarcinoma—provided that liver function is adequate. Accordingly the rate of simultaneous major liver resection in most recently published series is 90 % or higher, especially in patients operated within the last 5–10 years [1–22] (Table 20.1).

Even after a formal curative resection, loco-regional recurrence remains frequent and represents the most common site of recurrent disease. However, correct pathological diagnosis of R0 resection is extremely demanding. In analogy to pancreatic cancer, this is particularly due to difficulties in the pathological classification of an "R1" resection also in proximal bile duct cancers due to the complex three dimensional margin of the surgical specimen [23]. The result is a significant number of "occult" R1 resections. Anatomically, particularly in Corlett-Bismuth Type III or IV tumors occult or obvious R1 resection is most precarious at the following locations:

(a) the intrahepatic bile duct margin(s)—in case of procedures less than hemihepatectomies there is a doubled risk at the intrahepatic bile duct margin on both sides.
(b) the dorsal margin of the proximal common hepatic duct, where the right hepatic artery regularly traverses.
(c) the dorsal margin of the biliary confluence, which is situated ventrally to the portal vein bifurcation.

To limit the risk of incomplete tumor resection, it is essential to avoid these critical steps of surgical preparation if possible. For example during extended right hemihepatectomy with *en bloc* resection of the portal vein bifurcation, only one of these critical steps [the dissection of the proximal bile duct (a)] has to be performed. In contrast, during left hepatectomies, three critical steps are necessary (a–c), since the right hepatic artery and the right portal vein have to be dissected dorsal to the bile duct (Fig. 20.1). Procedures, where parts of both hepatic lobes are preserved bear the maximum risk for R1 resection, e.g. extrahepatic bile duct resection or central hepatectomies, since there is a risk of tumor dissemination or incomplete resection at the intrahepatic bile duct margin of both lobes—therefore these procedures are in our own practice only considered as "palliative" procedure for cases of severely impaired liver function. It is also accepted in most specialized centers, that hilar cholangiocarcinomas cannot be radically resected by local excision: this so-called "hilar resection" or extrahepatic bile duct resection is considered to be a palliative procedure for the reasons mentioned above. It has been shown to be associated with a recurrence rate of 80–100 % by several authors.

D. Seehofer, MD, PhD • P. Neuhaus, MD, PhD (✉)
Department of General-, Visceral- and Transplantation-Surgery, Charité – Universitätsmedizin Berlin, Berlin, Germany
e-mail: peter.neuhaus@charite.de

W.Y. Lau (ed.), *Hilar Cholangiocarcinoma*,
DOI 10.1007/978-94-007-6473-6_20, © Springer Science+Business Media Dordrecht and People's Medical Publishing House 2013

Table 20.1 Single center experiences of hilar cholangiocarcinoma published between 2005 and 2010: overview on surgical procedures, radicality and postoperative complications

Author	Center	Period	Number resected	Hepatectomies (HE) (%)	Right HE (%)	Left HE (%)	Hilar resection (%)	R0 resection (%)	Mortality (%)	Morbidity (%)]
Mansfield	Newcastle	1995–2003	18	**100**	**61**	**33**	0	72	17	50
Hemming	Gainsville, Fl	1997–2004	53	**98**	**68**	**30**	2	80	9	40
Lai	Hong Kong	1998–2002	26	**85**	**50**	**35**	15	73	8	42
Silva	Birmingham	1992–2003	45	**69**	**33**	**36**	31	51	9	42
Sano	Tokyo	2000–2004	102	**100**	**50**	**48**	0	61	0	50
Cheng	Shanghai	1997–2002	75	**77**	**33**	**44**	23		1	13
Witzigmann	Leipzig	1994–2004	59	**88**	**63**	**25**	12	70	12	52
Baton	Paris	1984–2003	59	**98**	**32**	**66**	0	46	5	42
Hasegawa	Kyoto	1990–2003	49	**90**	**47**	**43**	8	78	2	47
Otani	Miyazaki	1990–2005	27	**70**	**37**	**33**	30	74	0	37
Ito	Madison, Wi	1985–2006	38	**53**	**29**	**24**	47	63	3	26
Yubin	Guangzhou	1990–2004	115							20
Konstadoulakis	New York[a]	1988–2006	59	**86**	**34**	**49**	14	69	7	25
Murakami	Hiroshima	1990–2007	42	**86**	**43**	**42**	10	74	7	52
Lee	Seoul	2001–2008	302	**89**	**54**	**31**	11	71	2	43
Miyazaki	Chiba	2001–2008	107	**91**	**36**	**45**	9	59	2	
Rocha	New York[b]	2001–2008	60	**95**			5	80	5	35
Unno	Sendai	2001–2008	125	**100**	**59**	**41**	0	63	8	49
Young	Leeds	2001–2008	51	**92**	**45**	**47**	8	57	8	75
Hirano	Sapporo	2001–2008	146	**88**	**53**	**33**	12	88	3	44
Igami	Nagoya	2001–2008	298	**98**	**37**	**57**	2	74	2	43
van Gulik	Amsterdam	1998–2003	29	**72**	**38**	**35**	28	59	10	68

See Refs. [1–22]
In case of more than one publication the most recent is included
Bold values show the effect of the percentage of right and left hepatic resections on the radicality and postoperative morbidity/mortality
[a]Mount Sinai
[b]Memorial Sloan Kettering Cancer Center

If a hemihepatectomy is performed for hilar cholangiocarcinoma this means in most cases not an anatomical hemihepatectomy, because removal of the liver parenchyma adjacent to the hepatic hilum en bloc with the hilar plate is essential. Therefore, central parts of the segments 4, 5 and 8 respectively have to be resected in left hemihepatectomies as well as in right hemihepatectomies due to their close relation to the hilar plate and the biliary confluence. In addition, en bloc resection of the caudate lobe is mandatory in all forms of hepatectomies for hilar cholangiocarcinoma, because infiltration of the segment 1 bile ducts, which are joining the left hepatic duct close to the biliary confluence, is regularly seen. Therefore all hemihepatectomies for central bile duct cancers are more or less extended hemihepatectomies.

20.1.2 Consideration of the Surgical Procedure: Right vs. Left Hepatectomy

Bilateral surgical exploration of the hepatoduodenal ligament to determine the type of liver resection increases the risk of tumor cell dissemination and therefore opposes the oncological principle of a no touch technique. Thus, to achieve good oncological results it is recommendable to determine the general type of surgical procedure (i.e. right hepatectomy vs. left hepatectomy) early in the diagnostic workup for several reasons, which are outlined in the following.

The application of a specific operative procedure is based on tumor extension and the functional hepatic reserve. The ideal basis for initial evaluation is a MRCP. In our own practice an MRI including MRCP is performed before ERC or PTCD and decompression of cholestasis [24]. Local tumor extension, potential vascular involvement and the exact volume of both liver lobes are adequately shown by MRI and MRCP without any risk of cholangitis. In addition, biliary tumor extensions in both lobes are better demarcated with dilated bile ducts. This information is sufficient for a preliminary decision, if a right sided or a left sided hepatectomy is the adequate procedure in an individual case. However in some cases decision making might be demanding.

If permitted by local tumor extension and volume of the future liver remnant, a right sided hepatectomy is our preferred procedure, because of its higher oncological radicality

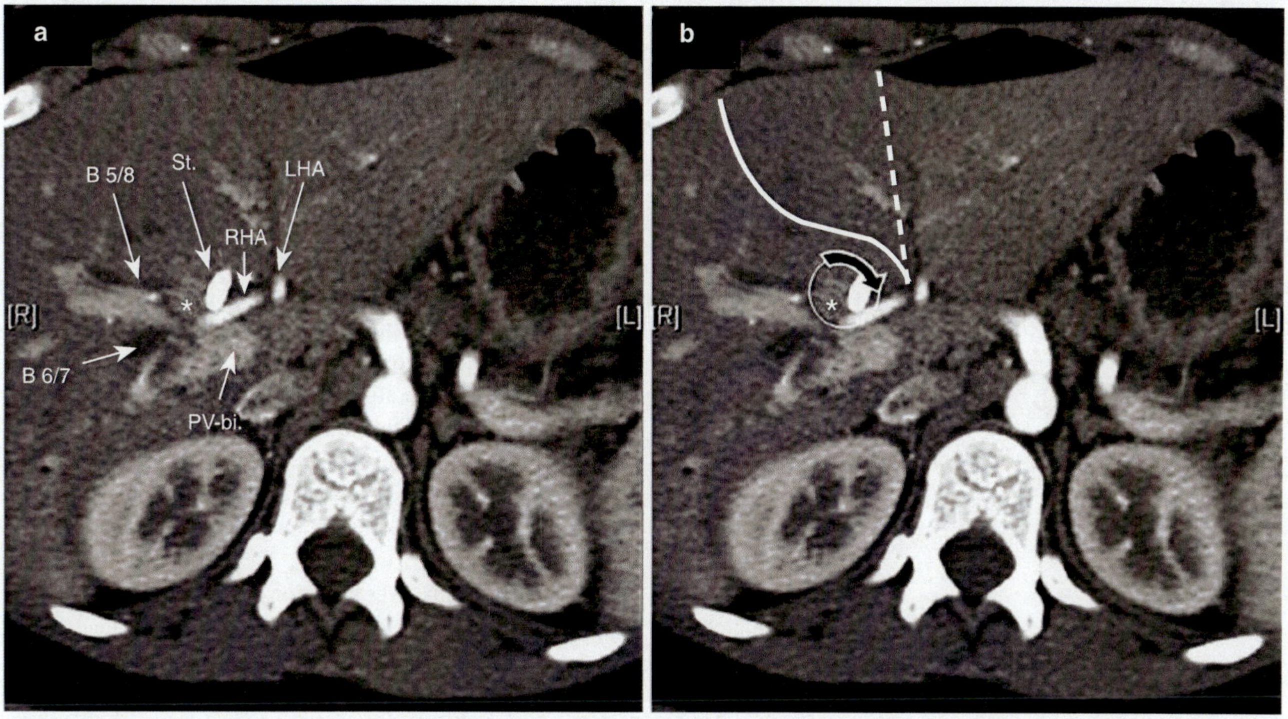

Fig. 20.1 (**a**) CT scan with representation of the close relation of a hilar cholangiocarcinoma (*) to the right hepatic artery (*RHA*) and the portal vein bifurcation (*PV-bi*); *St* biliary stent, *LHA* left hepatic artery, *B5/8* anterior sectoral duct to segments 5 and 8, *B 6/7* posterior sectoral duct to segments 6 and 7. (**b**) Schematic representation of the parenchymal dissection line during extended right hemihepatectomy for hilar cholangiocarcinoma (*solid line*) and right trisectionectomy (*dotted line*). The *curved arrow* represents the critical region, where the safety margin is markedly smaller during extended right hemihepatectomy compared to right trisectionectomy

based on a higher likelihood of an adequate safety margin. As described above, the right hepatic artery and the right portal vein have not to be separated from the bile duct and thereby the danger of tumor cell dissemination is avoided at these locations. Also the anatomy of the biliary tract favours achievement of a R0 resection in right hemihepatectomies, since the biliary confluence is located on the right side of the hepatoduodenal ligament. The right hepatic duct is normally short (<1 cm) or even absent. In contrast, the left hepatic duct has a relatively long and straight course between 2 and 5 cm until it traverses the left portal vein within the umbilical fissure and ramifies to the segments 2 and 3 branches. Branches to segment 4 which eventually join the left duct before the umbilical fissure can be resected by right trisectionectomy, if required. Thus, tumors invading the right sectoral ducts and the segmental ducts to segment 4—by definition type IV tumors—are still potentially resectable by right trisectionectomy.

In contrast, left hemihepatectomy or left trisectionectomy enables only a small safety margin within the biliary tree, since the sectoral and segmental bile ducts converge within the hilar region (Fig. 20.2). Thus, using left trisectionectomies rather than left hemihepatectomy, only a small additional safety margin can be gained by shifting the resectional plan further to the right (Fig. 20.2). Curative resection with an adequate safety margin is therefore more likely during right hepatectomies and these are accordingly associated with an

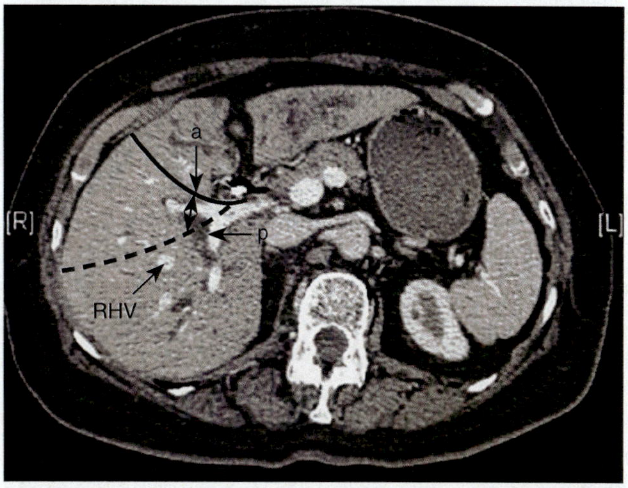

Fig. 20.2 CT scan showing the parenchymal dissection line during left hemihepatectomy (*solid line*) and during left trisectionectomy (*dotted line*) for hilar cholangiocarcinoma. The *double-arrow* (↔) is pointing to the narrowing gain of safety margin in the central region (*a* anterior sectoral duct, *p* posterior sectoral duct, *RHV* right hepatic vein)

increased rate of R0 resections compared to left hepatecomies (71 % vs. 33 % [25]). Also Miyazaki et al. reported a 50 % rate of R0 resection after left hepatectomy compared to 74 % after right hepatectomy [16]. The rate of R0 resections is not given seperately for right and left hemihepatectomies in most publications, however a positive correlation between the rate

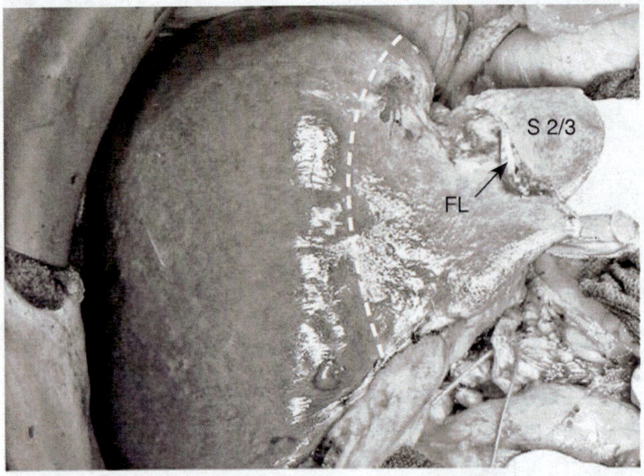

Fig. 20.3 Severe atrophy of the left lobe due to left portal vein occlusion precluding right hepatectomy. *FL* falciform ligament, *S 2/3* liver segments 2 and 3

of right hepatectomies and the rate of R0 resections is observed (Table 20.1). Nevertheless, there is no clear trend towards right hepatectomies in all centers, and good results are achievable by left hepatectomy as well.

In about one third of cases the left hepatic lobe is severely atrophic (Fig. 20.3) due to long-standing cholestasis and/or occlusion of the left portal branch, making right or extended right hemihepatectomy impossible. Also a severely impaired liver function might contraindicate extensive procedures like extended right hepatectomies. For these cases left hepatectomy is the alternative which is—adaequate experience provided—still associated with a high curative resection rate and good long term results (Table 20.1).

Apart from the oncological aspect with avoidance of bilateral hilar preparation, the additional reason, to decide for the type of hepatectomy early before surgery is the necessity of an optimal conditioning of the future liver remnant. This is a prerequisite for good postoperative results and a low rate of liver failure. It includes reversal of cholestasis and treatment of cholangitis. In addition, prior to extended right hepatectomies preoperative embolization of the right lobe is often advisable to lower the risk of postoperative liver failure. Since most of these issues are already described in earlier chapters, only some aspects, which are relevant for the choice of surgical procedure during extended resections are cursorily given in this chapter.

Extended right hemihepatectomy or right trisectionectomy in hilar cholangiocarcinoma patients is one of the most extensive resections because of the massive loss of functional liver volume. This results in a relatively small future liver remnant. Portal vein embolization is performed in almost all of these cases prior to surgery in the authors' own practice, although it might not be absolutely necessary in patients with a future liver remnant >40 %. However, the routine use of portal vein embolisation for patients with hilar cholangiocarcinoma even in patients with a future liver remnant of 50 % or less has recently been described with excellent postoperative results and a 0 in hospital mortality [5]. Despite all individual protocols for usage or omission of portal vein embolization, none of these is substantiated by prospective randomized trials. From a practical point of view, many patients do have to wait for surgery 1–3 weeks until relief of cholestasis and (almost) normalization of bilirubin values anyway. In our own practice, surgery is performed 2–4 weeks after embolization and consecutive hypertrophy of the left lobe with simultaneous adaptation of the portal blood flow to the future liver remnant. Due to a larger future liver remnant, preoperative portal vein embolization is generally not necessary prior to left hemihepatectomy, however it might be advisable before left trisectionectomy.

The final decision whether an extended right hepatectomy or a right trisectionectomy is feasible is based in our own practice on liver function tests. We routinely rely on the LiMAx (maximum liver function capacity) liver function test [26], which is used before all extended hepatectomies. Especially in patients with hilar cholangiocarcinoma this test might be superior to e.g. the ICG plasma disappearance rate, which is markedly influenced by obstructive jaundice [27]. On basis of the maximum liver function capacity (LiMAx) in combination with CT volumetry of the future liver remnant, it is decided, if a trisectionectomy is safe, or if parts of segment 4 have to be preserved to reduce the risk of liver failure. Also for the optimal timing of resection after portal vein embolization reliable liver function tests are useful.

Finally, local operability can be determined only during laparotomy. If not an extended liver resection is required (mainly in type I or type II tumors) previous embolization of one lobe gives away the flexibility of intraoperative decision for a right or left hepatectomy. This has to be weighed individually against the benefits of embolization.

20.1.3 Lymphadenectomy

Bismuth et al. have described positive regional lymph nodes in hilar cholangiocarcinoma to be of less prognostic significance than in other gastrointestinal cancers [28]. Even if several other experiences have found a markedly lower long term survival in lymph node positive patients (Table 20.2), still long term survival seems to be possible, in patients with positive regional lymph nodes. This is not true for patients with positive enlarged lymph nodes in the paraaortal region. Apart from this, the evidence for radical lymphadenectomy and particularly for its extent is very low. During en-bloc hilar resection the lymph nodes of the hepatoduodenal ligament are resected with the tumor anyway. In addition, we routinely perform a regional lymphadenectomy of the pancreatoduodenal and the coeliac lymph nodes for tumor staging. Data from Nagoya have shown that an extended lymphadenectomy including the

Table 20.2 Long term survival in single center experiences of hilar cholangiocarcinoma published between 2005 and 2010

Author	Center	Period	Number resected	Mortality (%)	5 year overall survival (%)	5 year survival R0 (%)	5 year survival R1 (%)	5 year survival N0 (%)	5 year survival N1 (%)
Mansfield	Newcastle	1995–2003	18	17	**21**			35	0
Hemming	Gainsville, Fl	1997–2004	53	9	**35**	45	0	45	21
Lai	Hong Kong	1998–2002	26	8	**12**	16	0	20	0
Silva	Birmingham	1992–2003	45	9		41	24	~ 33	~ 30
Sano	Tokyo	2000–2004	102	0	**44**				
Cheng	Shanghai	1997–2002	75	1	**12**				
Witzigmann	Leipzig	1994–2004	59	12	**22**	27	10		
Baton	Paris	1984–2003	59	5	**20**	28	6		
Hasegawa	Kyoto	1990–2003	49	2	**40**				
Otani	Miyazaki	1990–2005	27	0	**27**	~34	0	~34	0
Ito	Madison, Wi	1985–2006	38	3	**31**	~62	0		
Yubin	Guangzhou	1990–2004	115		**~25**				
Konstadoulakis	New York[a]	1988–2006	59	7	**35**		38	~43	~10
Murakami	Hiroshima	1990–2007	42	7	**30**				
Lee	Seoul	2001–2008	302	2	**33**	47	8	33	
Miyazaki	Chiba	2001–2008	107	2	**~28**	33	21	44 (only R0)	22 (only R0)
Rocha	New York[b]	2001–2008	60	5		~55	~20	~50	18
Unno	Sendai	2001–2008	125	8	**35**	46	19		
Young	Leeds	2001–2008	51	8	**20**	40			
Hirano	Sapporo	2001–2008	146	3	**36**				
Igami	Nagoya	2001–2008	298	2	**42**			62	21
van Gulik	Amsterdam	1998–2003	29	10	**34**				

See Refs. [1–22]
Bold values are to emphasize on the 5 year overall survival in the difference series
[a]Mount Sinai
[b]Memorial Sloan Cettering Cancer Center

paraaortic lymph nodes may be beneficial in patients with microscopic infiltration of these lymph nodes but without macroscopic signs of tumor infiltration [29]. However, clinical evidence for lymphadenectomy during extended resections remains low.

20.2 Surgical Technique: (Extended) Right Hemihepatectomy

During extended right hemihepatectomies or right trisectionectomies a no touch technique with simultaneous en bloc resection of the caudate lobe, the extrahepatic bile duct and the portal vein bifurcation is routinely performed at our centre to increase the oncological radicality [25]. However, in the following the technique with and without simultaneous portal vein resection is described.

20.2.1 Preparation of the Hepatoduodenal Ligament

The abdomen is explored for conditions precluding curative tumor resection (peritoneal seeding, distant metastases). In case of simultaneous portal vein resection, surgical preparation of the hepatoduodenal ligament proceeds only on its left side and distally along the duodenum and pancreas. Thereby, preparation is performed distant to the tumor bearing area resulting in a no-touch technique.

Dissection starts with a systematic lymphadenectomy along the common and proper hepatic artery and eventually the coeliac trunk. Thereby, the left side of the portal vein is exposed. The ramification of the hepatic artery is prepared, but the right hepatic artery is dissected and encircled close to its origin only. Further dissection of the right hepatic artery has to be avoided, and not to dissect close to the tumor region and risk tumor cell dissemination. Further preparation of the umbilical plate is ensued to clarify local operability. The left hepatic artery is completely dissected until its entrance in the liver parenchyma in the umbilical fissure at the left side of the left portal vein branch. The arterial branch to segment 4, which regularly arises from the left hepatic artery within the umbilical fissure is prepared close to its origin for trisectionectomies or completely for extended right hemihepatectomies, where it might be preserved (Fig. 20.4). The bridge of liver parenchyma connecting segments 3 and 4 is divided for assessment of local tumor extension in the left hepatic duct. Lowering of the hilar plate is to be avoided and the hepatic

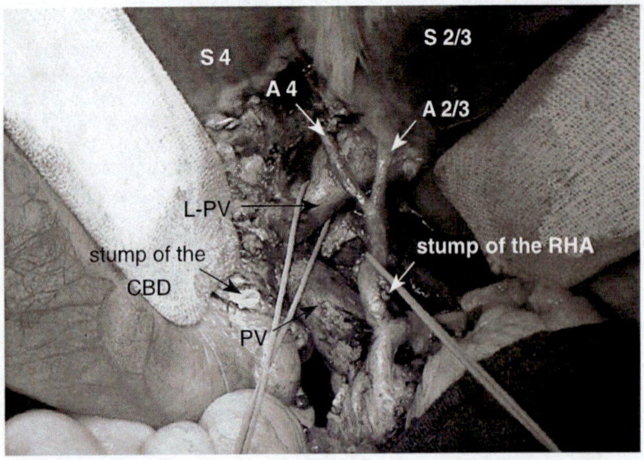

Fig. 20.4 Hilar preparation during extended right hemihepatectomy. The right hepatic artery (*RHA*) has been divided and the left hepatic artery (*LHA*) is pulled to the left. The common bile duct (*CBD*) has been divided at the upper level of the duodenum and the main trunk of the portal vein (*PV*) as well as the left branch of the portal vein (*L-PV*) have been prepared and encircled. To avoid further preparation close to the tumor region, the portal vein bifurcation might be resected and an end-to-end reconstruction of the PV and the L-PV can be performed. Alternatively, the portal vein bifurcation has to be further prepared and the right portal branch has to be divided. In case of right trisectionectomy the segment 4 branch of the left hepatic artery (*A 4*) is to be divided centrally and only the segment 2 and 3 branches of the artery (*A 2/3*) are to be preserved. If necessary the central part of the dotted line might be shifted further to the left

parenchyma surrounding the hilar plate is resected en bloc in order to comply with the principles of a no-touch technique.

Tumor extension within the left hepatic duct is palpated in the umbilical fissure. If the tumor clearly extends to the left side of the umbilical fissure, it is not likely to be resectable by right hepatic resection. However, identification of tumor boundaries is hardly possible by digital palpation or visualisation. On the one hand the tumor often extends up to 10 mm beyond the palpable margin due to submucosal or perivascular infiltration and on the other hand an inflammatory or desmoplastic reaction can mimic larger tumor extensions. Intraoperative tumor biopsies are to be avoided and a "macroscopic" surgical margin of 10 mm or more is intended, but especially in left hepatectomies often not achievable. Finally, tumor manifestation at the proximal margin can only be verified after division of the proximal bile duct by frozen section. If the margin is positive, additional resection is necessary to obtain R0 resection whenever possible.

The left branch of the portal vein is carefully prepared in the umbilical fissure. In case of planned portal vein resection it is to be encircled and taped proximal to the origin of the segmental portal vein branches of segment 2 and 3 (Fig. 20.4). One or more branches from the left portal vein to the caudate lobe and eventually to segment IV are carefully divided. Thereby the left portal branch is sufficiently mobilized over a distance of 1.5–2 cm to allow subsequent clamping and anastomosis.

If no portal vein resection is planned, all left sided caudate branches of the portal vein have to be divided for caudate lobe resection. In this case the portal vein bifurcation is than entirely prepared behind the bile duct and the right portal branch is centrally divided and ligated.

Regional lymph node dissection at the right side of the hepatodenal ligament is performed above the duodenum. A Kocher maneuver can be helpful for retropancreatic lymph node dissection. This exposes the right side of the portal vein, which can now be completely encircled above the pancreas. If the common and left hepatic artery as well as left portal vein and the proximal portal vein are not invaded by the tumor, no local contraindications for surgical resection exist and definitive steps can be undertaken.

The right hepatic artery is divided close to its origin and suture ligated. In case of planned trisectionectomy the segment 4 artery is divided as well. Now the left hepatic artery is retracted to the left by a vessel loop to facilitate further hilar preparation The distal common bile duct is divided close to the duodenum and the margin is sent for frozen section. Spillage of bile should be avoided, since it may contain tumor cells. In case of tumor infiltration of the distal bile duct margin an additional pancreatic head resection might be considered in selected patients who are otherwise curatively resected.

Now the right lobe is mobilized from the vena cava by division of the short hepatic veins and finally of the right hepatic vein. This enables further mobilisation of the caudate lobe from its right side under division of the short hepatic veins. Afterwards the liver is separated from the caval vein, and only the left and middle hepatic veins are preserved. The caudate lobe can now be retracted to the right to alleviate orientation during the parenchymal transection. The middle hepatic vein is divided intrahepatically during the parenchymal dissection.

20.2.2 Resection of the Portal Vein Bifurcation

The rational for portal vein resection as routine procedure during right hepatectomies for hilar cholangiocarcinoma has been discussed above. For further discussion of vascular resection see also the following chapter.

For portal vein resection the liver is lowered by placing abdominal packs between the right diaphragm and the liver to facilitate portal vein anastomosis. The main trunk of the portal vein and the left portal branch are clamped using vascular clamps. Both vessels are divided. Prolene 6/0 or 7/0 running suture is used for the end-to-end anastomosis. Differences in vessel diameter are adjusted during the anastomosis. Care is taken for correct orientation of both vessel stumps, especially the correct rotation is important. After placement of two corner sutures, the posterior wall is sutured from inside and the anterior wall from outside. Both running sutures are fixed with an air knot ("growth factor"), to avoid anastomotic stenosis. After reperfusion of the portal vein the abdominal packs are removed and the portal vein has a straight course. It is important to avoid mal-rotation of the portal vein stumps during portal vein anastomosis. If direct anastomosis of the portal stumps is not possible, a venous interposition graft might be created using the external iliac vein or a cryopreserved vein. However this is only necessary in cases with wide infiltration of the main portal trunk.

20.2.3 Parenchymal Dissection and Division of the Proximal Bile Duct

Negative ductal margins in hilar cholangiocarcinoma are achieved via a transhepatic approach only, therefore the proximal bile duct is to be divided after parenchymal transection. In general, dissection of the liver parenchyma starts anteriorly and proceeds to the base of the umbilical fissure. In our own practice parenchymal transection is routinely performed by using an ultrasound dissector with intermittent hilar occlusion if necessary, however other parenchymal dissection techniques are also possible [30]. Depending on the extent of hepatectomy the anterior dissection line starts either close to the falciform ligament (trisectionectomy) or varying degrees of segment 4 are preserved, if possible (extended right hemihepatectomy). If segment 4 is partially preserved it is important to deviate from the standard hemihepatectomy plane in the perihilar region by leaving the central parts of segment 4 and the hilar plate at the tumor (Fig. 20.1). This typically results in a kind of "hemi-Taij-Mahal" aspect of the resection surface (Fig. 20.1). The middle hepatic vein is divided during its intrahepatic course either centrally (trisectionectomy) or within the segment 4 (extended right hemihepatectomy). In case of partial preservation of segment 4 the dissection line has to drift dorsally of the middle hepatic vein in direction of the caudate lobe, in a way that the caudate lobe is left completely at the resected specimen. This might be eased by placing of a tape in along the ligamentum venosum between the left lateral lobe and the caudate lobe. By pulling the tape ventrally on the right side of the middle hepatic vein and on the right side of the left portal vein this results in a hanging maneuver which sometimes facilitates parenchymal transection. During extended right hepatectomies with partial preservation of segment 4, orientation within the segment 4 and especially ensuring of an appropriate three-dimensional safety margin is demanding in some cases (Fig. 20.1).

Partial preservation of segment 4 is the preferred technique in our own practice in case of marginal volume of the left lateral segments despite portal vein embolization and/or an impaired liver function, measured by the LiMAx liver function test [31], if this is enabled by tumor extensions. This increases the volume of the liver remnant and lowers the risk of postoperative liver failure. In case of a large volume of the left lateral segments 2 and 3 or a Bismuth type 4 tumor, trisectionectomy is the oncological procedure of choice. Also surgically, trisectionectomy can be performed in a more straightforward way than extended right hemihepatectomy (Fig. 20.1).

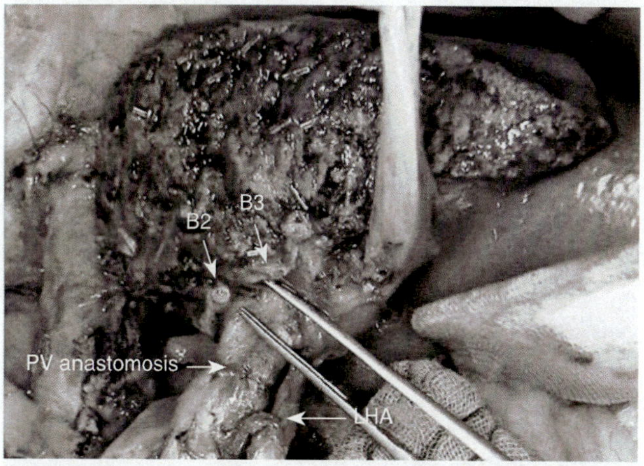

Fig. 20.5 Status after right trisectionectomy with portal vein reconstruction. The two biliary orifices to the segments 2 (*B2*) and 3 (*B3*) are shown. *LHA* left hepatic artery

Final step after complete parenchymal transection is the division of the intrahepatic proximal bile duct(s) at a presumptive tumor free position. The anatomy of the left hepatic duct is relatively constant, compared to the variations of the right hepatic duct. On the left side the relevant variations only concern the segment 4 ducts. These may merge the left hepatic duct at different levels between the biliary confluence and the umbilical fissure. Whereas in most cases after left trisectionectomy only one common or two segmental orifices have to be anastomosed (Fig. 20.5), after extended hepatectomies it might be necessary to perform an anastomoses with three or four orifices, since the oblique transection of the segment 4 may expose one or two additional ducts draining the segments 4a and 4b.

20.3 Surgical Technique: (Extended) Left Hemihepatectomy

In the following, the surgical techniques of left hemihepatectomy with en-bloc with caudate lobectomy and extrahepatic bile duct resection is described, possible technical modifications are additionally mentioned.

20.3.1 Hilar Preparation

For left hemihepatectomies preparation of the complete course of the common and proper hepatic artery as well as the

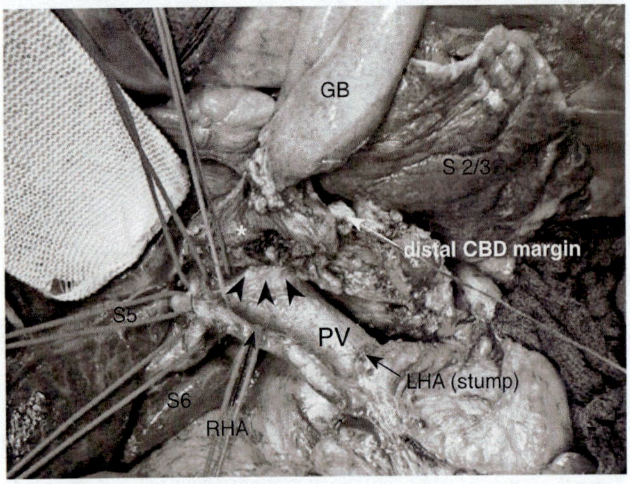

Fig. 20.6 Status after hilar preparation for left hemihepatectomy. The left hepatic artery (*LHA*) and the common bile duct (*CBD*) have been divided; the portal vein has been prepared, but it is infiltrated by the tumor at its bifurcation (*arrowheads*) necessitating portal vein resection. The right hepatic artery (*RHA*) and the segmental branches are prepared until the entrance in the parenchyma proximal to the hilar tumor (*). *S5* liver segment 5, *S6* liver segment 6, *GB* gallbladder, *S 2/3* liver segments 2 and 3

right hepatic artery is mandatory. For assessment of local tumor extension and lymphadenectomy we start preparation at the right side of the hepatoduodenal ligament. First, cholecystectomy is performed in an antegrade fashion starting at the fundus. The cystic duct is preserved in continuity. In the infundibular region preparation is continued by incision of the peritoneum immediately at the liver parenchyma. The complete cystic plate remains at the infundibulum of the gallbladder. Thereby the right hepatic artery and its ramification to the sector branches are exposed dorsally at the junction of the cystic and the hilar plate. The sectoral/segmental branches of the hepatic artery are further dissected until the entrance into the liver parenchyma dorsal to the left biliary system. At the same time the right portal branch is dissected dorsal to the arteries (Fig. 20.6). In case of an aberrant right hepatic artery from the superior mesenteric artery, this vessel is running dorsally to the portal vein and is hence less prone to tumor infiltration by hilar cholangiocarcinoma.

Now the proximal extent of the tumor should be assessed by palpation of the right hepatic duct and its assumed -intrahepatic course. Again, palpation might not adequately reflect tumor extensions as discussed above. Also for left hepatectomies lowering of the hilar plate is to be avoided and the hilar plate is resected en bloc with the surrounding liver parenchyma.

If the right hepatic artery and the right portal vein are not infiltrated and palpation of the proximal tumor extension does not preclude further resection, preparation is continued distally. The portal bifurcation and the main trunk of the portal vein are further dissected and thereby the right sided and dorsal lymph nodes are removed. A Kocher mobilization of the duodenum facilitates the dorsal retropancreatic lymph node dissection. The systematic regional lymphadenectomy is continued at the left side of the hepatoduodenal ligament. The common and proper hepatic artery are dissected until ramification to the right and left hepatic artery and the left margin of the portal vein is exposed.

If so far the preparation shows no contraindications for liver resection, division of the distal common bile duct at the upper border of the duodenum facilitates further preparation of the right hepatic artery. The common bile duct is divided and a frozen section is obtained. The common bile duct is elevated cranially and the course of the right hepatic artery is further prepared behind the common bile duct. The left hepatic artery is divided shortly after its origin. This exposes the left portal vein and two or more branches to the caudate lobe, which are divided. Afterwards the left branch of the portal vein is divided and ligated. In case of tumor infiltration of the portal vein bifurcation (Fig. 20.6) resection is either possible at this stage, but it is eventually easier after the parenchymal dissection and division of the right hepatic duct. However, due to early branching of the right portal vein the anastomosis might be technically demanding. General resection of the portal vein bifurcation during left hemihepatectomies is in our own practice not performed, since it does not provide significant additional oncological radicality, because the plane behind the common bile duct has to be dissected during preparation of the right hepatic artery. Thereby, the hilar plate is dissected anyway. If the artery is infiltrated by the tumor arterial resection might be considered in selected cases. Reconstruction is performed either by direct suture, by an interposition graft or arterial transposition [32]. If this not possible, arterioportal shunting might be considered [33].

The left hepatic lobe is now mobilized by dissection of the left triangular ligament and the Arantius ligament is divided close to the left hepatic vein. The caudate lobe is isolated from the caval vein by careful dissection of the short Spieghel-veins. Now the orifice of the left hepatic vein or the common trunk of the left and middle hepatic vein is properly exposed and can be divided and sutured.

20.3.2 Parenchymal Transection

Parenchymal transection proceeds cranially along the demarcation line of the right and left lobe (Cantlie line). In the hilar region, the plane of parenchymal dissection depends on local tumor extension. In every case, it is advisable to additionally remove central parts of segment 5 with the tumor to increase the safety margin. However, this safety margin has to be weighed against the number of bile duct orifices and the increasing risk of anastomotic leakage if dissection proceeds to far into the right lobe.

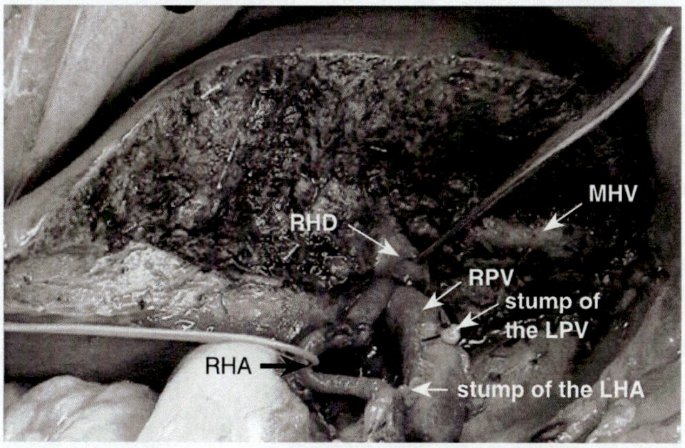

Fig. 20.7 Status after left hemihepatectomy for a Bismuth Corlette type IIIB tumor with division of the right hepatic duct (*RHD*) immediately before ramification to its sectoral branches. *RHA* right hepatic artery, *RPV* right portal vein, *LPV* left portal vein, *LHA* left hepatic artery, *MHV* middle hepatic vein

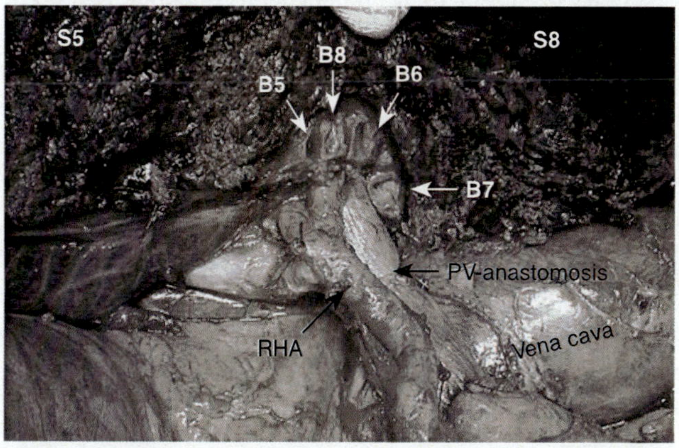

Fig. 20.8 Status after left hemihepatectomy for a Bismuth Corlette type IV tumor with atrophy of the left hepatic lobe with division of the biliary system at the level of the segmental bile ducts (*B5–B8*). The segmental ducts are situated in a semicircular manner around the portal vein. The portal vein bifurcation has been resected and a direct anastomosis of the main portal vein (*PV*) to the right portal branch has been performed (same case as in Fig. 20.6)

During parenchymal transection the middle hepatic vein is exposed and divided within the parenchyma (Fig. 20.7), if not done so extra-hepatically together with the left hepatic vein. After parenchymal transection the right hepatic duct (Fig. 20.7) or the right sectoral ducts are encircled in a presumably tumor free region, divided and the margin(s) is/are sent for frozen section. After left or extended left hemihepatectomy commonly two to four or even more bile duct orifices have to be reconstructed. The biliary orifices are mostly situated in a semicircular fashion around the right portal vein or its sectoral branches (Fig. 20.8). With it, in the majority of cases (>80 %) the posterior sectoral or segmental ducts run superiorly, dorsally, and then inferiorly to the right branch of the portal vein (Hjortsjö curve [34]). This should be kept in mind during final division of the biliary tree, and not to deviate from the dissection line, particularly during division of the postero-lateral ducts. This otherwise may result in a high number of orifices to be reconstructed. However, not only the number of orifices is the main concern, but also the increasing fragility of the bile duct wall within the liver parenchyma, which makes placing of sutures increasingly difficult and implies a significant risk of anastomotic leakage.

Further dissection dorsal to the bile duct and portal vein between the caudate process and segment 5 and 8 is easier after division of the proximal bile duct. In general, the resection line ends at the right border of the caval vein.

In case of tumor infiltration of the portal vein bifurcation or the portal trunk, the portal vein is now clamped above the pancreas and if possible at the right portal branch using vascular clamps. Both vessels are divided and reconstructed end to end using Prolene 6/0 or 7/0 running suture (Fig. 20.8). This procedure is technically demanding, because the right sectoral branches might not have a common trunk and vascular clamping might be difficult due to the short extrahepatic course before further ramification. In this case, total vascular exclusion of the liver might be performed by clamping of the caval vein supra- and infrahepatically. This allows suturing of the portal vein without clamping of the right branch at the hepatic side.

In case of tumor invasion along the right anterior sectoral duct, left hepatic trisectionectomy might be indicated in rare cases. However, the oncological advantage of shifting the parenchymal resection line to the right is limited, since it increases the safety margin centrally only slightly (Fig. 20.2). If a left trisectionectomy is planned, previous portal vein embolization might be useful. For left trisectionectomy dissection of the hepatoduodenal ligament is continued beyond the preparation for left hemihepatectomy and the anterior branch of the right hepatic artery and the right portal vein are divided. For further parenchymal transection mobilization of the right hepatic lobe is useful and further dissection of the short hepatic veins, preferentially from the left side, is mandatory. The liver is dissected along the demarcation line and finally the right posterior sectoral duct or the respective segmental ducts are divided.

Whereas left hemihepatectomy can be safely performed in patients with hilar cholangiocarcinoma, the perioperative morbidity and mortality of left trisectionectomy is thought to be considerably higher. For example, in the Leeds' experience a perioperative mortality of 23 % has been reported [35] and also the long term results were poor with no patient surviving more than 3 years. However, some other reports showed a more favorable postoperative outcome with low mortality rates [36, 37].

20.4 Biliary Reconstruction After Extended Resections

Biliary reconstruction after extended resections can be demanding and time consuming. If possible orifices might be merged using hepaticoplasty to minimize the number of anastomoses. For subtle anastomoses many surgeons prefer to insert a biliary drainage catheter to protect the anastomosis. In our own practice at least one catheter is placed as a transhepatic drain in the dominant bile duct(s). Therefore one (sub-) segmental bile duct is cannulated and the stab connected to the drain is pushed through the overlying parenchyma. Alternatively, a preoperatively placed PTC-drain can be used. Bilio-enteric anastomosis is performed using a Roux-en-Y jejunal limb. First the posterior row of the end-to-side hepaticojejunostomy is performed using interrupted 5-0 PDS suture, however running suture is also feasible, especially in large bile ducts to be anastomosed. If more than one duct is to be anastomosed, normally the posterior row of sutures of all ducts is placed first—however the technical concept has to be adapted individually. If applicable, afterwards the enteral portion of the transhepatic drain is pushed through the wall of the jejunal limb antimesenterially and secured by a suture or a Witzel's channel. The anterior wall of the bilioenteric anastomosis is completed and finally Roux en-Y reconstruction of the jejunum is performed.

20.5 Postoperative Complications and Management

Due to a considerably high postoperative mortality and morbidity surgical treatment of hilar cholangiocarcinoma still remains a challenge. Even in centres where many procedures are performed, postoperative complications are to be expected in every second to third patients (Table 20.1) and the in-hospital mortality is about 5–10 % (Table 20.1).

The most common and most relevant complications are bile leaks, temporary hepatic insufficiency, infectious complications (especially cholangitis) and vascular complications in case of vascular reconstruction. The possible association between preoperative biliary decompression and postoperative morbidity is discussed in detail earlier in this textbook. Whereas some authors reported a higher complication rate in jaundiced patients [38, 39] other routinely abstain from biliary decompression. This issue is clearly not finally solved, however, if an extended resection with a marginal future liver remnant is planned, biliary decompression might be more relevant than e.g. before left hemihepatectomy with resection of a severely atrophic left lobe. Especially after right trisectionectomy hepatic failure is a common cause of in-hospital death in patients with compromised liver function caused by obstructive jaundice. Risk factors for hyperbilirubinemia as one leading symptom of hepatic insufficiency have been analyzed by Hasegawa et al.: preoperative total bilirubin values of more than 2 mg/dl, postoperative major complications and extended surgery were independently associated with hyperbilirubinemia by multivariate analysis [9]. In a similar analysis form Sapporo prolonged operative time was identified as the only independent risk factor for postoperative complications [20]. Especially major postoperative complications, mainly infections, are thought to influence postoperative hepatic regeneration and liver function [40]. Schindl et al. have emphasized a reciprocal influence of postoperative hepatic dysfunction and postoperative infectious complications. This was particularly relevant in patients with a small residual liver volume. In this series, patients with a residual liver volume of 26.6 % or less had a 73 % risk of severe hepatic dysfunction in case of postoperative infections, whereas the risk was only 18 % in patients with the same residual volume but without infectious complications [41].

Aside from infectious complications the other major cofactors for the development of postoperative hepatic failure with an associated high risk of fatal outcome are vascular complications. Hirano et al. reported that 80 % of their cases of fatal liver failure were caused by vascular complications. These mainly included haemorrhage and subsequent occlusion of the hepatic artery associated with pancreatic leakage as well as impairment of portal venous flow due to distortion after portal reconstruction [20]. For early diagnosis of vascular occlusion, it is recommendable in patients with portal vein and/or arterial resection to monitor liver perfusion by Doppler ultrasound on a regular basis. In our own practice, this is performed once daily within the early postoperative days, because in case of early diagnosis successful thrombectomy might be possible. Nevertheless, the postoperative morbidity after hepatic artery reconstruction is higher than after portal vein resection and reconstruction, and for either vascular resection it is markedly higher than in patients without vascular reconstruction [42].

Naturally, special attention is given to biliary complications, which are observed in patients with hilar cholangiocarcinoma significantly more often than after liver resections for other reasons. For example in the Nagoya experience bile leaks manifested in more than 25 % of cases and cholangitis in 10 % of patients. In addition 10 % of patients developed intraabdominal or intrahepatic abscess formation [9]. Bile leaks might cause further severe complications like intra-abdominal haemorrhage, liver failure, infectious complications and postoperative death, which is often associated with infectious complications [43]. The incidence of an insufficient bilioenteric anastomosis clearly correlates with the number of orifices to be reconstructed. The risk of anastomotic leakage is significantly higher after an anastomosis with segmental ducts (Fig. 20.8) compared to anastomosis to the main hepatic duct (Fig. 20.7) [44].

Prophylaxis of biliary leakage is difficult. In the authors' own practice biliary drains are used routinely after liver resections for hilar cholangiocarcinoma, especially in patients with presumably fragile intrahepatic bilioenteric anastomoses. Additionally, these patients are not mobilized for 24 h after surgery. Five to seven days after surgery, the biliary drains are visualized by injecting contrast agent under fluoroscopic control. In case of minor leakage the drains may be left open to achieve continuous decompression of the bilioenteric anastomosis. Most cases of biliary leaks can be managed conservatively by drainage of the bilious secretion and if possible irrigation with sterile saline. Only in case of major leaks or further complications (e.g. haemorrhage due to vascular erosion) is operative revision indicated. However, due to the fragile nature of the intrahepatic bile ducts it might not be possible to improve the situation and adequate drainage is often the sole option in complicated cases.

Despite all efforts to decrease postoperative complications including decompression of jaundice for recovery of liver function, prophylaxis and treatment cholangitis and the use of preoperative portal vein embolization, the postoperative morbidity remains high after surgery for hilar cholangiocarcinoma. This operation clearly represents a high risk surgical procedure which should be reserved for experienced hepatobiliary centers. On the other side, the mortality has decreased using modern peri-operative regimens and therefore aggressive resection for hilar cholangiocarcinoma is justified despite the relatively high morbidity.

20.6 Long Term Results

Disease recurrence is still the most frequent cause of death after resection of hilar cholangiocarcinoma. Common sites of tumor recurrence are the peritoneum, the remnant liver and local lymph nodes [45]. Thereby, long term results of local resection without hepatectomy are significantly worse than after additional extended hepatectomies as shown in several retrospective series [22]. After hilar resection alone, long term cure can seldom be achieved [46, 47]. In contrast, extended hepatectomies offer a chance for cure of hilar cholangiocarcinoma. The 5 year overall survival (OS) rates of single center experiences, published since 2005 are reported between 20 and 40 % (Table 20.2). The median survival in these publications ranges between 20 [3] and 55 months [11]. Major determinants of long term outcome are analyzed in many series. In the given publications, several factors were significantly associated with an impaired survival in univariate analysis, but only in some studies. These included tumor stage (pT), left hepatectomy (vs. right hepatectomy), no postoperative chemotherapy, macroscopic tumor type (papillary vs. diffuse infiltrating), vascular invasion and positive lymph nodes (mainly positive coeliac lymph nodes).

It has been postulated already many years ago by Bismuth et al., that positive lymph nodes in hilar cholangiocarcinoma might be a less important prognostic factor than in other solid cancers of the upper GI-tract [28]. Therefore, regional lymph node metastases do not represent a contraindication for surgery and long term survival is possible in lymph node positive hilar cholangiocarcinoma as shown in several series (Table 20.2). One important prognostic factor is the lymph node ratio and the number of positive lymph nodes. It has been shown that patients with five or more positive lymph nodes have a significantly shorter survival, than patients with four or less positive lymph nodes [48]. Additionally long term results are influenced by the region of positive lymph nodes. Outcome is significantly impaired in case of positive nodes in the coeliac or paraaortal region [8]. Kitagawa et al. have reported, that particularly macroscopically detectable tumor infiltration of the para-aortic lymph nodes is associated with a poor long term prognosis (5 year survival rate 0 %), whereas in case of microscopically detectable infiltration a 5 year survival rate of 29 % was found [29].

In some but not all publications, the rate of R0 resections is higher in right hepatectomies than in left hepatectomies. However, the long term results of extended right hepatectomies are diminished by a higher postoperative mortality. In the experience reported by Kondo et al. a 0 postoperative mortality could be achieved and consequently long-term survival was significantly higher after right hepatectomy compared to left hepatectomy or caudate lobe resection [49].

In many retrospective analyses, several other determinants have been proven to be significantly associated with an impaired long term survival in multivariate analyses. Therefore, these have been accepted as negative factors for long term survival. These clearly include, poor differentiation of the tumor (G3), irresectability, incomplete tumor resection (R1 or even R2) and distant metastases, the latter three factors are normally associated with a 5 year survival of 0. However, after R1 resection long term survival seems to be achievable in a minority of patients. Whereas 5 year survival after R1 resection is 0 in many publications (Table 20.2), others have observed a 5 year survival of 10–20 % (Table 20.2) or even 38 % in a single publication [13]. However, as discussed above the incidence of R1 resection correlates with the accuracy of the pathological workup, and this might be an additional influential factor. In contrast, R0 resection is associated with a significantly improved 5 year survival rate of 30–50 % (Table 20.2).

References

1. Mansfield SD, Barakat O, Charnley RM, et al. Management of hilar cholangiocarcinoma in the North of England: pathology, treatment, and outcome. World J Gastroenterol. 2005;11:7625–30.

2. Hemming AW, Reed AI, Fujita S, et al. Surgical management of hilar cholangiocarcinoma. Ann Surg. 2005;241:693–9.
3. Lai EC, Lau WY. Aggressive surgical resection for hilar cholangiocarcinoma. ANZ J Surg. 2005;75:981–5.
4. Silva MA, Tekin K, Aytekin F, et al. Surgery for hilar cholangiocarcinoma; a 10 year experience of a tertiary referral centre in the UK. Eur J Surg Oncol. 2005;31:533–9.
5. Sano T, Shimada K, Sakamoto Y, et al. One hundred two consecutive hepatobiliary resections for perihilar cholangiocarcinoma with zero mortality. Ann Surg. 2006;44:240–7.
6. Cheng Q, Luo X, Zhang B, et al. Predictive factors for prognosis of hilar cholangiocarcinoma: postresection radiotherapy improves survival. Eur J Surg Oncol. 2007;33:202–7.
7. Witzigmann H, Berr F, Ringel U, et al. Surgical and palliative management and outcome in 184 patients with hilar cholangiocarcinoma: palliative photodynamic therapy plus stenting is comparable to R1/R2 resection. Ann Surg. 2006;244:230–9.
8. Baton O, Azoulay D, Adam DV, et al. Major hepatectomy for hilar cholangiocarcinoma type 3 and 4: prognostic factors and longterm outcomes. J Am Coll Surg. 2007;204:250–60.
9. Hasegawa S, Ikai I, Fujii H, et al. Surgical resection of hilar cholangiocarcinoma: analysis of survival and postoperative complications. World J Surg. 2007;31:1256–63.
10. Otani K, Chijiiwa K, Kai M, et al. Outcome of surgical treatment of hilar cholangiocarcinoma. J Gastrointest Surg. 2008;12:1033–40.
11. Ito F, Agni R, Rettammel RJ, et al. Resection of hilar cholangiocarcinoma: concomitant liver resection decreases hepatic recurrence. Ann Surg. 2008;248:273–9.
12. Yubin L, Chihua F, Zhixiang J, et al. Surgical management and prognostic factors of hilar cholangiocarcinoma: experience with 115 cases in China. Ann Surg Oncol. 2008;15:2113–9.
13. Konstadoulakis MM, Roayaie S, Gomatos IP, et al. Aggressive surgical resection for hilar cholangiocarcinoma: is it justified? Audit of a single center's experience. Am J Surg. 2008;196:160–9.
14. Murakami Y, Uemura K, Sudo T, et al. Gemcitabine-based adjuvant chemotherapy improves survival after aggressive surgery for hilar cholangiocarcinoma. J Gastrointest Surg. 2009;13:1470–9.
15. Lee SG, Song GW, Hwang S, et al. Surgical treatment of hilar cholangiocarcinoma in the new era: the Asan experience. J Hepatobiliary Pancreat Sci. 2010;17:476–89.
16. Miyazaki M, Kimura F, Shimizu H, et al. One hundred seven consecutive surgical resections for hilar cholangiocarcinoma of Bismuth types II, III, IV between 2001 and 2008. J Hepatobiliary Pancreat Sci. 2010;17:470–5.
17. Rocha FG, Matsuo K, Blumgart LH, et al. Hilar cholangiocarcinoma: the Memorial Sloan-Kettering Cancer Center experience. J Hepatobiliary Pancreat Sci. 2010;17:490–6.
18. Unno M, Katayose Y, Rikiyama T, et al. Major hepatectomy for perihilar cholangiocarcinoma. J Hepatobiliary Pancreat Sci. 2010; 17:463–9.
19. Young AL, Prasad KR, Toogood GJ, et al. Surgical treatment of hilar cholangiocarcinoma in a new era: comparison among leading Eastern and Western centers, Leeds. J Hepatobiliary Pancreat Sci. 2010;17:497–504.
20. Hirano S, Kondo S, Tanaka E, et al. Outcome of surgical treatment of hilar cholangiocarcinoma: a special reference to postoperative morbidity and mortality. J Hepatobiliary Pancreat Sci. 2010;17:455–62.
21. Igami T, Nishio H, Ebata T, Yokoyama Y, et al. Surgical treatment of hilar cholangiocarcinoma in the "new era": the Nagoya University experience. J Hepatobiliary Pancreat Sci. 2010;17(4):449–54.
22. van Gulik TM, Kloek JJ, Ruys AT, et al. Multidisciplinary management of hilar cholangiocarcinoma (Klatskin tumor): extended resection is associated with improved survival. Eur J Surg Oncol. 2011;37:65–71.
23. Verbeke CS. Resection margins and R1 rates in pancreatic cancer—are we there yet? Histopathology. 2008;52:787–96.
24. Vogl TJ, Schwarz WO, Heller M, et al. Staging of Klatskin tumours (hilar cholangiocarcinomas): comparison of MR cholangiography, MR imaging, and endoscopic retrograde cholangiography. Eur Radiol. 2006;16(10):2317–25.
25. Neuhaus P, Jonas S, Bechstein WO, et al. Extended resections for hilar cholangiocarcinoma. Ann Surg. 1999;230:808–18.
26. Stockmann M, Lock JF, Riecke B, et al. Prediction of postoperative outcome after hepatectomy with a new bedside test for maximal liver function capacity. Ann Surg. 2009;250:119–25.
27. Stockmann, Malinowski M, Lock JF, et al. Factors influencing the indocyanine green (ICG) test: additional impact of acute cholestasis? Hepatogastroenterology. 2009;56:734–8.
28. Bismuth H, Nakache R, Diamond T. Management strategies in resection for hilar cholangiocarcinoma. Ann Surg. 1992;215: 31–8.
29. Kitagawa Y, Nagino M, Kamiya J, et al. Lymph node metastasis from hilar cholangiocarcinoma: audit of 110 patients who underwent regional and paraaortic node dissection. Ann Surg. 2001;233: 385–92.
30. Pamecha V, Gurusamy KS, Sharma D, et al. Techniques for liver parenchymal transection: a meta-analysis of randomized controlled trials. HPB (Oxford). 2009;11:275–81.
31. Stockmann M, Lock JF, Malinowski M, et al. The LiMAx test: a new liver function test for predicting postoperative outcome in liver surgery. HPB (Oxford). 2010;12:139–46.
32. Nagino M, Nimura Y, Nishio H, et al. Hepatectomy with simultaneous resection of the portal vein and hepatic artery for advanced perihilar cholangiocarcinoma: an audit of 50 consecutive cases. Ann Surg. 2010;252:115–23.
33. Kondo S, Hirano S, Ambo Y, et al. Arterioportal shunting as an alternative to microvascular reconstruction after hepatic artery resection. Br J Surg. 2004;91(2):248–51.
34. Hjortsjö CH. The topography of the intrahepatic duct system. Acta Anat (Basel). 1951;11:599–615.
35. Nishio H, Hidalgo E, Hamady ZZ, et al. Left hepatic trisectionectomy for hepatobiliary malignancy: results and an appraisal of its current role. Ann Surg. 2005;242:267–75.
36. Shimada K, Sano T, Sakamoto Y, et al. Safety and effectiveness of left hepatic trisegmentectomy for hilar cholangiocarcinoma. World J Surg. 2005;29:723–7.
37. Lang H, Sotiropoulos GC, Brokalaki EI, et al. Left hepatic trisectionectomy for hepatobiliary malignancies. J Am Coll Surg. 2006; 203:311–21.
38. Cherqui D, Benoist S, Malassagne B, et al. Major liver resection for carcinoma in jaundiced patients without preoperative biliary drainage. Arch Surg. 2000;135:302–8.
39. Kanai M, Nimura Y, Kamiya J, et al. Preoperative intrahepatic segmental cholangitis in patients with advanced carcinoma involving the hepatic hilus. Surgery. 1996;119:498–504.
40. Seehofer D, Stockmann M, Schirmeier A, et al. Intraabdominal bacterial infections significantly alter regeneration and function of the liver in a rat model of major hepatectomy. Langenbecks Arch Surg. 2007;392:273–84.
41. Schindl MJ, Redhead DN, Fearon KCH, Edinburgh Liver Surgery and Transplantation Experimental Research Group (eLISTER), et al. The value of residual liver volume as a predictor of hepatic dysfunction and infection after major liver resection. Gut. 2005;54: 289–96.
42. Miyazaki M, Kato A, Ito H, et al. Combined vascular resection in operative resection for hilar cholangiocarcinoma: does it work or not? Surgery. 2007;141:581–8.
43. Nagino M, Nishio H, Ebata T, et al. Intrahepatic cholangiojejunostomy following hepatobiliary resection. Br J Surg. 2007;94:70–7.
44. de Castro SM, Kuhlmann KF, Busch OR, et al. Incidence and management of biliary leakage after hepaticojejunostomy. J Gastrointest Surg. 2005;9:1163–71.

45. Liu CL, Fan ST, Lo CM, et al. Improved operative and survival outcomes of surgical treatment for hilar cholangiocarcinoma. Br J Surg. 2006;93:1488–94.
46. Miyazaki M, Ito H, Nakagawa K, et al. Aggressive surgical approaches to hilar cholangiocarcinoma: hepatic or local resection? Surgery. 1998;123:131–6.
47. Jarnagin WR, Fong Y, DeMatteo RP, et al. Staging, resectability, and outcome in 225 patients with hilar cholangiocarcinoma. Ann Surg. 2001;234:507–17.
48. Hoang MP, Murakata LA, Katabi N, et al. Invasive papillary carcinomas of the extrahepatic bile ducts: a clinicopathologic and immunohistochemical study of 13 cases. Mod Pathol. 2002;15:1251–8.
49. Kondo S, Hirano S, Ambo Y, et al. Forty consecutive resections of hilar cholangiocarcinoma with no postoperative mortality and no positive ductal margins: results of a prospective study. Ann Surg. 2004;240:95–101.

Combined Liver Resection and Portal Vein Resection

21

K. Mekeel and A.W. Hemming

21.1 Introduction

Hilar cholangiocarcinoma is a difficult technical challenge for the hepatobiliary surgeon. Achieving negative surgical margins with tumor resection is demanding due to the close proximity of the bile duct bifurcation to the vascular inflow of the liver. As recently as 2001, patients with main portal vein involvement proximal to the bifurcation were considered to be unresectable [1]. However, as portal vein resection was employed in the resection of other hepatobiliary and pancreatic tumors with success, the same principles were extended to hilar cholangiocarcinoma. Although portal vein resection may increase the risks of the resection, this procedure increases the number of patients with potentially resectable disease, and remains the only hope for long-term survival in this uncommon cancer. This chapter will review the indications, surgical technique, and outcomes of portal vein resection for hilar cholangiocarcinoma, as well as a brief review of arterial resection.

As previously described, hilar cholangiocarcinoma is a relatively rare tumor, and only one third of patients diagnosed with cholangiocarcinoma are candidates for resection. With a small number of patients considered resectable, only a few surgeons at highly specialized centers have developed experience in the surgical management of this formidable disease. However, advances over the last two decades in hepatic surgical techniques have led to a more aggressive approach to the treatment of cholangiocarcinoma. Early reports of biliary resection and biliary enteric anastomosis have advanced to partial and subtotal hepatic resection, combined hepatopancreaticoduodenectomy, and vascular resection (Fig. 21.1), of either portal vein or hepatic artery, or even both. The first Western description of portal vein resection for hilar cholangiocarcinoma was by Hadjis and Blumgart, who suggested the need for portal vein resection in order to achieve tumor clearance [2]. The combination of extended right hepatic resection and portal vein resection was first described in the west by Klempnauer et al. in 1997 [3] and was taken further by Neuhaus et al. in 1999 [4] to include standard resection of the portal bifurcation in a "no touch" technique to minimize tumor dissemination at the time of surgery as well as to improve the rate of negative margin resections. This is often referred to as the Berlin concept [5].

The anatomic juxtaposition of the hepatic duct bifurcation to the bifurcation of the portal vein continues to be a technical challenge in resection of hilar cholangiocarcinoma due to tumor adherence or involvement of the portal vein at the bifurcation. In many cases the tumor may not have truly invaded the portal vein or hepatic artery, however the desmoplastic response to the tumor that is made up of fibrous tissue containing tumor cells extends to the vessel and cannot be

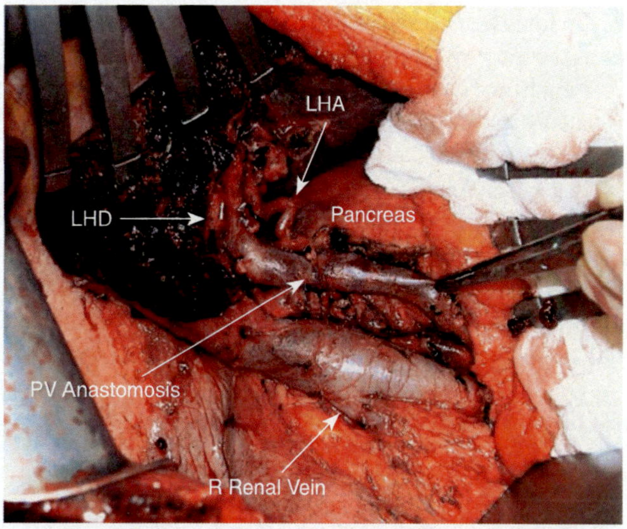

Fig. 21.1 Hepatopancreaticoduodenectomy with portal vein resection. *LHA* left hepatic artery, *LHD* left hepatic duct, *PV anastomosis* portal vein anastomosis, *R Renal vein* right renal vein

K. Mekeel, MD, FACS • A.W. Hemming, MD, FRCS, FACS (✉)
Division of Transplantation and Hepatobiliary Surgery,
University of California San Diego,
San Diego, CA, USA
e-mail: ahemming@ucsd.edu

W.Y. Lau (ed.), *Hilar Cholangiocarcinoma*,
DOI 10.1007/978-94-007-6473-6_21, © Springer Science+Business Media Dordrecht and People's Medical Publishing House 2013

separated from the vessel without potential injury and an increased probability of leaving tumor cells adherent to the exterior vessel wall. Portal vein resection may increase the ability to resect with negative margins and improve subsequent long-term survival, however the risk of the procedure may be increased and should not be minimized.

21.2 Indications for Portal Vein Reconstruction

1. The hilar cholangiocarcinoma tumor must meet standard criteria for an anatomic resection outside of portal vein involvement, including the potential for negative margins.
2. The future liver remnant (FLR) volume must be sufficient for post-operative hepatic function, usually 25 % or greater of total liver volume (TLV). Portal vein embolization should be considered in patients to increase FLR to >25 % TLV
3. Venous involvement can be central and at the bifurcation of the portal vein, however the distal portal vein on the liver remnant must have enough length clear of tumor to proceed with venous resection. On the left approximately 1 cm of left portal vein is required prior to segmental branching in order to have sufficient length for clamp placement. On the right, the right posterior branch needs to be clear of tumor. Venous anatomy to the right liver is more variable than the left and should be assessed by imaging prior to surgery. Arterial involvement and the potential for resection will be discussed below.
4. Extra-hepatic disease confined to porta hepatis or intrapancreatic portion of the bile duct. A complete portal lymphadenectomy should be completed at the time of resection. Portal lymph node spread decreases the chance of long term survival, but is not a contraindication to resection. Involvement of the common hepatic artery lymph node or aorto-caval lymph nodes is considered metastatic disease with less than 5 % 5-year survival. These patients likely should not be considered as candidates for resection. Intrahepatic metastases have a poor prognosis even if encompassed by hepatic resection and we would consider that a contraindication to resection.
5. Extrahepatic metastatic disease is a clear contraindication to resection.

21.3 Pre-operative Evaluation

The standard pre-operative work-up consists of a triphasic-computed tomography (CT) to assess biliary, portal, and hepatic arterial involvement as well as to perform liver volumetry and assess FLR. Patients are also staged with chest and abdominal CTs to exclude extra hepatic and metastatic disease. In many patients, potential resectability can be determined by this evaluation alone, however; additional information may be obtained in some patients with magnetic resonance cholangiopancreatography (MRCP) and contrast enhanced MRI to further delineate biliary anatomy and tumor extension.

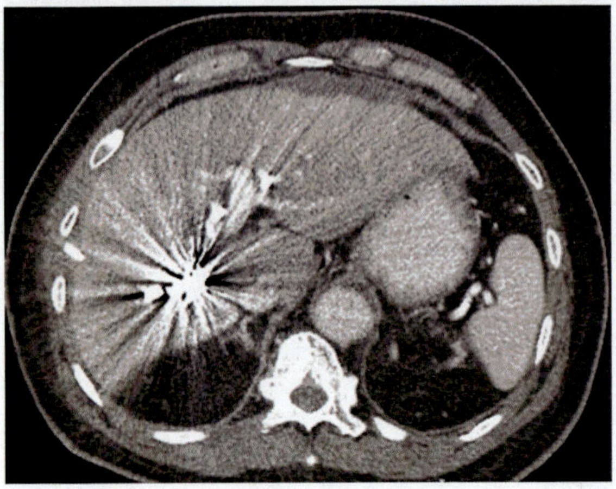

Fig. 21.2 Preoperative portal vein embolization of the right portal vein induces hypertrophy of the left lobe prior to resection

Although controversial, we feel that complete drainage and decompression of the remnant liver biliary tree is mandatory prior to resection, to decrease the risk of postoperative morbidity and mortality [6–8]. We consider an internally placed endoscopic cholangiopancreatography (ERCP) stent to be the first choice, but if adequate drainage is not achieved, percutaneous transhepatic drainage (PTCD) is required.

In many patients with hilar cholangiocarcinoma with vascular involvement, the FLR may already have experienced compensatory hypertrophy. However, if the hypertrophy has not occurred or if it is inadequate then pre-operative portal vein embolization should be performed (Fig. 21.2) on the side of the liver that is to be resected 4–6 weeks prior to surgery [9]. The importance of hypertrophy of the remnant liver in surgery for hilar cholangiocarcinoma has been demonstrated by multiple reports [10–14].

21.4 Procedure

21.4.1 Surgical Technique

1. The first step of this operation includes an abdominal exploration to detect disseminated abdominal disease. This may be completed using minimally invasive techniques such as laparoscopy, particularly for those patients with bulky portal disease [15], or a mini laparotomy using a portion of the potential incision. If no contraindications to resection are initially seen the incision is

widened and aorto-caval and common hepatic artery lymph nodes are sampled. If positive the patient is unlikely to benefit from resection.

2. Patients without disseminated disease undergo a standardized assessment of resectability, including an intraoperative ultrasound directed examination of the tumor and the relationship of the tumor to the major vascular structures.

3a. If the tumor is predominately right-sided and a right trisegmentectomy is contemplated, then dissection of the left hepatic duct and left portal vein at the base of the falciform ligament is performed. If the hepatic duct is clear at the segment 2/3 junction along with a patent left portal vein distally then a right trisegmentectomy can be performed. The left hepatic duct and left portal vein are accessible by dissecting the falciform ligament to the left portal vein capitalizing on the knowledge that the remnant of the umbilical vein (that during fetal circulation flowed into the left portal vein) runs within the round ligament of the falciform and will lead directly to the left portal vein at the portion just before the branching into segment 2, 3. This allows assessment of resectability before committing to bile duct division or hepatic resection. Even if the proximal portal vein and bile duct are involved, reconstruction can occur to the uninvolved distal structures.

3b. If the tumor is predominately left-sided and a left trisegmentectomy is contemplated, intraoperative ultrasound plays a more important role. In particular tumor involvement along the right posterior hepatic duct (segments 6/7) must be assessed. The bifurcation of the anterior and posterior branches of both the portal vein and hepatic ducts are relatively intrahepatic and is a difficult area to assess for definitive evidence of tumor by either ultrasound or by the manual and visual assessment of the surgeon. Although lowering of the hilar plate facilitates the assessment of the segment 6, 7, take off it is not recommended because of the potential to broach the tumor plane. There is no doubt that in many cases the surgeon must commit to resection and hepatic division without certainty regarding margins and vessel involvement which is more frequently encountered in performing a left trisegmentectomy than a right sided resection. An assessment of the portal venous anatomy as well an assessment of the position of the posterior branch of the hepatic artery and its position relative to the portal vein branches on the right should also be undertaken during intraoperative ultrasound examination.

4. After it has been determined that resection will proceed, the next step is dissection of the hepatic artery to ensure the hepatic arterial supply to the remnant liver is not involved by tumor. The common hepatic artery and left hepatic artery can be dissected out without committing

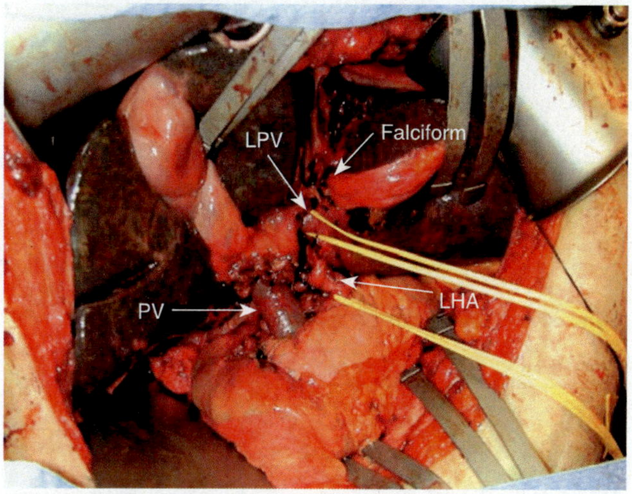

Fig. 21.3 Left portal vein dissected out at the base of the falciform ligament. The main portal vein and left portal vein are isolated without separating the hilar ductal structures from the portal bifurcation. *LHA* left hepatic artery, *LPV* left portal vein, *PV* portal vein

to resection by dissecting along the medial side of the artery. In general, involvement of the common hepatic artery or major hepatic branch to the remnant liver is considered a contraindication to resection, however; there has been some success reported with hepatic arterial resection in selected cases, which will be discussed later in this chapter. The right hepatic artery, if in a standard position anterior to the portal vein but posterior to the bile duct is difficult to dissect out until after the bile duct has been divided and flipped superiorly.

5. The common bile duct is then divided at the level of the pancreas and reflected superiorly (Fig. 21.3). A margin is sent from the distal common bile duct to assess for tumor involvement. Additional margin on the distal bile duct can be obtained by dissecting out the intra-pancreatic portion of the bile duct however pancreaticoduodenectomy may be considered if the margin is positive. A positive margin at this time requires a decision of how a negative distal margin can be obtained. If the patient is not a candidate for HPD then liver resection should not be considered in the face of a persistently positive distal margin. Lymph nodes of the hepatoduodenal ligament are resected either en-bloc with the bile duct as it is reflected superiorly along with the portal lymphatics or if the nodes must be removed separately then the level and position of the node is noted when the nodes are sent for permanent section . Reflecting the bile duct superiorly allows completion of the dissection of the right hepatic artery to its anterior/posterior division for a left sided resection and during that dissection possible involvement of the right hepatic artery or the posterior branch may preclude resection or necessitate resection

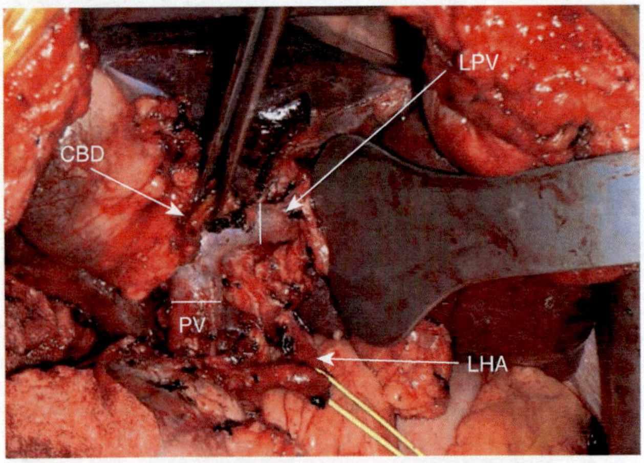

Fig. 21.4 The bile duct is flipped superiorly and the left lateral aspect of the portal vein dissected out. *Solid white lines* demonstrate where vascular clamps are placed to resect the portal vein confluence. *CBD* common bile duct, *LHA* left hepatic artery, *LPV* left portal vein, *PV* portal vein

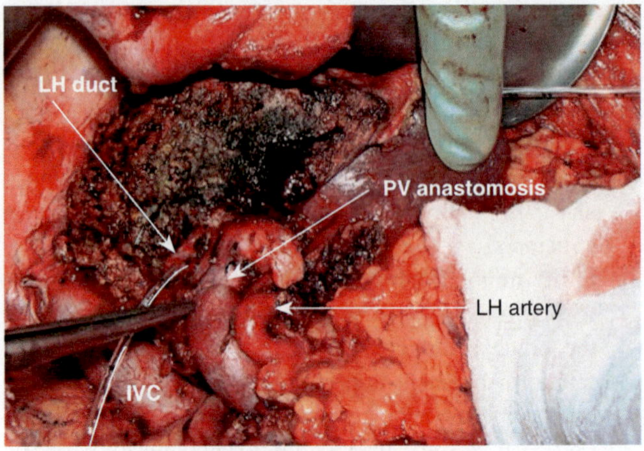

Fig. 21.5 Right trisegmentectomy with portal vein resection and reconstruction of main portal vein to left portal vein. *IVC* inferior vena cava, *LH artery* left hepatic artery, *LH duct* left hepatic duct, *PV anastomosis* portal vein anastomosis

and reconstruction. At this point the need for portal vein resection can be identified.

6. The portal vein resection can be performed at two different time points during the procedure depending on the extent of mobility of the portal vein, extent of tumor and accessibility in the patient. In the majority of patients undergoing right-sided trisegmentectomies where access is reasonable and the amount of portal vein expected to be resected relatively short, the portal vein resection and reconstruction can be performed prior to hepatic transection. After dissection of the left hepatic artery to its segmental branches and ligation of the right hepatic artery, the main portal vein below the tumor is isolated. The left portal vein above the tumor is dissected out past the transverse portion of the vein up to the ascending segment just before branching into main segmental branches. Multiple caudate branches require division in order to free up enough left portal vein to work with. The area of the main portal venous bifurcation is left en bloc with the tumor. Vascular clamps are placed on the main portal vein and left portal vein just before it's branching to main segmental branches (Fig. 21.4). The vein is then divided and left attached to the tumor. The left portal vein is then brought down to the main portal vein with a primary end to end anastomosis using 6-0 or 7-0 vascular sutures. Arterial perfusion can be maintained throughout the resection and reconstruction, minimizing ischemia to the FLR. The hepatic transection and specimen removal occurs after reconstruction with maintenance of both portal and hepatic arterial flow.

In some patients where access is difficult or the tumor extensive, the portal vein is dissected as much as possible to prior hepatic transection, however it is not divided until hepatic parenchymal transection is completed.

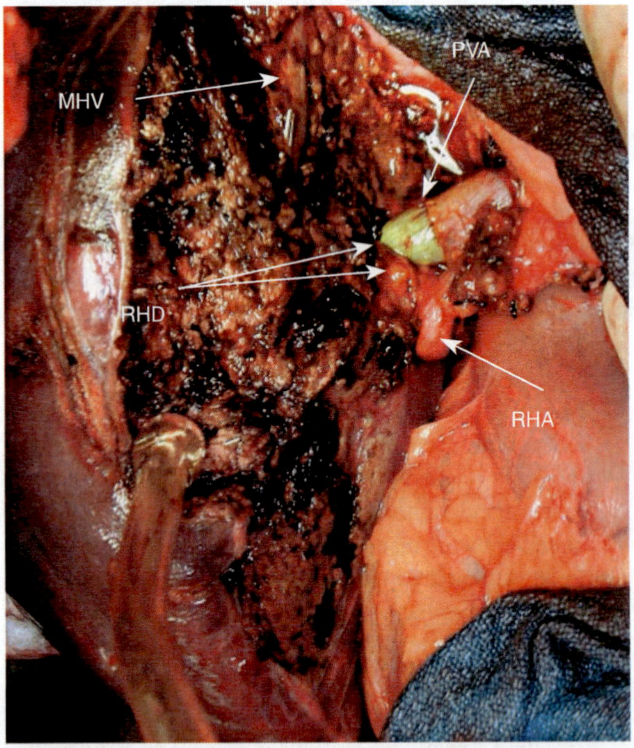

Fig. 21.6 Left hepatectomy with resection of portal vein bifurcation and anastomosis (*PVA*) of main portal vein to right portal vein. *MHV* middle hepatic vein, *RHA* right hepatic artery, *RHD* right hepatic duct at anterior and posterior division

Dividing the portal vein at this later stage mobilizes the specimen and allows a tremendous improvement in mobility of the hepatic side of the portal vein, which can be rotated down significantly from its original position to minimize tension on the venous anastomosis (Fig. 21.5). The majority of left sided (Fig. 21.6) resections with anastomosis of the main portal vein to either right portal vein branch or posterior sectoral portal vein

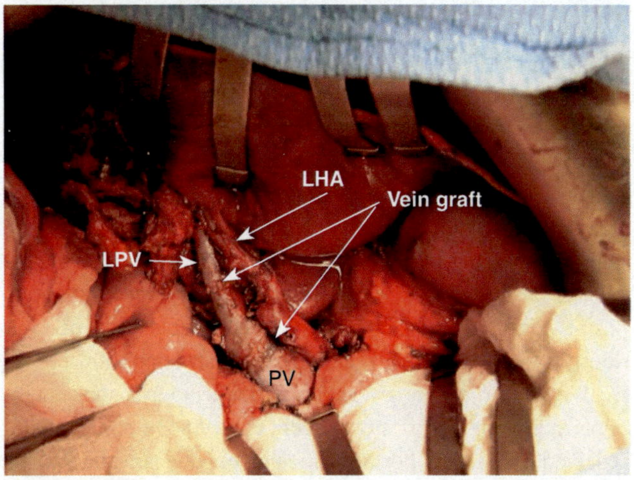

Fig. 21.7 Right hepatectomy with portal vein resection and reconstruction of the main portal vein to left portal vein. The right hepatic vein has been removed from the resected right lobe and used as an interposition graft. *LHA* left hepatic artery, *LPV* left portal vein, *PV* portal vein, *Vein graft* right hepatic vein used as an interposition graft

branch are more easily performed after hepatic parenchymal transection in our experience. In general the use of interposition grafts should not be required. If it appears that there will be excessive tension on the reconstruction by performing the reconstruction prior to hepatic parenchymal division then the reconstruction should be performed after the hepatic division when the additional mobility of the liver allows anastomosis. If even after hepatic transection a graft appears to be needed, hepatic vein from the resected side of the liver can be used to bridge the gap (Fig. 21.7) or if necessary the portion of the left renal vein between gonadal vein and IVC can be harvested and used as a graft. Both internal jugular vein and superficial femoral vein have been used as interposition grafts for the portal vein reconstruction, however the need for an interposition graft should be rare.

7. Liver resection should then be performed using techniques familiar to the operating surgeon. The general consensus is that the caudate lobe should be resected routinely. In general we attempt to perform the parenchymal transection with maintenance of flow in both portal vein and hepatic artery in attempts to limit ischemia to what is considered an "damaged" liver from biliary obstruction and because of the requirement of additional ischemia during the portal vein resection and reconstruction phase of the procedure. However if bleeding is encountered we have little hesitation in applying inflow occlusion to the liver irrespective of whether the portal vein resection is performed initially prior to parenchymal division, or it is done at the completion of the parenchymal transection. If inflow occlusion is required we apply occlusion for periods of 15 min followed by 5 min of reperfusion [16].
8. Frozen section analysis of margins should be used to guide resection, and if positive margins are encountered, additional resection should be performed if possible. Negative margins are the most important factor in long-term survival of this disease.
9. In the majority of right trisegmentectomies, left portal vein resection can be completed prior to completion of the hepatic transection if there is a sufficient length of intrahepatic left portal vein that is tumor free [11, 17]. In left trisegmentectomies and in right trisegmentectomies involving cases where the left portal vein is more substantially involved, venous resection and reconstruction can be completed after resection. Resection without immediate reconstruction is not recommended, as it leaves the remnant liver with prolonged ischemia.
10. Reconstruction is completed end to end with 5-0/6-0 running prolene suture, being careful to incorporate a growth factor as in liver transplantation. We generally "parachute" down the posterior wall to distribute tension along the venous anastomosis prior to bring the ends together and then run the anterior wall of the anastomosis. Alternatively the posterior wall can be parachuted down with a continuous suture and the front wall interrupted. As mentioned previously, if primary reconstruction is not feasible, hepatic vein from the side resected, left renal vein, superficial femoral vein or jugular vein can be considered for a conduit. Synthetic and cryopreserved grafts are not recommended due to the risk of infection and thrombosis. An important point is that arterial inflow to the remnant liver is maintained during reconstruction.
11. The biliary system should be reconstructed using a 60 cm roux-en-Y limb of jejunum.
12. Post-operative care is similar to a standard liver resection. Ultrasound should be used to confirm patency of the reconstructed vasculature, both intra- and post-operatively. At our center postoperative anticoagulation is reserved for patients at increased risk for thrombosis (hypercoaguable state, intraoperative thrombosis), complex reconstruction, or arterial reconstruction with small vessels (heparin, long-term aspirin). Other published series range from no anticoagulation [18] to catheters dripping heparin into the portal vein postoperatively [19].

21.5 Outcomes

21.5.1 Perioperative Morbidity and Mortality

21.5.1.1 Mortality

Early series with small numbers of patients with portal vein resection (PVR) for hilar cholangiocarcinoma had high mortality rates ranging from 8 to 33 %. This discouraged wide spread use of the described techniques [20–26]. In 2000,

Gerhards et al. [21] also found vascular reconstruction to be an independent predictor of increased mortality. With increasing experience with extended hepatectomies, vascular reconstruction, and living donor liver transplantation [27], the mortality rates at specialized high volume centers have decreased dramatically and are now equivalent to non-vascular resections. Recent series demonstrate mortality of 2 % or less with portal vein and combined resections [11, 13, 18, 28]. Nagino et al. [18] published a series of 50 combined hepatic artery resections with a perioperative mortality of 2 %, which is decreased significantly from a 9.6 % mortality from the same group in 2003 [24]. Lee et al. [27] also reported a mortality of 0 in 40 consecutive patients with PVR from 2005 to 2008 compared to 9.8 % from 1989 to 2005. The authors of both of these studies concluded that general improvement of technique, including use of microvascular techniques, and improved perioperative management utilizing portal vein embolization and remnant liver biliary drainage resulted in improved outcomes.

Hemming et al. [11, 14] demonstrated a trend toward decreased mortality in patients undergoing PVR. In 95 patients undergoing resection for hilar cholangiocarcinoma, 42 patients who underwent PVR had a perioperative mortality of 2 % compared to 8 % for the 53 patients undergoing resection alone. The authors postulated that portal vein involvement mimics portal vein embolization, creating hypertrophy of the remaining hepatic lobe, and decreasing the risk of post-operative liver failure. With experience, there was also a significant decrease in 30-day mortality as a consequence of improvements in perioperative management (portal vein embolization, biliary drainage of the future liver remnant). In the first half of the study the operative mortality was 10 % and subsequently there were no perioperative mortalities in the second half of the study ($P=0.04$) [14].

21.5.1.2 Morbidity

Despite improvement in mortality, these procedures continue to have a high morbidity, as do all major hepatic resections for hilar cholangiocarcinoma. Complications range from 43 to 100 % [13, 14, 25, 27]. Morbidity does not appear to differ between vascular and non vascular resections [23, 29], and in some cases may be decreased when compared to non vascular resections [19]. The most common complications are wound infection, bile leak, intra-abdominal abscess, sepsis, hemorrhage, reoperation and liver failure. The initial series demonstrated a high risk of postoperative liver insufficiency (defined in most series as hyperbilirubinemia, usually of serum bilirubin greater then 8–10 mg/dl) of up to 20 %. The more recent series using routine perioperative portal vein embolization showed liver failure to occur less frequently in 5–10 % of patients after resection [13], and most patients recovered with time.

The risk of complications directly related to vascular reconstruction is low. In one of the largest series of 111 patients who underwent portal vein reconstruction, five patients developed portal vein thrombosis intra- or post-operatively, and three requiring reoperation and thrombectomy. The paper reported four deaths from portal vein thrombosis and subsequent liver failure, but it is unclear if these were all related to portal vein resection and reconstruction [13]. Hirano et al. [19] reported 4 (10.8 %) intra-operative portal vein thromboses including two patients who received interposition grafts. All four were reconstructed intra-operatively without any long-term consequences. In a subsequent paper reporting on 50 more recent consecutive patients who received combined portal vein and hepatic arterial reconstructions by the same group, only one patient developed portal venous thrombosis postoperatively [18]. Hemming et al. [14] reported no anastomotic complications or thromboses in a review of 42 portal vein resections without the use of interposition grafts. There are several case reports of thrombosis with the use of interposition grafts [17, 19]. Although this is not a conclusive evidence, interposition grafts should only be used if absolutely necessary due to these concerns.

21.6 Survival

21.6.1 Overall Survival

The 1, 3, and 5-year survival after hepatic resection and portal vein resection have been reported in many series. It is clear that survival of patients undergoing vascular resection is higher than that of a cohort of unresectable tumors [13, 18, 23]. In addition, vascular resection increases the number of potentially resectable tumors [24]. These facts alone validate the use of vascular resection if technically feasible in suitable patients. Reports on long-term survival after portal vein resection for hilar cholangiocarcinoma are conflicting. When comparing patients who underwent portal vein resection to patients who underwent resection only, most studies showed inferior long-term survival [18, 23, 24, 26]. For example, Igmai et al. [13] found that the survival rates of patients undergoing portal vein resection were 37 % at 3 years and 23 % at 5 years, which were less than the survival of non vascular resections (42 % at 5 years, 52 % if R0), but it was still better than the survivals of R2/pM1 resections and unresectable disease, and the survival was equivalent to R1 resections.

Ebata et al. [24] also reported on a worse long-term survival in patients requiring portal vein resection. However multivariate analysis demonstrated that portal vein resection itself did not worsen survival, but it was the presence of transluminal tumor or positive margins that had a negative impact. In many series, multivariate analysis showed portal vein resection to be a negative prognostic factor [24, 26], but more recent studies demonstrated otherwise [19]. Using the "no touch" technique, Neuhaus et al. [30] reported improved survival when compared to standard hepatic resection, with portal vein resection being a positive predictor of long-term survival. With improvement in perioperative mortality as centers gain more experience with these procedures, the long-term survival is also improved. Dinant et al. [25] demonstrated an increased 2 year survival from 33 % (1998–1993) to 60 % (1998–2003) by adopting aggressive surgical techniques including trisectionectomies, vascular reconstruction, and caudate resection to achieve negative margins.

Obviously a decreased survival after portal vein resection may be secondary to invasion of the portal vein by tumor. Hilar cholangiocarcinomas typically manifest an intense fibrotic response around the hilar plate and vessels. Portal vein involvement may be directly related to tumor involvement, or indirectly related to entrapment in the fibrotic reaction. In most series, only 30–50 % of resected veins actually have microscopic or histologic tumor involvement [18, 24, 31, 32]. Other series reported up to 80 % involvement [14, 23], and there is obviously some difference between studies in the definition of histologic involvement. Whether or not histologic portal vein involvement influences survival is also controversial. Several series reported that histologic portal vein invasion is a negative prognostic factor for long-term survival [23, 32, 33], while other studies did not demonstrate this effect [14, 19]. A negative margin or R0 resection remains the best chance for long-term survival, and not surprisingly tumors requiring portal vein resection are also less likely to achieve an R0 resection [29].

In addition, several series have report on some patients surviving over 3 years [22, 34]. Nagino et al. [18] reported on six patients who lived longer than 3 years, and two patients who were alive after 5 years with combined portal vein and hepatic artery resection. Lee et al. [27] reported on ten patients who survived longer than 5 years after portal vein resection, including six patients who were alive and disease free at the time of publication, and they estimated that portal vein resection could offer long-term survival in more than one of ten patients with locally advanced hilar cholangiocarcinoma.

21.7 "No Touch" Resections

Some authors have advocated a "no touch" method resection for hilar cholangiocarcinoma [30, 31]. As mentioned above, hilar cholangiocarcinoma is challenging because of the proximity of the hepatic duct bifurcation to the major vascular inflow of the liver. Even if the portal vein is not directly involved with the tumor, the tumor may involve the perihilar lymphatics and neural tissue. To decrease the potential of locoregional recurrence for microscopic tumor spread and increase the likelihood of an R0 resection require an en bloc resection including right hepatectomy, caudate lobectomy, bile duct resection, and portal vein resection. Neuhaus et al. [30] championed this technique, with a 5-year survival of 72 % for patients who underwent en bloc vascular resection, which was significantly higher than patients undergoing non-vascular resection.

Subsequently, Hirando et al. [31] published a series of 64 patients, in which 25 patients underwent en bloc resection. Forty-three patients underwent conventional resection, including 18 patients with portal vein resection. Intra-operative thrombosis occurred in four patients, two patients in each of the portal vein resection and the en bloc groups. These were all revised intra-operatively and there were no post-operative portal vein complications. Two-year survival was not significantly different between the no resection, conventional, and en bloc groups (73.7 %/39.7 %/69.6 %), but trended down in the conventional resection group. Morbidity and in hospital mortality also did not differ between the groups. In contrast, Lee et al. [27] reported that in actual clinical practice, the "no-touch technique" for extensive surgical resection of hepatopancreatobiliary malignancies has failed to show a short-term survival benefit because of the high postoperative mortality [27]. Of course, the ultimate "no touch" technique is liver transplantation, which has encouraging results in very select patients [35].

21.8 Right Versus Left Resections

Some centers would argue that portal vein resection and aggressive liver resection for hilar cholangiocarcinoma should be limited to right trisegmentectomies, and left hepatectomies with left trisegmentectomies in particular to be avoided due to the anatomic differences in the right hepatic lobe [4, 36] and the difficulty in getting negative margins. In particular, the early ramifications of the right portal vein and biliary system require dissection that may broach microscopic tumor planes. The course of the right hepatic artery and in particular the position of the posterior right hepatic artery relative to both the posterior branches of the duct and relative position to the portal vein branches makes achieving a negative margin without broaching tumor planes more difficult. Left trisectionectomies have been reported to have an increased mortality, decreased R0 resections, and as a result decreased long term survival in some series when compared to right sided trisectionectomies [5].

However, as surgeons continue to push boundaries, experience with left sided hepatectomies for hilar cholangiocarcinoma with combined vascular resection continues to grow. Shimizu et al. [37] recently published a series of 224 patients of whom 88 underwent left hepatectomies and 84 underwent right hepatectomies. Portal vein resection was carried out in 23 of 88 left hepatectomies (26 %) and 25 of 84 right hepatectomies (30 %). Overall R0 resection, morbidity, and survival were equivalent between the two groups, except that left hepatectomies had an increased risk of bile leakage, and right hepatectomies had an increased risk of liver insufficiency and mortality as a result of the smaller remnant liver. However, there was a significantly decreased chance of an R0 resection with a left hepatectomy and portal vein resection compared to the right hepatectomy, and a subsequent decrease in long-term survival. If an R0 resection was achieved, survival was the same. There was also a significant increase in the use of partial wedge resections with vein patching versus a segmental vein resection and end-to-end venous anastomosis in left hepatectomies, due to the limited mobility and early ramifications of the right portal vein [37]. The authors concluded that while extended left or left trisegmentectomies are technically more demanding than right sided resections for hilar cholangiocarcinoma, in many cases they are the only option available to perform a curative resection.

21.9 Hepatic Artery Resection

Until recently hepatic arterial involvement was considered a contraindication to resection for hilar cholangiocarcinoma. However, as more experience is gained in these complex combined vascular and hepatic resections, aggressive centers are resecting and reconstructing both the right, left, and main hepatic artery with acceptable outcomes. These innovations may continue to extent the limits of resection with hilar cholangiocarcinoma, particularly in extended left trisegmentectomies where the right hepatic artery can often be involved with tumor as the artery runs close to the hepatic hilus.

Hepatic artery reconstructions can be completed in a segmental fashion with reconstruction using either an end-to-end anastomosis to the left gastric, right gastric or gastroduodenal or other alternative inflow, or an interposition graft (including greater saphenous vein or radial artery, or proximal splenic artery (Fig. 21.8)) [38]. As with portal vein resection, a distal hepatic artery clear of tumor is necessary. If portal vein resection is also required, hepatic arterial resection should be done in a sequential fashion before or after portal vein resection to protect the liver from ischemia. If this cannot be done, cold perfusion techniques may be necessary.

21.9.1 Combined Hepatic Artery and Portal Vein Resection

Early results from hepatic artery resection for hilar cholangiocarcinoma were dismal. Some early series including hepatic arterial resections with or without portal vein reconstruction had a high mortality of 33.3–55.6 % [23, 39, 40] with no long term survivors. Gerhards et al. [21] found in an univariate analysis that hepatic arterial resection increased mortality in extended liver resections for hilar cholangiocarcinoma. Miyazaki et al. [23] reported the results of nine combined hepatic artery and portal vein resections. There was no benefit in terms of survival (1- and 3-year survival rate; 17 % and 0, respectively) and it led to an increase in operative mortality (33 %) and morbidity (78 % compared to 36 %). A recent series comparing right and left hepatectomies found that hepatic arterial resection for both right and left hepatectomies (11 patients) decreased survival, and there were no survivors beyond 3 years [37].

However, recent advances in microsurgical techniques and increasing experience with vascular resections have improved outcomes in patients undergoing hepatic artery resection. Several series on portal vein reconstruction have included small numbers of patients with concomitant hepatic artery resection without any significant complications [11, 12, 32, 41]. In a series published by Yamanaka et al., 25 patients underwent major hepatic resection with vascular reconstruction for hilar cholangiocarcinoma. The series included: ten patients who underwent hepatic arterial reconstruction (nine right and one left hepatic artery) [20]. The reconstructions were all done in an end to end fashion to the proper hepatic artery or gastroduodenal artery, and 80 % were done using microsurgical techniques. Perioperative mortality was 8.8 %. Although survival was lower in the left trisegmentectomy group with vascular resections, the complications were not directly related to the vascular reconstruction. In a similar series, Shimada et al. looked at 39 patients with hilar cholangiocarcinoma and gallbladder cancer, of which 17 underwent hepatic arterial resection with or without portal vein resection [22]. Patency was achieved in

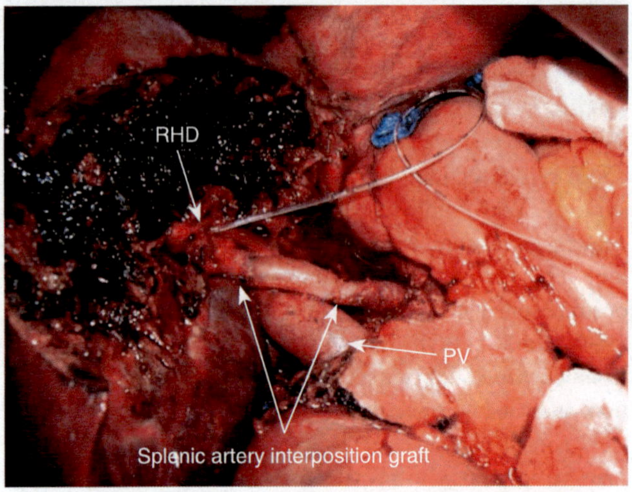

Fig. 21.8 Right hepatic artery reconstructed using the proximal splenic artery as an interposition graft. *PV* portal vein, *RHD* right hepatic duct

83 % of the reconstructed hepatic artery, and two patients developed multiple hepatic abscesses from hepatic arterial thrombosis. The results improved after they adopted microsurgical techniques. Perioperative mortality in the patients with vascular reconstruction was 13.3 % compared to 8.3 %, alone in the non-reconstruction cohorts. Two patients with combined HA/PV reconstruction survived more than 3 years.

In the largest series published to date, Nagino et al. [18] reported a series of 50 patients who underwent simultaneous resection of hilar cholangiocarcinoma, including 26 left trisegmentectomies, 23 left hepatectomies, and one right hepatectomy. R0 resection was achieved in 33 (66 %) patients. The 1, 3 and 5 year survivals were 78.9, 36.3, and 30.3 %, respectively. Twenty-seven (54 %) patients developed complications and one patient died perioperatively. All reconstructions were done with the assistance of a surgical microscope, and these included 32 end-to-end anastomoses, 11 greater saphenous vein or radial artery interpositions, and 2 reconstructions using the left or right gastric artery. Three patients were unable to be reconstructed. One patient with a vein graft thrombosed intra-operatively and was thrombectomized and revised without any complication. There were no long-term complications from the arterial reconstructions. The authors of this series believe that the microsurgical techniques offered an improvement over their earlier studies.

In some cases, reconstruction may not be necessary. Miyake et al. [42] reported a case where the right hepatic artery was unable to be reconstructed, but there was good collateral flow through the right phrenic artery and the patient recovered. If the branch of the hepatic artery supplying segment IV (or middle hepatic artery, which arises from the left hepatic artery in 75 % of cases) is the only artery which is involved by tumor, it can be resected without any significant complications, including biliary leaks and abscesses [19].

In preparation for hepatic arterial resection, some authors have advocated pre-operative hepatic arterial embolization to allow for the development of collaterals prior to resection. Yasuda et al. [34] described pre-operative embolization of the right hepatic artery to allow collateralization of the right liver remnant for left trisectionectomies with tumors involving the right and proper hepatic arteries. A series of six patients underwent left trisegmentectomy 3 weeks after arterial embolization for hilar cholangiocarcinoma. All six patients underwent R0 resection, and there were no liver failure or perioperative death. Two patients remain alive after 7 years.

In some cases, it may not be technically possible to reconstruct the hepatic artery, due to the extent of tumor involvement or its small caliber. In the largest series of hepatic arterial resection reported to date, Nagino et al. [18] described three patients in whom the artery was unable to be reconstructed. In one patient, it was a small segment 6 artery that did not require reconstruction. The other two patients underwent arterioportal shunting, which resulted in liver failure in one patient, and liver abscess in the other. Kondo et al. [43] reported better results in using arterioportal shunting in ten patients (6 HCCA and 4 GBCA). There were no deaths, and three patients developed complications including bile leakage and liver abscesses. Angiography performed 1 month after surgery showed shunt occlusion in 30 % of the patients. The remainder of the shunts was occluded by coil embolization after collateralization was confirmed.

Conclusion

Multiple series have now confirmed that an aggressive surgical approach to hilar cholangiocarcinoma is beneficial. Portal vein resection can be performed safely with low mortality and acceptable morbidity at high volume specialized centers. While routine en bloc portal vein resection of all hilar cholangiocarcinomas has been advocated by some centers it is difficult to recommend routine resection of the portal vein at this time. It is our recommendation that portal vein resection be carried out in cases where the portal vein cannot be separated from the tumor either because of direct tumor spread or peritumoral fibrosis. There is no doubt that combined portal vein resection offers improved survival when compared to no resection or a resection with positive margins. In selected patients, vascular resection increases the chance of obtaining negative resection margin, and may increase the number of patients who can be consider for resection. Recently the reported 5-year survival rate for hilar cholangiocarcinoma of 50 % exceeds the survival reported for pancreatic cancer. Portal vein resection for hilar cholangiocarcinoma in experienced hand should no longer be considered controversial. Hepatic arterial resection is also evolving and while it should not considered as routine at present, it may become a standard aggressive treatment of hilar cholangiocarcinoma in the future as techniques and experience continue to improve.

References

1. Jarnagin WR, Fong Y, DeMatteo RP, et al. Staging, resectability, and outcome in 225 patients with hilar cholangiocarcinoma. Ann Surg. 2001;234(4):507–17; discussion 17–9.
2. Hadjis NS, Blenkharn JI, Alexander N, et al. Outcome of radical surgery in hilar cholangiocarcinoma. Surgery. 1990;107(6):597–604.
3. Klempnauer J, Ridder GJ, Werner M, et al. What constitutes long-term survival after surgery for hilar cholangiocarcinoma? Cancer. 1997;79(1):26–34.
4. Neuhaus P, Jonas S, Bechstein WO, et al. Extended resections for hilar cholangiocarcinoma. Ann Surg. 1999;230(6):808–18; discussion 19.
5. Thelen A, Scholz A, Benckert C, et al. Microvessel density correlates with lymph node metastases and prognosis in hilar cholangiocarcinoma. J Gastroenterol. 2008;43(12):959–66.

6. Grandadam S, Compagnon P, Arnaud A, et al. Role of preoperative optimization of the liver for resection in patients with hilar cholangiocarcinoma type III. Ann Surg Oncol. 2010;17(12): 3155–61.
7. Nimura Y. Preoperative biliary drainage before resection for cholangiocarcinoma (Pro). HPB (Oxford). 2008;10(2):130–3.
8. Laurent A, Tayar C, Cherqui D. Cholangiocarcinoma: preoperative biliary drainage (Con). HPB (Oxford). 2008;10(2):126–9.
9. Hemming AW, Reed AI, Howard RJ, et al. Preoperative portal vein embolization for extended hepatectomy. Ann Surg. 2003;237(5): 686–91; discussion 91–3.
10. Kennedy TJ, Yopp A, Qin Y, et al. Role of preoperative biliary drainage of liver remnant prior to extended liver resection for hilar cholangiocarcinoma. HPB (Oxford). 2009;11(5):445–51.
11. Hemming AW, Kim RD, Mekeel KL, et al. Portal vein resection for hilar cholangiocarcinoma. Am Surg. 2006;72(7):599–604; discussion 604–5.
12. Lee SG, Lee YJ, Park KM, et al. One hundred and eleven liver resections for hilar bile duct cancer. J Hepatobiliary Pancreat Surg. 2000;7(2):135–41.
13. Igami T, Nishio H, Ebata T, et al. Surgical treatment of hilar cholangiocarcinoma in the "new era": the Nagoya University experience. J Hepatobiliary Pancreat Sci. 2010;17(4):449–54.
14. Hemming AW, Mekeel K, Khanna A, et al. Portal vein resection in the management of hilar cholangiocarcinoma. J Am Coll Surg. 2011;212(4):604–13; discussion 613–6.
15. D'Angelica M, Fong Y, Weber S, et al. The role of staging laparoscopy in hepatobiliary malignancy: prospective analysis of 401 cases. Ann Surg Oncol. 2003;10(2):183–9.
16. Petrowsky H, McCormack L, Trujillo M, et al. A prospective, randomized, controlled trial comparing intermittent portal triad clamping versus ischemic preconditioning with continuous clamping for major liver resection. Ann Surg. 2006;244(6):921–8; discussion 8–30.
17. Kondo S, Katoh H, Hirano S, et al. Portal vein resection and reconstruction prior to hepatic dissection during right hepatectomy and caudate lobectomy for hepatobiliary cancer. Br J Surg. 2003; 90(6):694–7.
18. Nagino M, Nimura Y, Nishio H, et al. Hepatectomy with simultaneous resection of the portal vein and hepatic artery for advanced perihilar cholangiocarcinoma: an audit of 50 consecutive cases. Ann Surg. 2010;252(1):115–23.
19. Hirano S, Kondo S, Tanaka E, et al. Safety of combined resection of the middle hepatic artery in right hemihepatectomy for hilar biliary malignancy. J Hepatobiliary Pancreat Surg. 2009;16(6):796–801.
20. Yamanaka N, Yasui C, Yamanaka J, et al. Left hemihepatectomy with microsurgical reconstruction of the right-sided hepatic vasculature. A strategy for preserving hepatic function in patients with proximal bile duct cancer. Langenbecks Arch Surg. 2001;386(5):364–8.
21. Gerhards MF, van Gulik TM, de Wit LT, et al. Evaluation of morbidity and mortality after resection for hilar cholangiocarcinoma—a single center experience. Surgery. 2000;127(4):395–404.
22. Shimada H, Endo I, Sugita M, et al. Hepatic resection combined with portal vein or hepatic artery reconstruction for advanced carcinoma of the hilar bile duct and gallbladder. World J Surg. 2003;27(10):1137–42.
23. Miyazaki M, Kato A, Ito H, et al. Combined vascular resection in operative resection for hilar cholangiocarcinoma: does it work or not? Surgery. 2007;141(5):581–8.
24. Ebata T, Nagino M, Kamiya J, et al. Hepatectomy with portal vein resection for hilar cholangiocarcinoma: audit of 52 consecutive cases. Ann Surg. 2003;238(5):720–7.
25. Dinant S, Gerhards MF, Rauws EA, et al. Improved outcome of resection of hilar cholangiocarcinoma (Klatskin tumor). Ann Surg Oncol. 2006;13(6):872–80.
26. Young AL, Prasad KR, Toogood GJ, et al. Surgical treatment of hilar cholangiocarcinoma in a new era: comparison among leading eastern and western centers, Leeds. J Hepatobiliary Pancreat Sci. 2010;17(4):497–504.
27. Lee SG, Song GW, Hwang S, et al. Surgical treatment of hilar cholangiocarcinoma in the new era: the Asan experience. J Hepatobiliary Pancreat Sci. 2010;17(4):476–89.
28. Miyazaki M, Kimura F, Shimizu H, et al. One hundred seven consecutive surgical resections for hilar cholangiocarcinoma of Bismuth types II, III, IV between 2001 and 2008. J Hepatobiliary Pancreat Sci. 2010;17(4):470–5.
29. Kurosaki I, Hatakeyama K, Minagawa M, et al. Portal vein resection in surgery for cancer of biliary tract and pancreas: special reference to the relationship between the surgical outcome and site of primary tumor. J Gastrointest Surg. 2008;12(5):907–18.
30. Neuhaus P, Jonas S, Settmacher U, et al. Surgical management of proximal bile duct cancer: extended right lobe resection increases resectability and radicality. Langenbecks Arch Surg. 2003;388(3): 194–200.
31. Hirano S, Kondo S, Tanaka E, et al. No-touch resection of hilar malignancies with right hepatectomy and routine portal reconstruction. J Hepatobiliary Pancreat Surg. 2009;16(4):502–7.
32. Hidalgo E, Asthana S, Nishio H, et al. Surgery for hilar cholangiocarcinoma: the Leeds experience. Eur J Surg Oncol. 2008;34(7):787–94.
33. Ebata T, Kamiya J, Nishio H, et al. The concept of perihilar cholangiocarcinoma is valid. Br J Surg. 2009;96(8):926–34.
34. Yasuda Y, Larsen PN, Ishibashi T, et al. Resection of hilar cholangiocarcinoma with left hepatectomy after pre-operative embolization of the proper hepatic artery. HPB (Oxford). 2010;12(2):147–52.
35. Heimbach JK, Haddock MG, Alberts SR, et al. Transplantation for hilar cholangiocarcinoma. Liver Transpl. 2004;10(10 Suppl 2):S65–8.
36. Kondo S, Hirano S, Ambo Y, et al. Forty consecutive resections of hilar cholangiocarcinoma with no postoperative mortality and no positive ductal margins: results of a prospective study. Ann Surg. 2004;240(1):95–101.
37. Shimizu H, Kimura F, Yoshidome H, et al. Aggressive surgical resection for hilar cholangiocarcinoma of the left-side predominance: radicality and safety of left-sided hepatectomy. Ann Surg. 2010;251(2):281–6.
38. Sakamoto Y, Sano T, Shimada K, et al. Clinical significance of reconstruction of the right hepatic artery for biliary malignancy. Langenbecks Arch Surg. 2006;391(3):203–8.
39. Ota T, Araida T, Yamamoto M, et al. Operative outcome and problems of right hepatic lobectomy with pancreatoduodenectomy for advanced carcinoma of the biliary tract. J Hepatobiliary Pancreat Surg. 2007;14(2):155–8.
40. Shimada K, Sano T, Sakamoto Y, et al. Clinical implications of combined portal vein resection as a palliative procedure in patients undergoing pancreaticoduodenectomy for pancreatic head carcinoma. Ann Surg Oncol. 2006;13(12):1569–78.
41. Madariaga JR, Iwatsuki S, Todo S, et al. Liver resection for hilar and peripheral cholangiocarcinomas: a study of 62 cases. Ann Surg. 1998;227(1):70–9.
42. Miyake H, Mizuno K, Iyomasa S, et al. Limited hepatectomy with left hepatic vein reconstruction for hepatocellular carcinoma on cirrhosis. Surgery. 2004;135(6):696.
43. Kondo S, Hirano S, Ambo Y, et al. Arterioportal shunting as an alternative to microvascular reconstruction after hepatic artery resection. Br J Surg. 2004;91(2):248–51.

The Hepatic Artery Reconstruction First Approach in Hilar Cholangiocarcinoma Type IIIb

22

E. de Santibañes, V. Ardiles, and F.A. Alvarez

22.1 Introduction

Even though recent advances in liver surgery have led to a more efficient approach to hilar cholangiocarcinoma (HC), resection with curative intent remains a challenge for hepatobiliary surgeons [1]. There is strong evidence to show better survival and long-term outcomes when microscopically tumor-free surgical margins are obtained in these patients [2]. En-bloc resections of liver parenchyma with the extrahepatic bile duct is mandatory to manage tumors with direct hepatic invasion, as well as to accomplish an R0 resection on tumors that frequently extend longitudinally out to involve the hepatic ducts [3–5].

Due to the close relation between the bile duct bifurcation and the vascular structures that enter the liver, tumor growth might rapidly compromise these structures. The achievement of negative surgical margins in these patients is technically demanding, requiring combined vascular resection and reconstruction [1–6]. Currently, resection of the portal vein (PV) is considered a routine procedure when it is compromised, concomitant resection of the hepatic artery remains controversial since it is associated with a higher operative mortality rate (33–55 %) [5, 7–10]. Several reasons might explain for these poor results, such as a greater duration of liver ischemia due to simultaneous portal vein resection in most cases, and pre-existing liver dysfunction due to obstructive jaundice and persistent cholangitis [9, 10]. These conditions are the key factors for the development of postoperative liver failure [7, 8, 11, 12].

In HC Bismuth-Corlette type IIIb, the tumor invades the left bile duct, and in some circumstances, compromises liver vascular structures [13]. Given the relationship of the right hepatic artery (RHA) is set in most cases behind the common hepatic duct and near the bifurcation, extension of the tumor posteriorly and to the right involves the RHA and the PV or its branches. Since HC type IIIb often requires a left hepatectomy extended to the anterior segments of the right liver, invasion of the RHA usually is a contraindication to perform these procedures with curative intent [2, 7, 11]. This leads to different treatment options to solve this problem.

Even though Majno et al. [14] consider that after resection of the hepatic artery, the remaining liver can function adequately with normal flow of the PV and collateral arteries, though the absence of arterial blood flow may cause liver necrosis, hepatic abscess formation and an increased risk of complications to the biliary anastomosis [14, 15]. Wang et al. [12] presented two patients with HC type IIIb with contralateral arterial invasion. They performed a left hepatectomy combined with RHA resection without reconstruction. The early postoperative results were satisfactory, however one patient developed liver necrosis and abscess 3 months later. Young et al. [16] reported using arterialization of the PV as a salvage procedure when arterial reconstruction was not possible. Miura et al. [17] and Yasuda et al. [18] reported resection of locally advanced HC after stepwise arterial embolization used to stimulate the development of neo-arterialization of the right liver so that the RHA could be resected without reconstruction.

As arterial vascular reconstruction is preferable to any of the techniques described above, other authors reported the use of arterial vascular reconstruction to increase the resectability of HC when tumor involvement of the hepatic artery became an obstacle to negative resection margins [7, 8, 19, 20]. In these series, arterial reconstruction was performed as the last step after the portal vein was reconstructed. When arterial reconstruction is performed at the end of the procedure, the surgeon may find it too late to realize that the distal artery of the future liver remnant (FLR) does not have enough length for reconstruction when oncological resection was completed. This is a critical situation which is not easy to solve [16].

E. de Santibañes, MD, PhD (✉) • V. Ardiles, MD
F.A. Alvarez, MD
General Surgery Service,
Hospital Italiano de Buenos Aires,
Buenos Aires, Argentina
e-mail: eduardo.desantibanes@hospitalitaliano.org.ar,
e.desantibanes@gmail.com

W.Y. Lau (ed.), *Hilar Cholangiocarcinoma*,
DOI 10.1007/978-94-007-6473-6_22, © Springer Science+Business Media Dordrecht and People's Medical Publishing House 2013

Since liver failure is the leading cause of death in these patients [8], to dissociate arterial and portal ischemia during vascular reconstruction to ensure the arterial blood supply to the remnant liver in the first surgical step might have a positive impact on early and late postoperative outcomes.

In this chapter we describe a novel surgical technique that allows an oncological clearance in patients with HC type IIIb with contralateral arterial invasion by performing arterial reconstruction as the first step of the surgical procedure.

22.2 Surgical Technique

We routinely use laparoscopic staging to rule out the presence of liver metastases or peritoneal carcinomatosis. After laparotomy, mobilization of the left liver is performed. Dissection of the hepatic pedicle starts from the duodenopancreas to the hilum. Complete lymphadenectomy of the celiac axis and its branches, the PV and the gastrohepatic ligament is then performed. This maneuver facilitates identification of the elements in the pedicle. During surgery, dissection should always be carried out away from the tumor. Once the presence of a HC type IIIb with contralateral arterial invasion is confirmed by palpation, visualization and intraoperative color-doppler ultrasound (IOUS), the next step is to isolate the posterior branch of the RHA (segments 6 and 7) inside the Rouviere's sulcus (Fig. 22.1). This artery, in most cases is free and away from the tumor and it can then be dissected easily. Once this step is accomplished, the distal common bile duct is transected as close as possible to its entrance into the pancreas. The edge of the transected duct is sent for fresh frozen pathological examination. As the left hepatic artery usually runs on the left edge of the hepatic pedicle and in most of the time it is not involved by the tumor, it can be mobilized and isolated along its full length. This allows enough length of the artery to reach the Rouviere's sulcus to perform an arterial reconstruction with the posterior branch of the RHA. The left hepatic artery is rotated 90° anti-clockwise in order to carry out an anastomosis with the arterial branch of segments 6 and 7 (Fig. 22.2). We prefer to perform the anastomosis using a microscope. It is important whenever possible to use the left hepatic artery because it has a similar diameter to the right posterior artery. Occasionally, the RHA is invaded by tumor and its proximal stump may also be used for arterial reconstruction with the posterior branch of the RHA (Fig. 22.3). Once the anastomosis is finished arterial blood supply to the FLR is ensured. Segment 1 is then mobilized to be included in the resection specimen. The left PV is divided and the liver parenchyma is transected (left trisectionectomy or extended left hepatectomy) (Fig. 22.4). If PV resection is required, it can be done after transection of liver parenchyma is completed, with the assurance that the remnant liver can tolerate portal clamping because it has good arterial vascularization. After vascular reconstruction is accomplished, the middle and left hepatic veins are divided and sutured. Finally the specimen is removed and biliary reconstruction is performed using a Roux-en-Y loop. At the end of the procedure, IOUS should always be done to confirm the adequacy vascularization of the liver remnant.

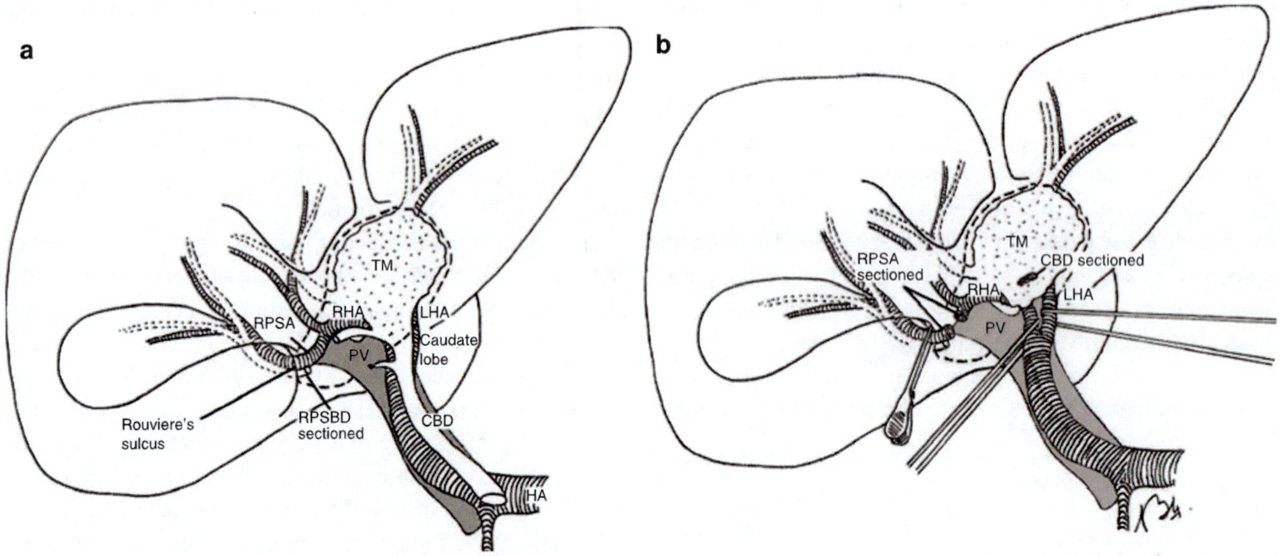

Fig. 22.1 (**a**) Once cholecystectomy is performed, the posterior branch of the right hepatic artery (*RHA*) is isolated within the Rouviere's sulcus. (**b**) The common bile duct (*CBD*) is divided distally and turned away from the operative field with the specimen. *TM* tumor, *LHA* left hepatic artery, *RPSA* right posterior segment artery, *HA* hepatic artery, *PV* portal vein, *RPSBD* right posterior segment bile duct

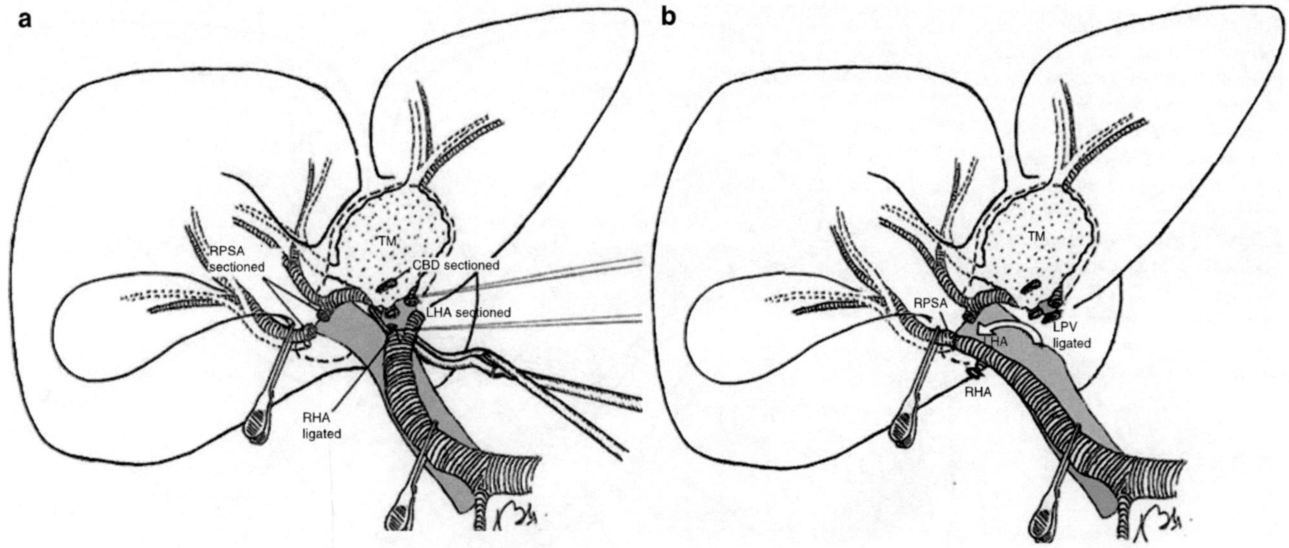

Fig. 22.2 (**a**) The right hepatic artery (*RHA*) and the left hepatic artery (*LHA*) are divided with tumor-free margins. (**b**) After this, the LHA is rotated to the right side of the porta hepatis. This maneuver allows arterial reconstruction between the LHA and the right posterior segment artery (*RPSA*). *LPV* left portal vein, *TM* tumor, *CBD* common bile duct (Reproduced with permission from *HPB: The Official Journal of the International Hepato Pancreato Biliary Association* [21])

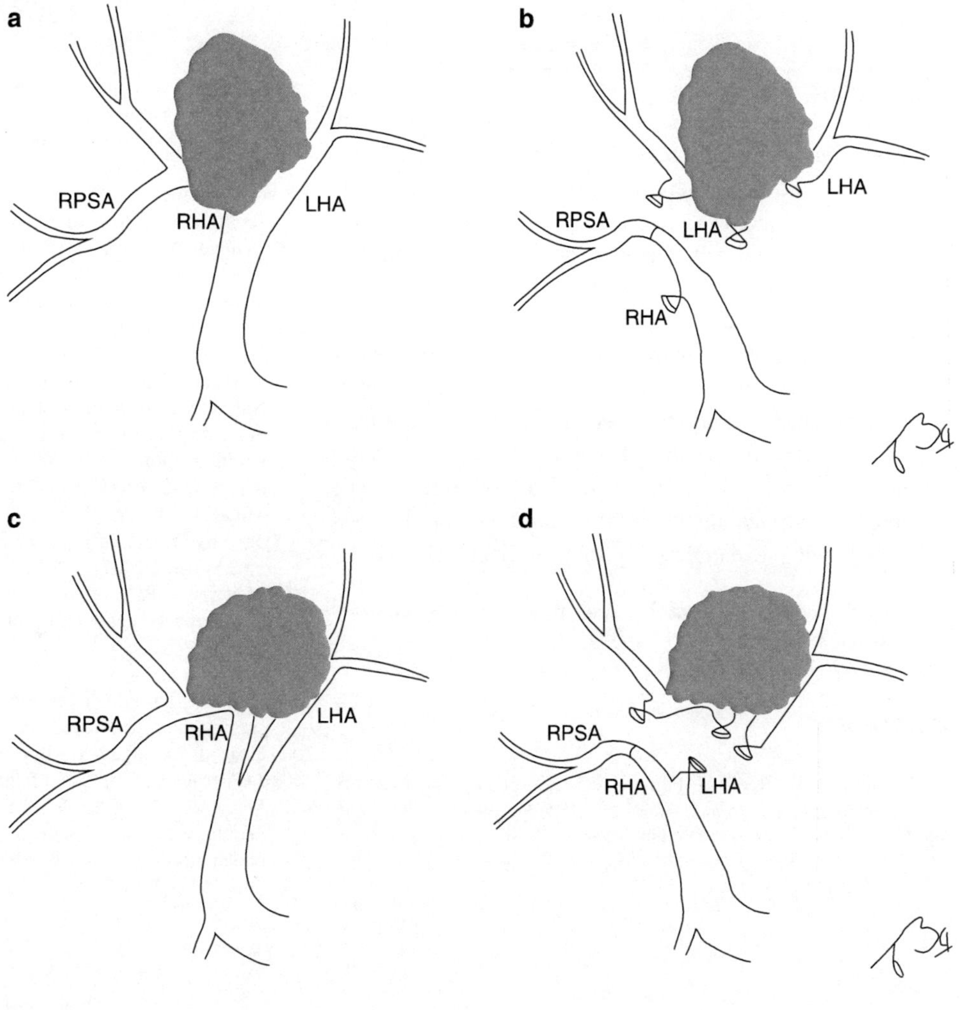

Fig. 22.3 This picture shows two possible intraoperative scenarios of arterial compromise and details the reconstructive alternatives with the right posterior segment artery (*RPSA*). (**a**) The right hepatic artery (*RHA*) is nearly totally invaded by the tumor before its bifurcation. (**b**) The reconstruction demands dividing the left hepatic artery (*LHA*) and its transfer to the right edge of the porta hepatis. By this means, the LHA can reach the posterior branch of the RHA and the anastomosis is performed. (**c**) The RHA is distally invaded by the tumor. (**d**) In this situation the reconstruction can be achieved with the proximal remnant of the common RHA

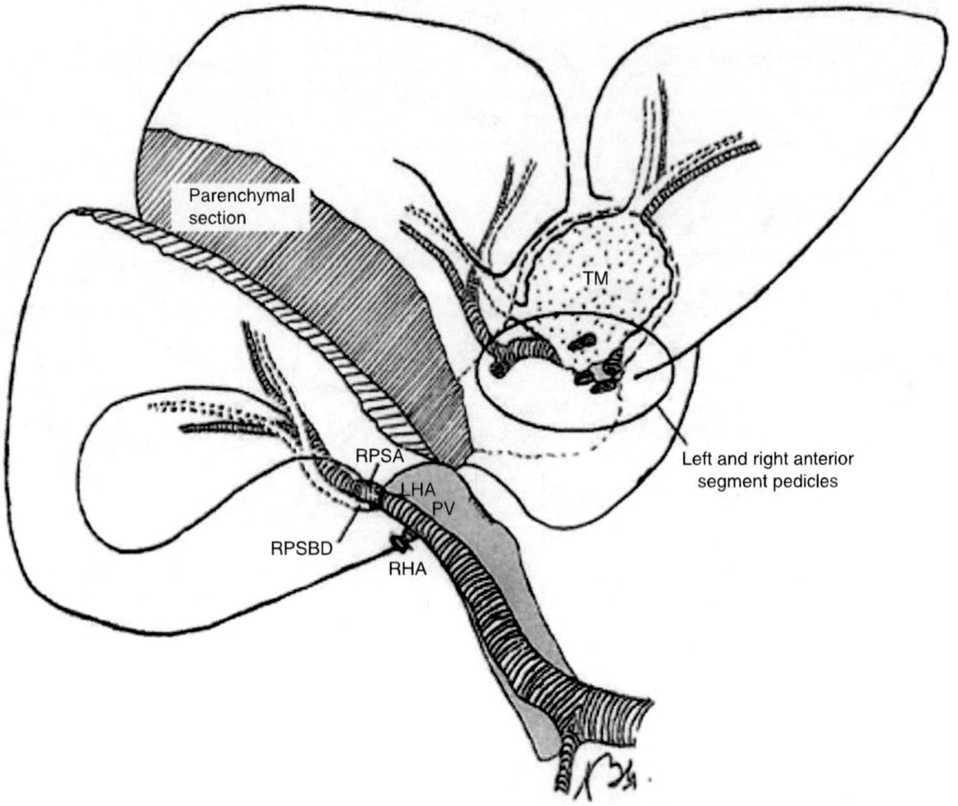

Fig. 22.4 After vascular reconstruction is completed and arterial blood flow is restored, the liver parenchyma is transected. *TM* tumor, *RHA* right hepatic artery, *LHA* left hepatic artery, *RPSA* right posterior segment artery, *PV* portal vein, *RPSBD* right posterior segment bile duct (Reproduced with permission from *HPB: The Official Journal of the International Hepato Pancreato Biliary Association* [21])

Conclusion

We described a novel surgical technique that allows performing an oncological resection in patients with HC type IIIb and contralateral arterial invasion that might otherwise be considered as unresectable. The technique is clinically and technically feasible [21]. In this technique, arterial anastomosis is carried out as the first surgical step to provide adequate arterial blood supply to the FLR before parenchymal transection. If additional PV resection is required, it can be done at the end of transection of the liver parenchyma. This ensures that the remnant liver can tolerate portal clamping because it has been arterially vascularizated. This novel approach offers these patients a hope of cure and might improve their outcomes by lessening the negative effects of prolonged liver ischemia.

Acknowledgements We thank Dr. Axel Beskow for the drawings included in this chapter.

References

1. Hemming AW, Reed AI, Fujita S, et al. Surgical management of hilar cholangiocarcinoma. Ann Surg. 2005;241:693–9.
2. Jarnagin WR, Fong Y, DeMatteo RP, et al. Staging, resectability, and outcome in 225 patients with hilar cholangiocarcinoma. Ann Surg. 2001;234:507–17.
3. Kosuge T, Yamamoto J, Shimada K, et al. Improved surgical results for hilar cholangiocarcinoma with procedures including major hepatic resection. Ann Surg. 1999;230:663–71.
4. Sano T, Shimada K, Sakamoto Y, et al. One hundred two consecutive hepatobiliary resections for perihilar cholangiocarcinoma with zero mortality. Ann Surg. 2006;244:240–7.
5. Neuhaus P, Jonas S, Settmacher U, et al. Surgical management of proximal bile duct cancer: extended right lobe resection increases resectability and radicality. Langenbecks Arch Surg. 2003;388:194–200.
6. Neuhaus P, Jonas S, Bechstein WO, et al. Extended resections for hilar cholangiocarcinoma. Ann Surg. 1999;230:808–18.
7. Nagino M, Nimura Y, Nishio H, et al. Hepatectomy with simultaneous resection of the portal vein and hepatic artery for advanced perihilar cholangiocarcinoma: an audit of 50 consecutive cases. Ann Surg. 2010;252:115–23.
8. Miyazaki M, Kato A, Ito H, et al. Combined vascular resection in operative resection for hilar cholangiocarcinoma: does it work or not? Surgery. 2007;141:581–8.
9. Madariaga JR, Iwatsuki S, Todo S, et al. Liver resection for hilar and peripheral cholangiocarcinomas: a study of 62 cases. Ann Surg. 1998;227:70–9.
10. Gerhards MF, van Gulik TM, de Wit LT, et al. Evaluation of morbidity and mortality after resection for hilar cholangiocarcinoma—a single center experience. Surgery. 2000;127:395–404.
11. Clary B, Jarnigan W, Pitt H, et al. Hilar cholangiocarcinoma. J Gastrointest Surg. 2004;8:298–302.
12. Wang WL, Tang XF, Yao MY, et al. Safety and efficiency of left hemihepatectomy combined with hepatic artery resection for hilar cholangiocarcinoma with artery infiltration: report of 2 cases. Can J Surg. 2008;51:305–7.

13. Bismuth H, Corlette MB. Intrahepatic cholangioenteric anastomosis in carcinoma of the hilus of the liver. Surg Gynecol Obstet. 1975;140:170–8.
14. Majno PE, Pretre R, Mentha G, et al. Operative injury to the hepatic artery. Consequences of a biliary-enteric anastomosis and principles for rational management. Arch Surg. 1996; 131(2):211–5.
15. Miyazaki M, Ito H, Nakagawa K, et al. Unilateral hepatic artery reconstruction is unnecessary in biliary tract carcinomas involving lobar hepatic artery: implications of interlobar hepatic artery and its preservation. Hepatogastroenterology. 2000;47:1526–30.
16. Young AL, Prasad KR, Adair R, et al. Portal vein arterialization as a salvage procedure during left hepatic trisectionectomy for hilar cholangiocarcinoma. J Am Coll Surg. 2008;207:e1–6.
17. Miura T, Hakamada K, Ohata T, et al. Resection of a locally advanced hilar tumor and the hepatic artery after stepwise hepatic arterial embolization: a case report. World J Gastroenterol. 2008; 14:3587–90.
18. Yasuda Y, Larsen PN, Ishibashi T, et al. Resection of hilar cholangiocarcinoma with left hepatectomy after pre-operative embolization of the proper hepatic artery. HPB (Oxford). 2010;12: 147–52.
19. Lee SG, Song GW, Hwang S, et al. Surgical treatment of hilar cholangiocarcinoma in the new era: the Asan experience. J Hepatobiliary Pancreat Sci. 2010;17:476–89.
20. Sakamoto Y, Sano T, Shimada K, et al. Clinical significance of reconstruction of the right hepatic artery for biliary malignancy. Langenbecks Arch Surg. 2006;391:203–8.
21. de Santibañes E, Ardiles V, Alvarez FA, et al. Hepatic artery reconstruction first for the treatment of hilar cholangiocarcinoma bismuth type IIIB with contralateral arterial invasion: a novel technical strategy. HPB (Oxford). 2012;14(1):67–70.

Local Resection Without Hepatectomy

23

L. Capussotti and L. Viganò

Abstract

In the last decades, surgical treatment of hilar cholangiocarcinoma has moved toward liver surgery in association with biliary resection in order to increase radicality and to achieve better survival results. In this chapter, results of isolated biliary resection in comparison with those of biliary and hepatic resection and its actual indications are analyzed in detail, considering our own experience and the literature presently available.

Local resection is not an adequate treatment for hilar cholangiocarcinoma involving the bile duct confluence (Bismuth-Corlette type II or more) and associated liver resection should be always recommended. In Bismuth-Corlette type Ihilar cholangiocarcinoma benefits of survival by association of biliary and liver resection have been reported, but further studies are necessary. At present, local resection should be scheduled only for small papillary Klatskin tumor without bile duct confluence involvement (type I) and confined to the bile duct wall (Tis and T1). Accurate preoperative staging is mandatory to correctly assess tumor extension and to plan adequate treatment strategy. Extension of treatment should always be decided according to patient conditions after an extensive evaluation of functional, volumetric and anaesthesiological parameters.

23.1 Introduction

In the last decades, surgical treatment of hilar cholangiocarcinoma has undergone a rapid evolution. \Before 1980, the majority of patients were not resected and in few cases local excision of the tumor was performed with low radicality and poor long-term outcomes. Since 1980, indications to resection have been progressively enlarged, and liver resection has been associated with bile duct resection to increase radicality and to achieve better survival results [1–4]. At present local resection seems to have a very narrow role in the management of Klatskin tumor, however its results in comparison with hepatectomy associated with bile duct resection and its actual indications have to be clarified.

L. Capussotti, MD (✉) • L. Viganò, MD
Department of HPB and Digestive Surgery,
Ospedale Mauriziano "Umberto I",
Largo Turati, Torino, Italy
e-mail: lcapussotti@mauriziano.it

In this chapter, we will consider the different aspects of surgery for hilar cholangiocarcinoma from our own experience and from the literature presently available, and we will try to establish if local resection has still a role for hilar cholangiocarcinoma and who are the good candidates to receive this treatment.

First of all it is important to underline that no randomized trials are available. All our considerations are based on retrospective studies and a few recent prospective studies including small number of patients. In 2007 the European HPB Association organized a consensus conference in Bruxelles on hilar cholangiocarcinoma. These Consensus conferences statements, based on complete literature review and invited expert experience at that time [5], will also be considered in this chapter.

First, we will briefly describe the technique of biliary resection without associated hepatectomy for hilar cholangiocarcinoma. Then, we will consider the pathologic characteristics of hilar cholangiocarcinoma, i.e. its spread and growth pattern, which are the unavoidable basis used for

W.Y. Lau (ed.), *Hilar Cholangiocarcinoma*,
DOI 10.1007/978-94-007-6473-6_23, © Springer Science+Business Media Dordrecht and People's Medical Publishing House 2013

planning an adequate treatment. Finally we will analyze the outcomes of isolated bile duct resection in comparison with those of bile duct resection associated with hepatectomy.

23.2 Surgical Technique

The surgical technique of biliary resection without associated hepatectomy for hilar cholangiocarcinoma may be slightly different in different centers. We will briefly depict the technique we adopt in our center.

Laparotomy is regularly preceded by explorative laparoscopy. The abdomen is completely explored for peritoneal deposits and superficial liver metastases. Laparoscopic hepatic ultrasonography is performed to confirm tumor site, its extension along bile ducts and its relationship with surrounding vascular structures and to exclude liver metastases (Fig. 23.1). Ultrasonographic exploration also evaluates the presence of enlarged lymph nodes along the hepatic pedicle, in the celiac and the retropancreatic area and in the interaortocaval space. If no contraindications to resection are disclosed, a right subcostal incision is performed. Complete exploration of the abdominal cavity and liver ultrasonography are repeated. The duodenum is mobilized to better evaluate the presence or absence of retropancreatic or interaorto-caval lymph-node metastases. Enlarged lymph nodes are removed and analyzed by frozen section. Lymph node metastases impact on treatment strategy as follows: interaorto-caval metastases are an absolute contraindication to resection; lymph node metastases in the celiac or retropancreatic area are a relative contraindication and decision should be made on case-by-case evaluation; lymph node metastases along the hepatic pedicle do not contraindicate the resection.

The gallbladder is mobilized and the right margin of the hepatic pedicle is dissected to identify and encircle the right hepatic artery and the portal trunk. Both are then cautiously dissected from the bile duct in order to exclude tumor infiltration. The hilar plate is lowered to better evaluate proximal extension of the tumor.

When resectability is established, the distal bile duct is encircled and sectioned at the superior margin of the pancreas. Distal bile duct margin is analyzed by frozen section. If neoplastic infiltration is demonstrated, further dissection and re-resection of the distal bile duct is attempted or duodenopancreatectomy is considered. A decision is based on both tumor characteristics and patient's conditions.

The sectioned bile duct is isolated up to the confluence. The right and left hepatic ducts are identified and sectioned as proximal as possible to achieve the widest margin. Bile ducts of segment 1 draining into the bile duct confluence are identified and sectioned. The proximal margins of both the right and left hepatic ducts are analyzed by frozen section. If neoplastic infiltration is demonstrated, further dissection and re-resection is attempted or the association of liver resection is considered. The decision has to be made according to liver function, future remnant parenchyma volumetry and patient performance status.

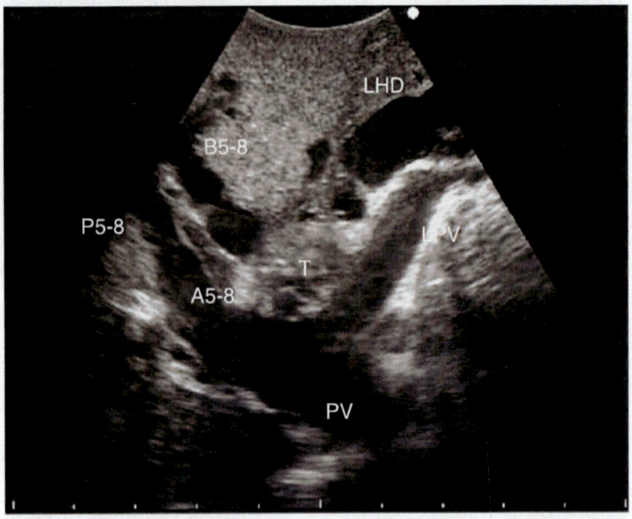

Fig. 23.1 Intraoperative liver ultrasonography in a patient affected by hilar cholangiocarcinoma. The Klatskin tumor (T) involves the bile duct confluence. The left hepatic duct (LHD) and the right anterior biliary duct (B5~8) are dilated. The tumor is in contact with the portal vein (PV) at its bifurcation and with the origin of the left portal branch (LPV) and of the right portal branch [the right anterior portal branch is visualized (P5~8)]. Infiltration of the origin of the right anterior arterial branch (A5~8) is suspected

Lymph node dissection of the hepatic pedicle, along the common hepatic artery and of the celiac and retropancreatic area is completed.

Bilio-enteric continuity is re-established by Roux-en Y cholangiojejunostomy. The anastomosis is performed by anastomosing the bile duct wall and the seromuscular layer of the intestine with 5–0 or 6–0 interrupted absorbable monofilament. Whenever possible, multiple intrahepatic bile ducts are grouped to form one anastomotic orifice. A transanastomotic biliary drainage, either transhepatic or transjejunal, is utilized according to the surgeon's preference. An abdominal retroanastomotic drain is usually used.

23.3 Pathologic Background

To establish the role of isolated bile duct resection for Klatskin tumor, some pathologic data have to be considered. In fact, pathologic characteristics of hilar cholangiocarcinoma have been widely studied in the last years and strongly impacted on its surgical management. Many data suggest that isolated bile duct resection is not an adequate treatment for Klatskin tumor.

First, cholangiocarcinoma is an aggressive neoplasm; extension along perineural sheath and associated with

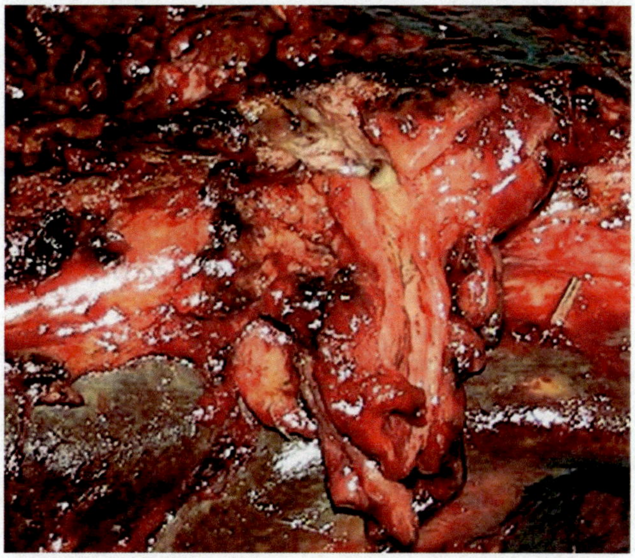

Fig. 23.2 Surgical specimen after bile duct and liver resection for hilar cholangiocarcinoma. The bile duct confluence and its first order branches have been sectioned. The longitudinal extension of the tumor along the hepatic ducts is evident. Liver resection is necessary to achieve negative margins

lymphangiosis carcinomatosa are commonly present [6, 7]. The definition of "early bile duct cancer" is not widely accepted because the submucosal layer of the bile duct is very thin and often lacking and the muscularis mucosae is absent in the bile duct; even small tumors may have aggressive behaviour and invasive pattern [8]. In 1999 Kayahara et al. reported neural invasion in no patient with mucosal tumor (Tis) and in 33 % of patients with neoplasm extended to the fibromuscular layer (T1) [7]. In this context, hilar cholangiocarcinoma rapidly reaches the surrounding vascular structures (the right hepatic artery and the portal trunk) which can be prematurely invaded by the tumor. This diffusion has been further underlined by the concept of radial margin. Some recent series analyzed completeness of resection not only considering proximal and distal biliary margins, but also evaluating the soft tissue surrounding the bile duct [9, 10]. The radial margin evaluation allowed to reclassify some cases as R1 resection and impacted on survival outcomes. These data do not preclude isolated bile duct resection, but remark that Klatskin tumor can be rarely considered as a localized lesion.

Second, in 2002 Ebata et al. reported that cholangiocarcinoma has both superficial and intramural extensions [11]. In order to completely remove an invasive neoplasm, a 10 mm margin is necessary. Further, margin should be 20 mm for removing all non-invasive components. The margin width required for a radical resection is still debated and the impact of non invasive neoplasm on surgical margin is uncertain [12]. However, it is clear that these wide margins can be achieved only by liver resection when cholangiocarcinoma involves the right or left hepatic duct (Fig. 23.2). These data will be further discussed in the section "radicality", when R0 resection rates after isolated bile duct resection and after associated biliary and liver resection are compared. Of note, it is important to remark that the reliability of intraoperative frozen section is poor: a high rate of false negative biliary margins have been reported [10]. It further underlines the need for an accurate preoperative treatment planning.

Finally, the bile duct confluence lies just in front of segment 1 and directly drains segment 1 biliary ducts [13]. For these anatomical reasons, segment 1 is often involved by the hilar cholangiocarcinoma. Segment 1 may be involved by bile duct invasion, by direct neoplastic infiltration or by perineural extension [2, 14–18]. In our experience, 82 patients underwent resection for hilar cholangiocarcinoma between 1989 and 2009. Segment 1 was resected in 71 patients and was invaded by Klatskin tumor in 16 (22.5 %). The risk of invasion increased with tumor extension: it was 10 % in Bismuth-Corlette type I~I Itumors vs. 25 % in type III~IV. The risk of segment 1 infiltration has been confirmed by high rates of tumor recurrence at this site after isolated bile duct resection [2, 14–18].

23.3.1 Isolated Biliary Resection vs. Biliary Resection Associated with Hepatectomy

To adequately compare isolated bile duct resection with bile duct resection plus hepatectomy, three topics have to be considered: short-term outcomes, radicality and survival.

23.3.1.1 Short-Term Outcomes

In the past, local resection has been widely considered to be safer than liver resection and with lower mortality rates [19–21]. In 1990 Boerma reviewed published papers and collected 581 patients who underwent resection for Klatskin tumor: considering the most relevant series, mortality was significantly lower after bile duct resection than after hepatectomy (8 % vs. 15 %) [22]. In the 1990s these data have been confirmed: in 1992 the Blumgart's group reported no mortality and 25 % morbidity after local excision in comparison with 8 % and 36 % respectively after extended procedures [23]; in 1996 Pichlmayr et al. reported mortality rates of 12.7 % after bile duct resection associated with liver surgery vs. 3.3 % after local excision [20]. The increased mortality rate after liver resection was considered as a clear indication to choose local resection: even if associated liver surgery can improve radicality, long-term benefits were lost because of high operative mortality rates [19].

In 2000 Launois et al. published different results: in a French survey mortality rates were higher but were similar in patients with and without liver resection (17 % vs. 14 %) [24]. These data were probably related to the collection of data from multiple centers. In fact, the same author reported

Table 23.1 Comparison of mortality rates after local resection (LR) vs. bile duct resection with associated hepatic resection (HR) in published series

		#		Mortality (%)		
Author	Year	LR	HR	LR	HR	P
Boerma [22]	1990	201	188	8.0	15.0	**<0.05**
Bismuth [45]	1992	10	13	0	0	n.s.
Baer [23]	1992	12	11	0	8.3	n.s.
Pichlmayr [20]	1996	30	95	3.3	12.7	n.s.
Miyazaki [21]	1998	11	65	0	15.0	n.s.
Launois [25]	1999	11	25	0	16.0	n.s.
Neuhaus [6]	1999	14	66	0	9.1	n.s.
Kosuge [43][a]	1999	13	52	7.7	9.6	n.s.
Nimura [49]	2000	8	100	0	6.0	n.s.
Launois [24] (French survey)	2000	51	47	14.0	17.0	n.s.
Jarnagin [40]	2001	18	62	6.0	11.0	n.s.
Capussotti [31]	2002	4	32	0	3.0	n.s.
Kondo [29]	2004	9	31	0	0	n.s.
Jang [42]	2005	25	23	0	0	n.s.
Dinant [3]	2006	60	37	13.1	26–17[b]	n.s.
Ito [35]	2008	18	20	0	0	n.s.
Shi [33]	2009	31	38	3.2	5.2	n.s.

[a]Local resection/limited hepatic resections vs major hepatectomies
[b]Results after right hepatectomy—left hepatectomy
Bold value indicate a significant in difference between LR and HR

in 1999 no mortality after isolated bile duct resection in their center [25].

The postoperative outcomes of liver surgery improved significantly in the last years, thanks to better patient selection, preoperative biliary drainage and portal vein embolization [26–29]. Almost all series reported mortality rates lower than 10 %, and in recent years these results further improved. This improvement left us to reconsider the association of liver resection with biliary resection. In 2000 Tsao et al. compared the results of surgical treatment in a Japanese centre (Nagoya) where liver resection was routinely performed with those of an American one (Lahey clinic) where isolated bile duct resection was preferred: short-term outcomes were good and were similar in the two groups, 4 % vs. 8 % mortality and 44 % vs. 51 % morbidity [30]. In 2002 our group published a paper including 36 patients resected for hilar cholangiocarcinoma with associated liver resection in 32 (88.9 %): the mortality and morbidity rates were 2.8 % and 47.2 % respectively [31]. Many other recent papers reported excellent results after biliary and liver resection and some of them even achieved zero mortality [26, 28, 29, 32–35]. Short-term outcomes of the largest published series are summarized in Table 23.1.

According to these data, operative risk should no longer be considered a contraindication to biliary and liver resection. However, despite these enthusiastic results, liver surgery for Klatskin tumor has still to be considered with caution. Postoperative outcomes are worse than those reported after liver resection for other indications. The patient capability to tolerate the required extended liver resections has to be accurately assessed by combining functional, volumetric and anaesthesiological evaluations. A strict patient selection is mandatory. In selected patients, who cannot tolerate liver surgery, a local resection could be considered if a complete resection can be achieved.

23.3.1.2 Radicality

We previously considered pathologic characteristic of Klatskin tumor and reported the longitudinal and radial diffusion of the tumor. These data let us consider local excision not to be adequate for a radical resection. This has been confirmed by surgical series: the rate of radical resections increased with the rate of associated liver resections (Fig. 23.3) [1]. R0 resection rates ranged from 15 % in Cameron series with 20 % of hepatectomy to 56 % in Blumgart series with 60 % of liver resections and reached 80 % when liver resection was associated in about 80 % of cases [36–39]. Nimura et al. performed liver resection in 98 % of cases and his radicality rate was 83 % [16]; our centre had similar results: 89 % of liver resections and 89 % of radicality [31]. Many studies reported that R0 resections are significantly less common after local excision than after associated liver surgery [3, 6, 9, 21, 33, 35, 40]. In 2000 Tsao et al. compared the results of Klatskin tumor resection at Nagoya University and at Lahey Clinic: the former centre performed liver resection in 89 % of cases and R0 resection was achieved in 79 %, the latter performed hepatectomy only in 16 % of patients and the radicality significantly decreased to 28 % [30]. This concept has been further strengthened by a recent paper from Van Gulik et al.: in their center management of Klatskin tumor changed in the last 25 years and the proportion of local resection decreased from 91 % before 1993 to 28 % between 1998 and 2003 [41]. The R0 resection rate radically improved from 13 % to 59 %.

A comparison of the radicality rates after isolated bile duct resection and after combined biliary and hepatic resection in the largest published series is summarized in Table 23.2.

Anyway, liver resection is not always necessary to reach negative margins: in 2004 Kondo et al. published a series of 40 consecutive patients with radical resection including nine cases treated by isolated bile duct resection according to the tumor site [29]. Similarly, in our series 7 out of 82 patients had isolated bile duct resection, including 6 Bismuth-Corlette type I~II tumors: only one patient had a R1 resection (positive proximal bile duct margin at final pathology). These data could be in favor of local resection in selected cases, but long-term outcomes have to be considered.

23.3.1.3 Survival

Many published series did not show any evidence of statistical difference in the survival between local resection and

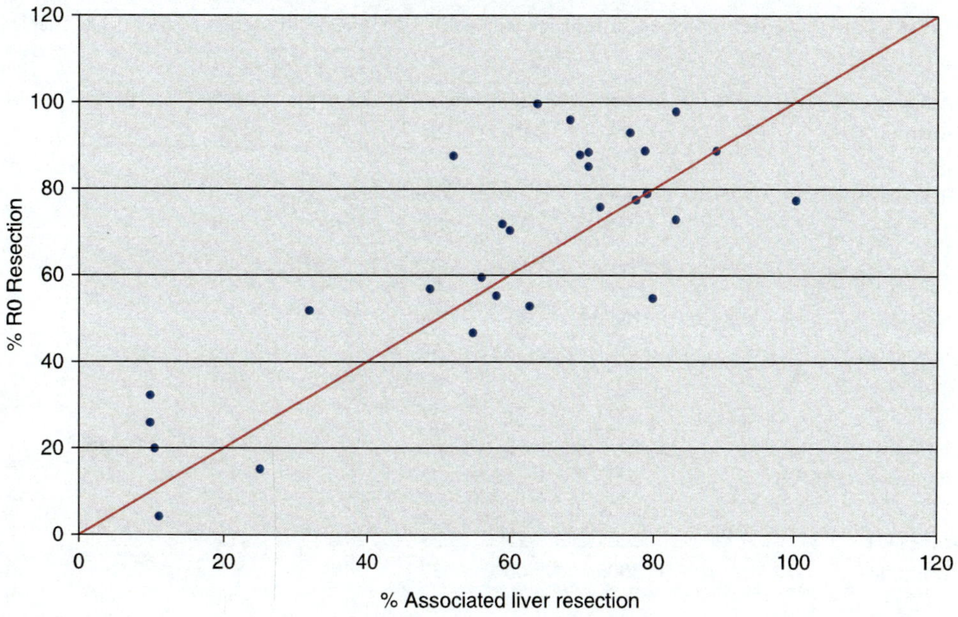

Fig. 23.3 Relationship between associated liver resection rate and R0 resection rate for hilar cholangiocarcinoma across the available surgical series in the literature

Table 23.2 Comparison of radicality rates after local resection (LR) vs. bile duct resection with associated hepatic resection (HR) in published series

		#		Radicality (%)		
Author	Year	LR	HR	LR	HR	P
Bismuth [45]	1992	10	13	30.0	46.1	n.s.
Miyazaki [21]	1998	11	65	45.0	75.0	**<0.05**
Neuhaus [6]	1999	14	66	29.0	61.0	**<0.05**
Kosuge [43] [a]	1999	13	52	38.5	55.8	n.s.
Jarnagin [40]	2001	18	62	56.0	84.0	**<0.05**
Capussotti [31]	2002	4	32	75.0	90.6	n.s.
Kondo [29]	2004	9	31	100	100	n.s.
Dinant [3]	2006	60	37	14.8	42–37[b]	**<0.05**
Ito [35]	2008	18	20	39	85	**<0.05**
Shi [33]	2009	31	38	41.9	74.2	**<0.05**

[a]Local resection/limited hepatic resections vs. major hepatectomies
[b]Results after right hepatectomy—left hepatectomy
Bold values indicate a significant in difference between LR and HR

extended surgery [2, 4, 19–21, 23, 24, 42–44]. Launois et al. published in 1999 a series of 40 consecutive resected patients: survival outcomes after local resection were significantly higher than those after associated hepatectomy (5-year survival rates 27 % vs. 6 %) [25]. These data could be related to the fact that the treatment was planned according to the tumor location and that liver resection was scheduled for patients with more extended disease.

Considering patients with a similar disease extension, in 2000 Tsao et al. compared Oriental and US experiences and reported significantly better survival in Japanese patients with more aggressive surgical strategy (5- and 10-year survival rates were 16 % and 12 % vs. 7 % and 0) [30]. Van Gulik et al., looking at their results in the last 25 years, observed that an increased proportion of liver resection was associated with survival improvement (5-year survival was 20 % when liver resection rate was 9 % vs. 33 % when it became 72 %) [41].

Some studies clearly demonstrated that associated biliary and hepatic resection significantly improve survival. In detail:

- In the Boerma review published in 1990 the survival was significantly decreased after local resection (5-year survival rate 7 % vs. 17 %) [22].
- In 2001 Jarnagin et al. analyzed 80 consecutive patients and reported actuarial 5-year survival rate of 37 % in patients with liver resection and 0 % in patients without it. In order to exclude that the difference in survival was related to the radicality rates, the analysis was repeated only on R0 patients and the results were confirmed [40].
- In 2004 Kondo et al. reported the long-term results in 40 consecutive patients with R0 resection. Nine patients who received isolated bile duct resection had a significantly decreased survival in comparison with 17 patients who received right hepatectomy [29].
- In 2008 Ito et al. observed higher overall and disease-free survival rates in 20 patients who received liver resection vs. 18 who received isolated bile duct resection [35].
- In 2009 Shi et al. reported a higher early recurrence rate after local resection in comparison with associated hepatectomy (at 1 year 74.2 % vs. 28.9 %) [33]. Survival results of the largest published series are summarized in Table 23.3.

All these data are concerned with hilar cholangiocarcinoma with different extensions into the bile ducts. Probably patients who received local resection had tumors without, or with, a minimal involvement of the bile duct confluence, although this is not clearly defined in the majority of papers.

Table 23.3 Comparison of survival after local resection (LR) vs. bile duct resection with associated hepatic resection (HR) in published series

		#		5-year survival (%)			Median survival (months)		
Author	Year	LR	HR	LR	HR	p	LR	HR	p
Boerma [22]	1990	201	188	7.0	17.0	**<0.05**			
Baer [23]	1992	12	11				36	32	n.s.
Pichlmayr [20]	1996	30	95	28.9	26.3	n.s.			
Miyazaki [21]	1998	11	65	16.0	33.0	n.s.			
				3 years	3 years				
Launois [25]	1999	11	25	27.3	6.0	**<0.05**			
Neuhaus [6]	1999	14	66	0	28–57[a]	n.s.			
Kosuge [43][b]	1999	13	52				38.6	27.0	n.s.
Nimura [49]	2000	8	100	16.0	26.0	n.s.			
Launois [24] (*French survey*)	2000	51	47				23	24	n.s.
Jarnagin [40]	2001	18	62	0	37.0	**<0.05**			
Capussotti [31]	2002	4	32	0[c]	54.5[c]	**<0.05**[c]			
Kondo [29]	2004	9	31				20.8[d]	NA[d]	**<0.05**[d]
Jang [42]	2005	25	23	28.0	47.8	n.s.			
Dinant [3]	2006	60	37				21.5	38–69[e]	n.s.
Ito [35]	2008	18	20	0	50	**<0.05**	31	65	**<0.05**

[a]Different survival rates according to type of hepatectomy
[b]Local resection/limited hepatic resections vs major hepatectomies
[c]Only BC I-II included
[d]Local resection/caudate segmentectomy/left hepatectomy vs right hepatectomy
[e]Results after right hepatectomy—left hepatectomy
Bold values indicate a significant in difference between LR and HR

To clarify if local resection may have a role in these patients, we focused on the results in Bismuth-Corlette type I~II hilar cholangiocarcinoma.

Two French papers suggested that local resection could be indicated in selected patients [25, 45]. Bismuth et al. in 1992 reported three patients with Bismuth-Corlette type I tumors undergoing isolated bile duct resection: two cases with R0 resection had long-term survivals without recurrence; one case with a R1 resection had recurrence, but a long survival was achieved after reresection [45]. On the contrary all patients with local resection for Bismuth-Corlette type II tumor had recurrence. In 1999 Launois et al. reported four patients with Bismuth-Corlette type I tumor (undergoing local resection in three cases) and four patients with Bismuth-Corlette type II (local resection in three) [25]. Five-year survival results were good (type I 20 %; type II 25 %), similar to those reported for other types. Patients with local resection had mainly Tis and T1 tumors. Two long-survivors have been reported: one Bismuth-Corlette type I T1bN0M0 and one Bismuth-Corlette type II TisN0M0.

Different results have recently been published with poor outcomes. In the Neuhaus series published in 1999 radicality of isolated local resection was 33 % (2/6) in Bismuth-Corlette type I tumors and 25 % (1/4) in Bismuth-Corlette type II; among them no patient survived 5 years [6]. Similar results have been reported after local resection by Su et al. in 1996 (25 % R0 resection rate for Bismuth-Corlette type Itumors) and van Gulik et al. in 1999 (19 % R0 resection rate for Bismuth-Corlette type I~II tumors) [46, 47]. In 2005 Jang et al. reported 25 patients undergoing isolated bile duct resection for Bismuth-Corlette type I~II or common hepatic duct cancer [42]. Seven patients (28 %) survived 5 years or more but three of them were alive with recurrence despite their early stage (T1N0 in 2 and T2N0 in 1). In Kondo series in 2004, nine patients (six Bismuth-Corlette type I and three Bismuth-Corlette type II) underwent local resection: even if all had radical resection, their survival rates were significantly lower than those patients with associated liver surgery (median survival 19 vs. 21 months) [29]. In our experience, 20 patients affected by Bismuth-Corlette type I~II hilar cholangiocarcinoma have been resected (Fig. 23.4), including six receiving isolated bile duct resection. R0 resection was achieved in all but one cases (one Bismuth-Corlette type II with proximal bile duct neoplastic infiltration after isolated bile duct resection). Despite a high radicality rate, the survival of Bismuth-Corlette type I~II tumors was significantly lower in the patients with isolated bile duct resection (six cases) than those with associated liver resection [14]: no patient with bile duct resection was alive at 3 years vs. 51.4 % at 5 years for those receiving biliary and hepatic resection (Fig. 23.5). On the other hand, Makuuchi's group in 2003 reported a series of patients with systematic liver resection: the mean survival was 42 months in nine patients with Bismuth-Corlette type I and 51 months in eight with Bismuth-Corlette type II [28].

At present, only one paper specifically focused on Bismuth-Corlette type I and II hilar cholangiocarcinoma. It has been published by the Nagoya group in 2007 [48].

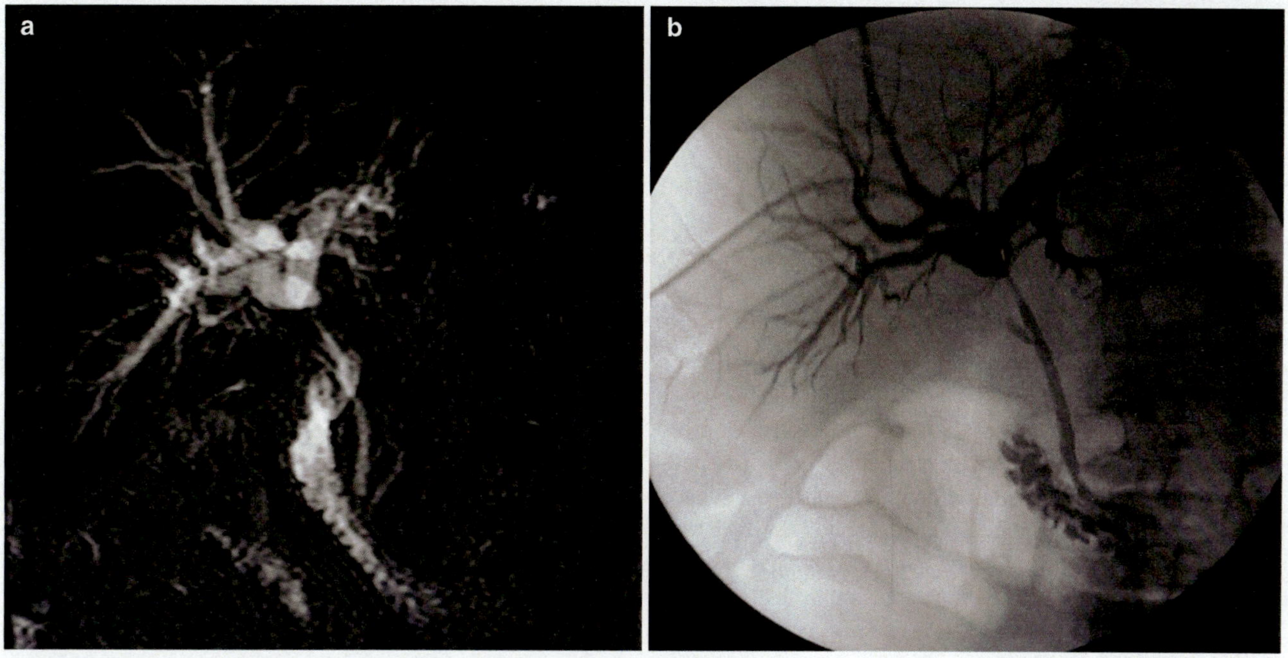

Fig. 23.4 MRCP (**a**) and PTC (**b**) imaging in a patient affected by Bismuth-Corlette type I Klatskin tumor

Fig. 23.5 Survival curves of patients affected by Bismuth-Corlette type I~II hilar cholangiocarcinomas undergoing resection in our center between 1989 and 2009 (20 patients). Patients are stratified according to received treatment: isolated bile duct resection (n=6) vs. biliary and liver resection (n=14)

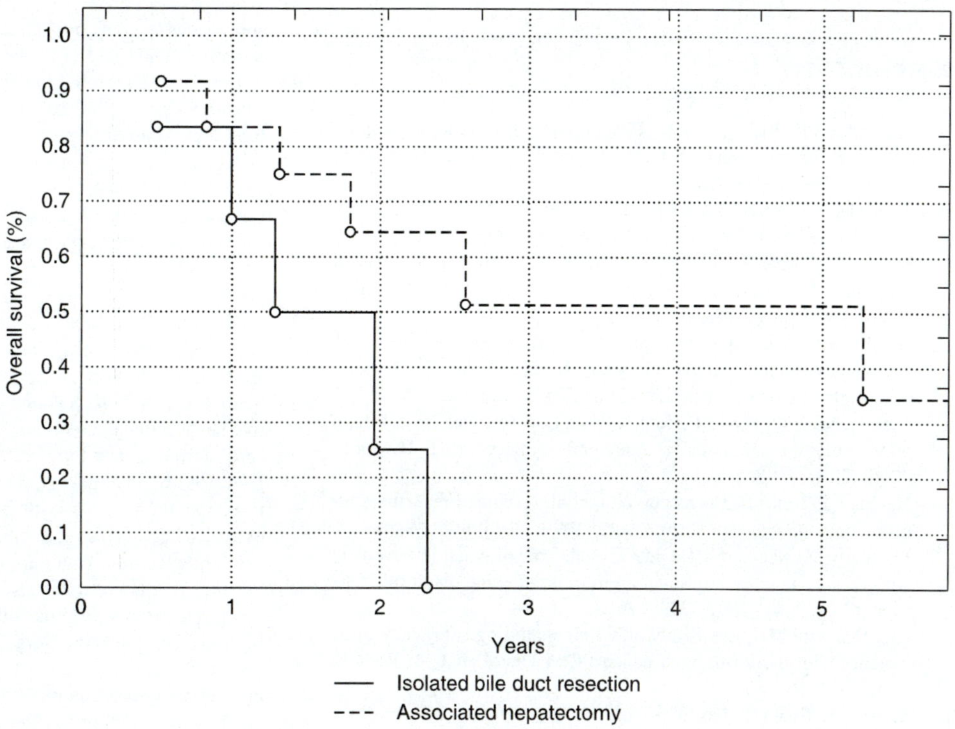

Fifty-four patients were collected. In 14 isolated bile ducts resection was performed. Unfortunately, the study analyzed the outcomes of right hepatectomies with caudate lobectomy compared with those of more limited resections, and few data are available about isolated bile duct resection without hepatectomy. The authors suggested a surgical approach based on cholangiographic tumor type. Extended hepatectomy was always recommended in the event of a nodular or infiltrating tumor [49]. Seven patients with a nodular or infiltrating tumor had isolated bile duct resection and four were not radical. On the contrary, bile duct resection with or without limited hepatectomy was considered adequate in the case of papillary tumor without superficial cancer spreading. Regardless, further studies are needed to better define these indications, mainly because only two patients of the papillary group have been treated by isolated local resection.

Conclusion

Local resection is not an adequate treatment for hilar cholangiocarcinoma involving the bile duct confluence (Bismuth-Corlette type II or more) and associated liver resection should always be recommended. In Bismuth-Corlette type I hilar cholangiocarcinoma the benefits of survival by association of biliary and liver resection have been reported, but further studies are necessary. At present, local resection should be scheduled only for small papillary Klatskin tumor without bile duct confluence involvement (type I) and confined to the bile duct wall (Tis and T1). Accurate preoperative staging is mandatory to correctly assess the tumor extension and to plan an adequate treatment strategy. An extension of the treatment should always be decided according to the patient's condition after an extensive evaluation of functional, volumetric and anaesthesiological parameters.

References

1. Saldinger PF, Blumgart LH. Resection of hilar cholangiocarcinoma—a European and United States experience. J Hepatobiliary Pancreat Surg. 2000;7(2):111–4.
2. Tabata M, Kawarada Y, Yokoi H, et al. Surgical treatment for hilar cholangiocarcinoma. J Hepatobiliary Pancreat Surg. 2000;7(2):148–54.
3. Dinant S, Gerhards MF, Rauws EA, et al. Improved outcome of resection of hilar cholangiocarcinoma (Klatskin tumor). Ann Surg Oncol. 2006;13(6):872–80.
4. DeOliveira ML, Cunningham SC, Cameron JL, et al. Cholangiocarcinoma: thirty-one-year experience with 564 patients at a single institution. Ann Surg. 2007;245(5):755–62.
5. Capussotti L, Vigano L, Ferrero A, et al. Local surgical resection of hilar cholangiocarcinoma: is there still a place? HPB (Oxford). 2008;10(3):174–8.
6. Neuhaus P, Jonas S, Bechstein WO, et al. Extended resections for hilar cholangiocarcinoma. Ann Surg. 1999;230(6):808–18.
7. Kayahara M, Nagakawa T, Ohta T, et al. Role of nodal involvement and the periductal soft-tissue margin in middle and distal bile duct cancer. Ann Surg. 1999;229(1):76–83.
8. Cha JM, Kim MH, Lee SK, et al. Clinicopathological review of 61 patients with early bile duct cancer. Clin Oncol (R Coll Radiol). 2006;18(9):669–77.
9. Shingu Y, Ebata T, Nishio H, et al. Clinical value of additional resection of a margin-positive proximal bile duct in hilar cholangiocarcinoma. Surgery. 2010;147(1):49–56.
10. Endo I, House MG, Klimstra DS, et al. Clinical significance of intraoperative bile duct margin assessment for hilar cholangiocarcinoma. Ann Surg Oncol. 2008;15(8):2104–12.
11. Ebata T, Watanabe H, Ajioka Y, et al. Pathological appraisal of lines of resection for bile duct carcinoma. Br J Surg. 2002;89(10):1260–7.
12. Wakai T, Shirai Y, Moroda T, et al. Impact of ductal resection margin status on long-term survival in patients undergoing resection for extrahepatic cholangiocarcinoma. Cancer. 2005;103(6):1210–6.
13. Abdalla EK, Vauthey JN, Couinaud C. The caudate lobe of the liver: implications of embryology and anatomy for surgery. Surg Oncol Clin N Am. 2002;11(4):835–48.
14. Mizumoto R, Kawarada Y, Suzuki H. Surgical treatment of hilar carcinoma of the bile duct. Surg Gynecol Obstet. 1986;162: 153–62.
15. Suzuki M, Takahashi T, Ouchi K, et al. The development and extension of hepatohilar bile duct carcinoma. A three-dimensional tumor mapping in the intrahepatic biliary tree visualized with the aid of a graphic computer system. Cancer. 1989;64:658–66.
16. Nimura Y, Hayakawa N, Kamiya J, et al. Hepatic segmentectomy with caudate lobe resection for bile duct carcinoma of the hepatic hilus. World J Surg. 1990;14:535–44.
17. Ogura Y, Mizumoto R, Tabata M, et al. Surgical treatment of carcinoma of the hepatic duct confluence: analysis of 55 resected carcinomas. World J Surg. 1993;17:85–92.
18. Sugiura Y, Nakamura S, Iida S, et al. Extensive resection of the bile ducts combined with liver resection for cancer of the main hepatic duct junction: a cooperative study of the Keio bile duct cancer study group. Surgery. 1994;115:445–51.
19. Nakeeb A, Pitt HA, Sohn TA, et al. Cholangiocarcinoma. A spectrum of intrahepatic, perihilar, and distal tumors. Ann Surg. 1996;224(4):463–73.
20. Pichlmayr R, Weimann A, Klempnauer J, et al. Surgical treatment in proximal bile duct cancer. A single-center experience. Ann Surg. 1996;224(5):628–38.
21. Miyazaki M, Ito H, Nakagawa K, et al. Aggressive surgical approaches to hilar cholangiocarcinoma: hepatic or local resection? Surgery. 1998;123(2):131–6.
22. Boerma EJ. Research into the results of resection of hilar bile duct cancer. Surgery. 1990;108(3):572–80.
23. Baer HU, Stain SC, Dennison AR, et al. Improvements in survival by aggressive resections of hilar cholangiocarcinoma. Ann Surg. 1993;217(1):20–7.
24. Launois B, Reding R, Lebeau G, et al. Surgery for hilar cholangiocarcinoma: French experience in a collective survey of 552 extrahepatic bile duct cancers. J Hepatobiliary Pancreat Surg. 2000;7(2):128–34.
25. Launois B, Terblanche J, Lakehal M, et al. Proximal bile duct cancer: high resectability rate and 5-year survival. Ann Surg. 1999;230(2):266–75.
26. Sano T, Shimada K, Sakamoto Y, et al. One hundred two consecutive hepatobiliary resections for perihilar cholangiocarcinoma with zero mortality. Ann Surg. 2006;244(2):240–7.
27. Kawasaki S, Imamura H, Kobayashi A, et al. Results of surgical resection for patients with hilar bile duct cancer: application of extended hepatectomy after biliary drainage and hemihepatic portal vein embolization. Ann Surg. 2003;238(1):84–92.
28. Seyama Y, Kubota K, Sano K, et al. Long-term outcome of extended hemihepatectomy for hilar bile duct cancer with no mortality and high survival rate. Ann Surg. 2003;238(1):73–83.
29. Kondo S, Hirano S, Ambo Y, et al. Forty consecutive resections of hilar cholangiocarcinoma with no postoperative mortality and no positive ductal margins: results of a prospective study. Ann Surg. 2004;240(1):95–101.
30. Tsao JI, Nimura Y, Kamiya J, et al. Management of hilar cholangiocarcinoma: comparison of an American and a Japanese experience. Ann Surg. 2000;232(2):166–74.
31. Capussotti L, Muratore A, Polastri R, et al. Liver resection for hilar cholangiocarcinoma: in-hospital mortality and longterm survival. J Am Coll Surg. 2002;195(5):641–7.

32. Lee SG, Song GW, Hwang S, et al. Surgical treatment of hilar cholangiocarcinoma in the new era: the Asan experience. J Hepatobiliary Pancreat Sci. 2010;17(4):476–89.
33. Shi Z, Yang MZ, He QL, et al. Addition of hepatectomy decreases liver recurrence and leads to long survival in hilar cholangiocarcinoma. World J Gastroenterol. 2009;15(15):1892–6.
34. Igami T, Nishio H, Ebata T, et al. Surgical treatment of hilar cholangiocarcinoma in the "new era": the Nagoya University experience. J Hepatobiliary Pancreat Sci. 2010;17(4):449–54.
35. Ito F, Cho CS, Rikkers LF, et al. Hilar cholangiocarcinoma: current management. Ann Surg. 2009;250(2):210–8.
36. Cameron JL, Pitt HA, Zinner MJ, et al. Management of proximal cholangiocarcinomas by surgical resection and radiotherapy. Am J Surg. 1990;159(1):91–7.
37. Hadjis NS, Blenkharn JI, Alexander N, et al. Outcome of radical surgery in hilar cholangiocarcinoma. Surgery. 1990;107(6):597–604.
38. Klempnauer J, Ridder GJ, Werner M, et al. What constitutes long-term survival after surgery for hilar cholangiocarcinoma? Cancer. 1997;79(1):26–34.
39. Burke EC, Jarnagin WR, Hochwald SN, et al. Hilar Cholangiocarcinoma: patterns of spread, the importance of hepatic resection for curative operation, and a presurgical clinical staging system. Ann Surg. 1998;228(3):385–94.
40. Jarnagin WR, Fong Y, DeMatteo RP, et al. Staging, resectability, and outcome in 225 patients with hilar cholangiocarcinoma. Ann Surg. 2001;234(4):507–17.
41. van Gulik TM, Kloek JJ, Ruys AT, et al. Multidisciplinary management of hilar cholangiocarcinoma (Klatskin tumor): extended resection is associated with improved survival. Eur J Surg Oncol. 2011;37(1):65–71.
42. Jang JY, Kim SW, Park DJ, et al. Actual long-term outcome of extrahepatic bile duct cancer after surgical resection. Ann Surg. 2005;241(1):77–84.
43. Kosuge T, Yamamoto J, Shimada K, et al. Improved surgical results for hilar cholangiocarcinoma with procedures including major hepatic resection. Ann Surg. 1999;230(5):663–71.
44. Witzigmann H, Berr F, Ringel U, et al. Surgical and palliative management and outcome in 184 patients with hilar cholangiocarcinoma: palliative photodynamic therapy plus stenting is comparable to r1/r2 resection. Ann Surg. 2006;244(2):230–9.
45. Bismuth H, Nakache R, Diamond T. Management strategies in resection for hilar cholangiocarcinoma. Ann Surg. 1992;215(1):31–8.
46. Su CH, Tsay SH, Wu CC, et al. Factors influencing postoperative morbidity, mortality, and survival after resection for hilar cholangiocarcinoma. Ann Surg. 1996;223(4):384–94.
47. van Gulik TM, Gerhards M, de Vries J, et al. Local resection of biliopancreatic cancer. Ann Oncol. 1999;10 Suppl 4Suppl 4:243–6.
48. Ikeyama T, Nagino M, Oda K, et al. Surgical approach to bismuth type I and II hilar cholangiocarcinomas: audit of 54 consecutive cases. Ann Surg. 2007;246(6):1052–7.
49. Nimura Y, Kamiya J, Kondo S, et al. Aggressive preoperative management and extended surgery for hilar cholangiocarcinoma: Nagoya experience. J Hepatobiliary Pancreat Surg. 2000;7(2):155–62.

Ex Situ Ex Vivo Resection and Autotransplantation

24

A.K.K. Chui

24.1 Introduction

Cholangiocarcinoma represents a difficult cancer with poor prognosis. It is not a common disease, and may occur anywhere along the intrahepatic or extrahepatic biliary tree. Cholangiocarcinoma usually presents with painless jaundice, and this diagnosis should be considered in every case of obstructive jaundice. These bile duct cancers are best classified according to the anatomical location into three board groups: (a) intrahepatic, (b) hilar or perihilar, and (c) distal [1]. Intrahepatic cholangiocarcinomas occur with the lowest frequency and are usually managed with liver resection, as are other resectable liver tumors. Distal type cholangiocarcinomas are the second most common type accounting for about 25 %. Depending on whether the extrahepatic bile duct is involved above or below the upper border of duodenum, treatment is usually with extrahepatic bile duct resection with or without pancreatoduodenectomy. Tumor that involves the confluence of the right and left hepatic ducts (hilar cholangiocarcinoma) is the most common. It accounts for about 60 % of all cholangiocarcinoma cases [2, 3]. Bismuth and Corlette further classified the hilar cholangiocarcinomas into four subtypes [4]. Regardless of the biliary locations or the subtypes of cholangiocarcinomas, surgical resection of the tumor, whenever possible, is the preferred treatment and is the only effective treatment modality that is capable of offering a chance of cure. However, for many patients with metastatic or peritoneal spread, surgical tumor clearance is not possible and is not recommended.

For locally advanced tumor, frequently surgical resection is not possible for technical reasons. This is especially the case for hilar cholangiocarcinomas (or Klatskin tumor) due to its anatomical close proximity to crucial structures. Even for those patients who have undergone surgical resection, long-term survivals of only 27–32.8 % are reported in most series. Negative resection margin and tumor clearance is the most important factor in achieving long term survival [5]. Therefore, aggressive surgical management including complex liver resections has been advocated to increase the resectability and the subsequent survival. Meanwhile, there are no effective and curative non-surgical treatment modalities, in selected cases of locally advanced cholangiocarcinomas that are considered unresectable with conventional techniques, ex situ ex vivo resection and autotransplantation as a last resource is being discussed.

24.2 Impact of Liver Transplantation on Ex Situ Ex Vivo Resection and Autotransplantation

Since the first successful human orthotopic liver transplantation took place in 1963 [6], liver transplantation has reached a new height. Not only the number of liver transplants performed worldwide has significantly increased, the mortality rate among elective transplant cases has decreased to less than 10 % [7]. There are many reasons for the improved outcomes, but surgical innovations have contributed a great deal. The development of veno-venous bypass during the anhepatic phase was a significant milestone in the evolution of liver transplantation surgery [8]. This stabilizes the hemodynamic conditions of the patient during caval and portal vein clamping. The bypass helps to reduce venous congestion, thereby the blood loss and blood transfusion requirements. The bowel is less congested and the renal function is better preserved afterwards. It eases pressure on the surgical team to rapidly perform difficult vascular anastomoses and encourage trainees to undertake the procedure during the learning curve. Although used routinely in the past, veno-venous bypass is now used selectively by most units, based on the individual physiological parameters encountered during the surgery. In another modification, the full length of the

A.K.K. Chui, MBBS(NSW), FRCS(Ed), FRACS, FCSHK, FHKAM(Surg), MD(UNSW)
Private Practice, Suite 604, Wing On Central Building, 26 Des Voeux Road, Central, Hong Kong
e-mail: akkchui@pacific.net.hk

W.Y. Lau (ed.), *Hilar Cholangiocarcinoma*,
DOI 10.1007/978-94-007-6473-6_24, © Springer Science+Business Media Dordrecht and People's Medical Publishing House 2013

recipient inferior vena cava (IVC) was preserved, and the new liver was placed "piggyback" onto its anterior surface. A particularly appealing feature of the piggyback operation in children or some adults for whom veno-venous bypass might not be feasible was that vena caval occlusion could be avoided during hepatectomy and sewing in of the graft. The technique had been used in some of the earliest patients, but the formal description and widespread use of the piggyback operation took place much later [9]. This technique has simplified the graft implantation procedure. The donor supra hepatic cava is anastomosed end to side to the recipient's IVC. This further reduces the need for veno-venous bypass, as caval clamping can be removed after only one anastomosis. Another landmark improvement in organ transplantation in general came from the introduction of the University of Wisconsin (UW) preservation solution by Belzer and colleagues [10]. The UW solution has increased safe cold storage of the liver graft up to 24 h. The significantly longer preservation time allows for a less hurried operation with much greater flexibility and precision in the planning and execution of liver transplantation. All these have been instrumental to the development of ex situ ex vivo liver resection and partial autotransplantation.

Allograft liver transplantation in patients with hepatic malignant conditions remains highly controversial, mainly because of the shortage of donor organs. If not conducted properly, this can become a divisive issue in the transplantation community about the allocation of organs. In the allograft transplant settings, organ recipients after transplantation are required to be on long term immunosuppression which is bad for the recipient's immunity against tumor growth and recurrence. In fact, allograft liver transplantation for cholangiocarcinoma has been shown to deliver very poor results and is not justifiable [11]. Most transplant centers have abandoned transplanting cholangiocarcinoma in light of poor outcomes and donor organ shortage [12]. Ex situ ex vivo liver resection and autotransplantation has the advantage of not requiring a donor liver graft, and can circumvent the need and the inherent complications of long term immunosuppression.

The persistent ongoing shortage of organs in allograft transplantation has led surgeons to develop innovative surgical techniques to expand the donor pool. With respect to allograft liver transplantation, these techniques include reducing adult-sized livers for children or small sized recipients, split liver transplantation by which a single donor liver is split into two grafts for two recipients, and living related/unrelated donor liver transplantation. All of these procedures involve ex vivo or bench surgery that are based on clear understanding of the detailed segmental anatomy of the liver. With exception of living donor transplantation, in which only part of the liver is removed from the live donor, otherwise, during these procedures, the liver is completely removed from the donor and is flushed with cold preservation solution. A bloodless transection of hepatic parenchyma can then be performed allowing complex reconstruction of hepatic veins, portal structures after which the liver graft is implanted into the recipient. Such techniques, together with the knowledge of hypothermic organ perfusion in organ preservation have made possible the technique of ex situ ex vivo resection and autotransplantation. In this setting, the entire liver is first removed from the patient. The liver then undergoes bench surgery of resection and reconstruction. Afterwards, a portion of the liver considered disease free will be re-implanted back into the same patient. Indeed, such an approach was pioneered by Rudolph Pichlmayr and his team in 1988 [13]. Application of these techniques allows liver surgeons today to redefine indications for resectional surgery and possibly expand the group of patients with liver tumors to whom a chance for cure may be offered.

Parallel to the refinement of the surgical techniques, there was more effective monitoring of intra-operative coagulopathy, using thromboelastographs, the advent of rapid infusion device and blood autotransfusion. The bleeding problem associated with liver transplantation was largely overcome. Meanwhile, improvements in various surgical and monitoring equipments, advances in anesthesia and intensive care medicine have reduced the risk of morbidities and mortalities from liver transplantation. Many of these are applicable to complicated hepatic surgery.

24.3 Technical Aspects in Ex Situ Ex Vivo Resection and Autotransplantation

In many ways, the procedure is similar to that of living donor liver transplantation in that only portion of a healthy liver is implanted. The difference is that there is no donor required. As such, there is no issue concerning organ rejection and immunosuppression is not necessary. However, the medical team needs to ensure that the liver portion to be implanted should have an adequate functional mass in spite of injury from bench resection and preservation. There is a lot of data and discussion in the field of living donor liver transplantation in the literature on what a minimum liver mass should be. In general, the graft/ recipient's body weight ratio should be >0.8 % [14], or the liver graft volume should not be <30 % of the standard liver volume [15]. These rules should act as guidance and best be respected during the process of assessment before autotransplantation. While there is no concern of on- going injury from rejection after the surgery, the technical challenge from reconstructions of vessels and bile ducts in ex situ ex vivo surgery is probably more difficult and can be more complicated. This type of surgery should only be performed in specialized centre where surgeons are familiar with all aspects of both complex hepato-biliary surgery and liver transplantation.

24.3.1 Initial Exploration and Dissection

Like in standard allograft liver transplantation, the routine approach is through a bilateral transverse incision in the upper abdomen with an upper midline extension upwards to the xiphoid sternum (Mercedes-Benz incision). A retractor which is able to lift up the costal margins bilaterally and cephalically is crucial in order to provide adequate exposure and access. Although tumor extent has been carefully evaluated by various radiological means before the surgery, a thorough examination of the abdominal cavity at the beginning of the surgery is mandatory. The liver is completely freed of its ligamentous attachments for easy access and accurate assessment. The extent of intrahepatic involvement by the tumor and possible unexpected tumor spread is assessed by palpation and intra-operative ultrasound. Only when there is no contraindication such as metastatic tumors and there is a reasonable chance of achieving resection with tumor free margins should one proceed with the complex procedure.

The diaphragm is first detached from the suprahepatic IVC. The dissection at this site is a useful technique to achieve an extra length of IVC for extrapericardial or intrapericardial caval clamping during vascular exclusion for total hepatectomy. This can also facilitate caval anastomoses during implantation of the liver later on. For oncological and diagnostic reasons, as well as for improved exposure, usually all the lymphatic, neural, and connective tissue from the hepatoduodenal ligament should be removed entirely in most cases. In case there is no need to resect the common bile duct, then the adjacent tissue with its blood supply around the duct should be preserved. Obviously, in such situation, the duct is to be shortened and biliary drainage will be reconstituted by hepatico- jejunostomy. Lymphadenectomy is usually extended along the hepatic artery up to the celiac trunk. Depending on the location of the tumor and its involvement to the IVC, the liver may be dissected away from the cava, or can be removed en bloc together with the cava. If the IVC is involved by the tumor as in the latter scenario, the IVC will need to be reconstructed afterwards.

24.3.2 Veno-venous Bypass

The main aim of veno-venous bypass is to lower the portal venous pressure and thereby minimize bleeding, hemodynamic instability, venous hypertension and intestinal edema during the anhepatic phase. The duration of the anhepatic period is expected to be long in ex situ ex vivo resection and autotransplantation. Different to cases in allograft liver transplantation for often cirrhosis, patients in autotransplantation do not have significant portal collateral circulation, veno-venous bypass is therefore almost always necessary in ex situ ex vivo resection and autotransplantation.

The veno-venous bypass allows venous return without interruption via the axillary vein (alternative is via internal jugular vein) from the trunk and the lower limbs during caval clamping. Up to 50 % of the cardiac output can be returned to the heart from the lower body and the viscera through the bypass. The bypass is applied exactly the same as in allograft liver transplantation [16], with bypass from the portal circulation and the left femoral vein to the left axillary vein using heparin- coated shunts (Gott) and a roller pump. The Y shunt and the blood pump are first primed with normal saline containing a small amount of heparin (500 U/L). Blood is taken from the iliac vein by means of a cannula inserted via the left saphenous vein (the left limb of the Y) and from the portal vein or the inferior mesenteric vein via a cannula (forming the right limb of the Y). The blood passes through a centrifugal blood pump (with an "air" alarm) and is delivered to the left axillary vein thereby returning blood to the heart. Blood flow via the bypass can vary from 1 to 2 L/min. This can be adjusted according to the patient's condition. Hypothermia of the patient is prevented using a heat exchanger.

All portal triad structures are individually dissected free. The liver is fully mobilized and is attached only by the main vascular pedicles. In order to get the veno-venous bypass working prior to cross clamping, the portal vein may or may not be transected. The bypass shunt may be inserted into the proximal end of the portal vein (in case of transection) or into the inferior mesenteric vein (in case of portal vein clamping). In any case, the arterial blood supply to the liver is maintained until cold perfusion of the liver is ready, just before and removal of the organ.

Veno-venous bypass is not without complications. These include unique problems including air embolism, thromboembolic complications and mechanical injury associated with global capillary leak, leading to third- spacing of fluid after surgery [17]. Therefore, the duration of the veno-venous bypass should be shortest possible. Surgically creation of a temporary an end-to-side porto-caval shunt replacing portal part of the veno-venous bypass shunt whenever possible during surgery is a good strategy. This helps to reduce the duration and the degree of dependence on the machanical shunt, and its associated complications. At this stage, due to the scarcity of performing ex situ ex vivo surgery, the experience gathered in any single unit may not be enough to propose selective utilization of veno-venous bypass.

24.3.3 Hypothermic Perfusion

The UW solution is commonly used as the preservation solution in allograft liver transplantation. However, in autotransplantation, the preservation solution histidine-tryptophan-ketoglutarate (HTK) solution is preferred [18]. This is because of its relatively low potassium content as compared to other preservation fluids, which minimizes the risk of cardio- circulatory complications after liver re-perfusion. This solution also has added advantage of having a low viscosity, which allows fast and homogeneous perfusion of the organ.

In ex situ ex vivo surgery, the exact approach may depend somewhat on the circumstances. The hepatic side of portal vein can be cannulated with a shunt in preparation for flushing and cooling. Blood circulation from the hepatic artery and the IVC are still being maintained until this stage. When the veno-venous bypass is working and both the hepatic arteries are divided, hypothermic liver perfusion is started in situ immediately after clamping of the suprahepatic and infrahepatic IVC. In other words, the liver is now in a state of total vascular exclusion. Outflow of preservation fluid is provided by an opening at any of the hepatic vein or on the cava. This cold outflow fluid should be effectively removed by suction to minimize hypothermia. After the initial flushing and cooling, the entire liver is removed from the patient. Cooling is continued and maintained during the time when bench surgical procedures including resection of tumor, reconstruction of vessels, and repair of leakage from vessels and the resection plane are performed.

24.3.4 Bench Surgery and Implantation

After the liver is thoroughly perfused with HTK solution, the resection on bench is performed similar to that in liver allograft reduction or splitting into two liver grafts. The liver is placed in a bowl containing iced perfusion fluid. At this stage, the gall bladder would have been removed already and much of the dissection around the vessels would have been performed. Also similar to conventional liver resection surgery, Cavitron Ultrasonic Aspirator (CUSA; Valley Lab) is used for parenchymal transection. The liver transection is totally bloodless. In all cases, the liver segmental planes are followed as much as possible in order to preserve the viability of liver parenchyma. Individual vicryl ties are preferred for ligations, the vessels and bile ducts crossing the resection line can also be closed with prolene sutures, or with the aid of titanium hemoclips, depending on their size. Ultrasound mapping of important structures including the tumor margin may be useful. Frozen section tissue biopsy may be done at this stage to confirm tumor free margin whenever it is indicated.

After the tumor bearing part of the liver is removed, perfusion of the healthy liver portion is repeated to identify any potential leakage of bile or blood. All these potential sources from the resection plane are carefully repaired with prolene sutures. The resection surface may be sealed with fibrin glue. Likewise, any small branches from the arteries and veins are perfused and any small branches that are left untied are ligated or sutured with a 6/0 prolene at this stage. Vessels reconstructions are to be performed next. In contrast to allograft liver transplantation, there is no luxury of long vessel length, vessel patch, or spare vessels available as in cadaveric liver transplantation, or to a lesser degree as in living donor transplantation. Therefore, extra care and precision during dissection and re-anastomoses of vessels is required in this procedure. The principles of implantation of the remnant liver and the anastomoses of vessels are performed exactly the same way as in living donor transplantation.

During this hypothermic period, complicated reconstructions of vessels are almost always required prior to re-implantation of the liver (partial autotransplantation). For vascular reconstruction of the hepatic artery, portal vein, hepatic veins, and the IVC, autologous veins are preferred and should be used whenever possible. Some of these can be obtained from the liver specimen itself such as the portal vein or the hepatic veins provided that the vessels are far away from the tumor. Other convenient sites to obtain autologous veins should include the internal jugular vein from the neck and the saphenous veins from the thighs. Prosthetic material such as Gortex may have to be used if autologous veins are not available or are not suitable.

24.3.5 Anesthesia

Patient's physiological parameters may fluctuate widely during the time of total vascular exclusion. The anesthetic team has an important role to stabilize the hemodynamic conditions of the patient. Because of the long duration of the anhepatic phase, and the subsequent implantation of a reduced sized and dysfunctioned liver, the risk of severe bleeding can be a problem [19]. Coagulopathy is caused by marked fibrinolysis and the depletion of hemostatic factors. The situation can be improved by early and prophylactic replacement of fresh frozen plasma and platelets. Acidosis is common and can be alleviated by sodium bicarbonate and hyperventilation. Because the cold perfusion of the liver takes place while it is still in vivo, patient should be protected from hypothermia. Anesthetists should be experienced in all aspects of liver transplantation. Close intraoperative monitoring is an integral part of the entire procedure. In fact, many of these treatments and stringent measures should be continued till at least after the initial post- operative phase when the patient has become stable.

24.4 Liver Tumors that May Be Suitable for This Procedure

Surgical resection has been an effective treatment option for liver tumors, be it benign or malignant, primary or secondary. The good outcome would be more assured if complete removal of all tumor tissue is achieved. For malignant cases, the role of surgery is even more important as untreated patients are destined for a poor prognosis with short survival.

However, there is a small group of patients having tumors that are unresectable due to its size, its local extension or its location in close proximity to critical structures. Under such circumstances, resection using conventional techniques could be either too risky or even impossible. Besides the technical difficulties in vascular control trying to control bleeding and without causing too much ischemic damage to the liver, the inability to achieve adequate resection margin are the main concerns. For unresectable tumors that have no effective non-surgical treatment, ex situ ex vivo resection and autotransplantation represents a possible viable option.

24.4.1 Tumors that Involve the IVC

Until the recent past, patients with tumor involvement of the inferior vena cava (IVC) were considered contraindicated for standard liver resection. However, it is now known that the IVC can be partially or segmentally resected when tumor involvement occurs. After resection, depending on the size of the defect, available reconstruction methods include simple suture, patch repair with synthetic materials including Dacron and polytetrafluoroethylene (PTFE, Gortex) or with autologous veins or pericardium. Whole segment of IVC can be substituted with autologous vein in the form of a composite graft. The IVC can also been replaced with synthetic material such as ringed PTFE or Dacron tube graft [20–22]. If prosthetic materials are used, anticoagulation after surgery to reduce the risk of vascular graft thrombosis would be required.

Nowadays, with advances in surgical techniques, ex situ ex vivo resection and autotransplantation approach is seldom required for tumors involving the IVC. There are many approaches that enable resection of the tumor and the involved cava. Total vascular exclusion that involves a Pringle maneuver with clamping of the IVC above and below the liver is a good relatively simple method. Both the vascular control and repair of the caval defect can be safely achieved [23]. The normothermic ischemia imposed by this technique only allows for a quick resection/ repair that last for a short time. Veno-venous bypass may or may not be introduced. However, in extremely rare situations where tumor resection can only be achieved with prolonged clamping of both the suprahepatic and infrahepatic IVC, or the IVC resection would involve the confluence of hepatic veins (described below), hypothermic liver perfusion approaches including ex situ ex vivo surgery may have to be considered [20].

24.4.2 Tumors at Hepatic Hilum or at the Hepatic Veins and IVC Confluence

Selected cases of liver tumors located at or near the bifurcation of the portal pedicle, or tumors in close proximity to the confluence of the IVC and hepatic veins are probably the types of tumors that are most commonly considered for ex situ ex vivo resection and autotransplantation so far [24]. For tumors in such locations, there is currently no other way that one can technically resect the tumor safely with a margin and at the same time overcome the problems of vascular control and ischemic damage to the remaining liver (as mentioned above). Nevertheless, the overall number reported of such cases having undergone ex situ ex vivo surgery is small. The reasons for the rarity are easily understood. Firstly, tumors with such characteristics are genuinely uncommon. Secondly, such surgery is complex and only a few sophisticated centers are willing to perform such procedures. Most other cases are probably discarded as inoperable. Thirdly, in the surgical community, the usefulness of this approach, given the costs and the risks, is yet to be confirmed. Although the number reported is small, this technique has been applied for a variety of tumors including cholangiocarcinoma, hepatocellular carcinoma, liver metastasis from colorectal cancer or renal cell carcinoma, leiomyosarcoma, neuroendocrine tumors and benign tumors. It is accepted that such an approach offers a way to resect tumors radically and provides a better, if not the only, chance for complete resection. It also does it without the need for allograft liver transplantation in which a donor liver graft would be required. Nevertheless, ex situ ex vivo surgery being a costly and complicated technique should be justifiable by the outcomes.

24.5 Variations to the Ex Situ Ex Vivo Technique

As described above, the main problems in major liver surgery are bleeding and warm ischemic insults to the liver. The time period allowed by conventional vascular clamping and resulting ischemia is too short to allow complex liver resections and lengthy vascular reconstructions, as well as re-implantation. In order to overcome such problem, cooling the liver with chilled preservation solution (HTK solution) would enhance tolerance of the remnant liver to cold ischemia. Besides the ex situ ex vivo technique in which the liver is completely removed from the abdominal cavity by transection of both afferent and efferent vessels, there are two other similar approaches but with difference:

1. In situ surgery [25]—the liver, albeit completely mobilized, remains in the right hypochondrium and the integrity of both afferent and efferent vessels is conserved.
2. Ex situ in vivo surgery [26]—the efferent vessels i.e. all three hepatic veins, or the vena cava (after fully mobilized from its dorsal attachments) above the confluence of the hepatic veins are transected. The afferent vessels, included in the portal pedicle, remain intact and in vivo. The

additional mobility of the liver allows it to be exteriorized from the abdominal cavity (ex situ).

Including the ex situ ex vivo technique, all three approaches involve total vascular exclusion as well as cold perfusion of the liver. A long period of total vascular exclusion which includes occlusion of IVC is frequently necessary. The consequential venous congestion in patients without pre-existing collateral circulation may cause major problem. Therefore, the veno-venous bypass is usually indispensable to avoid any pressure of time during the delicate procedure in all three approaches.

For the in situ technique, the portal vein does not need to be transected. The vessel may be clamped below the incision and the portal limb of the veno-venous bypass shunt can be inserted into the inferior mesenteric vein. The inflow of preservation fluid can be given via cannulation through an incision of the portal vein above the portal vein clamp. The outflow is let out through a drain placed through a vena cavotomy inferior to the liver. In the ex situ in vivo technique, the liver remnant, after resection and sometime after reconstruction, needs to be re-implanted onto the IVC. The main difference between the three approaches is the extent of liver mobilization. However, if the surgery involves complicated resection and reconstruction, these two in vivo approaches do not support a prolonged anhepatic period as well as what can be provided by the ex situ ex vivo approach. Therefore in vivo approaches by comparison have been used even less frequently.

24.6 Outcomes of Ex Situ Ex Vivo Surgery and Autotransplantation

24.6.1 Overall Results

Pichlmayr et al. first performed ex situ ex vivo liver resection and autotransplantation in 1988 [27]. This group in Germany has the largest experience with such technique of surgery in the world to-date. In their most recent publication, 24 cases of ex vivo liver resection performed between 1988 and 1998 [21]. The procedure was completed in 22 of 24 cases. In two, the completed back- table work left the liver remnant unsuitable for auto transplantation, so both of these patients underwent cadaveric transplant 17 and 19 h after hepatectomy. In 4 out of the 22 patients, liver failure ensued following the procedure, also requiring cadaveric liver transplantation. Fifteen patients survived the postoperative period and were discharged after 36.5 ± 16 days. The median survival time of the six patients who had colorectal metastases was 21 months. The two patients with benign disease were alive 5 and 9 years after the procedure. From this experience, it becomes apparent that the procedure carries high postoperative mortalities and morbidities.

There are other isolated cases of ex situ ex vivo resection reported in the literature [22, 28]. Although these reports focused primarily on the technical aspect of the procedure, the gathered results showed that benign tumor or less malignant tumor types such as neuroendocrine tumor do reasonably well after such treatment [29]. The procedure can be quite worthwhile for such selected cases. Among patients with malignant tumors, some tumor types do better than others. However, the overall long term results can best be described as modest. For some malignant tumors like cholangiocarcinoma, the results have been disappointing. Early tumor recurrence seemed to be a common problem for these patients. This remains a major concern for applying such technique in malignant tumors, and therefore thorough consideration and careful selection of tumor types are warranted.

24.6.2 Cholangiocarcinoma

Curative treatment of patients with localized cholangiocarcinoma is only possible with complete resection [5]. This can be difficult to achieve as reflected by the suboptimal long-term survival after conventional resectional surgery. The difficulty becomes much more paramount in advanced cases of hilar cholangiocarcinoma in which, for example, the tumor has invaded the portal vein or the hepatic artery or the tumor has involved second order biliary branches. Under these circumstances, conventional surgical approach cannot effectively circumvent the problems of bleeding and ischemic insult to the liver while the same time to achieve tumor clearance. Ex situ ex vivo resection and partial liver autotransplantation is able to overcome the two problems and offers a much better chance of securing clear resection margins.

Among hilar cholangiocarcinomas, Bismuth type IV cholangiocarcinoma in particular has a very poor prognosis [4]. Although ex situ ex-vivo resection and autotransplantation represent a viable treatment option, only six cases of autotransplantation for hilar cholangiocarcinoma have ever been performed and reported in the English literature. According to the world's largest experience from the Pichlmayr's center, Oldhafer [21] reported the long term outcomes of 22 patients. Among them, those who had hilar cholangiocarcinoma and required this surgery were among the worst results. According to their experience, three out of four hilar cholangiocarcinoma patients treated with this procedure did not survive the operation. The other remaining patient survived the surgery but died of early tumor recurrence. Oldhafer also suggested that ex situ ex vivo liver surgery should be avoided in patients with cholestasis, thinking that long- standing cholestasis may reduce the liver's tolerance to ischemia.

There have been no other long term results reported in the literature for hilar cholangiocarcinoma treated with this

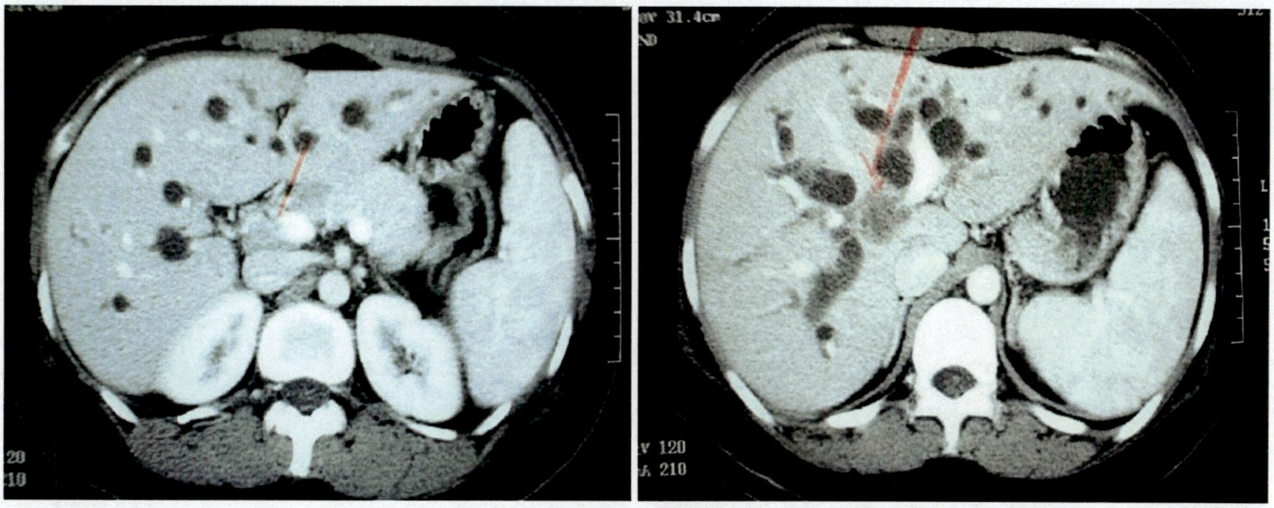

Figs. 24.1–24.2 Preoperative CT scan demonstrating a mass at the portal confluence and intrahepatic ductal dilatation

technique except for one patient treated by the author (described below) with a 17 month survival without recurrent disease [30]. This patient had done well in spite of presence of pre-operative cholestasis. At the time of reporting, this was the first successful case with the longest tumor free survival in the world after such treatment for a locally advanced hilar cholangiocarcinoma. For about 2 years after the surgery, she was able to return to work and lived a normal productive life. Sadly, she also developed tumor recurrence at 2 years and subsequently died 2 ½ years from the time of surgery.

In the literature, there was another successful case report of a long term tumor free survival [31]. This case involved a 41 year old patient who had an advanced intrahepatic, a non-hilar type, cholangiocarcinoma involving the left lobe of liver. Again, the tumor could not be resected by conventional technique. After surgical treatment of ex situ ex vivo resection and autotransplantation, the patient was still alive and tumor free 23 months afterward.

Case Illustration—The technique is being exemplified by the following patient.

The patient was a 26 years old female with no past medical history. She presented to her primary care physician with a history of jaundice and tea-colored urine. She did not have any fever, chills, or abdominal pain. Laboratory investigation revealed elevations in her bilirubin (334 μmol/L), alkaline phosphatase, and liver transaminases. Hepatitis serologies were negative. Ultrasound examination of her abdomen revealed gross biliary ductal dilatation with abrupt truncation at the ductal confluence. The gall bladder was normal, and no gallstones were seen. An endoscopic retrograde cholangiopancreatography was performed but failed cannulation of the common bile duct. Marked dilatation of right and left intrahepatic ducts (IHD) down to the level of the porta hepatis were shown on CT scan (Figs. 24.1–24.2) and on the magnetic resonance cholangiogram.

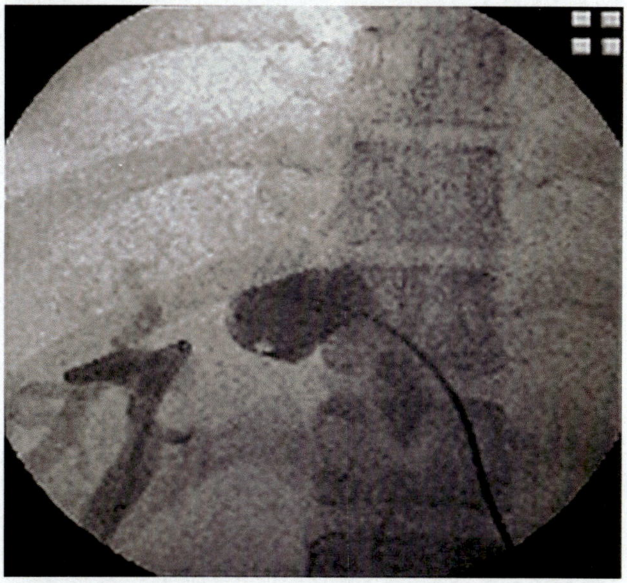

Fig. 24.3 Percutaneous cholangiogram showing that segment IV duct was involved by the tumor

A percutaneous cholangiogram (Fig. 24.3) was performed and showed right side dilated IHD with obstruction at the ductal confluence. She was initially managed with percutaneous transhepatic biliary drainage (PTBD), one on either side of the biliary tree. She was complicated by an episode of hemobilia from the right PTBD. A hepatic angiogram showed no active bleeding but a hypovascular tumor with portal vein involvement. Hemobilia settled after the original PTBD was replaced with a new one. In addition to a 2.3 cm hilar mass, an MRI scan (Fig. 24.4–24.5) showed bilateral tumor involvements up to the origins of the left medial and lateral segmental ducts, and the origins of the right anterior and posterior segmental ducts (Bismuth type IV hilar cholangiocarcinoma). The confluence of the portal vein was also involved

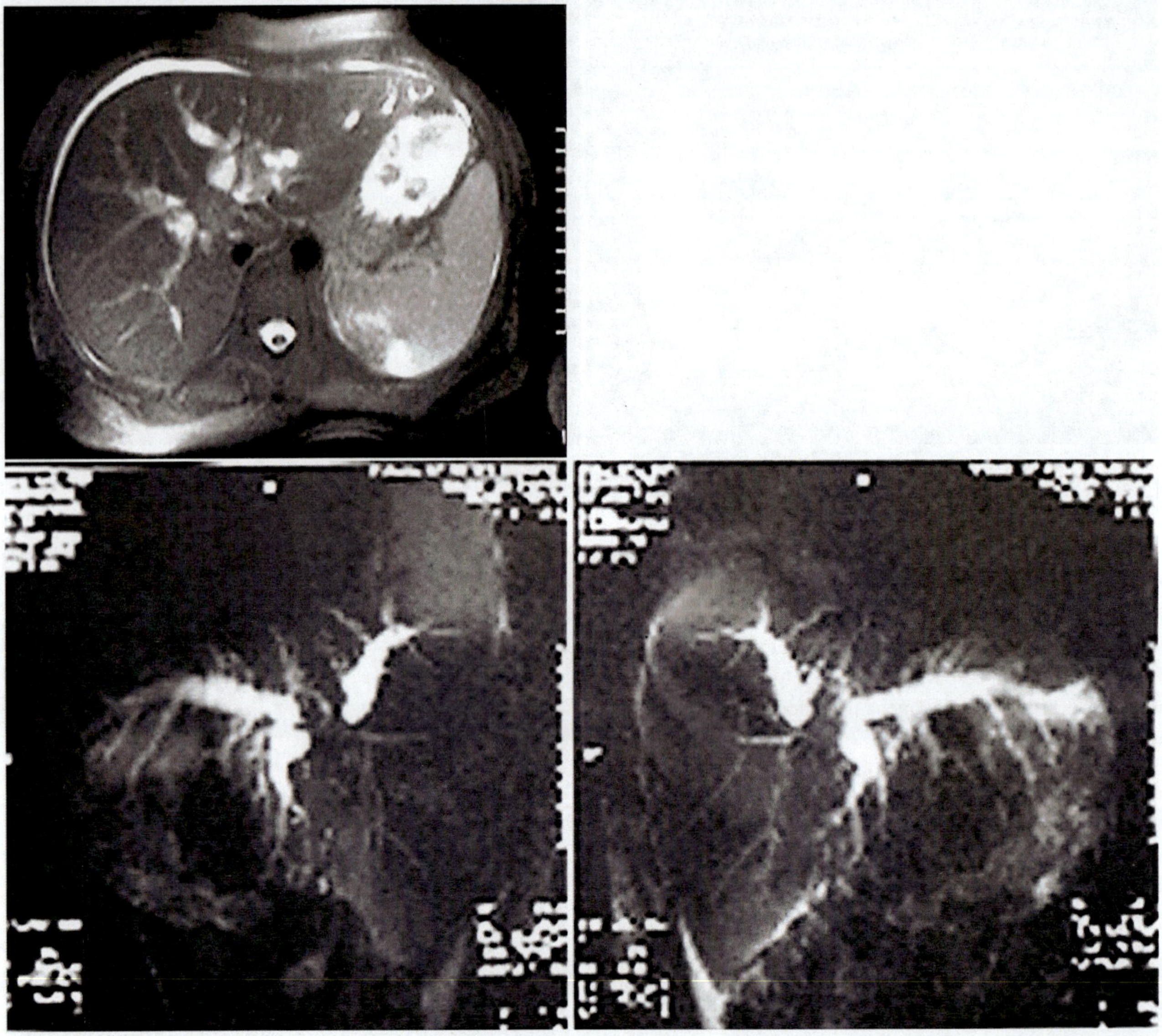

Fig. 24.4–24.5 Magnetic resonance cholangiogram demonstrating the location of the tumor within the biliary system

by the tumor. FNA of the lesion showed suspicion of cholangiocarcinoma. Laparoscopy and laparoscopic ultrasound confirmed that the confluence of the portal vein and the right hepatic artery had been encased by the tumor. The rest of the abdomen was clear of tumor. In view of the patient's young age and that there was no other more effective treatment, after careful consideration and deliberation with the patient and her family, consent was obtained and an ex situ and ex vivo liver resection with partial liver autotransplantation was performed on 10 May 2001.

24.6.3 The Surgical Procedure

The surgery lasted for 15½h with an anhepatic period of 5½h. Segments 1, 5, 6, 7, 8 and part of segment 4 were resected on bench. A veno-venous bypass was used initially during hepatectomy until an end to side portocaval shunt was established while the patient was anhepatic (Fig. 24.6). The harvested right internal jugular vein was used to reconstruct the now short left portal vein (Fig. 24.7). The harvested right hepatic vein was used to lengthen the left hepatic vein (Fig. 24.8). Before implantation, repeated (three times) frozen sections on the margins of the segments 2, 3 and 4 biliary ducts were performed until tumor clearance was ensured. Liver remnant composed of segments 2, 3 and part of 4 was autotransplanted in a piggyback fashion. A roux-en-Y loop was fashioned and anastomosed individually to the segment 2, 3 and 4 bile ducts (Fig. 24.9). The resected specimen weighed 1,160 g (Fig. 24.10). Final histology reported a 3 cm well differentiated mucinous adenocarcinoma, accompanied by perineural invasion and portal vein infiltration however the intima of the

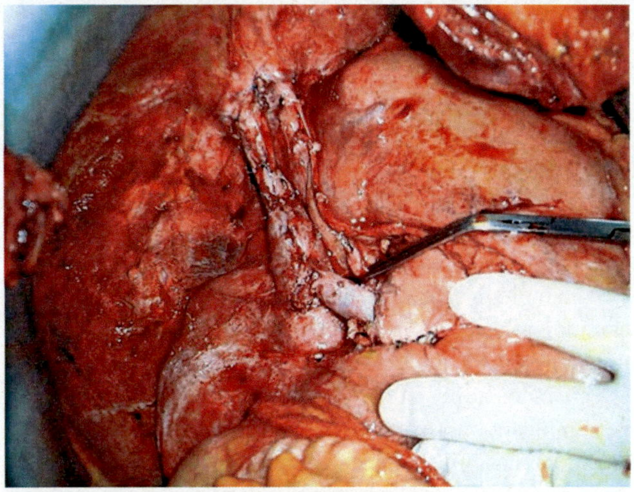

Fig. 24.6 Porto-caval shunt, clamp was on the hepatic artery

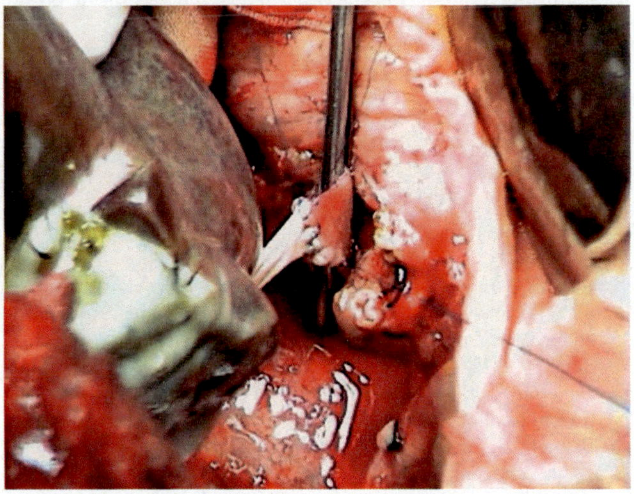

Fig. 24.7 Internal jugular vein has lengthened the left portal vein for anastomosis

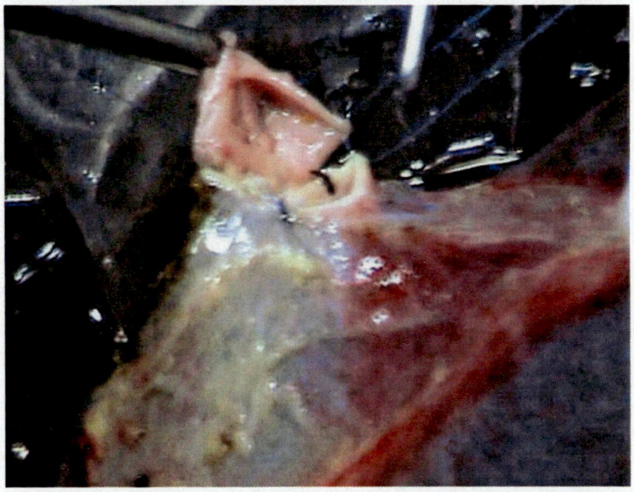

Fig. 24.8 Harvested right hepatic vein to lengthen left hepatic vein

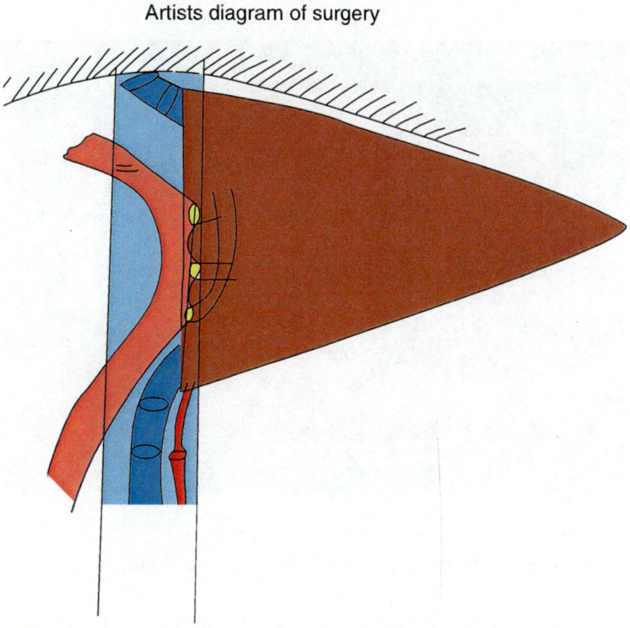

Fig. 24.9 Illustration of surgery. A roux-en-Y loop was fashioned and anastomosed individually to the segment 2, 3 and 4 bile ducts

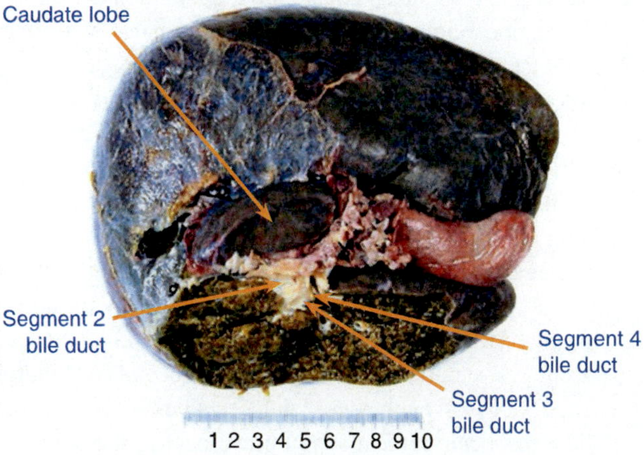

Fig. 24.10 The resected specimen weighed 1,160 g

portal vein was spared. The resection margins were all clear of tumor. Post- operatively, the patient was cholestatic with large ascitic output for a prolonged period. She was discharged on day 45. MRI scan at 3 months and CT scans at 6 (Fig. 24.11) and 9 months showed a regenerated liver without any evidence of tumor recurrence.

24.7 Summary

Technical improvements and organ preservation in the field of liver transplantation have added to the success in the development of ex situ ex vivo surgery. Experience with reduced sized, split liver and living related liver transplantation has

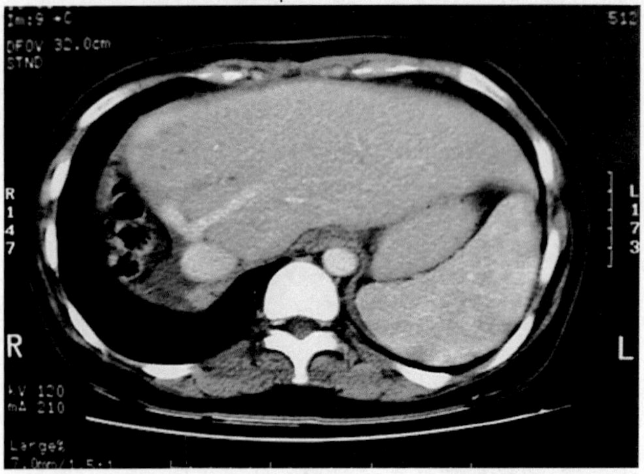

Fig. 24.11 Postoperative CT scan taken at 6 months. The scan demonstrates regeneration of the left lobe and no evidence of tumor recurrence

provided the skill available for bench surgery and complex reconstructions required for partial liver autotransplantation. The use of vein grafts taken from the resected liver as well as patient's own veins can make portal vein or hepatic vein reconstruction feasible and make the implantation easier.

Cholangiocarcinomas generally are associated with one of the worst prognosis, especially if surgical resection is not possible. Unfortunately, patients frequently present late and are considered inoperable at the time of diagnosis. For localized cholangiocarcinomas, surgery achieving a negative resection margin is by far the most important independent predictor of outcome. Although many experts have recommended aggressive surgical approach to these patients, often traditional techniques of liver resection prove difficult if not impossible. Hilar cholangiocarcionomas with involvement of vascular structures or extension into secondary biliary branches are usually considered unresectable.

There has been tremendous improvement in the surgical technical aspects with ex situ ex vivo surgery and auotransplantation over the years. Many of the technical difficulties have been overcome. Tumors usually considered for such treatment are those involving the hepatic hilum or the proximal hepatic veins. There is no doubt that the ex situ ex vivo resection and autotransplantation technique will continue to improve. There will be more patients benefited from this surgery to remove otherwise unresectable tumors. However, taken into account the cost, the complex surgical procedure and the associated morbidities and mortalities, perhaps only the young or highly selected otherwise healthy patients should be considered for this procedure.

Previous results have shown that benign and some malignant tumors do reasonably well after such treatment. The results for cholangiocarcinoma have been less than satisfactory so far. There has been some improvement, as evident by two reported successful cases in recent years. In absence of effective treatment for advanced cholangiocarcinoma besides surgery, ex situ ex vivo surgical approach may be considered as a last resort for highly selected cases. Continual surgical advances will encourage more attempts to treat advanced cholangiocarcinoma with this technique. Reduction in surgical morbidities and mortalities will further improve the outcomes. There is still a long way off before it should become a recommended treatment.

The biological and the oncological aspects of cholangiocarcinoma have yet to be fully understood. Until we have breakthroughs in the field of non-surgical treatments such as effective neo adjuvant or adjuvant treatments, there will not be significant improvement in long term survival despite the technical feasibility of such complex procedure. As a treatment for cholangiocarcinoma, its future role depends on availability of effective non-surgical treatment. On one hand, the application of ex situ ex vivo surgery could be much more frequent. On the other hand, the technique could become unnecessary.

References

1. Nakeeb A, Pitt HA, Sohn TA, et al. Cholangiocarcinoma: a spectrum of intrahepatic, perihilar, and distal tumors. Ann Surg. 1996; 224:463–75.
2. Burke EC, Jarnagin WR, Hochwald SN, et al. Hilar cholangiocarcinoma – patterns of spread, the importance of hepatic resection for curative operation, and a presurgical clinical staging system. Ann Surg. 1998;228(3):385–94.
3. Nagorney DM, Donohue JH, Farnell. Outcomes after curative resections of cholangiocarcinoma. Arch Surg. 1993;128:871–9.
4. Bismuth H, Corlette MB. Intrahepatic cholangioenteric anastomosis in carcinoma of the hilus of the liver. Surg Gynecol Obstet. 1975;140:170–8.
5. Jarnagin WR, Fong Y, DeMatteo RP, et al. Staging, resectability, and outcome in 225 patients with hilar cholangiocarcinoma. Ann Surg. 2001;234(4):507–19.
6. Starzl TE, Marchioro TL, Kaula KN, et al. Homotransplantation of human liver. Ann Surg. 1963;177:659–76.
7. Belghiti J, Makuuchi M. Technical progress in liver transplantation. HPB Off J Int Hepato Pancreato Bil Assoc. 2004;6(2):67–8.
8. Griffith BP, Shaw BW, Hardesty RL, et al. Veno-venous bypass without systemic anti-coagulation for transplantation of human liver. Surg Gynecol Obstet. 1985;160:271–2.
9. Tzakis A, Todo S, Starzl TE. Orthotopic liver transplantation with preservation of the inferior vena cava. Am Surg. 1989;210:649–52.
10. Kalayoglu M, Sollinger HW, Stratta RJ, et al. Extended preservation of the liver for clinical transplantation. Lancet. 1988;1:617–9.
11. Meyer C, Penn I, James L. Liver transplantation for cholangiocarcinoma: results in 207 patients. Transplantation. 2000;69(8):1633–7.
12. Marsh JW, Geller DA, Finkelstein SD, et al. Role of liver transplantation for hepatobiliary malignant disorders. Lancet Oncol. 2004; 5(8):480–8.
13. Pichlmayr R, Bretschneider HJ, Kircchner E, et al. Ex- situ operation an der Leber. Eine neue Moeglichkeit in der Leberchirurgie. Langenbecks Arch Chir. 1988;373(2):122–6.
14. Inomata Y, Kiuchi T, Lim ID, et al. Auxillary partial orthotopic living donor liver transplantation as an aid for small-for-size grafts in larger recipients. Transplantation. 1999;67:1314–9.

15. Park KM, Lee SG, Lee YJ, et al. Adult-to-adult living donor liver transplantation at Asian medical center, Seoul, Korea. Transplant Proc. 1999;31:456–8.
16. Shaw Jr BW, Martin DJ, Marquez JM, et al. Venous bypass in clinical liver transplantation. Ann Surg. 1984;200:524–34.
17. Khoury GF, Mann ME, Porot MJ, et al. Air embolism associated with veno-venous bypass during orthotopic liver transplantation. Anesthesiology. 1987;67:848–51.
18. Hatano E, Tanaka A, Shinohara H, et al. Superiority of HTK solution to UW solution for tissue oxygenation in living related liver transplantation. Transplant Proc. 1996;28:1880–1.
19. Grosse H, Pichlmayr R, Hausen B, et al. Anaesthetic problems in ex situ resection of the liver. Anaesthesia. 1990;45:726–31.
20. Hemming AW, Cattral MS. Ex vivo resection with replacement of the inferior vena cava and hepatic vein replacement by transposition of the portal vein. J Am Coll Surg. 1999;189(5):523–6.
21. Oldhafer KJ, Lang H, Schlitt HJ, et al. Long term experience after ex situ liver surgery. Surgery. 2000;127(5):520–7.
22. Yagyu T, Shimizu R, Nishida M, et al. Reconstruction of the hepatic vein to the prosthetic inferior vena cava in right extended hemihepatectomy with ex situ procedure. Surgery. 1994;115:740–4.
23. Lodge JP, Ammori BJ, Prasad KR, et al. Ex vivo and in situ resection of inferior vena cava with hepatectomy for colorectal metastases. Ann Surg. 2000;231(4):471–9.
24. Raab R, Schlitt HJ, Oldhafer KJ, et al. Ex-vivo resection techniques in tissue- preserving surgery for liver malignancies. Langenbecks Arch Surg. 2000;385(3):179–84.
25. Fortner JG, Shin MH, Kinne DW, et al. Major hepatic resection using vascular isolation and hypothermic perfusion. Ann Surg. 1974;180:644–52.
26. Hannoun L, Panis Y, Balladur P, et al. "Ex situ in vivo" liver surgery. Principle and first results. Lancet. 1991;337:1616–7.
27. Pichimayr R, Grosse H, Hauss J, et al. Technique and preliminary results of extracorporeal liver surgery (bench procedure) and of surgery on the in situ perfused liver. Br J Surg. 1990;77(1):21–6.
28. Belghiti J, Dousset B, Sauvanet A, et al. Preliminary results with "ex situ" surgery for hepatic tumors: an alternative between palliative treatment and liver transplantation? Gastroenterol Clin Biol. 1991;15:449–53.
29. Hemming AW, Chari RS, Cattral MS. Ex vivo liver resection. Can J Surg. 2000;43(3):222–4.
30. Chui AK, Island ER, Rao AR, et al. The longest survivor and first potential cure of an advanced cholangiocarcinoma by ex vivo resection and autotransplantation: a case report and review of the literature. Am Surg. 2003;69(5):441–4.
31. Gruttadauria S, Marsh J, Bartlett DL, et al. Ex situ rresection techniques and liver autotransplantation: last resource for otherwise unresectable malignancy. Dig Dis Sci. 2005;50(10):1829–35.

Liver Transplantation

25

J.C. Hong and R.W. Busuttil

25.1 Background

Hilar cholangiocarcinoma (CCA) is a rare but devastating malignancy that presents late and is notoriously difficult to diagnose due to lack of effective screening tests. Treatment of hilar CCA is similarly challenging because of the lack of effective adjuvant therapy, aggressive infiltrative and longitudinal growth pattern of CCA, and location of the tumor in close proximity to vital structures. Historically, the usual management for these patients was palliative despite the absence of distant metastasis at initial presentation and the prognosis has been poor. The development and evolution of liver surgery including orthotopic liver transplantation (OLT) over the past four decades has significantly improved the surgical management of CCA. A complete extirpation of tumor including all microscopically detectable disease (R0 resection) offers the only possibility of long-term survival in patients with CCA. Unfortunately, many patients present with unresctable hilar CCA due to the presence of advanced liver disease and/or tumor extension to hepatic parenchyma and/or major vessels (hepatic artery and portal vein) of both right and left hemilivers, metastasis to regional lymph nodes or insufficient future liver remnant volume (Table 25.1).

J.C. Hong, MD, FACS
Division of Liver and Pancreas Transplantation,
Department of Surgery, The Pfleger Liver Institute,
Ronald Reagan-UCLA Medical Center,
Los Angeles, CA, USA

Department of Surgery, David Geffen School of Medicine,
Dumont-UCLA Transplant and Liver
Cancer Centers, University of California,
Los Angeles, CA, USA

R.W. Busuttil, MD, PhD, FACS (✉)
Department of Surgery, David Geffen School of Medicine,
Dumont-UCLA Transplant and Liver
Cancer Centers, University of California,
Los Angeles, CA, USA
e-mail: rbusuttil@mednet.ucla.edu

25.2 Orthotopic Liver Transplantation for Hilar Cholangiocarcinoma

While earlier studies on long-term survival outcomes with radical resection of early stage hilar tumors report a 5-year survival rate of up to 34 % [1], outcomes for CCA with aggressive features, including multifocality and large tumor size >2 cm remain poor due to the limitations of resection as treatment modality in achieving clear margins [2–5]. For tumors that are locally unresectable, total hepatectomy with regional lymphadenectomy and OLT addresses all relevant resection margins and treats the underlying liver disease. Historical experience with OLT for CCA was disappointing because of the universal recurrence of the disease and subsequent mortality (Table 25.2) [6–8] and has led many centers to consider CCA as a contraindication for OLT until the introduction of a multidisciplinary approach of neoadjuvant chemoradiation therapy followed by OLT [9].

The early reports from Thomas Jefferson University and the Mayo Clinic indicated the potential utility of radiation and chemotherapy in palliative therapy of CCA [10, 11]. Patients with unresectable CCA who received at least 55 Gy of radiation treatment demonstrated a 2-year survival of 48 % compared to 0 for those without radiation treatment [10]. Furthermore, 14 % of the patients who received radiation therapy survived for 5 years or more. The University of

Table 25.1 Contraindications for surgical resection for hilar cholangiocarcinoma

Bilateral tumor extension involving left and right secondary biliary radicals
Unilobar involvement with encasement of contralateral portal vein or hepatic artery
Bilateral vascular involvement
Distant metastases
Underlying liver disease (advanced fibrosis, cirrhosis)
Future liver remnant (FLR) <30 % and absence or inadequate FLR volume increase after portal vein occlusion
Severe co-morbidities

W.Y. Lau (ed.), *Hilar Cholangiocarcinoma*,
DOI 10.1007/978-94-007-6473-6_25,

Table 25.2 Collected series of liver transplantation for cholangiocarcinoma

Author	Period	n	Adjunctive therapy	Recurrence rate, %	Patient survival, % 2 years	3 years	5 years
Steiber [24]	1980–1988	10	Adjuvant	60	30	–	–
Goldstein [25]	1984–1992	17	Adjuvant	78	21	–	–
Meyer [6]	1968–1997	207	Adjuvant	51	48	–	23
Shimoda [27]	1984–2000	25	Adjuvant	41	–	35	–
Sudan [12]	1987–2000	11	Neoadjuvant	18	–	–	30
Robles [7]	1988–2001	59	Adjuvant	46	–	–	42 (Intrahepatic) 30 (Hilar)
Ghali [8]	1996–2003	10	None	80	–	30	–
Heimbach [15]	1993–2006	65	Neoadjuvant	17	–	–	76
Becker [28]	1987–2005	280	–	–	–	–	38
Morris-Stiff [29]	1981–2004	13	–	–	–	–	46
Hong [18]	1985–2009	38		41	52	38	32
			None	40	27	20	20
			Neoadjuvant + Adjuvant	28	88	75	47
			Adjuvant	50	58	33	33

Nebraska pioneered the use of neoadjuvant radiation therapy before OLT [12]. Their protocol used only intrabiliary brachytherapy delivered through iridium-192 wires, to a total dose of 6,000 cGy followed by daily intravenous 5-flurouracil until the time of transplantation. Patients with extrahepatic malignancy discovered during exploratory laparotomy were ineligible for liver transplantation. The tumor-free survival of 45 % was observed with a median follow up of 7.5 years after OLT [13].

25.2.1 Mayo Protocol for Hilar CCA

With the apparent benefits of chemotherapy and radiation therapy before OLT, the group from the Mayo Clinic developed a protocol with the intent of treating a highly select group of patients with hilar CCA with a strict regimen of preoperative staging and neoadjuvant treatment followed by OLT [9]. The inclusion criteria for patients with CCA involve a strict selection of patients with early stage CCA either deemed locally unresectable or arising in the setting of underlying PSC (Table 25.1). Patients with hilar CCA were included only if there was no mass lesion below the level of the cystic duct (Table 25.3). The presence of microscopic disease suspected below this level and the absence of any other contraindication for OLT, warranted an addition of pancreaticoduodenectomy at the time of liver transplantation. Vascular encasement of the hilar structures was not a contraindication to transplantation. The upper limit of tumor size was 3 cm when the mass was visible on cross-sectional imaging studies, and there must be no evidence of intrahepatic or extrahepatic metastases by any imaging studies. The protocol specifically excluded patients with intrahepatic (peripheral) CCA or gallbladder cancer. Surgical intervention and percutaneous biopsy were avoided to minimize peritoneal seeding. Candidates must have no active infections or medical conditions that preclude neoadjuvant therapy or liver transplantation. Since 2002, an endoscopic ultrasound-guided regional lymph node aspiration has been routinely done in all patients before beginning neoadjuvant therapy [14]. The identification of lymph node metastases obviated the need for staging exploratory laparotomy and disqualified the patients from subsequent liver transplantation.

Table 25.3 Mayo Clinic criteria for liver transplantation for hilar cholangiocarcinoma [30]

Candidates must satisfy diagnostic criteria for hilar CCA: malignant-appearing stricture on cholangiography, and biopsy cytology results demonstrating malignancy, carbohydrate antigen 19-9 > 100 U/ml, or aneuploidy
Unresectable hilar CCA
Tumor size <3 cm on cross-sectional imaging studies (CT scan, ultrasound, MRI)
No intra- and extrahepatic metastases on surveillance every 3 months
No regional hepatic lymph node involvement and peritoneal metastases

In the Mayo protocol, patients receive external beam radiotherapy to a target dose of 4,500 cGy followed by transcatheter radiation (2,000~3,000 cGy) with iridium-192 wires. These wires are placed by endoscopic retrograde cholangiography or percutaneous transhepatic cholangiography. Systemic 5-flurouracil is given during radiation treatment followed by oral capecitabine (Xeloda) after radiation therapy until the day of transplantation. Before transplantation, all patients undergo a scheduled staging laparotomy including biopsy of at least one lymph node along the proper hepatic artery and another along the common bile duct as well as any lymph nodes or nodules suspicious for tumor. Only patients with negative staging operation remain eligible for transplantation. The first published result of this protocol showed a patient survival rate of 100 % among the transplanted patients with a median follow up of 44 months and only one case of tumor-recurrence. However, among the 19 patients enrolled who received neoadjuvant therapy, only 12 patients remained eligible for OLT; 1 died from biliary sepsis while 6 patients (33 %) had tumor progression that precluded transplantation. Since the application of the Mayo protocol, the survival analysis of patients with CCA has yielded 1- and 5-year patient survival rates of 91 % and 76 %, respectively; and 5-year recurrence-free survival of 60 % [15]. Predictors for tumor recurrence include older patients, CA19-9 levels >100 U/ml on the day of transplantation, prior cholecystectomy, mass on cross-sectional imaging, tumor grade, and residual tumor >2 cm as well perineural invasion in explant.

25.2.2 Complications of Neoadjuvant Radiation Therapy

The survival benefits with this protocol were associated with significant morbidity. Cholangitis, intrahepatic abscess and sepsis were frequent infectious complications related to indwelling stent alone, neoadjuvant radiation-induced tumor necrosis, or in conjunction with other treatment-related neutropenia [9]. Severe inflammatory changes and dense fibrosis in the porta hepatis attributable to radiation therapy may lead to difficulty in identifying and isolating the portal structures during transplantation. The greatest concern, however, is the risk for long-term vascular complications after transplantation. The overall late vascular complication rate after transplantation was 41 % in the Mayo Clinic series; 21 % of the patients developed hepatic arterial complications while 20 % experienced portal venous complications [16]. These vascular events have been attributed to the late effects of vascular tissue injury from radiation therapy leading to fibrosis and chronic ischemic injury. In order to avoid using the irradiated native hepatic artery, an infrarenal interposition arterial graft was routinely used to reconstruct arterial inflow to all deceased donor grafts while the native hepatic artery was used in living donor graft. The native portal vein was used in deceased donor transplants, whereas in living donor transplants, a portal vein interposition graft was constructed using a blood-group compatible third party iliac vein. In this analysis, hepatic arterial complications were more prevalent in recipients of living donor partial grafts who received neoadjuvant chemoradiation therapy for CCA than with recipients transplanted with living donor grafts for other indications. For patients who received deceased donor whole-organ grafts reconstructed with interposition infrarenal aortic conduit, the rates of hepatic arterial complication were similar to those of recipients transplanted for other indications who did not received neoadjuvant chemoradiation therapy. In contrast, late portal vein stenosis was more prevalent in both deceased donor whole-graft and living donor partial graft with CCA when compared with controls. Most vascular complications were managed with a percutaneous endovascular approach and these complications were reported not to have adversely affected patient and graft survival.

25.2.3 The University of California Los Angeles (UCLA) Criteria and Treatment Protocol for CCA

While the application of strict Mayo Clinic patient selection criteria, regimen of preoperative staging and neoadjuvant chemoradiation treatment followed by OLT have resulted in excellent long-term recurrence free survival outcomes [17], only 58 % of the patients had histologically proven cancer on explanted liver. Proponents for expansion of OLT criteria for CCA argue patient inclusion guidelines restricted to hilar tumors based only on size may exclude patients with locally advanced hilar CCA, Stage IIA, IIB, and III (American Joint Committee on Cancer, 6th Edition) from a potentially curative procedure despite the absence of metastatic disease. Hong and Busuttil have recently reported that survival benefits can also be achieved in patients with locally advanced CCA (>3 cm in size, tumor extension to hepatic parenchyma, branches of the portal vein and/or hepatic artery, and presence of perineural and lymphovascular invasion) utilizing a similar neoadjuvant and adjuvant protocol [18]. The 5-year disease recurrence-free survival was 47 % in patients who received OLT in combination with neoadjuvant and adjuvant therapies compared to zero in the resection group.

The UCLA group proposed a post OLT tumor-recurrence risk stratification system to identify patients with locally advanced intrahepatic and hilar CCA who would benefit from OLT. Independent multivariate predictors were assigned risk score points based on the log of the hazard ratio for tumor recurrence after OLT (Table 25.4). The risk score points were summed and patients stratified into three predictive

Table 25.4 The UCLA Prognostic Scoring System for tumor-recurrence after liver transplantation for cholangiocarcinoma [31]

Risk factors	Risk score points
Multifocality	4
Perineural invasion	4
Infiltrative tumor growth pattern	3
No neoadjuvant therapy	3
History of primary sclerosing cholangitis	2
Hilar CCA	1
Lymphovascular invasion	1

Reprinted from JACS [32]; with permission from Elsevier

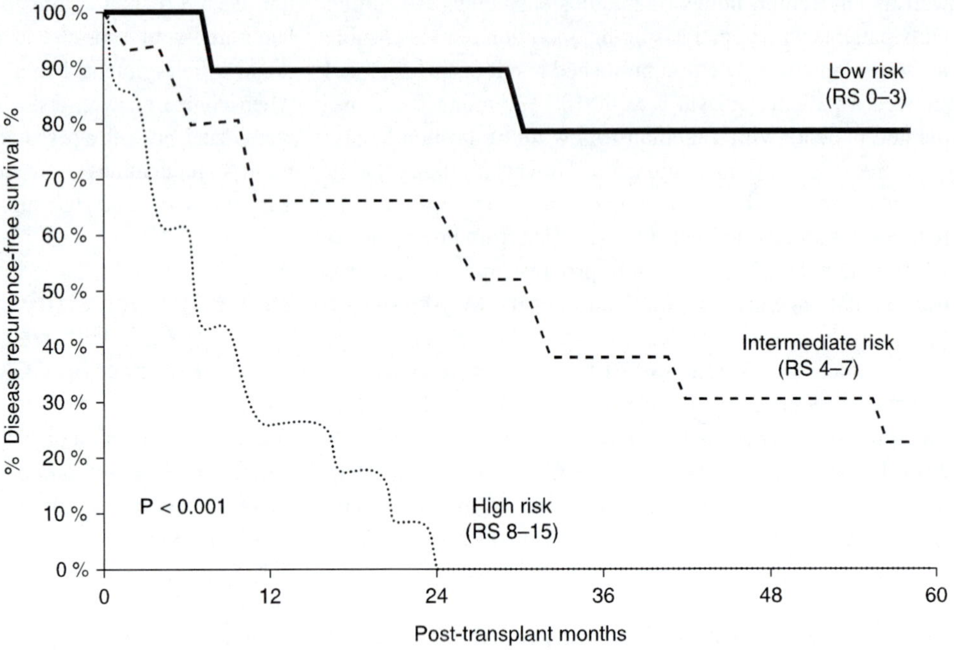

Fig. 25.1 Disease recurrence-free survival in locally advanced cholangiocarcinoma by risk categories (Reprinted from JACS [32]; with permission from Elsevier)

index category: low, intermediate and high risk groups. The 5-year tumor recurrence-free patient survival was significantly higher in LR (78 %) compared to IR (19 %) and HR (0) groups ($P<0.001$); survival benefit was also seen in IR compared to HR groups (Fig. 25.1).

Inclusion criteria for the UCLA treatment protocol for unresectable CCA include tumor size ≤8 cm for intrahepatic and ≤3.5 cm for hilar CCA in patients, disease confined within the confines of the operative field for total hepatectomy and regional lymphadenectomy for OLT, and absence of distant metastasis. Figure 25.2 shows our treatment algorithm. A tumor biopsy is used prior to neoadjuvant therapy in all patients. Our neoadjuvant treatment protocol utilizes locoregional followed by chemotherapy for locally advanced intrahepatic and hilar CCA. Intrahepatic CCA ≤6 cm or hilar tumors are treated with stereotactic body radiation therapy (SBRT) for a total dose of 40 Gy, fractionated into five treatment sessions over 7~12 days [19, 20]. The short locoregional treatment course allows the administration of full, uncompromised doses of chemotherapy as early as 10~14 days from the last radiation session. For intrahepatic tumors >6 cm, transarterial chemoembolization is given instead of SBRT [21]. Neoadjuvant chemotherapy includes a 5-fluorouracil or capecitabine-based regimen until the time of transplantation. Other agents include oxaliplatin, leucovorin, and gemcitabine [22–25]. Surveillance of tumor progression includes imaging with computed tomography or magnetic resonance imaging of the chest and abdomen as well as determination of serum tumor marker carbohydrate antigen (CA) 19-9 levels regularly every 3 months. Positron emission tomography scan is used selectively in patients

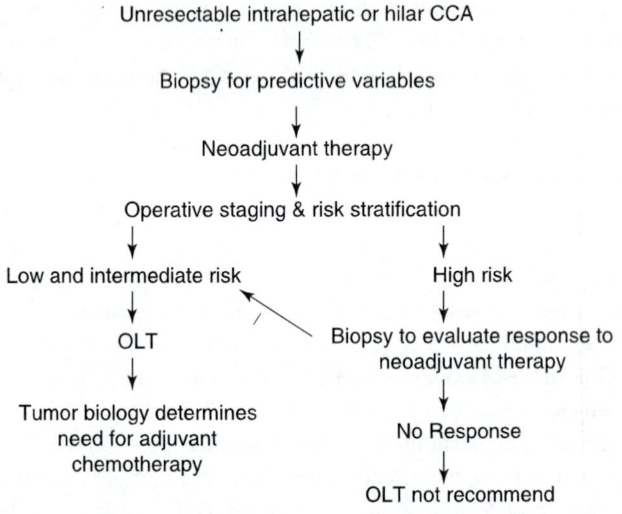

Fig. 25.2 Flow diagram of the UCLA treatment protocol for OLT candidates with hilar cholangiocarcinoma (Reprinted from JACS [32]; with permission from Elsevier)

with suspicion of metastasis on routine imaging. Progression of disease beyond the confines of the operative field of total hepatectomy and regional lymphadenectomy for OLT, identified during neoadjuvant treatment or in pre-OLT surgical staging laparotomy, precludes transplantation.

Patients in the low and intermediate risk groups would receive OLT. This protocol includes patients deemed to have intermediate risk for tumor recurrence after OLT because only 27 % of the patients in the intermediate risk group received neoadjuvant therapy in the retrospective study. The potential utility of neoadjuvant therapies to achieve a survival rate of >50 % at 5 years after OLT in the intermediate group is currently being evaluated in a prospective study. For high-risk patients, another biopsy of the tumor is performed after completion of neoadjuvant therapy to evaluate response to treatment. While OLT may still be considered for patients who exhibit disease down-staging, definitive surgical therapy is not recommended in the absence of a favorable tumor response to neoadjuvant treatments.

Adjuvant chemotherapy is given based upon tumor biology determined in pre-treatment biopsy and in explanted specimen. While the survival benefit with adjuvant chemotherapy after resection is unproven, post-OLT adjuvant chemotherapy may have a role in reducing the risk for tumor recurrence by controlling potential occult disease in the face of impaired immune surveillance of the patient from immunosuppressive therapy. Furthermore, we use a sirolimus-based maintenance immunosuppression regimen in our treatment protocol because of its antiproliferative and antiangiogenic properties [22, 23, 26].

25.3 Summary

The management for CCA remains challenging because of the rarity and aggressive nature of the disease, lack of effective adjuvant therapy, as well as the diverse locations of tumor. In contrast to HCC, there has been no effective screening test for CCA such that patients oftentimes present with unresectable disease. Surgical extirpation of the tumor is the only chance for potential cure. During the last two decades, an R0 resection has constantly been reported the most important predictor of prolonged survival. Although outcomes after radical bile duct resection with partial hepatectomy for hilar CCA have improved compared to two-decades ago, the long-term survival remains low. OLT in combination with neoadjuvant therapy provides tumor recurrence-free survival in a select group of patients.

References

1. Chen XP, Lau WY, Huang ZY, et al. Extent of liver resection for hilar cholangiocarcinoma. Br J Surg. 2009;96:1167–75.
2. Endo I, Gonen M, Yopp AC, et al. Intrahepatic cholangiocarcinoma: rising frequency, improved survival, and determinants of outcome after resection. Ann Surg. 2008;248:84–96.
3. Jonas S, Thelen A, Benckert C, et al. Extended liver resection for intrahepatic cholangiocarcinoma: a comparison of the prognostic accuracy of the fifth and sixth editions of the TNM classification. Ann Surg. 2009;249:303–9.
4. Dinant S, Gerhards MF, Rauws EA, et al. Improved outcome of resection of hilar cholangiocarcinoma (Klatskin tumor). Ann Surg Oncol. 2006;13:872–80.
5. DeOliveira ML, Cunningham SC, Cameron JL, et al. Cholangiocarcinoma: thirty-one-year experience with 564 patients at a single institution. Ann Surg. 2007;245:755–62.
6. Meyer CG, Penn I, James L. Liver transplantation for cholangiocarcinoma: results in 207 patients. Transplantation. 2000;69:1633–7.
7. Robles R, Figueras J, Turrion VS, et al. Spanish experience in liver transplantation for hilar and peripheral cholangiocarcinoma. Ann Surg. 2004;239:265–71.
8. Ghali P, Marotta PJ, Yoshida EM, et al. Liver transplantation for incidental cholangiocarcinoma: analysis of the Canadian experience. Liver Transpl. 2005;11:1412–6.
9. De Vreede I, Steers JL, Burch PA, et al. Prolonged disease-free survival after orthotopic liver transplantation plus adjuvant chemoirradiation for cholangiocarcinoma. Liver Transpl. 2000;6: 309–16.
10. Alden ME, Mohiuddin M. The impact of radiation dose in combined external beam and intraluminal Ir-192 brachytherapy for bile duct cancer. Int J Radiat Oncol Biol Phys. 1994;28:945–51.
11. Foo ML, Gunderson LL, Bender CE, et al. External radiation therapy and transcatheter iridium in the treatment of extrahepatic bile duct carcinoma. Int J Radiat Oncol Biol Phys. 1997;39:929–35.
12. Sudan D, DeRoover A, Chinnakotla S, et al. Radiochemotherapy and transplantation allow long-term survival for nonresectable hilar cholangiocarcinoma. Am J Transplant. 2002;2:774–9.
13. Patel T. Increasing incidence and mortality of primary intrahepatic cholangiocarcinoma in the United States. Hepatology. 2001;33: 1353–7.
14. Gleeson FC, Rajan E, Levy MJ, et al. EUS-guided FNA of regional lymph nodes in patients with unresectable hilar cholangiocarcinoma. Gastrointest Endosc. 2008;67:438–43.
15. Heimbach JK, Gores GJ, Haddock MG, et al. Predictors of disease recurrence following neoadjuvant chemoradiotherapy and liver transplantation for unresectable perihilar cholangiocarcinoma. Transplantation. 2006;82:1703–7.
16. Mantel HT, Rosen CB, Heimbach JK, et al. Vascular complications after orthotopic liver transplantation after neoadjuvant therapy for hilar cholangiocarcinoma. Liver Transpl. 2007;13:1372–81.
17. Rea DJ, Heimbach JK, Rosen CB, et al. Liver transplantation with neoadjuvant chemoradiation is more effective than resection for hilar cholangiocarcinoma. Ann Surg. 2005;242:451–8. discussion 8–61.
18. Hong JC, Jones CM, Duffy JP, et al. Comparative analysis of resection and liver transplantation for intrahepatic and hilar cholangiocarcinoma: a 24-year experience in a single center. Arch Surg. 2011;146:683–9.
19. Tse RV, Hawkins M, Lockwood G, et al. PhaseI study of individualized stereotactic body radiotherapy for hepatocellular carcinoma and intrahepatic cholangiocarcinoma. J Clin Oncol. 2008;26: 657–64.
20. Rusthoven KE, Kavanagh BD, Cardenes H, et al. Multi-institutional phase I/II trial of stereotactic body radiation therapy for liver metastases. J Clin Oncol. 2009;27:1572–8.
21. Gusani NJ, Balaa FK, Steel JL, et al. Treatment of unresectable cholangiocarcinoma with gemcitabine-based transcatheter arterial chemoembolization (TACE): a single-institution experience. J Gastrointest Surg. 2008;12:129–37.
22. Toso C, Merani S, Bigam DL, et al. Sirolimus-based immunosuppression is associated with increased survival after liver transplantation for hepatocellular carcinoma. Hepatology. 2010;51: 1237–43.
23. Zimmerman MA, Trotter JF, Wachs M, et al. Sirolimus-based immunosuppression following liver transplantation for hepatocellular carcinoma. Liver Transpl. 2008;14:633–8.
24. Stieber AC, Marino IR, Iwatsuki S, et al. Cholangiocarcinoma in sclerosing cholangitis. The role of liver transplantation. Int Surg. 1989;74:1–3.
25. Goldstein RM, Stone M, Tillery GW, et al. Is liver transplantation indicated for cholangiocarcinoma? Am J Surg. 1993;166:768–71. discussion 71–72.

26. Okada T, Sawada T, Kubota K. Rapamycin inhibits growth of cholangiocarcinoma cells. Hepatogastroenterology. 2009;56: 6–10.
27. Shimoda M, Farmer DG, Colquhoun SD, et al. Liver transplantation for cholangiocellular carcinoma: analysis of a single-center experience and review of the literature. Liver Transpl. 2001; 7:1023–33.
28. Becker NS, Barshes NR, Aloia TA, et al. Analysis of recent pediatric orthotopic liver transplantation outcomes indicates that allograft type is no longer a predictor of survivals. Liver Transpl. 2008; 14:1125–32.
29. Morris-Stiff G, Bhati C, Olliff S, et al. Cholangiocarcinoma complicating primary sclerosing cholangitis: a 24-year experience. Dig Surg. 2008;25:126–32.
30. Gores GJ, Gish RG, Sudan D, et al. Model for End-stage Liver Disease (MELD) exception for cholangiocarcinoma or biliary dysplasia. Liver Transpl. 2006;12:95–7.
31. Hong JC, Petrowsky H, Kaldas FM, et al. Predictive index for tumor recurrence after liver transplantation for locally advanced intrahepatic and hilar cholangiocarcinoma. J Am Coll Surg. 2011;212:514–20. discussion 20–21.
32. JACS. 2011;212(4):514–20.

Neoadjuvant/Adjuvant Therapy for Liver Resection and Transplantation

26

B.K.P. Goh and C.B. Rosen

26.1 Introduction

Long-term control of hilar cholangiocarcinoma (CCA) and extrahepatic cholangiocarcinoma (CCA) in general can only be obtained with complete surgical removal of all neoplastic tissue in toto either via surgical resection or transplantation [1]. Most investigators have demonstrated that complete surgical resection with negative margins (R0 resection) is the most important determinant of survival in hilar CCA [2, 3]. However, only a minority of patients are able to receive an oncologic resection [4]. Moreover, even after complete resection with negative margins the overall survival of patients with hilar CCA has been reported to range from 30 % to 52 % [5]. Murakami et al. [6] suggested that patients with UICC stage II and III CCAs to receive adjuvant therapy due to the high recurrence rate compare to Stage I tumors. The most common site of first recurrence after oncologic resection of hilar CCA is locoregional which often leads to potentially fatal complications such as biliary obstruction, sepsis and liver failure [4, 7, 8]. Only approximately 10–15 % of patients develop distant metastases before locoregional recurrence [7].

In an effort to improve the results after surgical resection, neoadjuvant and adjuvant treatment using various modalities including chemotherapy (CT), radiotherapy (RT) and chemoradiotherapy (CRT) have been administered before and after surgical resection of extrahepatic CCA. Presently, there is lack of robust data supporting or refuting the use of neoadjuvant or adjuvant therapy. Most of the studies reported in the literature have been limited to small retrospective series, and prospective data are scarce [2, 4, 7]. A major limitation in performing a study analyzing the effectiveness of neoadjuvant and adjuvant therapy in hilar CCA is the rarity of the disease. This is further compounded by the fact that only a minority of patients are able to undergo a potentially curative resection [1, 4]. Hence, it is not surprising that most investigators combine their analyses of hilar CCA and distal CCA together as extrahepatic CCA [9–14]. In earlier studies, many investigators even combined their analysis of extrahepatic CCA with intrahepatic CCA and gallbladder cancers [15–17].

Before the twentieth century, the role of non-surgical therapy such as CT or RT was controversial and had been thought to be largely ineffective and possibly even detrimental [1]. Effective chemotherapy for bile duct cancers was limited by the absence of agents and combination of agents with adequate antitumoral activity [1]. At present, there remains no established adjuvant treatment for bile duct cancers, although newer chemotherapeutic agents such as gemcitabine and S-1 have proven to be promising in unresectable cancers [18]. It is highly anticipated that adjuvant treatment with these drugs may potentially be useful.

Presently, only data analyzing the potential benefit of adjuvant RT, CT and concurrent CRT have come predominantly from relatively small retrospective series [2, 4, 7]. All these studies are limited by small patient numbers, different tumor stages, uncontrolled heterogeneous patient characteristics, selection bias and non-uniform treatment methods [4]. No prospective randomized controlled trial has been performed to date to address this issue. The rationale for adjuvant treatment in hilar CCA is the low potential for complete R0 resection and the poor survival rates associated with incompletely resected or unresectable cancers. Recurrence patterns in hilar CCA and other extrahepatic CCA are most frequently locoregional [8] emphasizing the importance of good locoregional adjuvant treatment especially after incomplete surgical resection.

B.K.P. Goh, MBBS, MMed, MSc, FRCS(Ed)
Department of Surgery, Singapore General Hospital, Outram Road, Singapore 169608, Singapore

C.B. Rosen, MD (✉)
Division of Transplantation Surgery, Mayo Clinic and Mayo Clinic College of Medicine, Rochester, MN, USA
e-mail: rosen.charles@mayo.edu

W.Y. Lau (ed.), *Hilar Cholangiocarcinoma*,
DOI 10.1007/978-94-007-6473-6_26, © Springer Science+Business Media Dordrecht and People's Medical Publishing House 2013

26.2 Treatment Modalities

26.2.1 Radiation Therapy (RT)

Although, bile duct tumors were initially thought to be radioresistant [15], this hypothesis is not correct. RT has been used for the primary treatment of CCA, palliative treatment of advanced CCA as well as neoadjuvant or adjuvant therapy with surgical resection with varying degrees of success. Several series have demonstrated prolonged survival in patients with advanced, unresectable CCA who undergo RT [19–22]. As a result, RT has subsequently been used as adjuvant or neoadjuvant treatment. The theoretical benefits of RT are that it may destroy tumor cells not removed during surgery when used as adjuvant therapy; and avoid intraoperative tumor dissemination and increase tumor clearance when used as neoadjuvant therapy.

Various techniques have been used to administer radiotherapy including external beam radiation therapy (EBRT), intraoperative radiation therapy (IORT) or intraluminal brachytherapy (ILBT) via percutaneously or endoscopically placed biliary stents containing iridium-192 [1, 15]. Newer modalities using charged particles such as helium, proton and neon have also been reported [2, 23]. Charged particles offer the advantage over conventional photon energy of a more highly localized energy disposition [2].

The optimal RT dose and schedule remains unclear as a wide range of doses and techniques have been reported in the literature [4]. An example of a typical RT regime is 45~50 Gy via EBRT over about 5 weeks with IORT of 15~20 Gy or ILBT of 20~30 Gy [24, 25]. It is logical that the higher the radiation dose, the more effective RT is in destroying tumor cells. However, the dose of RT is limited by the tolerance of normal surrounding tissues such as the liver, stomach, duodenum, kidney and spinal cord [26]. Radiation doses beyond 50~55 Gy can result in bowel ulceration, perforation or obstruction from fibrosis [2, 4]. In general, most studies have reported a low incidence of severe acute toxicity associated with RT [7].

ILBT enables delivery of higher doses of irradiation to the tumor with minimal risk to adjacent normal tissue. This can be performed via radiation seeds inserted into a catheter within the bile duct [4]. The main limitation of ILBT is that the dose is effective only to a depth of 0.5~1 cm [4].

26.2.2 Chemotherapy (CT)

Strategies for adjuvant chemotherapy for extrahepatic CCA are derived from treatment experiences with unresectable tumors. 5-FU, as a single agent or in combination with other chemotherapeutic agents, has been studied extensively in unresectable CCA [27]. Most of these trials were small and uncontrolled and overall response rates were only 0~40 % [27]. 5-FU has been used in combination with various drugs such as cisplatin, epirubicin, IFN-α, capecitabine and S1 [18]. More recently, single-agent gemcitabine has been shown to be effective in bile duct malignancies [27]. The newer drugs appear to be more effective than those used in the past [16] and combinations of gemcitabine with other agents such as cisplatin have demonstrated response rates of 9–50 % [27].

An extensive literature review of 65 clinical trials in 1998 revealed no survival benefits of CT in either the adjuvant or palliative settings for extrahepatic CCA [1]. Randomized controlled trials [28–30] comparing different CT regimens did not demonstrate superiority of any CT regimen for advanced CCA. However, a more recent pooled analysis of 104 studies involving 2,810 patients suggested that gemcitabine combined with cisplatin or oxaliplatin resulted in the best response rates for CCA and gallbladder carcinoma [4, 23, 31]. A randomized, controlled trial by Glimelius et al. [32] demonstrated improved survival and quality of life compared to best supportive care in patients with advanced unresectable CCA, and CT is now commonly administered to eligible patients with unresectable CCA. The best response rates are obtained with gemcitabine combined with platinum-based agent regimens [23].

26.2.3 Chemoradiation Therapy (CRT)

Preclinical studies support combination of RT with radiosensitizing agents such as 5-FU, mitomycin and cisplatin [1, 15]. This strategy arose from the benefit seen with radiosensitization in the treatment of other gastrointestinal cancers such rectal and pancreatic cancers [1, 4]. Most studies have demonstrated that adjuvant CRT is well-tolerated in patients with CCA [33].

26.2.4 Photodynamic Therapy (PDT)

PDT is a treatment modality composed of two-steps. First, a photosensitizing agent is administered intravenously (usually) and preferentially accumulates in cancer cells. Subsequently, light of a specific wavelength is delivered directly to the malignant tissue. The light activates the agent resulting in tumor necrosis. PDT is effective for palliation of unresectable CCA. A prospective randomized trial demonstrated superiority of PDT with stenting compared to stenting alone with improvements in both survival and quality of life [34]. PDT has much fewer side-effects compared to traditional CT and RT. The major limitation of PDT is that it is only effective to a depth of 4–6 mm [5]. PDT has also recently been used as neoadjuvant treatment before resection [35].

26.3 Adjuvant Treatment

26.3.1 Radiation Therapy (RT)

The rationale for adjuvant RT is the high likelihood of having microscopic or gross residual disease after resection. Moreover, the pattern of recurrence after CCA has been shown to be predominantly loco-regional [8]. Adjuvant RT is administered to control the small remaining tumor load with the hope that improved loco-regional control will ultimately improve overall patient survival [4]. Initial concerns about toxicity and morbidity [7] have been obviated by experience. Most of the complications from RT in the literature have not been severe and could be classified as GradeIor II based on the RTOG criteria [36].

Most of the data available in the literature on the use of adjuvant RT is limited to small retrospective series [10, 11, 17, 37–41] and a single prospective case-controlled study [42] (Table 26.1). The data supporting use of adjuvant RT in hilar CCA is equivocal. Some studies demonstrate a survival benefit [25, 38, 39, 41, 43] whereas others show none [15, 37, 40, 42]. In general, adjuvant RT after R0 resection has not been shown to be beneficial [37, 39, 40], whereas there may be a survival advantage for patients with positive resection margins [3, 11, 25, 43, 44]. Data from most retrospective studies also suggest a benefit of adjuvant RT after dose-scaling irradiation [45, 46]. Stein et al. provided further evidence in support of adjuvant therapy by achieving similar patient survival for patients with R1 resection and adjuvant RT to those with R0 resection (median survival 21.5 months versus 26 months, $P = 0.45$) in patients with node negative cholangiocarcinoma [44].

Nonetheless, the only prospective study [42] to date from the Johns Hopkins failed to demonstrate a survival benefit with adjuvant RT [12, 47]. The study showed similar survival between 14 patients who underwent resection with adjuvant RT versus 31 patients who had resection alone (median survival of 20 months in both groups). A major criticism of the study was the low radiation dose (median dose of 45 Gy) and only 8 of 31 patients received a radiation boost of 13 Gy [38]. RT dose is important [45, 46]; patients who receive cumulative doses more than 45 Gy are more likely to benefit than patients receiving less than 45 Gy [38].

Proponents [33] of adjuvant treatment argue that several of the studies suggesting no benefit with adjuvant RT [15, 33, 42, 48] in actual fact do indeed demonstrate a benefit. They point out that patients in the RT groups had more aggressive tumors so that the similar survival in both groups actually suggests that adjuvant RT is beneficial. In the study by Nakeeb et al. [15], 43 % of patients in the RT group had palliative surgery and there was a far higher rate of hepatic and portal vein invasion compared to the surgery only group [33]. On the other hand, it could be argued that in many of these retrospective studies, patients who were more fit with better performance status were selected for adjuvant treatment such as CT or RT whereas those who did not received adjuvant therapy were probably deemed to ill. Hence, prolonged survival in the treated group might be due to selection of healthier patients.

Further complicating matters, three recent larger studies utilizing the SEER database demonstrated conflicting results (Table 26.1) [49–51]. In the study by Fuller et al., there was neither a benefit with adjuvant RT in patients who had total resection nor subtotal resection of their tumors [49]. The survival curves seem to suggest an early survival advantage with RT but the advantage seemed to dissipate over time [49]. Vern-Gross et al. found similar results showing no survival benefit with adjuvant RT in either patient with local or regional disease [51]. In contrast, the study by Shinohara et al. demonstrated a survival benefit in patients who had adjuvant RT compared to resection alone (16 vs. 9 months, $P < 0.0001$) [50]. A major difference in methodology could account for this difference. Patients who had follow-up of less than 3 months were excluded in the Vern-Gross study to allow patients an opportunity to undergo RT [51]. It is also important to note that after adjusting for confounders using the propensity score, no significant survival benefit was associated with the use of adjuvant RT in the study by Shinohara et al. [50] Studies using the SEER database share numerous limitations common to population databases such as incorrect data entry and important uncaptured data such as margin status and use of chemotherapy [49–51].

In summary, the majority of recent data from small retrospective studies suggest that improved survival may be obtained with adjuvant RT especially in patients with positive margins and with dose escalation [2, 4, 7, 47]. However, there was no survival benefit demonstrated from the only well-controlled prospective study to date. Data from large population-based studies also failed to demonstrate a survival benefit with adjuvant RT. It is obvious that more prospective studies ideally conducted in a randomized fashion are needed to investigate the role of adjuvant RT after resection of hilar CCA.

26.3.2 Chemotherapy (CT)

Although the majority of initial recurrences after resection of hilar CCA occur locally and regionally [8]; distant metastases do develop and are an important cause of mortality [6]. Hasegawa et al. reported that 60 % of patients who underwent R0 resection of hilar CCA developed systemic recurrences in the peritoneum and liver [52]. Presently, data on adjuvant CT for hilar CCA is scarce (Table 26.2) [4], and most of the studies are on patients with advanced unresectable tumors. The most commonly used CT agents reported in

Table 26.1 Summary of recent series studying the survival outcomes of adjuvant radiation therapy after surgical resection vs. surgical resection alone

Author, institution, year	Tumor type	Patients	Radiation	R0 resection	Median survival, months	P-value
Cameron, J Hopkins, 1990 [37]	53 HiCCA	38 SRT	EBRT ± ILBT	39 (74 %)	21 % 3years OS	NS
		15 S			21 % 3years OS	
Gonzalez, EORTC, 1990 [41]	55 HiCCA	38 SRT	EBRT ± ILBT	4 (7 %)	19 m	0.0005
		17 S			8 m	
Schoenthaler, UCSF, 1994 [10]	HiCC + OEHCCA	6 SRT	EBRT/CP ± CT	6 (22 %)	21.5 m	NA
		6 SCP			61 m	
		15 S			16 m	
		6 SRT		0 (0 %)	21.5 m	0.011
		6 SCP			61 m	0.0005
		9 S			11 m	
Pitt, J Hopkins, 1995 [42]	31 HiCCA	14 SRT	EBRT + IR-102 seeds	9 (29 %)	20 m	NS
		17 S			20 m	
Zlotecki, U Florida, 1998 [17]	GBCa + HiCCA + OEHCCA	8 SRT	EBRT + ILBT	10 (59 %)	43.4 m	NA
		9 S			26.1 m	
Todoroki, Tsukuba, 2000 [25]	47 HiCCA	28 SRT	IORT ±/or EBRT	0	32 m	0.0141
		19 S			10 m	
Heron, Pittsburgh, 2003 [38]	28 HiCCA	23 SRT	EBRT	12 (43 %)	24 m	0.023
		5 RT			13 m	
Gerhards, Amsterdam, 2003 [39]	91 HiCCA	71 SRT	EBRT+/–ILBT	11 (15 %)	24 m	<0.01
		20 S		2 (10 %)	8 m	
Itoh, Kanazawa, 2005 [11]	10 HiCCA	11 SRT	EBRT	8 (42 %)	17 m	0.49
	9 OEHCCA	8 S			16 m	
		7 SRT	EBRT	0	NA	0.035
		2 S			NA	
Sagawa, Hokkaido, 2005 [40]	69 HiCCA	39 SRT	EBRT ± ILBT	21 (54 %)	23 m	0.554
		30 S		13 (43 %)	20 m	
Cheng, Shanghai prospective, 2007 [43]	75 HiCCA	23 SRT	EBRT	NA	NA	0.02
		18 SCT	5-FU			0.66
		34 S				
Fuller, SEER, 2009 [49]	1,569 HiCCA + OEHCCA	Total resec	NA	NA		NS
		275 SRT			26 m	
		464 S			25 m	
		Subtotal resec	NA	R2		NS
		75 SRT			24 m	
		120 S			21 m	
Shinohara, SEER, 2009 [50]	HiCCA + OEHCCA	701 SRT	NA	NA	16 m	<0.0001
		1,372 S			9 m	
Vern-Gross, SEER, 2010 [51]	HiCCA + OEHCCA	Localized	NA	NA		0.038
		86 SRT			28 m	
		325 S			36 m	
		Regional				0.80
		387 SRT			18 m	
		693 S			18 m	

Sagawa: Stage III/IVa, RT had improved survival over S, $P=0.042$
Schoenthaler: 22 % of surgical resection patients had CRT with no effect on survival, 11 m vs. 7 m, $P=0.227$)
6 S with R0 resection, MOS–39 m
EBRT external beam radiotherapy, *HiCCA* hilar cholangiocarcinoma, *ILBT* intraluminal brachytherapy, *IORT* intraoperative radiotherapy, *m* months, *NA* not available, *NS* not significant, *OEHCCA* other extrahepatic cholangiocarcinoma, *OS* overall-survival, *S* surgery, *SCP* surgery + charged particles, *SCT* surgery + adjuvant chemotherapy, *SRT* surgery + adjuvant radiotherapy

Table 26.2 Summary of recent studies reporting the survival outcomes of surgical resection alone versus surgical resection and adjuvant chemotherapy

Author, institution, year	Tumor	Patients	Chemotherapy	R0 resection	Median OS	P-value
Takada, Japan (RCT), 2002 [13]	HiCCA	58 CT	MMC + 5-FU	34 (59 %)	27 % 5-years	NS
	OEHCCA	60 S		38 (63 %)	24 % 5-years	
Cheng, Shanghai prospective, 2007 [43]	75 HiCCA	23 SRT	EBRT	NA	Improved	0.02
		18 SCT	5-FU		No difference	0.66
		34 S				
Yubin, Guandong, 2008 [53]	HiCCA	48 CT	5-FU + MMC + Epi + hydro/Gem + Oxa + Cap	92 (44 %)	43 m	<0.05
		67 S			37 m	
Murukami, Hiroshima, 2009 [18]	HiCCA	18 CT	Gem ± S1	13 (72 %)	57 % 5-years	0.026
		20 S		15 (75 %)	23 % 5-years	

Takada: no difference in 5-year OS in patients with curative resection (41 % vs 28 %, P=0.482) or noncurative resection (8 % vs. 16 %, P=0.303)
Yubin: some patients received RT
Murukami: only adjuvant CT was independent prognostic factor on multivariate analysis
CT chemotherapy, *EBRT* external beam radiotherapy, *HiCCA* hilar cholangiocarcinoma, *ILBT* intraluminal brachytherapy, *IORT* intraoperative radiotherapy, *m* months, *NA* not available, *NS* not significant, *OEHCCA* other extrahepatic cholangiocarcinoma, *OS* overall-survival, *S* surgery, *SCT* surgery + adjuvant chemotherapy, *SRT* surgery + adjuvant radiotherapy

the literature have been gemcitabine and 5-FU [4]. These have been used as single agents or in combination with other agents such as oxaliplatin, epirubicin, capecitabine, cisplatin and leucovorin [4].

A large Japanese multi-institution randomized controlled trial of adjuvant chemotherapy using 5-FU for bile duct cancer demonstrated no survival benefit at 5 years [12]. The large phase III trial enrolled 508 patients with pancreatico-biliary cancers, including 139 patients with CCA. Patients were randomized to receive surgical resection alone or resection with adjuvant CT. Adjuvant CT was two courses of mitomycin C plus infusion of 5-FU, followed by oral administration of 5-FU until tumor progression. There was no survival benefit of adjuvant CT in either patients who underwent curative resection (41 % 5 year survival with adjuvant therapy versus 28 % with resection only, $P=0.48$) or those who underwent non-curative resection (5 year survival, 8 % with adjuvant therapy versus 16 % for those treated with resection only, $P=0.30$). Adjuvant CT was only found to be beneficial in patients with gallbladder carcinoma.

A prospective study subsequently conducted by Cheng et al. in 75 patients with hilar CCA also failed to demonstrate an improvement in survival with adjuvant CT [43]. They compared three groups of patients who underwent surgery alone, adjuvant CT and adjuvant RT. Choice of whether to receive adjuvant therapy or type of therapy was made by the patients. The study showed an improvement in survival with adjuvant RT but not with adjuvant CT. However, two more recent retrospective studies from China and Japan have suggested a survival benefit with adjuvant CT. In the study by Yubin et al. of 115 resected patients, addition of adjuvant CT improved (mean or median) 5 year survival from 37 to 43 months, $P<0.05$ [53]. Some of the patients also received adjuvant RT but its contribution was not analyzed. Murukami et al. in a small study of 42 patients also demonstrated a survival advantage in patients receiving adjuvant CT with gemcitabine and S-1 [18]. Moreover, they demonstrated that adjuvant CT was the only independent prognostic factor of survival after resection of hilar CCA.

In summary, data on adjuvant CT after resection of hilar CCA is scarce and results from the only randomized controlled trial demonstrated no benefit. Hence, adjuvant CT alone cannot be recommended at present [4, 47] outside the setting of a clinical trial.

26.3.3 Chemoradiation Therapy (CRT)

Adjuvant CRT for CC has been shown to be effective for patients with distal CCA [9, 14], but not hilar CCA [2, 9, 14, 33, 54, 55] (Table 26.3). In a historical case-controlled study at Johns Hopkins, patients who underwent resection for distal extrahepatic CCA with adjuvant CRT using 5-FU alone or in combination with other agents and EBRT had a median overall survival of 36.9 months with postoperative CRT (n=34) versus 22 months with surgical resection alone (n=30), $P=0.04$ [5, 14]. All 34 patients received CRT as part of a prospective institutional policy. A more recent study from MD Anderson in hilar CCA and distal CCA also demonstrated promising results; patients with a high risk of loco-regional recurrence (who had an R1 resection or nodal involvement) treated with adjuvant CRT had similar survival to patients with a standard risk of loco-regional recurrence (who had an R0 surgical resection without nodal involvement) treated with adjuvant CRT [33]. Kim et al. in an uncontrolled study of 84 patients who had adjuvant CRT also reported similar findings [56]. Patients who underwent an R1 resection had a similar survival compared to those who

Table 26.3 Recent studies comparing outcomes after surgical resection vs surgical resection and adjuvant chemoradiation therapy

Author, institution, year	Tumor	Patients	CRT	R0 resection	Median OS, months	P-value
Serafini, S Florida, 2001 [9]	47 HiCCA	SCRT	EBRT	NA	Mean 39 m	NS
		S	5-FU		32 m	
	34 OEHCCA	SCRT	EBRT	NA	Mean 41 m	0.04
		S	5-FU		25 m	
Nakeeb, Wisconsin, 2002 [54]	72 HiCCA	42 SCRT	EBRT	44 resected	16.4	<0.02
	15 OEHCCA	12 SCT	5-FU/Gem	33 R0	10.7	
	29 GBCa	13 SRT			7.8	
	24 IHCCA	73 S			6.7	
Kelley, S Florida, 2004 [55]	52 I/HiHCCA	34 SCRT	EBRT	67 (71 %)	41	<0.05
	42 OEHCCA	53 S	5-FU		24	
Hughes, J Hopkins, 2007 [14]	34 OEHCCA	34 SCRT	EBRT	8 (24 %)	36.9 m	<0.04
		30 S	5-FU ± Leu ± Cisp ± IFN-a	23 (77 %)	22 m	
Borghero, MDACC, 2008 [33]	36 HiCCA	42 SCRT	EBRT ± ILBT ± IORT	15 (36 %)	32 m	0.6
	29 OEHCCA	23 S	5 FU/Gem ± Cisp ± Cap	23 (100 %)	31 m	

Serafini—distal tumors 41 m vs. 25 m, $P=0.05$
Nakeeb—multivariate analysis in resected patients: adjuvant CRT, $P<0.08$
EBRT external beam radiotherapy, *HiCCA* hilar cholangiocarcinoma, *ILBT* intraluminal brachytherapy, *IORT* intraoperative radiotherapy, *m* months, *NA* not available, *NS* not significant, *OEHCCA* other extrahepatic cholangiocarcinoma, *OS* overall-survival, *S* surgery, *SCT* surgery + adjuvant chemotherapy, *SRT* surgery + adjuvant radiotherapy

underwent an R0 resection (median survival, 24 vs. 25 months, $P=0.78$). Hence, data from retrospective studies suggest that adjuvant CRT is beneficial in patients with extrahepatic CCA, especially those with distal CCA. However, the data presently available for hilar CCA is less clear.

26.4 Neoadjuvant Treatment

Neoadjuvant treatment has the theoretical advantage of improving tumor resectability and minimizing perioperative tumor dissemination [51]. Experience with neoadjuvant treatment for CCA before surgical resection is limited [23]. McMasters et al. [57] reported a series of 40 patients with resected extrahepatic CCA. Nine patients received neoadjuvant CRT, and there was a complete pathologic response in three patients and negative resection margins in all nine patients. There was no difference in the survival of patients who received surgery alone (n = 11), neoadjuvant CRT (n = 9), adjuvant RT (n = 2) and adjuvant CRT (n = 18). More recently, Nelson et al. reported the results of neoadjuvant and adjuvant CRT in 45 patients with resected extrahepatic CCA [13]. Twelve patients with more advanced disease received neoadjuvant therapy and their survival was 53 % at 5 years vs. 23 % for the 33 patients that only received adjuvant CRT ($P=0.16$) [13]. The authors concluded that neoadjuvant therapy may be superior to adjuvant treatment.

Small series in the literature have described the use of PDT as neoadjuvant treatment before surgical resection. In a phase II study of seven patients with advanced HiCC, R0 resection was achieved in all patients after neoadjuvant PDT and the 1 year recurrence-free survival was 83 % [35]. Subsequent studies have also confirmed the safety of PDT in the neoadjuvant setting and its ability to downstage tumors [58, 59].

Liver transplantation for hilar CCA remains controversial. Early experiences with liver transplantation alone for hilar CCA showed very poor results with recurrence rates of >50 % and 5 year survival of only 10–20 % [60, 61]. The Mayo Clinic has combined neoadjuvant radiotherapy with chemotherapy, careful selection of patients with early stage disease, operative staging to rule-out patients with regional lymph node involvement and extrahepatic disease, and subsequent liver transplantation. Results are promising with 56 % 5 year survival after beginning of neoadjuvant therapy and 74 % 5 year survival after transplantation. Approximately 30 % of patients would have findings at the staging operation which precluded liver transplantation, but this percentage is now less than 15 % with routine use of endoscopic ultrasound directed aspiration of regional lymph nodes prior to beginning neoadjuvant therapy [62–64]. Diagnosis of CCA requires presence of a malignant appearing lesion on cholangiography and at least one of the following: elevation of CA-19.9 >100, polysomy by FISH, malignant cytology or histology, or a mass on cross-sectional imaging. Patients with tumors extending below the cystic duct or >3 cm in radial diameter are not eligible for treatment. Also excluded are patients with transperitoneal tumor biopsy or aspiration (due to seeding), intrahepatic and extrahepatic metastases. Vascular encasement does not preclude treatment. All patients have either unresectable disease or CCA arising in the setting of primary sclerosing cholangitis. Neoadjuvant therapy includes EBRT (40~45 Gy), followed by ILBT (20~30 Gy) with iridium wires placed preferentially by

ERCP. All patients undergo operative staging with biopsy of an hepatic arterial lymph node and a pericholedochal lymph node prior to transplantation. Transplantation is performed with either a living donor or deceased donor graft.

26.4.1 Future Developments

Newer RT techniques such as computer tomographic-based RT with more precise tumor targeting, proton therapy and 4-D treatment techniques may result in better results [2, 4]. Furthermore, cytotoxic agents as gemcitabine based multi-agent therapies have proved promising in the treatment of CCA [31]. In addition to traditional adjuvant and neoadjuvant treatment modalities with CT and RT, molecular targeted therapy is currently probably the fastest growing treatment modality in the field of oncology. Tumor expression profiles studied in CCA may be used as sites for possible targeted therapy as well as prognostication. Epidermal growth factor receptors (EGFR) such as ErbB2 and/or ErbB1has been shown to be over-expressed in CCA cells [4, 47] and EGFR inhibitors may be useful in the treatment of CCA [64]. Erlotinib has demonstrated promising results in a recent Phase II study and sorafenib which is currently used in the palliative treatment of hepatocellular carcinoma has also demonstrated growth suppression of CC cells [4, 65].

Conclusion

At present, data supporting the use of adjuvant and neoadjuvant treatment for surgical resection of hilar CCA are equivocal. Hence, the efficacy and usefulness of neoadjuvant and adjuvant treatments remain debatable [23]. However, most centers treating CC would administer some sort of adjuvant treatment if the patient is deemed fit. A worldwide survey of 331 authorities from 262 centers in 32 countries by Nakeeb and Pitt [15, 66] revealed that adjuvant CRT is administered in most centers, especially in Americas (71 %). The latest National Comprehensive Cancer Network (NCCN) guidelines also recommend adjuvant CRT for patients with high risk of recurrence after surgical resection which includes patients with positive margins and lymph nodes [67]. In lower risk patients, the guidelines suggest either observation after surgery or treatment with adjuvant CRT. Currently, it is almost universally agreed that the use of neoadjuvant CRT before liver transplantation for hilar CCA is mandatory and that liver transplantation alone should not knowingly be done for patient with CCA. In conclusion, strong level 1 evidence demonstrating the benefits of adjuvant and neoadjuvant therapy in CCA are not available. Large multi-institutional phase III trials are needed to clarify the role of adjuvant and neoadjuvant therapy in patients with CCA.

References

1. Hejna M, Pruckmayer M, Raderer M. The role of chemotherapy and radiation in the management of biliary cancer: a review of the literature. Eur J Cancer. 1998;34:977–86.
2. Czito BG, Anscher MS, Willett CG. Radiation therapy in the treatment of cholangiocarcinoma. Oncology (Williston Park). 2006; 20:873–84.
3. Aljifri M, Walsh MJ, Molinari M. Advances in diagnosis, treatment and palliation of cholangiocarcinoma: 1990–2009. World J Gastroenterol. 2009;15(34):4240–62.
4. Anderson C, Kim R. Adjuvant therapy for resected extrahepatic cholangiocarcinoma: a review of the literature and future directions. Cancer Treat Rev. 2009;35:322–7.
5. Aljiffry M, Abdulelah A, Walsh M, et al. Evidence-based approach to cholangiocarcinoma: a systemic review of the current literature. J Am Coll Surg. 2009;208:134–47.
6. Murakami Y, Uemura K, Hayasidani Y, et al. Indication for postoperative adjuvant therapy in biliary carcinoma based on analysis of recurrence and survival after surgical resection. Dig Dis Sci. 2009; 54:1360–4.
7. Macdonald OK, Crane CH. Palliative and postoperative radiotherapy in biliary tract cancer. Surg Oncol Clin N Am. 2002;11:941–54.
8. Jarnargin WR, Ruo L, Little SA, et al. Patterns of initial disease recurrence after resection of gallbladder carcinoma and hilar cholangiocarcinoma: implications for adjuvant therapeutic strategies. Cancer. 2003;98:1689–700.
9. Serafini FM, Sachs D, Bloomston M, et al. Location, not staging, of cholangiocarcinoma determines the role for adjuvant chemoradiation therapy. Am Surg. 2001;67:839–43.
10. Schoenthaler R, Phillips TL, Castro J, et al. Carcinoma of the extrahepatic bile ducts. The University of California at San Francisco experience. Ann Surg. 1994;219:267–74.
11. Itoh H, Nishijima K, Kurosaka Y, et al. Magnitude of combination therapy of radical resection and external beam radiotherapy for patients with carcinomas of the extrahepatic bile duct and gallbladder. Dig Dis Sci. 2005;50:2231–42.
12. Takada T, Amano H, Yasuda H, et al. Is postoperative adjuvant chemotherapy useful for gallbladder carcinoma? A phase III multicenter prospective randomized controlled trial in patients with resected pancreaticobiliary carcinoma. Cancer. 2002;95:1685–95.
13. Nelson JW, Ghafoori P, Willett CG, et al. Concurrent chemoradiotherapy in resected extrahepatic cholangiocarcinoma. Int J Radiat Oncol Biol Phys. 2009;73:148–53.
14. Hughes MA, Frassica DA, Yeo CJ, et al. Adjuvant concurrent chemoradiation for adenocarcinoma of the distal common bile duct. Int J Radiat Oncol Biol Phys. 2007;68:178–82.
15. Nakeeb A, Pitt HA. Radiation therapy, chemotherapy and chemoradiation in hilar cholangiocarcinoma. HPB. 2005;7:278–82.
16. Ben-David MA, Griffith KA, Abu-Isa E, et al. External-beam radiotherapy for localized extrahepatic cholangiocarcinoma. Int J Radiat Oncol Biol Phys. 2006;66:772–9.
17. Zlotecki RA, Jung LA, Vauthey JN, et al. Carcinoma of the extrahepatic biliary tract: surgery and radiotherapy for curative and palliative intent. Radiat Oncol Investig. 1998;6:240–7.
18. Murakami Y, Uemura K, Sudo T, et al. Gemcitabine-based adjuvant chemotherapy improves survival after aggressive surgery for hilar cholangiocarcinoma. J Gastrointest Surg. 2009;13:1470–9.
19. Qian XJ, Zhai RY, Dai DK, et al. Treatment of malignant biliary obstruction by combined percutaneous transhepatic biliary drainage with local tumor treatment. World J Gastroenterol. 2006; 12:331–5.
20. Takamura A, Saito H, Kamada T, et al. Intraluminal low-dose-rate 192 Ir brachytherapy combined with external beam radiotherapy and biliary stenting for unresectable extra hepatic bile duct carcinoma. Int J Radiat Oncol Biol Phys. 2003;57:1357–65.

21. Singh V, Kapoor R, Solanki KK, et al. Endoscopic intraluminal brachytherapy and metal stent in malignant hilar biliary obstruction: a pilot study. Liver Int. 2007;27:347–52.
22. Zhai R, Qian X, Dai D, et al. Malignant biliary obstruction: treatment with interventional radiology. Chin Med J (Engl). 2003; 116:888–92.
23. Alvaro D, Cannizzaro R, Labianca R, et al. Cholangiocarcinoma: a position paper by the Italian Society of Gastroenterology (SIGE), the Italian Association of Hospital Gastroenterology (AIGO), the Italian Association of Medical Oncology (AIOM) and the Italian Association of Oncological Radiotherapy (AIRO). Dig Liver Dis. 2010;42(12):831–8.
24. Foo ML, Gunderson LL, Bender CE, et al. External radiation therapy and transcatheter iridium in the treatment of extrahepatic bile duct carcinoma. Int J Radiat Oncol Biol Phys. 1997;39:929–35.
25. Todoroki T, Ohara K, Kawamoto T, et al. Benefits of adjuvant radiotherapy after radical resection of locally advanced main hepatic duct carcinoma. Int J Radiat Oncol Biol Phys. 2000;46:581–7.
26. Gunderson LL, Haddock MG, Foo ML, et al. Conformal irradiation for hepatobiliary malignancies. Ann Oncol. 1999;10(S4):S221–5.
27. Thongprasert S. The role of chemotherapy in cholangiocarcinoma. Ann Oncol. 2005;16(S2):ii93–6.
28. Rao S, Cunningham D, Hawkins RE, et al. Phase III study of 5-FU, etoposide and leucovorin (FELV) compared to epirubicin, cisplatin and 5-FU (ECF) in previously untreated patients with advanced biliary cancer. Br J Cancer. 2005;92:1650–4.
29. Ducreux M, Van Cutsem E, Van Laethem JL, et al. A randomized phase II trial of weekly high-dose 5 fluorouracil with and without folinic acid and cisplatin in patients with advanced biliary tract carcinoma: results of the 40955 EORTC trial. Eur J Cancer. 2005;41:398–403.
30. Kornek GV, Schuell B, Laengle F, et al. Mitomycin C in combination capecitabine or biweekly high-dose gemcitabine in patients with advanced biliary tract cancer: a randomized phase II trial. Ann Oncol. 2004;15:478–83.
31. Eckel F, Schmid RM. Chemotherapy in advanced biliary tract carcinoma: a pooled analysis of clinical trials. Br J Cancer. 2007; 96:896–902.
32. Glimelius B, Hoffman K, Sjoden PO, et al. Chemotherapy improve survival and quality of life in advanced pancreatic and biliary cancer. Ann Oncol. 1996;7:593–600.
33. Borghero Y, Crane CH, Szlaruk J, et al. Extrahepatic bile duct adenocarcinoma: patients at high-risk for local recurrence treated with surgery and adjuvant chemoradiation have an equivalent overall survival to patients with standard-risk treated with surgery alone. Ann Surg Oncol. 2008;15:3147–56.
34. Ortner ME, Caca K, Berr F, et al. Successful photodynamic therapy for nonresectable cholangiocarcinoma: a randomized prospective study. Gastroenterology. 2003;125:1355–63.
35. Wiedmann M, Caca K, Berr F, et al. Neoadjuvant photodynamic therapy as a new approach to treating hilar cholangiocarcinoma: a phase II pilot study. Cancer. 2003;97:2783–90.
36. Hermann T, Knorr A, Dorner K. The RTOG/EORTC classification criteria for early and late radiation reactions. Radiobiol Radiother (Berl). 1987;28:519–28.
37. Cameron JL, Pitt HA, Zinner MJ, et al. Management of proximal cholangiocarcinomas by surgical resection and radiotherapy. Am J Surg. 1990;159:91–7.
38. Heron DE, Stein DE, Eschelman DJ, et al. Cholangiocarcinomas: the impact of tumor location and treatment strategy on outcome. Am J Clin Oncol. 2003;26:422–8.
39. Gerhards MF, van Gulik TM, Gonzalez Gonzalez D, et al. Results of postoperative radiotherapy for resectable hilar cholangiocarcinoma. World J Surg. 2003;27:173–9.
40. Sagawa N, Kondo S, Morkiwa T, et al. Effectiveness of radiation therapy after surgery for hilar cholangiocarcinoma. Surg Today. 2005;35:548–52.
41. González González D, Gerard JP, Maners AW, et al. Results of radiation therapy in carcinoma of the proximal bile duct (Klatskin tumor). Semin Liver Dis. 1990;1:131–41.
42. Pitt HA, Nakeeb A, Abrams RA, et al. Perihilar cholangiocarcinoma. Postoperative radiotherapy does not improve survival. Ann Surg. 1995;221:788–97.
43. Cheng Q, Luo X, Zhang B, et al. Predictive factors for prognosis of hilar cholangiocarcinoma: postresection radiotherapy improves survival. Eur J Surg Oncol. 2007;33:202–7.
44. Stein DE, Heron DE, Rosato EL, et al. Positive microscopic margins alter outcome in lymph node-negative cholangiocarcinoma when resection is combined with adjuvant radiotherapy. Am J Clin Oncol. 2005;28:21–3.
45. Alden ME, Mohiuddin M. The impact of radiation dose in combined external beam and intraluminal ir-192 brachytherapy for bile duct cancer. Int J Radiat Oncol Biol Phys. 1994;28:945–51.
46. Kamada T, Saitou H, Takamura A, et al. The role of radiotherapy in the management of extrahepatic bile duct cancer: an analysis of 145 consecutive patients treated with intraluminal and/or external beam radiotherapy. Int J Radiat Oncol Biol Phys. 1996; 34:767–74.
47. Gatto M, Bragazzi MC, Semeraro R, et al. Cholangiocarcinoma: update and future perspectives. Dig Liver Dis. 2010;42:253–60.
48. Urego M, Flickenger J, Car B, et al. Radiotherapy and multimodality management of cholangiocarcinoma. Int J Radiat Oncol Biol Phys. 1999;44:121–6.
49. Fuller CD, Wang SJ, Choi M, et al. Multimodality therapy for locoregional extrahepatic cholangiocarcinoma. A population-based analysis. Cancer. 2009;115:5176–83.
50. Shinohara ET, Mitra N, Guo M, et al. Radiotherapy is associated with improved survival in adjuvant and palliative treatment of extrahepatic cholangiocarcinomas. Int J Radiat Oncol Biol Phys. 2009;74:1191–8.
51. Vern-Gross TZ, Shivnani AT, Chen K, et al. Survival outcomes in resected extrahepatic cholangiocarcinoma: effect of adjuvant radiotherapy in a surveillance, epidemiology and end results analysis. Int J Radiat Oncol Biol Phys. 2011;81(1):189–98.
52. Hasegawa S, Ikai I, Fujii H, et al. Surgical resection of hilar cholangiocarcinoma: analysis of survival and postoperative complications. World J Surg. 2007;31:1256–63.
53. Yubin L, Chihua F, Zhixiang J, et al. Surgical management and prognostic factors of hilar cholangiocarcinoma: experience with 115 cases in China. Ann Surg Oncol. 2008;15:2113–9.
54. Nakeeb A, Tran KQ, Black MJ, et al. Improved survival in resected biliary malignancies. Surgery. 2002;132:555–63.
55. Kelley ST, Bloomston M, Serafini F, et al. Cholangiocarcinoma: advocate an aggressive operative approach with adjuvant chemotherapy. Am Surg. 2004;70:744–9.
56. Kim S, Kim SW, Bang YJ, et al. Role of postoperative radiotherapy in the management of extrahepatic bile duct cancer. Int J Radiat Oncol Biol Phys. 2002;54:414–9.
57. McMasters KM, Tuttle TM, Leach SD, et al. Neoadjuvant chemoradiation for extrahepatic cholangiocarcinoma. Am J Surg. 1997; 174:605–9.
58. Witizigmann H, Berr F, Ringel U, et al. Surgical and palliative management and outcome in 184 patient with hilar cholangiocarcinoma. Palliative photodynamic therapy plus stenting is comparable to R1/R2 resection. Ann Surg. 2006;244:230–8.
59. Kiesslich T, Wolkersdorfer G, Neureiter D, et al. Photodynamic therapy for unresectable perihilar cholangiocarcinoma. Photochem Photobiol Sci. 2009;8:23–30.

60. Ito F, Cho CS, Rikkers LF, et al. Hilar cholangiocarcinoma: current management. Ann Surg. 2009;250:210–8.
61. Meyer CG, Penn I, James L. Liver transplantation for cholangiocarcinoma: results in 207 patients. Transplantation. 2000;69:1633–7.
62. Rea DJ, Heimbach JK, Rosen CB, et al. Liver transplantation with neoadjuvant chemoradiation is more effective than resection for hilar cholangiocarcinoma. Ann Surg. 2005;242:451–61.
63. Rosen CB, Heimbach JK, Gores GJ. Liver transplantation for cholangiocarcinoma. Transpl Int. 2010;23:692–7.
64. Rosen CB. Personal communication. 2011.
65. Socoteanu MP, Mott F, Alpini G, et al. C-Met targeted therapy of cholangiocarcinoma. World J Gastroenterol. 2008;14:2990–4.
66. Pitt HA, Broelsch C, Fong Y, et al. Adjuvant therapy for biliary malignancies: international trends and possibilities. J Gastrointest Surg. 2003;7:309A.
67. Benson AB 3rd, Abrams TA, Ben-Josef E, et al. NCCN clinical practice guidelines in oncology: hepatobiliary cancers. J Natl Compr Canc Netw. 2009;7:350–91.

Palliative Surgical Treatment

27

E.C.H. Lai, S.H.Y. Lau, and W.Y. Lau

27.1 Introduction

Tumors at the biliary confluence at the hilum of the liver (also called Klatskin tumors) comprise 40–60 % of all cholangiocarcinomas. The preoperative evaluation of a patient with suspected hilar cholangiocarcinoma is directed toward the following four primary objectives: (1) an assessment of the extent and level of biliary tract and vascular involvement including portal vein and hepatic artery involvement; (2) an assessment of the liver for evidence of lobar atrophy or concomitant liver pathology; (3) an assessment of the extent or presence of nodal disease and/or distant metastases; and (4) an assessment of the patients overall fitness for operation. The three primary goals in the surgical management of hilar cholangiocarcinoma are complete tumor excision with negative histological margins, relief of symptoms relating to biliary obstruction, and restoration of bilioenteric continuity [1, 2]. However, these are only achievable in the minority of patients (20~30 %). When advanced local disease, or obvious extrahepatic metastases are identified preoperatively or at the time of laparotomy, therapeutic interventions are directed toward the relief of biliary obstruction and its associated symptoms and complications such as itching, cholangitis, and liver failure in order to improve the quality of life. Different modalities are currently available to drain the biliary system and include endoscopic, percutaneous, and surgical bypass. The best technique remains controversial. Endoscopic biliary drainage can be achieved by plastic (polyethylene) or metallic stents. However, endoscopic stenting for hilar malignancies is associated with a high failure rate. Percutaneous insertion of a biliary stent can be preferable for hilar cholangiocarcinoma as the stent placement is more predictable than with an endoscopic approach. Intrahepatic biliary-enteric bypass has an advantage in this regard since the anastomosis can be placed some distance from the primary tumor, but requires a major operative procedure with associated morbidity. Surgery is associated with greater early morbidity and mortality but greater long-term patency and a lower incidence of recurrent jaundice. Percutaneous transhepatic biliary drainage (PTBD) is the preferred method if unresectability is determined before surgery. If unresectability or the presence of metastatic disease is identified at laparotomy, palliative options include postoperative placement of transhepatic stents, operatively placed transtumoral stents, or the performance of an operative bilioenteric bypass. When deciding among these options, the general physical condition, age of the patient, and predicted life expectancy must be considered. Within the literature, there have been insufficient data to show whether a surgical or a non-surgical approach provides the more cost effective and better palliation [3, 4]. The lack of randomized data and the heterogeneity within studies makes any direct comparisons difficult. These studies need to be interpreted with caution also. The study population between the surgical and nonsurgical groups was dissimilar with the better risk patients receiving operative palliation and those with poor risk, advanced disease or severe co-morbidities referred for nonoperative biliary drainage.

E.C.H. Lai, MBChB(CUHK), MRCS(Ed), FRACS, FCSHK, FHKAM(Surgery)
Department of Surgery,
Pamela Youde Nethersole Eastern Hospital,
Chai Wan, Hong Kong

Department of Surgery, The Chinese University of Hong Kong,
Shatin, New Territories, Hong Kong

S.H.Y. Lau, MBChB(CUHK), MRCS(Ed)
Department of Surgery,
Queen Elizabeth Hospital,
Kowloon, Hong Kong

W.Y. Lau, MD(CUHK), DSc(CUHK), FRCS, FACS, FRACS(Hon) (✉)
Faculty of Medicine,
The Chinese University of Hong Kong,
Shatin, New Territories, Hong Kong
e-mail: josephlau@cuhk.edu.hk

W.Y. Lau (ed.), *Hilar Cholangiocarcinoma*,
DOI 10.1007/978-94-007-6473-6_27, © Springer Science+Business Media Dordrecht and People's Medical Publishing House 2013

27.2 Different Types of Surgical Biliary Bypass

For patients with unresectable hilar cholangiocarcinomas, several surgical techniques have been described for biliary bypass [5]. Palliative biliary bypass can be performed by: (1) exposing the left hepatic duct by opening the umbilical fissure, elevating the base of the quadrate lobe and lowering the left hepatic ductal system from the undersurface of the quadrate lobe; (2) exposing branches of the left hepatic ducts by dissection at the base of the ligamentum teres.; (3) by partial excision of the left lateral segment and performing a biliary-enteric anastomosis to the openings in branches of the left hepatic duct (Longmire procedure); or (4) Cahow's intrahepatic cholangiojejunostomy—this is an alternative approach to dissect out a peripheral bile duct to perform a bilioenteric bypass if the approach to the left hepatic duct or its branches is technically impossible due to the tumor growth. Biliary bypass can also be performed to the right sectoral ducts. The type of bypass is usually dictated by the location of the tumor. In general, segment III bypass is performed unless the left liver is atrophic or is heavily involved with tumors or the primary lesion extends to the umbilical fissure of the liver. Internal biliary bypass to either the right or the left sided biliary system is enough for the jaundice to subside. Unless there is a special reason, e.g. cholangitis, bypass is usually done to one side of the biliary system.

27.2.1 Approach to Left Hepatic Duct

The Longmire procedure of intrahepatic cholangiojejunostomy after partial hepatectomy was first described by Longmire and Sanford in 1948 [6, 7]. Little was known about the anatomy of the liver at that time. The classic studies of Healey and Schroy were not to be published until 1953 [8]. Couinaud in 1955 first described the exposure of the left hepatic duct, and specifically the bile duct to segment III, by dissection of the round ligament and anterior division of the umbilical fissure [9]. In 1956, Hepp, in coauthorship with Couinaud, published an account of the first two intrahepatic biliary-enteric anastomoses approaching the left duct by detaching the hilar plate of the liver [10]. Subsequently, in 1957, Soupault and Couinaud proposed a trans-scissural approach to identify the segment III duct, by following the round ligament into the recessus of Rex in the umbilical fissure and construct an anastomosis between the left duct and a defunctionalized jejunal loop [11, 12]. This technique has become known as the "round ligament approach". The procedure was later popularized by Bismuth and Corlette [13], and Blumgart and Kelly [14].

27.2.1.1 Extrafascial Approach to the Left Hepatic Duct

This approach may not be applicable to patients with hilar cholangiocarcinoma if the tumor is infiltrative to the hepatic plate and to the liver. It can be done occasional for an unresectable tumor which is located mainly at the confluence and the right hepatic duct.

The ligamentum teres is divided and then elevated. The liver is elevated so as to expose its undersurface. An incision is made at the posterior edge of segment IV where Glisson's capsule is attached to the hilar plate. The upper surface of the hilar plate can then be separated from the hepatic parenchyma and, by lifting the segment IV upwards, display of the left hepatic duct, sometimes up to the bile duct confluence which is always extrahepatic, can be effected. A side-to-side left duct to jejunum mucosa to mucosa anastomosis can then be made. In case of unresectable hilar or right ductal carcinoma, the hilar plate can be opened at the anterosuperior surface to identify the left hepatic duct. A side-to-side left duct to jejunum mucosa to mucosa anastomosis can then be made. This approach is also called the extrafascial approach to the left duct up to the confluence (i.e. approaching the left hepatic duct up to the confluence of the bile duct outside of the Glissonian sheath and the liver plate).

In the rare occasion when the extrafascial approach is hazardous because of the extent of the tumor, especially when anatomical deformity has been created by atrophy/hypertrophy of liver segments, and in patients where there appears to be a very deep hilus which is displaced upwards and rotated laterally, a simultaneous opening of the deepest portion of the gallbladder fossa and the umbilical fissure gives good exposure to the biliary confluence and the left duct without the necessity for full hepatectomy or liver resection. This procedure simply represents mobilization of the inferior portion of segment IV from the midplane (principal fissure) to the intersectional plane (umbilical fissure) to expose the left duct and the confluence of the bile duct.

The maneuver is of particular value when in exposing the extrahepatic segment of the left hepatic duct since it has a long course beneath segment IV. It is not effective in exposing the extrahepatic right duct or its secondary branches, which are short.

27.2.1.2 Ligamentum Teres (Round Ligament) Segment III Approach

Segment III biliary bypass was the most studied surgical procedure in the past. The procedure is performed by using the round ligament approach to the duct of segment III in the base of the umbilical fissure. The ligamentum teres is divided and then elevated. The liver is elevated so as to expose its undersurface. The segment III duct is exposed by first

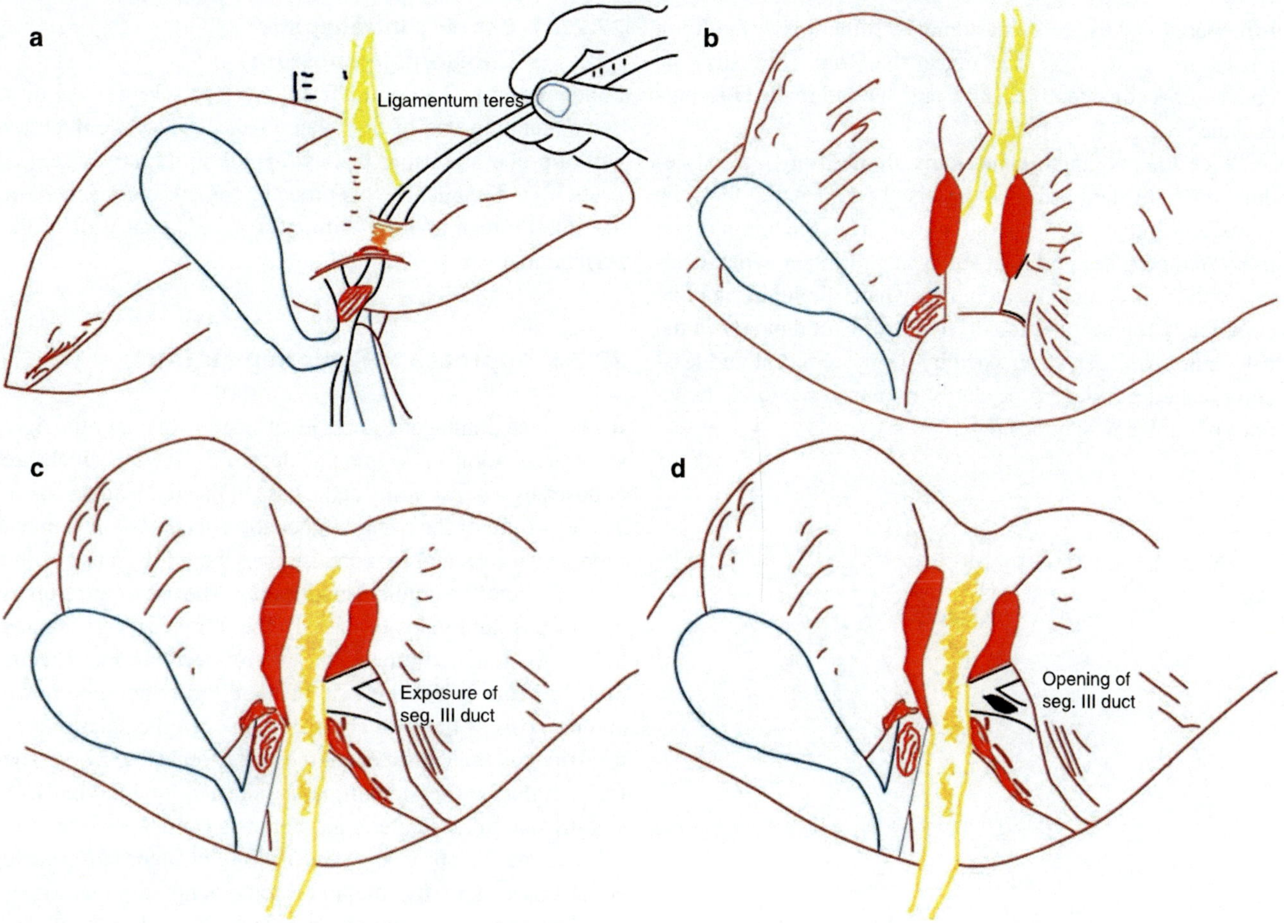

Fig. 27.1 Ligamentum teres (round ligament) segment III approach

dividing the bridge of liver tissue (if present) connecting segment III to the quadrate lobe. The ligament teres is then pulled downwards. Incision of the overlying peritoneum and division of the vessels radiating from the round ligament into the umbilical fissure exposes the segment III duct in a location posterosuperior to the segment III portal vein. The segment III duct is exposed. The depth of liver tissue which needs to be opened will vary depending on the degree of left lobe hypertrophy. It is usually necessary to open the umbilical fissure to a depth of 5–6 cm to expose the segment III duct. The Cavitron Ultrasonic Surgical Aspirator (CUSA) or Water jet dissector can facilitate the dissection. The duct is opened longitudinally in preparation for side to side anastomosis with a Roux-en-Y jejunal limb (Fig. 27.1). Segment III bypass is technically easier and preferred, because of the more constant anatomy and long extrahepatic course of the left hepatic duct, and because the anastomosis can be made away from the hilar tumor.

The anatomical basis for Segment III duct bypass was investigated by Vellar and his colleagues in Australia by dissection of 54 normal livers removed at autopsy [15]. In 64.8 % of the anatomical dissections, the findings were favourable for a segment III cholangiojejunostomy. In these specimens the segment III duct bypass would have drained segments II, III and IV. In 35.2 % of the specimens the anatomical disposition was potentially unfavorable, mainly due to the segment II or IV ducts joining close to the confluence and therefore liable to obstruction by the tumor. In 9 of the 54 specimens the true left hepatic duct was less than 6 mm in length, making it unsuitable for a bypass procedure to drain the left liver. Several surgical series show that segment III bypass can be performed with peri-operative mortality and morbidity rates varying between 0~11.5 % and 13~45 %, respectively. Relief of jaundice can be obtained in 73~100 % of patients undergoing bypass [16–20].

27.2.2 Longmire Procedure

The left liver is completely mobilized by division of the left triangular ligament. The mid-portion of the left lateral sector is then divided so as to expose the segment II duct and occasionally the segment III duct. A Roux-en-Y loop of jejunum is prepared and used for anastomosis. If there is difficulty in identifying a suitable sized duct, the Roux loop may be opened up a considerable length and sutured to the Glisson's capsule (Fig. 27.2).

Since the cholangiojejunostomy in the Longmire procedure is established utilizing the distal left hepatic duct, the dissection and anastomosis is far away from the hilum of the liver. Avoiding the porta hepatis is an advantage when dealing with hilar cholangiocarcinoma where the hilum may be completely replaced by tumor. It was used commonly in the past, but it has been superseded by the more recent and less-complicated surgical procedures of non-resectional hepatico- or cholangio-jejunostomy.

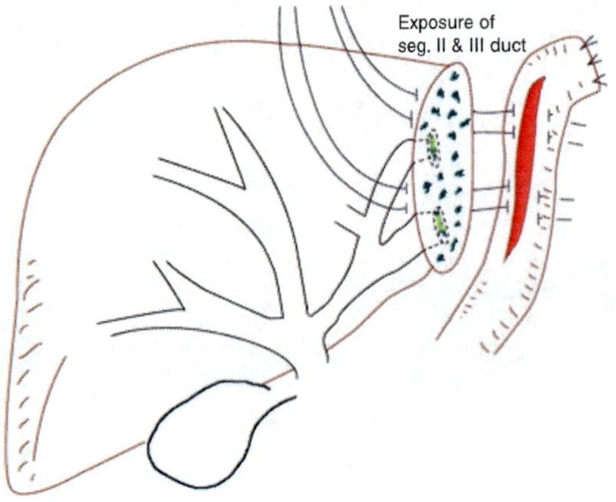

Fig. 27.2 Longmire procedure

27.2.2.1 Cahow's Intrahepatic Cholangiojejunostomy

Cahow described an anterior approach to a segmental duct by cannulating one of the dilated subcapsular bile ductules with a probe and using this as a guide to the larger central ducts [21]. Technically this procedure is difficult because of the small lumen and the thin and fragile ductal wall of the peripheral ducts.

27.2.3 Approach to Right Hepatic Duct

Right-sided drainage requires identification of either the right anterior sectoral or segmental ducts (V or VI), which are exposed by a hepatotomy at the base of the gall bladder fossa. The exposure of the right intrahepatic ductal system is much more hazardous and less precise than the left because of the lack of precise anatomical land-marks. The use of intra-operative ultrasound helps to identify the intrahepatic structures better. Anatomically the right anterior sectoral duct and its branches run on the left side of the corresponding vein. In essence, part of the liver is resected to open the anterior sectoral duct on the left aspect of the portal vein (Fig. 27.3). The relevant duct is then identified and opened longitudinally. A side-to-side biliary-enteric anastomosis is then performed to a Roux-en-Y loop of jejunum using interrupted absorbable sutures. An alternative method is to open into the segment V duct through the gallbladder fossa (Fig. 27.4). The tip of segment V/VI of the right liver can also be removed to expose

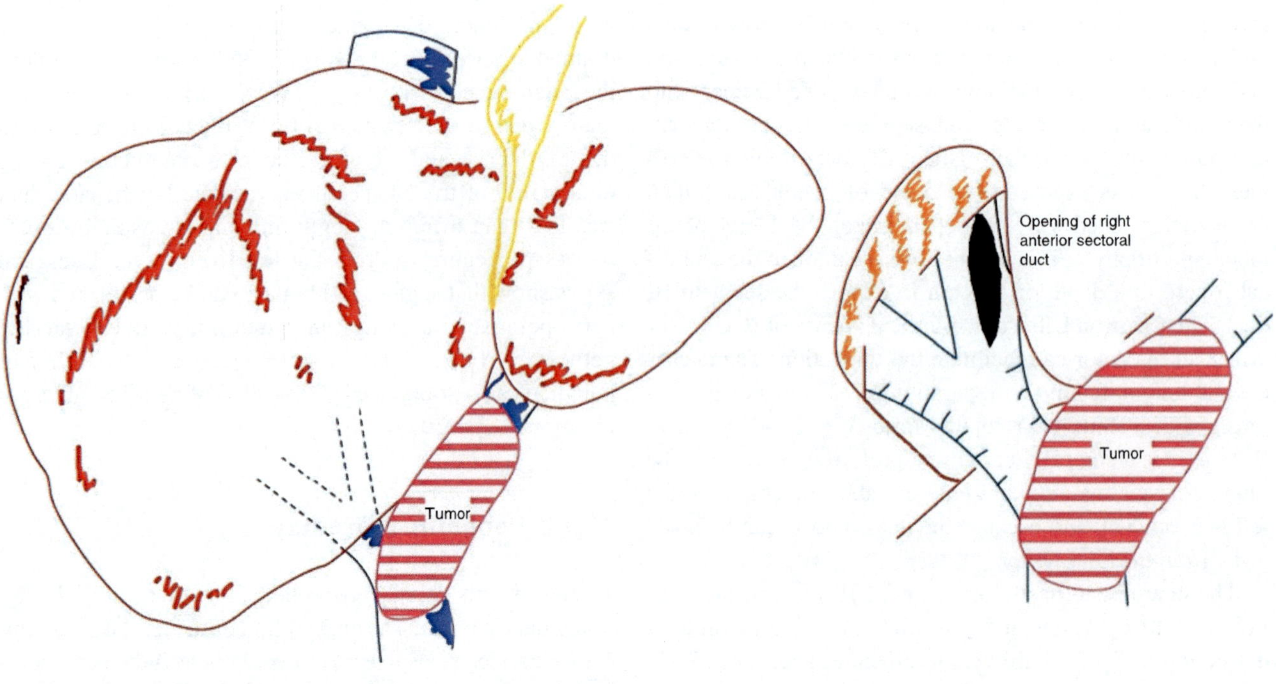

Fig. 27.3 Part of the liver is resected to open the anterior sectoral duct

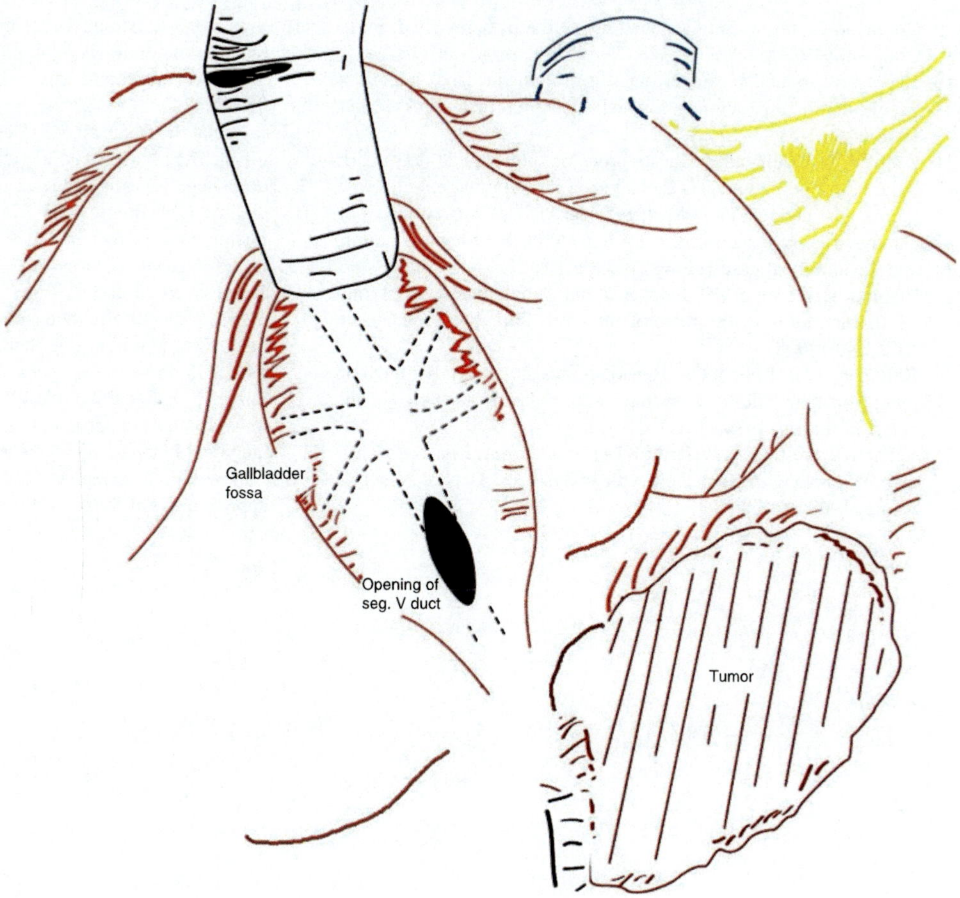

Fig. 27.4 Open into the segment V duct through the gallbladder fossa

the bile duct for anastomosis. This is very rarely done because the ducts exposed are peripheral, with thin walls and small lumens which make the anastomosis technically difficult.

Conclusion

In conclusion, the majority of patients who are diagnosed with hilar cholangiocarcinoma require a palliative approach. The type of bypass is usually dictated by the location of the tumor. In general, segment III bypass is performed unless the left lobe is atrophic or heavily involved with tumor or if the primary lesion extends to the umbilical fissure of the liver. Surgery is associated with greater early morbidity and mortality but greater long-term patency and a lower incidence of recurrent jaundice. Percutaneous transhepatic biliary drainage (PTBD) is the preferred method if unresectability is determined before surgery. There is a need for randomized controlled data to identify the optimal approach for the various subgroups of patients, particularly with improvements in endoscopic and radiological prostheses. Such trials must include quality of life assessment since this is frequently ignored in previously reported series.

References

1. Jarnagin WR, Shoup M. Surgical management of cholangiocarcinoma. Semin Liver Dis. 2004;24:189–99.
2. Lai EC, Lau WY. Aggressive surgical resection for hilar cholangiocarcinoma. ANZ J Surg. 2005;75:981–5.
3. Nordback IH, Pitt HA, Coleman J, et al. Unresectable hilar cholangiocarcinoma: percutaneous versus operative palliation. Surgery. 1994;115:597–603.
4. Wongkonkitsin N, Phugkhem A, Jenwitheesuk K, et al. Palliative surgical bypass versus percutaneous transhepatic biliary drainage on unresectable hilar cholangiocarcinoma. J Med Assoc Thai. 2006;89:1890–5.
5. Lau WY. Intrahepatic Glissonian Triad: anatomy relevant to liver resection and liver transplantation//Applied anatomy in liver resection and liver transplantation. Beijing: People's Meidical Publishing House; 2010. p. 45–59. Chapter 6.
6. Longmire WP, Sandford MC. Intrahepatic cholangiojejunostomy with partial hepatectomy for biliary obstruction. Surgery. 1948;24:264–76.
7. Cameron JL, Gayler BW, Harrington DP. Modification of the Longmire procedure. Ann Surg. 1978;187:379–82.
8. Healey JE, Schroy PC. Anatomy of the biliary ducts within the human liver: analysis of the prevailing pattern of branching and the major variations of the biliary ducts. Arch Surg. 1953;66: 599–616.

9. Couinaud C, editor. Surgical anatomy of the liver revisited. Paris: Couinaud; 1989.
10. Hepp J, Couinaud C. Eabord et l'utilisation du canal hepatique gauche dans la reparation de la voie biliaire principale. Presse Med. 1956;64:947–8.
11. Soupauh R, Couinaud C. Sur un proce'de' nouveau de de'rivation biliare intra-he'patique, les cholangio-je'junostomies gauches sans sacrifice he'patique. Press Med. 1957;65:1157–9.
12. Couinaud C. Exposure of the left hepatic duct through the hilum and the umbilical fissure. Surgery. 1989;105:21–7.
13. Bismuth H, Corlette MB. Intrahepatic cholangioenteric anastomosis in carcinoma of the hilus of the liver. Surg Gynecol Obstet. 1975;140:170–8.
14. Blumgart LH, Kelley CJ. Hepaticojejunostomy in benign and malignant high bile duct stricture: approaches to the left hepatic ducts. Br J Surg. 1984;71:257–61.
15. Vellar ID, Banting SW, Hardy KJ. The anatomical basis for segment III cholangiojejunostomy with analysis of 13 cases. Aust N Z J Surg. 1998;68:498–503.
16. Traynor O, Castaing D, Bismuth H. Left intrahepatic cholangioenteric anastomosis (round ligament approach): an effective palliative treatment for hilar cancers. Br J Surg. 1987;74: 952–4.
17. Jagannath P, Bhansali MS, Desouza LJ, et al. Palliative segment III biliary bypass (left cholangio-jejunostomy) in malignant block at porta hepatis. Indian J Gastroenterol. 1992;11:71–2.
18. Guthrie CM, Banting SW, Garden OJ, et al. Segment III cholangiojejunostomy for palliation of malignant hilar obstruction. Br J Surg. 1994;81:1639–41.
19. Jarnagin WR, Burke E, Powers C, et al. Intrahepatic biliary enteric bypass provides effective palliation in selected patients with malignant obstruction at the hepatic duct confluence. Am J Surg. 1998;175:453–60.
20. Suzuki S, Kurachi K, Yokoi Y, et al. Intrahepatic cholangiojejunostomy for unresectable malignant biliary tumors with obstructive jaundice. J Hepatobiliary Pancreat Surg. 2001;8:124–9.
21. Cahow CE. Intrahepatic cholangiojejunostomy: a new simplified approach. Am J Surg. 1979;137:443–8.

Palliation by Endoscopic Approach

28

J. Toouli and S.G. Barreto

28.1 Introduction

Endoscopic retrograde cholangiopancreatography (ERCP) with stenting has been used in the palliation of malignant obstructive jaundice for nearly three decades [1–3]. The initial success of endoscopic internal biliary drainage [1, 2], coupled with its low invasiveness [4] as a form of palliation, led to the suggestion that it represented the treatment of choice for unresectable cholangiocarcinomas [2] over the percutaneous or surgical alternatives. Endoscopic stenting of malignant hilar strictures, however, remains a technically challenging prospect. This, along with advances in interventional radiology over the years amongst other reasons, has precluded the development of clear delineation of the ideal technique for palliating hilar cholangiocarcinomas. In most instances, the extent of the obstruction, the anatomical arrangement of the intrahepatic ducts and the available local expertise shall determine the approach.

An advanced hilar cholangiocarcinoma could lead to a unilateral or bilateral obstruction of the biliary tree at the hilum with resultant obstructive jaundice and pruritus, cholangitis, and reduced quality of life. Ideally, palliation would thus aim at relieving all the obstructed systems thereby preventing the sequelae of biliary stasis with the potential added benefit of improved survival [5].

The use of endoscopy as a form of palliation affords the benefits of lower morbidity as well as the added benefits of permitting the delivery of adjuvant therapies including radiotherapy and photodynamic therapy. Stenting may also be done at the time of ERCP when this procedure has been undertaken for the diagnosis of jaundice. However, certain limitations exist; catheterizing the intrahepatic biliary tree may be technically impossible if the tumour has produced total blockage. Furthermore, placement of multiple stents is technically challenging [6].

This chapter will provide an overview of the results of endoscopy in palliation of hilar cholangiocarcinomas, the indications for this approach and the problems, as well as future perspectives.

J. Toouli, MBBS, PhD, FRACS (✉)
S.G. Barreto, MBBS, MS, PhD
Department of Surgery, Flinders University, Adelaide, SA, Australia
e-mail: jim.toouli@flinders.edu.au

28.2 Technique

28.2.1 Stents

Stents for biliary drainage are primarily classified into plastic and metallic. Table 28.1 provides a list of the available stents. Metal stents are also classified into coated (with polytetrafluoroethylene–fluorinated ethylene propylene) or uncoated (Fig. 28.1).

Metallic stents are associated with significantly higher patency rates than plastic stents. The difference may be as long as 4 months after insertion [7]. However, the cost of metal stents is higher when compared to plastic stents. On the other hand, an advantage of metallic stents over plastic stents is the ability to permit drainage of the side branches of the biliary tree through the mesh [8].

Table 28.1 Classification of endo-biliary stents

Plastic
Carey-Coons stent (Percuflex; Meditech/Boston Scientific)
Silicone stents (Malecot; Cook, Inc)
Metal
Self-expandable
Gianturco-Rosch Z stent (Cook,. Bloomington, IN)
Wallstent (Boston Scientific; Natick, Mass)
Luminex stent (Bard; Tempe, Ariz)
Smartstent (Cordis Endovascular; Miami, Fla)
Balloon-mounted
Palmaz stent (Johnson & Johnson/Cordis, New Brunswick, NJ)
Self-expandable requiring balloon dilatation after deployment
Strecker stent (BSIC Co, Hilden, Germany)

W.Y. Lau (ed.), *Hilar Cholangiocarcinoma*,
DOI 10.1007/978-94-007-6473-6_28, © Springer Science+Business Media Dordrecht and People's Medical Publishing House 2013

28.3 Results of Endoscopy in the Palliation of Hilar Cholangiocarcinomas

Endoscopic biliary stenting for hilar cholangiocarcinomas has been shown to have a success rate ranging from 41 to 91 % [9–12] in terms of early palliation. The need for reintervention is correspondingly higher for plastic stents compared to metallic stents. Issues which arise when considering stenting include the following (Fig. 28.2a, b):

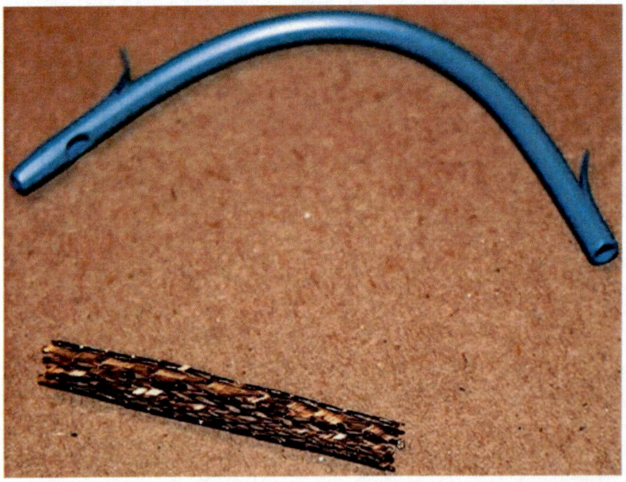

Fig. 28.1 Stents used for drainage of hilar obstruction: a Cotton-Leung plastic biliary® stent 10Fr/7 cm and a Zilver® self-expanding metal stent 10Fr/4 cm (Courtesy Cook Medical)

28.3.1 Stage of the Cholangiocarcinoma

Devierre et al. [2] demonstrated a successful endoscopic intubation rate of 89 % including Bismuth type III lesions. They were able to show that achieving complete drainage was associated with low rates of cholangitis and mortality. While the benefit of endoscopic stenting in type I and II lesions is widely accepted, its role in more advanced lesions is uncertain. A number of studies compared the outcomes of endoscopic versus percutaneous stenting in more advanced tumours (type III and IV). The findings from these studies indicate that while successful complete biliary drainage may be achieved endoscopically in type III lesions, in some type III and most type IV lesions, the percutaneous route may provide higher initial success rate and low level of procedure-related cholangitis [13, 14].

28.3.2 Endoscopy Versus Percutaneous Approach

The diagnosis of a hilar cholangiocarcinoma is often made at the time of ERCP. The endoscopist then has a choice of whether to proceed with insertion of an endoscopic stent or stop the procedure for a choice to be made on the form of drainage. The decision is not easy as it is well known that the procedure itself, i.e. the ERCP, may lead to infection proximal to the obstruction. In general, the weight of evidence

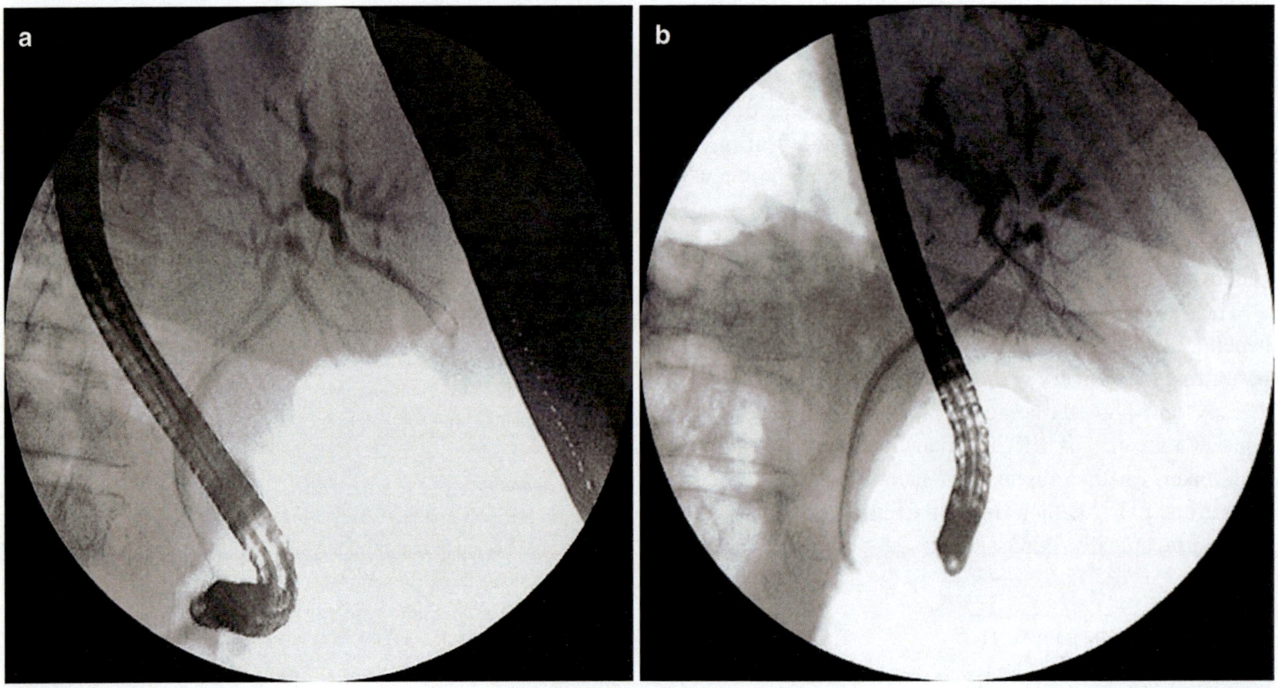

Fig. 28.2 (**a**) ERCP image showing a Bismuth type IV hilar obstruction. A wire is threaded through the obstruction into the dominant right hepatic duct. (**b**) A plastic stent has been inserted endoscopically through the stricture, thus draining the right hepatic duct

would support drainage via an endoscopic stent during the same procedure. In this scenario, percutaneous intervention would only be used if the endoscopic approach does not result in adequate drainage.

The first randomised trial comparing endoscopic versus the percutaneous approach for treating malignant biliary obstruction demonstrated a higher success and lower mortality rate for the endoscopic approach [4]. This trial was criticised for the use of a rigid transhepatic catheter for the percutaneous approach as it led to problems associated with liver puncture (haemorrhage and bile leaks). The only other randomised trial comparing the two approaches was performed by Pinol et al. [15]. 54 patients were randomised to receive a percutaneous self-expandable metallic stent (SEMS) (n=28) or a 12-F endoscopic polyethylene prosthesis (n=26). While the technical success rates of both techniques were similar, therapeutic success (71 % vs. 42%; $P<0.03$) as well as the median survival (3.7 vs. 2.0 months; $P<0.02$) was higher in the percutaneous group. This was attributed to the metal stents being used in the percutaneous group as opposed to plastic stents in the endoscopic group. Major complications (related to bacterial infection), however, were more common in the percutaneous group (61 % vs. 35 %; $P<0.09$). The SEMS alone was identified as an independent predictor of survival based on Cox regression analysis.

In a recent retrospective study, Paik et al. [14] demonstrated a higher success rate for biliary decompression in patients with type III and IV lesions using percutaneously-inserted SEMS as compared to endoscopic stents. There was no difference in procedure-related complications between the two groups. So long as biliary drainage could be successfully achieved, median survival and stent patency rates were not different in the two groups.

The complementary use of the two approaches for hilar cholangiocarcinomas has also been described [16, 17]. In instances where an endoscopically-placed stent was required, percutaneous access allowed the passage of a wire through the liver and through the obstructing tumour. An endoscopic stent then could be introduced over the wire.

28.3.3 Unilateral Versus Bilateral

While a single stent is sufficient to drain the obstructed liver above type I tumours or tumours obstructing a single ductal system, multiple stents are required to drain the liver in type II, III and IV tumours. The data on unilateral versus bilateral drainage is far less convincing with studies reporting conflicting results. It has been shown that drainage of 25 % of the liver volume is needed to achieve biochemical improvement and relief of symptoms [18].

The studies favouring unilateral only drainage have based their conclusions on the higher success rates at stent insertion and complete drainage coupled with lower rates of post-procedural cholangitis [10, 19]. One study comparing unilateral versus bilateral endoscopic insertion of plastic stents for type II and III lesions demonstrated no difference in mortality or survival [20]. In contrast, bilateral drainage in tumours obstructing both ducts, although technically demanding, has been shown to be feasible associated with a lower incidence of cholangitis, lower 30-day mortality, and even improved survival [2, 21–23]. It is widely accepted that the injection of contrast at the time of ERCP into the biliary tree would predispose to cholangitis and even septicaemia from bacterial contamination of an undrained segment.

The only randomised trial comparing unilateral versus bilateral endoscopic drainage in hilar cholangiocarcinomas was published in 2001 [19] and utilised plastic stents in tumours that were Bismuth type I to III. No type IV tumours were included in this study. The study revealed a significantly lower success rate for bilateral stent insertion as opposed to unilateral stent insertion ($P<0.041$) and a higher rate of early complications in patients with bilateral stents owing to a higher incidence of cholangitis. Other parameters such as successful drainage, 30-day mortality and median survival were not different between the two groups of patients. Despite these findings including the technical difficulty of endoscopic bilateral stenting, the perceived advantage of bilateral drainage continues to be advocated [2, 21–23].

Endoscopic bilateral drainage, when feasible, would be considered ideal in a bilaterally obstructed system. To facilitate bilateral stenting newer stents such as the Y stent (Niti-S Biliary Y stent; Taewoong, Seoul, Korea), a hybrid of spiral and Z stents have been developed. The feasibility of this stent has been demonstrated in smaller studies [24]. However, results from further, larger studies are awaited. Slimmer, open cell design stents [25] have also been developed. In addition, the triple lumen catheter [26] to facilitate selective cannulation of multiply obstructed ducts has also been developed.

28.3.4 Plastic Versus Metal

The only randomised trial published to date [27] comparing metal versus plastic stenting in 20 patients with hilar cholangiocarcinomas demonstrated a higher incidence of cholangitis, higher stent failure rates and consequently a higher number of re-interventions in patients with plastic stents. However, plastic stents are considerably cheaper than SEMS. On the other hand, the cost-related benefits of plastic stents were offset by an overall longer hospital stay required due to multiple stent changes for the plastic stents.

So while the available evidence [10, 12, 27, 28] supports the use of SEMS over plastic stents in patients in whom the survival is expected to be more than 6 months (advanced disease but not metastatic to the liver), there do exist specific indications when plastic stents would be preferred. For instance, a plastic stent may be advantageous in patients requiring stent of both the right and left biliary systems as the use of plastic stents in this scenario is technically easier, as well as in those who are planned for photodynamic therapy [29, 30]. In the latter instance the metal stents cannot be used as the metal in the stents interferes with the therapy.

28.3.5 Quality of Life Benefits Following Endoscopic Stenting

One of the few studies [31] that assessed quality of life following biliary drainage for malignant biliary obstruction found that jaundice appeared to be prolonged in patients with hilar lesions as compared to distal bile duct lesions. However, in 80 % of patients, adequate symptomatic relief could be achieved. Although not specifically studied in patients with hilar cholangiocarcinoma, endoscopic stent insertion in patients with malignant biliary obstruction, besides reducing pruritus and anorexia, has been shown to improve the quality of life parameters assessed by emotional, cognitive and global health scores [32, 33]. Similarly, the endoscopic relief of biliary obstruction in patients with pancreatic cancer has been demonstrated to reverse the negative metabolic effects and deranged T- and B-cell functions [34].

28.4 Complications

Complications following endoscopic stenting can be classified into those related to the procedure (early) and those specific to the stent (late). Table 28.2 provides a list of these complications.

The injection of contrast at the time of ERCP with failure to achieve complete drainage of the obstructed segments thereafter predisposes to the development of early cholangitis. The use of air as a contrast agent (air contrast cholangiography) instead of iodine-based contrast medium has been suggested to reduce the incidence of immediate post procedural cholangitis [35, 36]. Larger comparative studies are needed to evaluate this technique.

The 30-day mortality rate following endoscopic stenting has been reported to be as high as 18 % [11]. This is not surprising considering that these patients are often in a terminal state due to the burden of their malignancy.

Table 28.2 Classification of complications [6, 40, 41]

Early/procedure-related
Perforation
Cholangitis
Haemorrhage
Pancreatitis
Late/stent-related
Plastic stent
Migration
Premature occlusion by encrustation and tumour overgrowth
Metal stent
Obstruction secondary to tumour ingrowth or overgrowth
Sludge formation

28.5 Widening the Scope of Endoscopy as a Palliative Tool

In recent years two centres have reported biliary drainage via intrahepatic duct puncture and stent placement under endosonographic (EUS) guidance [37, 38]. Will et al. [37] have used this approach in two patients with hilar cholangiocarcinomas. The utility of this approach is in instances where the endoscopist is unable to reach the papilla owing to pyloric or duodenal stenosis or inability to introduce the catheter into the bile duct [37]. The limitations of this procedure would include the need for multiple stenting as may be the case in complex hilar strictures as EUS may not be able to accurately define such complex strictures [39]. Further studies are clearly required before its wider use.

Conclusion

Endoscopic palliation of jaundice in patients with hilar cholangiocarcinomas is best achieved in patients in whom preoperative drainage was achieved endoscopically. At the present time, percutaneous drainage of the biliary system is a useful tool in patients in whom endoscopic drainage cannot be achieved due to technical reasons or for non-availability of advanced endoscopic facilities. The two techniques should not be regarded as mutually exclusive but rather as complementary with the choice of procedure dependant on the technique most suitable to give the best outcome. Endoscopic stent insertion is a valuable tool to facilitate delivery of other forms of adjuvant therapy including brachytherapy and photodynamic therapy. The development of newer stents and techniques for deployment as well as the rapidly emerging applications of EUS could widen the scope of endoscopy as a palliative tool in hilar cholangiocarcinomas.

Acknowledgements The authors wish to acknowledge the help of Dr. Christopher Worthley who provided the ERCP images.

References

1. Cotton PB. Endoscopic methods for relief of malignant obstructive jaundice. World J Surg. 1984;8(6):854–61.
2. Deviere J, Baize M, de Toeuf J, et al. Long-term follow-up of patients with hilar malignant stricture treated by endoscopic internal biliary drainage. Gastrointest Endosc. 1988;34(2):95–101.

3. Soehendra N, Reynders-Frederix V. Palliative bile duct drainage—a new endoscopic method of introducing a transpapillary drain. Endoscopy. 1980;12(1):8–11.
4. Speer AG, Cotton PB, Russell RC, et al. Randomised trial of endoscopic versus percutaneous stent insertion in malignant obstructive jaundice. Lancet. 1987;2(8550):57–62.
5. Schmassmann A, von Gunten E, Knuchel J, et al. Wallstents versus plastic stents in malignant biliary obstruction: effects of stent patency of the first and second stent on patient compliance and survival. Am J Gastroenterol. 1996;91(4):654–9.
6. Wilson M. The application of metallic stents in malignant biliary obstruction. Tech Vasc Interv Radiol. 1999;2(1):39–52.
7. Moss AC, Morris E, Leyden J, et al. Do the benefits of metal stents justify the costs? A systematic review and meta-analysis of trials comparing endoscopic stents for malignant biliary obstruction. Eur J Gastroenterol Hepatol. 2007;19(12):1119–24.
8. Cipolletta L, Rotondano G, Marmo R, et al. Endoscopic palliation of malignant obstructive jaundice: an evidence-based review. Dig Liver Dis. 2007;39(4):375–88.
9. Cheng JL, Bruno MJ, Bergman JJ, et al. Endoscopic palliation of patients with biliary obstruction caused by nonresectable hilar cholangiocarcinoma: efficacy of self-expandable metallic Wallstents. Gastrointest Endosc. 2002;56(1):33–9.
10. De Palma GD, Pezzullo A, Rega M, et al. Unilateral placement of metallic stents for malignant hilar obstruction: a prospective study. Gastrointest Endosc. 2003;58(1):50–3.
11. Liu CL, Lo CM, Lai EC, et al. Endoscopic retrograde cholangiopancreatography and endoscopic endoprosthesis insertion in patients with Klatskin tumors. Arch Surg. 1998;133(3):293–6.
12. Peters RA, Williams SG, Lombard M, et al. The management of high-grade hilar strictures by endoscopic insertion of self-expanding metal endoprostheses. Endoscopy. 1997;29(1):10–6.
13. Lee SH, Park JK, Yoon WJ, et al. Optimal biliary drainage for inoperable Klatskin's tumor based on Bismuth type. World J Gastroenterol. 2007;13(29):3948–55.
14. Paik WH, Park YS, Hwang JH, et al. Palliative treatment with self-expandable metallic stents in patients with advanced type III or IV hilar cholangiocarcinoma: a percutaneous versus endoscopic approach. Gastrointest Endosc. 2009;69(1):55–62.
15. Pinol V, Castells A, Bordas JM, et al. Percutaneous self-expanding metal stents versus endoscopic polyethylene endoprostheses for treating malignant biliary obstruction: randomised clinical trial. Radiology. 2002;225(1):27–34.
16. Moorthy S, Prabhu N, Sreekumar K, et al. Hilar cholangiocarcinoma: results of percutaneous stenting with self-expandable metal stents. Indian J Radiol Imaging. 2004;14:45–51.
17. Neal CP, Thomasset SC, Bools D, et al. Combined percutaneous-endoscopic stenting of malignant biliary obstruction: results from 106 consecutive procedures and identification of factors associated with adverse outcome. Surg Endosc. 2010;24(2):423–31.
18. Dowsett JF, Vaira D, Hatfield AR, et al. Endoscopic biliary therapy using the combined percutaneous and endoscopic technique. Gastroenterology. 1989;96(4):1180–6.
19. De Palma GD, Galloro G, Siciliano S, et al. Unilateral versus bilateral endoscopic hepatic duct drainage in patients with malignant hilar biliary obstruction: results of a prospective, randomised, and controlled study. Gastrointest Endosc. 2001;53(6):547–53.
20. Polydorou AA, Chisholm EM, Romanos AA, et al. A comparison of right versus left hepatic duct endoprosthesis insertion in malignant hilar biliary obstruction. Endoscopy. 1989;21(6):266–71.
21. Chang WH, Kortan P, Haber GB. Outcome in patients with bifurcation tumors who undergo unilateral versus bilateral hepatic duct drainage. Gastrointest Endosc. 1998;47(5):354–62.
22. Dumas R, Demuth N, Buckley M, et al. Endoscopic bilateral metal stent placement for malignant hilar stenoses: identification of optimal technique. Gastrointest Endosc. 2000;51(3):334–8.
23. Naitoh I, Ohara H, Nakazawa T, et al. Unilateral versus bilateral endoscopic metal stenting for malignant hilar biliary obstruction. J Gastroenterol Hepatol. 2009;24(4):552–7.
24. Lee JH, Kang DH, Kim JY, et al. Endoscopic bilateral metal stent placement for advanced hilar cholangiocarcinoma: a pilot study of a newly designed Y stent. Gastrointest Endosc. 2007;66(2):364–9.
25. Kim JY, Kang DH, Kim HW, et al. Usefulness of slimmer and open-cell-design stents for endoscopic bilateral stenting and endoscopic revision in patients with hilar cholangiocarcinoma (with video). Gastrointest Endosc. 2009;70(6):1109–15.
26. Kim JY, Kang DH, Choi CW, et al. Selective intrahepatic duct cannulation by using a triple-lumen catheter for endoscopic bilateral stenting in hilar cholangiocarcinoma. Gastrointest Endosc. 2010;72(1):192–8.
27. Wagner HJ, Knyrim K, Vakil N, et al. Plastic endoprostheses versus metal stents in the palliative treatment of malignant hilar biliary obstruction. A prospective and randomised trial. Endoscopy. 1993;25(3):213–8.
28. Kaassis M, Boyer J, Dumas R, et al. Plastic or metal stents for malignant stricture of the common bile duct? Results of a randomised prospective study. Gastrointest Endosc. 2003;57(2):178–82.
29. Ortner ME, Caca K, Berr F, et al. Successful photodynamic therapy for nonresectable cholangiocarcinoma: a randomised prospective study. Gastroenterology. 2003;125(5):1355–63.
30. Zoepf T, Jakobs R, Arnold JC, et al. Palliation of nonresectable bile duct cancer: improved survival after photodynamic therapy. Am J Gastroenterol. 2005;100(11):2426–30.
31. Cheung KL, Lai EC. Endoscopic stenting for malignant biliary obstruction. Arch Surg. 1995;130(2):204–7.
32. Ballinger AB, McHugh M, Catnach SM, et al. Symptom relief and quality of life after stenting for malignant bile duct obstruction. Gut. 1994;35(4):467–70.
33. Luman W, Cull A, Palmer KR. Quality of life in patients stented for malignant biliary obstructions. Eur J Gastroenterol Hepatol. 1997;9(5):481–4.
34. Siegel JH, Snady H. The significance of endoscopically placed prostheses in the management of biliary obstruction due to carcinoma of the pancreas: results of nonoperative decompression in 277 patients. Am J Gastroenterol. 1986;81(8):634–41.
35. Pisello F, Geraci G, Modica G, et al. Cholangitis prevention in endoscopic Klatskin tumor palliation: air cholangiography technique. Langenbecks Arch Surg. 2009;394(6):1109–14.
36. Singh V, Singh G, Gupta V, et al. Contrast-free air cholangiography-assisted unilateral plastic stenting in malignant hilar biliary obstruction. Hepatobiliary Pancreat Dis Int. 2010;9(1):88–92.
37. Will U, Thieme A, Fueldner F, et al. Treatment of biliary obstruction in selected patients by endoscopic ultrasonography (EUS)-guided transluminal biliary drainage. Endoscopy. 2007;39(4):292–5.
38. Yamao K, Bhatia V, Mizuno N, et al. EUS-guided choledochoduodenostomy for palliative biliary drainage in patients with malignant biliary obstruction: results of long-term follow-up. Endoscopy. 2008;40(4):340–2.
39. Geller A. Klatskin tumor–palliative therapy: the jury is still out or may be not yet in. Gastrointest Endosc. 2009;69(1):63–5.
40. Hausegger KA, Kleinert R, Lammer J, et al. Malignant biliary obstruction: histologic findings after treatment with self-expandable stents. Radiology. 1992;185(2):461–4.
41. Mueller PR, Ferrucci Jr JT, Teplick SK, et al. Biliary stent endoprosthesis: analysis of complications in 113 patients. Radiology. 1985;156(3):637–9.

Percutaneous Palliation of Cholangiocarcinoma

29

P.D. Peng, J.F.H. Geschwind, and M.A. Choti

29.1 Introduction

Cholangiocarcinomas are malignant tumors arising from the biliary tract and have an worldwide incidence of 0.5~2.0/100,000 [1]. Complete resection of early stage tumors can be curative [2]. In cases when the disease is unresectable, the prognosis is generally poor with a 1 year survival of 53 % and 5 year survival of less than 5 % [3–6].

As most patients present with unresectable disease, palliation is a central goal in management of patients with cholangiocarcinoma. Over 75 % of cholangiocarcinomas are extrahepatic, which includes both hilar and distal bile duct tumors, and the most common presenting symptom with these tumors is painless jaundice from biliary obstruction, occurring in up to 90 % of patients [7]. Associated symptoms accompanying obstructive jaundice can include pruritus, weight loss, nausea, abdominal pain, and malabsorptive diarrhea. Additionally, biliary obstruction increases the risk for cholangitis, especially after procedural interventions, and also leads to metabolic and synthetic liver dysfunction. The natural clinical course of unresectable cholangiocarcinoma progresses with biliary obstruction followed by death from liver failure or cholangitis within 12 months [8]. In patients who progress with intrahepatic cholangiocarcinoma, they typically develop liver failure and local tumor symptoms or develop symptoms from distant disease, with biliary obstruction typically presenting later in the disease.

P.D. Peng, MD • M.A. Choti, MD, FRCS (✉)
Department of Surgery, Johns Hopkins
University School of Medicine,
John Hopkins Hospital, Baltimore, MD, USA
e-mail: mchoti@jhmi.edu

J.F.H. Geschwind, MD
Department of Radiology, Johns Hopkins
University School of Medicine,
John Hopkins Hospital,
Baltimore, MD, USA

29.2 Goals of Palliation

Palliative care, as defined by the World Health Organization, is an approach which improves the quality of life of patients facing life-threatening illness [9]. In advanced cholangiocarcinoma, palliation should focus on relief from the symptoms of biliary obstruction, and thus biliary decompression is critical to symptomatic palliation. Obstructive jaundice can also be accompanied by refractory pruritus, anorexia, malabsorptive diarrhea, and progressive malnutrition, all of which can lead to generalized wasting. If left untreated, biliary obstruction can result in cholangitis or metabolic and synthetic liver dysfunction that can precipitate early death. For these reasons, decompression of biliary obstruction leads to a dramatic improvement in the overall medical condition that contributes to a prolongation of comfortable survival.

A recent prospective cohort study evaluating patient quality-of-life before and after decompression of malignant biliary obstruction determined that 84 % of patients demonstrated improvement in serum bilirubin levels and this was associated with significant improvements in both social function and mental health [10]. Another study demonstrated biliary decompression following stent placement improved appetite and reduced abdominal pain, in addition to relieving jaundice and pruritus [11]. Biliary decompression can be accomplished through endoscopic, percutaneous, or operative methods. While each technique has its advantages and should be considered complimentary rather than competitive, the percutaneous approach has proven to be an effective modality when palliating biliary obstruction from cholangiocarcinoma.

29.3 Distal Cholangiocarcinoma

When comparing methods for biliary decompression, perihilar and distal tumors should be considered differently due to both technical and anatomic differences. For jaundiced patients with definitively unresectable distal tumors found on preoperative evaluation, nonoperative palliative therapy is

W.Y. Lau (ed.), *Hilar Cholangiocarcinoma*,
DOI 10.1007/978-94-007-6473-6_29, © Springer Science+Business Media Dordrecht and People's Medical Publishing House 2013

generally indicated. Since its clinical inception in 1980, the use of endoscopically placed biliary endoprostheses has continued to evolve and now serves as the predominant modality for palliating obstructive jaundice. With experience and standardized equipment, biliary drainage can be accomplished successfully with a 10Fr endoprosthesis in over 90 % of patients during endoscopic retrograde cholangiopancreatography (ERCP). A randomised trial in 1994 compared endoscopic and surgical bypass in malignant low bile duct strictures. This study revealed a lower procedural-related mortality (3 % vs. 14 %) and major complication rate (11 % vs. 29 %) rate in the endoscopic group compared to the operative approach, yet recurrent jaundice occurred more frequently in the endoscopic group (38 % vs. 2 %) [12]. No difference in survival was seen between groups. The lower morbidity of the non-operative approach favored the less invasive technique in patients with limited life expectancy and the introduction of metallic stents increased the patency rate for endoscopic drainage.

A prospective, randomised trial of endoscopically placed metallic stents vs. polyethylene stents for distal malignant biliary obstruction found prolonged patency of the metallic stent group (273 vs. 126 days) [13]. As stent occlusion in bare metallic stents was often due to tumor in-growth, a number of trials compared covered stents with the bare metal stents and found no difference in the patency rate. However, the covered metal stents were associated with a higher complication rate of stent migration [14, 15]. With increased experience at tertiary centers, standardized equipment, and the use of self-expanding bare metallic stents for increased patency, endoscopic biliary drainage is now successful in over 90 % of patients and is the preferred approach for distal cholangiocarcinoma [16, 17]. In cases when this approach is unsuccessful, technical failures usually result from tumor infiltration into the duodenal wall that prevents access to the ampulla. In the event that endoscopic management is unsuccessful or not possible, percutaneous transhepatic cholangiography and stent placement should be performed to accomplish external biliary drainage.

29.4 Hilar Cholangiocarcinoma

Perihilar cholangiocarcinomas account for two-thirds of the tumors and present most frequently in the sixth or seventh decades. The most commonly used Bismuth-Corlette classification accounts for extent of biliary ductal involvement: Type I tumors involve only the common hepatic duct and not the confluence of the left and right hepatic ducts, Type II tumors involve the bifurcation but do not extend into the left or right segmental hepatic ducts, Type III tumors extend into either the left OR right segmental hepatic ducts, and Type IV tumors extend into both the left and right segmental hepatic ducts from the confluence. The involvement of the bifurcation of the left and right biliary systems in addition to proximal segmental extension in Type III~IV can provide challenges for effective endoscopic drainage. Anatomic variations can introduce further complexity into strategies for biliary decompression.

While the palliation of periampullary tumors has been well-studied, the evidence comparing methods of palliation for perihilar tumors is currently evolving. In general, the success rate of endoscopic stent decompression is only approximately 50 % and largely reflects technical experience. Despite technical difficulty, insertion of a plastic biliary endoprosthesis is the most common method used by experienced endoscopists to palliate hilar obstruction. Two randomised studies comparing endoscopic versus percutaneous biliary decompression in malignant biliary obstruction have been reported with conflicting results. An early randomised trial comparing endoscopic and percutaneous rigid polyethylene stent insertion in patients with malignant obstructive jaundice demonstrated that the endoscopic approach had a significantly higher success rate for relief of jaundice (81 % vs. 61 %) and a lower 30-day mortality (15 % vs. 33 %) [18]. Introduction of internal self-expanding metallic stents which are associated with longer patency lead to a more recent randomised study compared percutaneous self-expanding metal stents vs. endoscopic 12-Fr polyethylene endoprostheses for treating malignant biliary obstruction and found that while technical success rates were similar, the therapeutic success rate was higher in the percutaneous group (71 % vs. 42 %) [19]. Both studies were limited by combining both distal and perihilar tumors. In addition, the introduction of self-expanding metal stents in the second trial complicates direct comparison, however the studies suggest that percutaneous introduction of metal stents was associated with higher clinical success rate when compared with endoscopically placed polyethylene stents.

The choice of stent material remains contentious, regardless of the approach. Silastic biliary catheters or stents require repeat manipulations to maintain patency and prevent cholangitis. It is for this reason that primary or delayed placement of a self-expanding metallic stent has become preferable for unresectable patients with in whom palliative interventions alone are appropriate. Although metallic stents afford significantly better long-term patency compared to endoprostheses, occlusions can occur with tumor ingrowth. In such cases, reaccess to the biliary tree can be more problematic. For this reason, novel biliary stents, incorporating an impermeable sheath or cytotoxic compounds, have recently been developed to avoid complications of re-occlusion. Furthermore, most clinicians feel uncomfortable placing metallic biliary stents during the initial endoscopic or percutaneous procedure, particularly if a definitive opinion regarding resectability has not been rendered. In most circumstances, metallic stents are deployed at the time of a re-manipulation of an existing biliary drainage catheter. Another advantage of bare metal over plastic stents for the management of hilar tumors is the open mesh design which has the potential for permitting continued patency of the contralateral ducts which would otherwise be occluded by the closed-wall stent.

A small prospective trial directly comparing endoscopically placed metallic vs. polyethylene stents was underpowered for statistical significance but found a trend toward greater long-term (>30 days) stent failure in the polyethylene group (43 % vs. 22 %) with a statistically significant higher incidence of cholangitis (36 % vs. 15 %) [20, 21]. Findings from a multicenter observational cohort study supported the superiority of metal stents with fewer adverse outcomes (which included cholangitis, stent occlusion or migration, and need for unplanned endoscopic procedures) [22]. Again these studies demonstrate that self-expanding metal stents are superior in maintaining biliary drainage for disease palliation when compared to plastic stents.

A recent multicenter retrospective study compared percutaneous to endoscopic placement of self-expandable metal stents in patients with Bismuth III and IV hilar cholangiocarcinoma [23]. Baseline characteristics were similar in the two groups, but the rate of successful biliary decompression was significantly higher in the group with percutaneously placed metal stents (93 % vs. 77 %). Median survival was significantly higher in those patients with successful biliary decompression (8.7 months vs. 1.8 months). Stent patency was comparable in the two groups. This non-randomised study suggested that hilar cholangiocarcinoma may be best palliated through percutaneous introduction of bare metal stents. However as we await results from randomised clinical trials, palliation of biliary obstruction from hilar cholangiocarcinoma may currently be best approached with a multidisciplinary strategy accounting for institutional expertise.

29.5 Techniques of Percutaneous Transhepatic Biliary Drainage

Percutaneous biliary decompression evolved from initial procedures for percutaneous transhepatic cholangiography [24]. Development of catheters with side holes allow percutaneous drains to traverse into the duodenum, allowing for external stent capping and internal biliary drainage [25]. The introduction of self-expanding metallic stents has potential advantages associated with drainage of intervening segments and longer patency rates [26].

Percutaneous transhepatic biliary drainage can provide internal or external drainage. The goal is percutaneous placement of an external or internal biliary drainage polyethylene catheter or internal biliary metallic stent for biliary decompression. External drainage is commonly performed under ultrasound guidance as a temporizing measure in patients preoperatively prior to resection, patients failing endoscopic drainage, or during episodes of acute cholangitis for biliary decompression and further medical management. In the latter two situations, the patients can undergo eventual internalization of drainage by clamping the external catheter or exchange for an internal stent. Preoperative imaging through MRCP or CT allows assessment of tumor location and hepatic biliary dilation. The general technique involves ultrasound or CT radiographic guided placement of a thin Chiba needle into the liver. Aspiration of bile confirms placement in the biliary system. Antegrade cholangiogram is then generally performed to localize site of obstruction allowing a 0.014-in. guidewire to be passed across the stricture. Catheter placement over the guidewire with tip extending into duodenum allows internal and external bile drainage.

A retrospective review comparing endoscopically placed 10-Fr and 8-Fr biliary stents found that the larger stent was associated with fewer episodes of cholangitis and increased patency due to the larger diameter [27]. When 10-Fr stents were compared with 11.5-Fr stents in a retrospective study, there was no difference in patency of the two stent sizes [28]. These data suggest that 10-Fr stents are large enough to provide adequate drainage. In practice, recurrent symptoms of pain or cholangitis with a percutaneously placed 10-Fr stent may be an indication for PTBD stent upsizing.

Self-expanding metallic stents, as previously mentioned can be associated with high patency rates under fluoroscopic guidance. Technical advances now allow deployment of the metallic stents through 7-Fr catheters minimizing hepatic injury during placement and deployment. The catheter can then be left in place for several days and removed allowing for internalization of biliary drainage.

29.6 Unilateral Versus Bilateral Drainage

Biliary obstruction by hilar cholangiocarcinoma generally results in two separately obstructed systems—left and right. Literature from operative palliation of malignant hilar biliary obstruction compared those patients with free communication and those with no communication between the right and left draining systems after operative unilateral drainage through an intrahepatic biliary enteric bypass. There was no difference in median survival, decrease in serum bilirubin, or symptomatic palliation between the two groups indicating that unilateral drainage was sufficient for palliation [29].

A prospective, randomised controlled study examined the role of unilateral vs. bilateral endoscopic hepatic duct drainage in patients with malignant hilar biliary obstruction. The unilateral group had a higher rate of technical success (89 % vs. 77 %). Surprisingly, unilateral stents also had a lower rate of both complications (19 % vs. 27 %) and cholangitis (9 %

vs 17 %) [30]. A retrospective review of patients undergoing endoscopic stent placement for palliation of unresectable malignant hilar biliary obstruction found no difference between right or left hepatic ductal drainage in terms of technical success, complications, 30-day mortality, and patency [31]. Taken together, unilateral drainage of malignant hilar biliary obstruction appears to provide adequate palliation, at least when performed through the endoscopic route. It remains to be determined in patients undergoing percutaneous stent placement for palliation whether unilateral access is sufficient or whether bilateral internalized stents afford improved and more durable palliation.

29.7 Intrabiliary Therapies for Palliation

While decompression of biliary obstruction is the primary goal of palliation for unresectable cholangiocarcinoma, the introduction of percutaneous catheter-based therapies are being investigated for local tumor control in order to provide more durable palliation and improved survival.

29.7.1 Photodynamic Therapy

Photodynamic therapy (PDT) involves the introduction of a photosensitizer to the target tissue. When the tissue is locally illuminated with a corresponding wavelength of light, the photosensitizer undergoes a type II photochemical reaction and generates cytotoxic oxygen-derived free radicals, which then mediates apoptotic and necrotic cell death. Three compounds are currently being used as photosensitizers in cholangiocarcinoma: Photofrin (Axcan Pharma, Canada), Photosan (SeeLab, Germany), and Delta-aminolevulinic acid (Medac, Germany) [32].

Promising results have been reported from a number of preliminary studies of PDT for palliation of cholangiocarcinoma [33–38]. Two recent prospective, randomised trial reported significant survival advantage with PDT. In the first multicenter trial, 39 patients with unresectable hilar cholangiocarcinoma were randomised to two groups: biliary stenting followed by PDT with Photofrin versus stenting alone [39]. Only patients with successful biliary stenting through, either endoscopy or percutaneously, fulfilled inclusion criteria. The study found that addition of PDT resulted in a significant survival advantage (493 vs. 98 days). The second randomised clinical trial accrued 32 patients with unresectable bile duct cancer [40]. Both groups had undergone previous biliary stenting through endoscopic or percutaneous means. The experimental group underwent PDT with Photosan resulting in a mean survival of 21 months compared to the control group which had a median survival of 7 months. While these two small randomised trials are promising, larger controlled trials are needed to confirm the efficacy and applicability of PDT for the palliation of unresectable cholangiocarcinoma.

29.7.2 Intraluminal Brachytherapy

Patients with unresectable disease are candidates for radiotherapy. Although external beam radiotherapy is the most common application, the introduction of intraluminal brachytherapy has been studied in advanced cholangiocarcinoma [41–44]. The intraluminal radiotherapy is performed by loading a percutaneous biliary catheter with Iridium-192 strands to the level of the malignant stricture. A single small prospective trial randomised 21 patients with unresectable cholangiocarcinoma to percutaneous biliary stenting alone versus biliary stenting followed by intraluminal Ir-192 brachytherapy (30 Gy) and external radiotherapy (50 Gy) [45]. This study found an improvement in median survival from 298 days in the control to 388 days in the group undergoing radiation therapy. The addition of external beam radiotherapy is a confounding factor which may have influenced the survival difference, however further studies may clarify the role of intraluminal brachytherapy in the palliation of cholangiocarcinoma.

29.8 Summary

While relatively uncommon, cholangiocarcinoma can be associated with some of the most challenging patients to successfully palliate. Although complete surgical resection with negative margins can result in cure, only approximately 20 % of patients may be candidates for curative-intent therapy. Moreover, compared to other hepatobiliary malignancies, these patients are often markedly symptomatic and difficult to manage. Thus palliation is an important issue in disease management in unresectable and recurrent patients. Symptoms of cholangiocarcinoma are primarily related to biliary obstruction, and include jaundice, pruritus, weight loss, nausea, and abdominal pain. Additionally, patients are at an increased risk of developing cholangitis, especially after instrumentation. Endoscopic, percutaneous, and operative approaches to biliary decompression are effective. For distal cholangiocarcinomas, endoscopic stenting has a high success rate and is generally the primary approach, with percutanous transhepatic biliary stenting reserved for endoscopic failures. In contrast, hilar cholangiocarcinoma is more often managed via a percutaneous approach. There is evidence that unilateral stenting is adequate for palliation. Self-expanding bare metal stents are associated with increased patency when compared to polyethylene plastic stents. Covered stents have a comparable patency rate to bare metal stents, however are associated with a high rate of complication and stent migration.

Intrabiliary therapies for palliation include photodynamic therapy and intraluminal brachytherapy. Photodynamic therapy is emerging as a promising option for palliative therapy. There is limited evidence regarding the role of intraluminal brachytherapy. Both approaches remain, at this time, investigational for cholangiocarcinoma palliation. What is clear is that optimal management of patients with cholangiocarcinoma requires a multidisciplinary team of dedicated clinicians, including surgeons, interventional and diagnostic radiologists, gastroenterologists, and hepatologists.

References

1. Parkin DM, Whelan SL, Ferlay J, et al. Cancer incidence in five continents, vol. VII. Lyon: IARC Press; 2002.
2. Lazaridis KN, Gores GJ. Cholangiocarcinoma. Gastroenterology. 2005;128(6):1655–67.
3. Khan SA, Thomas HC, Davidson BR, et al. Cholangiocarcinoma. Lancet. 2005;366(9493):1303–14.
4. Jarnagin WR, Fong Y, DeMatteo RP, et al. Staging, resectability, and outcome in 225 patients with hilar cholangiocarcinoma. Ann Surg. 2001;234(4):507–17. discussion 517–519.
5. Pitt HA, Nakeeb A, Abrams RA, et al. Perihilar cholangiocarcinoma. Postoperative radiotherapy does not improve survival. Ann Surg. 1995;221(6):788–97. discussion 797–798.
6. Pitt HA, Dooley WC, Yeo CJ, et al. Malignancies of the biliary tree. Curr Probl Surg. 1995;32(1):1–90.
7. Burke EC, Jarnagin WR, Hochwald SN, et al. Hilar cholangiocarcinoma: patterns of spread, the importance of hepatic resection for curative operation, and a presurgical clinical staging system. Ann Surg. 1998;228(3):385–94.
8. Farley DR, Weaver AL, Nagorney DM. "Natural history" of unresected cholangiocarcinoma: patient outcome after noncurative intervention. Mayo Clin Proc. 1995;70(5):425–9.
9. WHO National Cancer Control Programmes 2002.
10. Abraham NS, Barkun JS, Barkun AN. Palliation of malignant biliary obstruction: a prospective trial examining impact on quality of life. Gastrointest Endosc. 2002;56(6):835–41.
11. Ballinger AB, McHugh M, Catnach SM, et al. Symptom relief and quality of life after stenting for malignant bile duct obstruction. Gut. 1994;35(4):467–70.
12. Smith AC, Dowsett JF, Russell RC, et al. Randomised trial of endoscopic stenting versus surgical bypass in malignant low bile duct obstruction. Lancet. 1994;344(8938):1655–60.
13. Davids PH, Groen AK, Rauws EA, et al. Randomised trial of self-expanding metal stents versus polyethylene stents for distal malignant biliary obstruction. Lancet. 1992;340(8834–8835): 1488–92.
14. Kullman E, Frozanpor F, Soderlund C, et al. Covered versus uncovered self-expandable nitinol stents in the palliative treatment of malignant distal biliary obstruction: results from a randomised, multicenter study. Gastrointest Endosc. 2010;72(5):915–23.
15. Telford JJ, Carr-Locke DL, Baron TH, et al. A randomised trial comparing uncovered and partially covered self-expandable metal stents in the palliation of distal malignant biliary obstruction. Gastrointest Endosc. 2010;72(5):907–14.
16. Baron TH. Palliation of malignant obstructive jaundice. Gastroenterol Clin North Am. 2006;35(1):101–12.
17. England RE, Martin DF. Endoscopic and percutaneous intervention in malignant obstructive jaundice. Cardiovasc Intervent Radiol. 1996;19(6):381–7.
18. Speer AG, Cotton PB, Russell RC, et al. Randomised trial of endoscopic versus percutaneous stent insertion in malignant obstructive jaundice. Lancet. 1987;2(8550):57–62.
19. Pinol V, Castells A, Bordas JM, et al. Percutaneous self-expanding metal stents versus endoscopic polyethylene endoprostheses for treating malignant biliary obstruction: randomised clinical trial. Radiology. 2002;225(1):27–34.
20. Knyrim K, Wagner HJ, Pausch J, et al. A prospective, randomised, controlled trial of metal stents for malignant obstruction of the common bile duct. Endoscopy. 1993;25(3):207–12.
21. Wagner HJ, Knyrim K, Vakil N, et al. Plastic endoprostheses versus metal stents in the palliative treatment of malignant hilar biliary obstruction. A prospective and randomised trial. Endoscopy. 1993; 25(3):213–8.
22. Perdue DG, Freeman ML, DiSario JA, et al. Plastic versus self-expanding metallic stents for malignant hilar biliary obstruction: a prospective multicenter observational cohort study. J Clin Gastroenterol. 2008;42(9):1040–6.
23. Paik WH, Park YS, Hwang JH, et al. Palliative treatment with self-expandable metallic stents in patients with advanced type III or IV hilar cholangiocarcinoma: a percutaneous versus endoscopic approach. Gastrointest Endosc. 2009;69(1):55–62.
24. Kaude JV, Weidenmier CH, Agee OF. Decompression of bile ducts with the percutaneous transhepatic technic. Radiology. 1969;93(1):69–71.
25. Molnar W, Stockum AE. Relief of obstructive jaundice through percutaneous transhepatic catheter—a new therapeutic method. Am J Roentgenol Radium Ther Nucl Med. 1974;122(2):356–67.
26. Neuhaus H, Hagenmuller F, Classen M. Self-expanding biliary stents: preliminary clinical experience. Endoscopy. 1989;21(5):225–8.
27. Speer AG, Cotton PB, MacRae KD. Endoscopic management of malignant biliary obstruction: stents of 10 French gauge are preferable to stents of 8 French gauge. Gastrointest Endosc. 1988;34(5):412–7.
28. Pereira-Lima JC, Jakobs R, Maier M, et al. Endoscopic biliary stenting for the palliation of pancreatic cancer: results, survival predictive factors, and comparison of 10-French with 11.5-French gauge stents. Am J Gastroenterol. 1996;91(10):2179–84.
29. Baer HU, Rhyner M, Stain SC, et al. The effect of communication between the right and left liver on the outcome of surgical drainage for jaundice due to malignant obstruction at the hilus of the liver. HPB Surg. 1994;8(1):27–31.
30. De Palma GD, Galloro G, Siciliano S, et al. Unilateral versus bilateral endoscopic hepatic duct drainage in patients with malignant hilar biliary obstruction: results of a prospective, randomised, and controlled study. Gastrointest Endosc. 2001;53(6):547–53.
31. Polydorou AA, Chisholm EM, Romanos AA, et al. A comparison of right versus left hepatic duct endoprosthesis insertion in malignant hilar biliary obstruction. Endoscopy. 1989;21(6):266–71.
32. Ortner MA, Dorta G. Technology insight: photodynamic therapy for cholangiocarcinoma. Nat Clin Pract Gastroenterol Hepatol. 2006;3(8):459–67.
33. Ortner MA, Liebetruth J, Schreiber S, et al. Photodynamic therapy of nonresectable cholangiocarcinoma. Gastroenterology. 1998;114(3): 536–42.
34. Berr F, Wiedmann M, Tannapfel A, et al. Photodynamic therapy for advanced bile duct cancer: evidence for improved palliation and extended survival. Hepatology. 2000;31(2):291–8.
35. Rumalla A, Baron TH, Wang KK, et al. Endoscopic application of photodynamic therapy for cholangiocarcinoma. Gastrointest Endosc. 2001;53(4):500–4.
36. Harewood GC, Baron TH, Rumalla A, et al. Pilot study to assess patient outcomes following endoscopic application of photodynamic therapy for advanced cholangiocarcinoma. J Gastroenterol Hepatol. 2005;20(3):415–20.

37. Dumoulin FL, Gerhardt T, Fuchs S, et al. Phase II study of photodynamic therapy and metal stent as palliative treatment for nonresectable hilar cholangiocarcinoma. Gastrointest Endosc. 2003;57(7):860–7.
38. McCaughan Jr JS, Mertens BF, Cho C, et al. Photodynamic therapy to treat tumors of the extrahepatic biliary ducts. A case report. Arch Surg. 1991;126(1):111–3.
39. Ortner ME, Caca K, Berr F, et al. Successful photodynamic therapy for nonresectable cholangiocarcinoma: a randomised prospective study. Gastroenterology. 2003;125(5):1355–63.
40. Zoepf T, Jakobs R, Arnold JC, et al. Palliation of nonresectable bile duct cancer: improved survival after photodynamic therapy. Am J Gastroenterol. 2005;100(11):2426–30.
41. Leung JT, Kuan R. Intraluminal brachytherapy in the treatment of bile duct carcinomas. Australas Radiol. 1997;41(2):151–4.
42. Leung J, Guiney M, Das R. Intraluminal brachytherapy in bile duct carcinomas. Aust N Z J Surg. 1996;66(2):74–7.
43. Vallis KA, Benjamin IS, Munro AJ, et al. External beam and intraluminal radiotherapy for locally advanced bile duct cancer: role and tolerability. Radiother Oncol. 1996;41(1):61–6.
44. Takamura A, Saito H, Kamada T, et al. Intraluminal low--dose-rate 192Ir brachytherapy combined with external beam radiotherapy and biliary stenting for unresectable extrahepatic bile duct carcinoma. Int J Radiat Oncol Biol Phys. 2003;57(5):1357–65.
45. Valek V, Kysela P, Kala Z, et al. Brachytherapy and percutaneous stenting in the treatment of cholangiocarcinoma: a prospective randomised study. Eur J Radiol. 2007;62(2):175–9.

Photodynamic Therapy

30

M.A. Ortner and C. Jost

30.1 Introduction

The majority of patients with cholangiocarcinoma (CCA) present with advanced disease. Therefore, complete resection with negative margins (R0), the only treatment with the potential for cure, is achievable in less than 40 % of patients [1–5]. Since the majority of patients present with nonresectable disease at the time of diagnosis, palliative modalities play a crucial role in the treatment of CCA.

Inoperable patients with advanced cholangiocarcinoma typically present with obstructive jaundice. Therefore, the primary standard goal of treatment is to relieve cholestasis by endoscopic or percutaneous biliary stenting. Although insertion of endoprosthesis improves jaundice in the majority of patients and may provide a better quality of life [6–10], it seems to prolong survival only slightly [2, 11, 12]. Particularly in hilar cholangiocarcinoma invading multiple intrahepatic bile ducts, tumors greater than 3 cm and metastatic tumors, survival is short. These patients survive for less than 100 days and die of liver failure and cholangitis [13–15].

The second goal of treatment is the prolongation of survival by reducing tumor burden. The classical methods are palliative chemo-and radiotherapy. Response rates of chemo- and radiotherapy are low. The only randomised trial comparing chemotherapy with best supportive care in patients with cholangiocarcinoma did not show a survival advantage [16]. For a long time no chemotherapeutic agent has been classified to improve survival in advanced cholangiocarcinoma. However, chemotherapy seems to provide a clinical benefit with improvement of quality of life in half of the patients treated [17]. Recently it has been shown that gemcitabene combined with platinum demonstrates the highest response rates and improves survival compared to gemcitabene alone [18, 19].

Results with radiotherapy in nonresectable cholangiocarcinoma are conflicting. A retrospective comparison of stenting alone with stenting plus radiotherapy did not show a survival advantage of radiotherapy [20]. There seemed to be a survival advantage in the radiotherapy group in the first 9 months after diagnosis, but the length of hospital stay was considerably longer in the patients receiving radiotherapy. A prospective randomised trial indicated a survival advantage of brachytherapy in addition to stenting [21]. However, in the group with stenting alone, only patients with Bismuth type III and IV tumors were included, whereas in the group with additional radiotherapy, one third of patients had Bismuth type I and II tumors. Furthermore only 8 of 21 patients were treated with brachytherapy alone. Stereotactic body radiotherapy for unresectable cholangiocarcinoma seems to be a promising new option for patients with nonresectable cholangiocaricnoma; this treatment warrants further investigation [22, 23].

Despite improvement of radio- and chemotherapy, the outcome with both modalities is still not satisfying. In the last few years it crystallized that photodynamic therapy (PDT) is an auspicious treatment option for nonresectable extrahepatic cholangiocarcinoma. This chapter describes the mechanism of action of PDT and gives an overview of the experience with this new local treatment of cholangiocarcinoma.

30.2 Photodynamic Therapy

30.2.1 History of Photodynamic Therapy

The first reports of photodynamic therapy date back to the Egyptians. It experienced a rebirth in the twentieth century. The use of combined dye and illumination for the treatment of skin disease was first proposed in 1903 by Tappeiner and Jesonik and the Nobel Prize was awarded to Niels Finsen in

M.A. Ortner, MD (✉)
Department of Gastroenterology,
University Hospital Zuerich, Zuerich, Switzerland
e-mail: ma.ortner@bluewin.ch

C. Jost, MD
Department of Gastroenterology,
University Hospital Bern,
Bern, Switzerland

W.Y. Lau (ed.), *Hilar Cholangiocarcinoma*,
DOI 10.1007/978-94-007-6473-6_30, © Springer Science+Business Media Dordrecht and People's Medical Publishing House 2013

1903 for his work on phototherapy. Photodynamic therapy at this time was limited to skin diseases. In 1961, Lipson et al. reported the development of hematoporphyrin derivative, a mixture of porphyrins, for tumor localization [24]. Application in the GI-tract was not possible before the development of fiberendoscopes and laser technology. The first reported application of photodynamic therapy in the gastrointestinal tract was by Kato et al. in 1986 [25].

Today photodynamic therapy is an approved anticancer treatment (brain tumor, lung cancer, head and neck cancer, esophageal cancer, pancreatic cancer, urinary bladder cancer, prostate cancer, various types of skin cancer, cutaneous recurrence of breast cancer). In the gastrointestinal tract it is furthermore approved for treatment of Barrett's esophagus. Non-cancer indications of photodynamic therapy include age-related macular degeneration and cardiovascular disorders (restenosis).

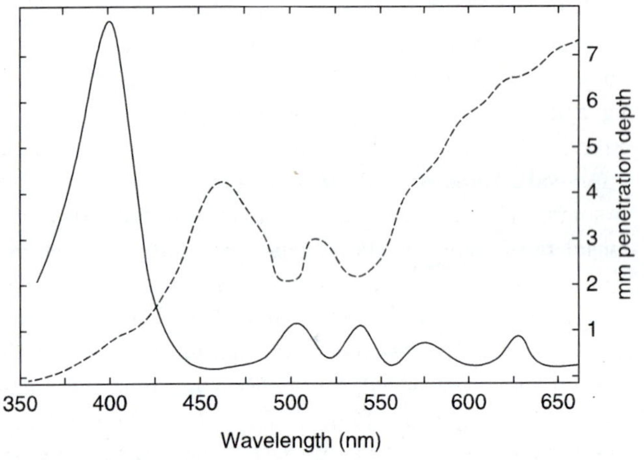

Fig. 30.1 Absorption and penetration depth of porphyrins. __ excitation wavelength. ---penetration depth

30.2.2 Principle of Photodynamic Therapy

Photodynamic therapy utilizes two individually non-toxic components. A photosensitizing chemical called photosensitizer and light are applied in sequence [26].

The first step is local or systemic administration of a photosensitizing drug. This nontoxic photosensitizer is preferably uptaken by the tumor tissue. This targeted lesion is then illuminated with light. Its wavelength corresponds to the absorption spectra of the photosensitizer. Most photosensitizers are activated by several wavelengths. For tumor treatment usually the longest of the wavelengths is used since depth of necrosis correlates with wavelength (Fig. 30.1). The photochemical process is then initiated by illumination of the targeted lesion with light (Fig. 30.2).

In the presence of oxygen molecules various cytotoxic species are generated (e.g. singlet oxygen and other reactive oxygen species). Singlet oxygen is generated by a photochemical process type II (Fig. 30.2). The photosensitizer in its ground state absorbs a photon of light and is thereby boosted into the activated singlet state [27]. This singlet state can fall back in the ground state and light is liberated as fluorescence. For the photodynamic effect the singlet state has to be transformed to the triplet state by intersystem crossing. The likelihood of triplet formation increases with the life-span of the singlet state. The life span of the triplet state (half-life milliseconds) is considerably longer than the life span of the singlet state (<1 μs) since optical transitions to the ground state are rare. This allows contact to a lot of molecules of the surrounding. If the photosensitizer in the triplet state hits another molecule whose ground state is a triple state, energy transfer is possible and both molecules merge

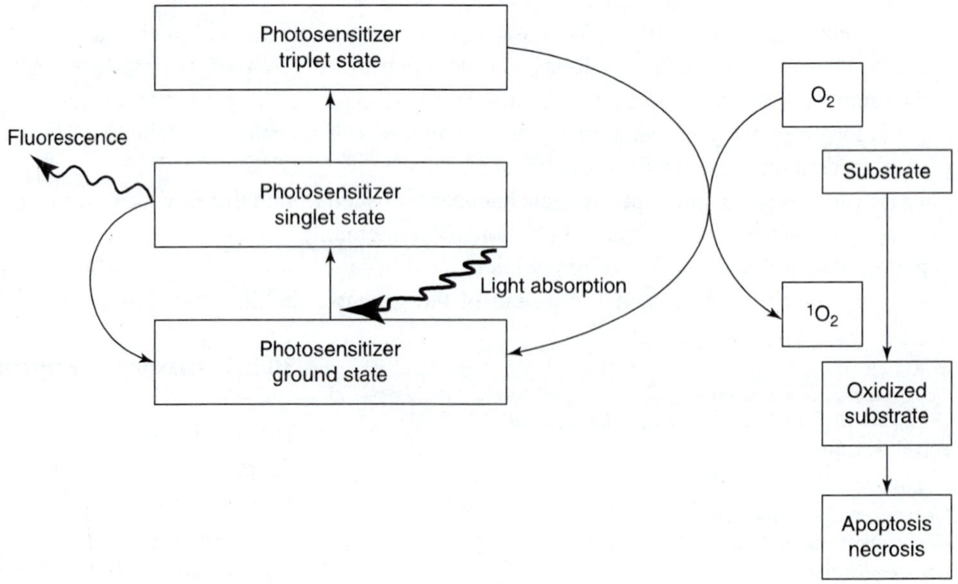

Fig. 30.2 Photochemical reaction type II

to their singlet state. One of the few molecules with a triplet ground state is molecular oxygen. Since the energy of the activated photosensitizer is greater than required for transformation of the oxygen to singlet oxygen, this energy transfer can proceed. The photosensitizer returns to its ground state after transfer of electron energy to the oxygen. Singlet oxygen has a long life span concerning its crossover to the ground state. Due to its responsiveness it is able to oxygenize cell elements. Cellular sites of damage are membranes, mitochondria, microtubules or lysosomes. Quantity and location of photodynamic therapy induced cytotoxic species determine the nature and consequence of photodynamic therapy such as apoptosis and necrosis of tumor cells.

The alternative photochemical reaction type I leads to a direct interaction of the photosensitizer in its triplet state with other biomolecules by electron or hydrogen transfer. This interaction results in generation of free radicals. These radicals can interact with molecular oxygen to form hydroxyl radicals, hydrogen peroxide and superoxide anions [28, 29]. Photochemical reaction type I play a less important role in the mechanism of photodynamic therapy.

Photodynamic therapy also has a vascular "anti-angiogenic" effect. It damages tumor endothelial cells and thus induces the release of vasoactive molecules. This leads to an increase of vascular permeability and also to platelet aggregation, leukocyte adhesion, vessel constriction and blood flow stasis. The consequences are tumor hypoxia and ischemic death of tumor cells via deprivation of oxygen and nutritient [30].

Finally, PDT induces dose-dependent immune responses. At high doses, as applied for tumor treatment, damages of cellular membranes and the blood vessel wall lead to recruitment of neutrophils, monocytes/macrophages and activation of pro-inflammatory cytokines like interleukin IL-1β, IL-2 and tumor necrosis factor TNF-α [31, 32]. This enhancement of the host immune system plays an important role in secondary cytotoxicity and tumor control. Serum IL-6, a bile duct epithelium growth factor correlating with tumor burden in cholangiocarcinoma, decreases after PDT [33].

Since photosensitizers accumulate also in the skin, the major side effect of PDT is cutaneous photosensitivity.

30.3 Photodynamic Therapy for Hilar Cholangiocarcinoma

30.3.1 Photosensitizers

Three types of photosensitizers are currently used for photodynamic therapy in cholangiocarcinoma: Exogenous hematoporphyrin derivates (Photofrin® and Photosan®), the prodrug of an endogenous porphyrin derivate (Gliolan®) and meso-tetrahydroxyphenylchlorine (Foscan®).

The most frequently used photosensitizer is the hematoporphyrin derivate Photofrin® (Axcan Pharma Inc., Mount-Saint-Hilaire, Canada). Human bile duct carcinomas grown in nude mice are highly sensitive to PDT with hematoporphyrin derivates [34]. Hematoporphyrin derivates reduce tumor volume and decrease regrowth rate. Quantitative fluorescence microscopy and digital image analysis has shown that Photofrin® preferentially accumulates in bile duct neoplasm's, reaching peak values during the first 2 days [35]. The ratios of fluorescence in tumour versus normal tissue were 1.7 ± 0.7 and 2.3 ± 1.2 (mean ± SD) at days 1 and 2 after photosensitizer administration, respectively.

Photofrin®, a complex mixture of porphyrin oligomers synthesized from hematoporphyrin dihydrochloride, is supplied as a powder. It is manufactured at a label strength of 75 and 15 mg/vial. The 75 mg/vial is reconstituted with 31.8 ml 0.9 % sodium chloride or 5 % dextrose and each 15 mg/vial with 6.6 ml, respectively. For treatment of cholangiocarcinoma it is administered intravenously at a dosage of 2 mg/kg body weight usually 48 h before laser light illumination. With activation at 630 nm wavelength and an energy dose of 180 J/cm^2, a decrease of tumor thickness between 4 and 6 mm is obtained [2, 36]. The major side effect is skin photosensitization. The photosensitivity reactions are mostly mild to moderate with erythema. Swelling, pruritus, burning sensation, blisters, increased hair growth, skin discoloration, skin nodules and increased skin fragility occur seldomly and only if reasonable precautions for light exposure are not taken. Patients should be advised to stay indoors, away from bright light, for 3~4 days and then can cautiously increase exposure to sunlight. Strong sunlight has to be avoided for 4~6 weeks. No interaction studies of Photofrin® and other drugs have been performed. However, it is possible that other photosensitizing agents (e.g. tetracyclines, sulfonamides, phenotiazines, sulfonylurea, hypoglycemic agents, thiazide diuretics, griseofulvin and fluoroquinolones) could increase the risk of photosensitivity reactions. Therefore, these drugs should, if possible, be avoided during the first 7 days of photodynamic therapy.

Compounds that quench active oxygen species or scavenge radicals, such as dimethly sulfoxide, β-carotene, ethanol, formate and mannitol can be expected to decrease photodynamic therapy activity. Preclinical data also suggest that allopurinol, calcium channel blockers and some prostaglandin synthesis inhibitors could interfere with Photofrin® therapy. Furthermore, drugs that decrease clotting, vasoconstriction or platelet aggregation e.g. thromboxane A 2 inhibitors could decrease the efficacy of photodynamic therapy. Glucocorticoids given before or concomitant with photodynamic therapy are known to decrease the effect.

Other rare side effects reported are mild constipation, coughing, nausea, pain/swelling at injection site, mood changes (e.g. anxiety), fever and tachycardia.

Photodynamic therapy with Photofrin® displays a safe profile even with a second treatment session within 45 days [37].

Another hematoporphyrin derivate used is Photosan® (SeeLab, Wesselburneerkoog, Germany) [38, 39]. So far the excitation wavelength used, drug dosage and the dose-light interval was the same as with Photofrin®. However, light dosage was slightly different with 200 J/cm length of stenosis. Reported side effects are similar to those with Photofrin®. Additionally, a metallic taste, liver-toxicity and anaphylaxis are reported with Photosan® [40].

Delta-aminolevulinic acid (Gliolan®, Medac, Hamburg, Germany), an amino acid produced in every nucleated cell, is a prodrug [41]. Delta-aminolevulinic acid is a precursor of heme, and its enzymatic conversion to protoporphyrin IX is regulated by feedback inhibition. Following administration of an excess of exogenous delta-aminolaevulinic acid the natural regulatory mechanism is bypassed. Protoporphyrin IX accumulates, since the enzyme ferrochelatase, catalyzing chelation of ferrous ion into the protoporphyrin molecule, is decreased in malignant tissue. Endogenously generated protoporphyrin IX is an excellent photosensitizing agent. Delta-aminolevulinic acid accumulates also in bile duct tumor cell lines [42].

For treatment of cholangiocarcinoma, a drug dose of 60 mg/kg bodyweight is administered orally in orange juice. The activation wave length is the same as with the exogenous porphyrins, namely 630 nm. Light dose used was 200 J/cm^2 [43]. Photosensitivity plays a minor role with Gliolan® lasting only 1~2 days. Other systemic side effects, such as abnormal liver function, hypotension, and vomiting, can occur. Due to a penetration depth of less than 2 mm it cannot be recommended for the treatment of cholangiocarcinoma.

Another photosensitizing agent is meso-tetrahydroxyphenyl chlorine (mTHPC, temoporfin, Foscan®, Biolitec AG, Jena, Germany). The solvent- based formulation mTHPC (Foscan®) as well as a liposomal (water soluble) formulation (Foslip®, Biolitec AG, Jena, Germany) turned both out to be potent photosensitizing agents killing about 90 % of cholangiocarcinoma cancer cells [44]. Cell lines with low cytokeratin-19, high vimentin and high proliferative phenotype preferentially show higher uptake of mTHPC [45].

In cholangiocarcinoma, photoactivation is performed with non-thermal light at 652 nm 72 h after intravenous administration of 0.15 mg/kg body weight of Foscan® [46]. Photosensitivity is gradually getting back to normal after day 15 onward and people will be able to go back to their normal routine light exposure by day 22. As with porphyrins there is a potential for exacerbation of skin photosensitivity if other photosensitizing agents are administered. Such a reaction has been reported with topical 5-fluorouracil. Other reported side effects are: injection site pain, pain sensation in the treated tumor area, hemorrhage, fever, constipation, vomiting, anemia, nausea and giddiness.

Phototoxicity is 100~200 times stronger than with Photofrin® leading to deeper tumor necrosis.

30.3.2 Technical Aspects of PDT in Hilar Cholangiocarcinoma

Lasers light producing high energy monochromatic light of a specific wavelength is used for intraluminal illumination. As light source, an argon dye laser or diode lasers can be used. Up until now cylindrical diffuser fibers have been used to deliver light to the target side. Theoretically, balloon diffusers could be used as well. Fibers can be positioned into the bile duct strictures with the help of a standard cannula or a cholangioscope [47, 48]. Even and circumferential illumination is only obtained when the fiber is not covered by the cannula or an endoprosthesis. For adequate positioning the cylindrical laser diffuser should be equipped with radiopaque markers. In Europe, fibers specifically designed for PDT in the bile duct are available. Plastic fibers (Medlight SA, Ecublens, Switzerland) can be smoothly introduced into the bile duct, whereas intubation is more difficult with the quartz fibers (Ceram Optec, Bonn, Germany). In the United States only quartz fibers for the esophagus (Fibers Direct, Andover, MA) are approved by the US Food and Drug Administration (FDA). Due to the stiffness of the esophageal fibers breakage has been a problem and treatment could generally only be performed in the main hepatic ducts. Light doses used for PDT in the bile duct ranged between 154 and 242 J/cm^2. Photoactivation is often performed under continuous saline perfusion and concurrent oxygen administration (4 l/min) via a nasal catheter [47, 48]. However, the effect of these additional measurements has not been evaluated and needs further investigation.

After PDT, plastic endoprosthesis are inserted to ensure biliary drainage. PDT can also be performed through metal stents [39, 46, 49, 50] and percutaneously [47, 51]. However, it has to be taken into account that metal threads and joints of the stent cause a shadow effect leading to light absorption, thereby diminishing efficacy [50]. Therefore, light dose has to be adjusted to counteract the reduction of light transmittance caused by the metal stent. Since the endoluminal light irradiation is often carried out at the maximal power output allowed for the diffuser fiber, the light irradiation time has to be adjusted to compensate for the reduction of light transmittance caused by the stent materials.

30.3.3 Photodynamic Therapy as Palliative Treatment for Nonresectable Hilar Cholangiocarcinoma

The first hint that photodynamic therapy may be a treatment option for advanced nonresectbale hilar cholangiocarcinoma (Table 30.1) came from uncontrolled studies [43, 46, 47,

Table 30.1 Uncontrolled trials of photodynamic therapy in nonresectable hilar cholangiocarcinoma

Author	Photosensitizer	Median survival time
Ortner et al. [47]	Photofrin®	439 days
Berr et al. [52]	Photofrin®	330 days
Rumalla et al. [53]	Photofrin®	Not reported
Zoepf et al. [43]	Gliolan®	Not reported
Harewood et al. [54]	Photofrin®	276 days
Shim CS et al. [51]	Photofrin®	558 days
Pereira et al. [46]	Foscan®	Not reported

52–54]. In all trials with haematoporphyrin derivates and the trial with mTHPC tumor regression and bile duct recanalization was seen after PDT.

Thirty-day mortality between 0 % and 16 %, procedure related mortality of 0, median survival time between 276 and 558 days, 6 month survival times between 89 % and 91 % and 1-year survival between 45 % and 78 % were remarkably good.

Observed side effects with Photofrin® were phototoxicity (4~25 %), stenosis (0~10 %), cholangitis (0~25 %), bilioma (0.3 %), abscess formation (0.2 %), biliary leakage (0.2 %) and hemobilia (2 %). With Gliolan® cholangitis was observed in 50 % of patients and hypotension in 25 % and with Foscan® cholangitis in 15 %, gallbladder emypema in 8 %, liver abscesses in 8 % and hemobilia in 15 %.

In one retrospective trial [49], metal stent insertion plus photodynamic therapy was compared with a historical control group treated with metal stents alone. The authors did not observe a beneficial effect of PDT. This failure of photodynamic therapy could be caused by insufficient drainage in the photodynamic therapy group, since in only 45 % of patients with hilar cholangiocarcinomas, two metal stents could be inserted. Another explanation could be that light dose was not adjusted to the reduction of light transmittance caused by the stent materials. The incomplete follow-up data of the historical controls is a further problem of this trial.

All other comparative trials showed a survival advantage for photodynamic therapy (Table 30.2). A recently published paper [39] from the same group demonstrated a survival advantage of photodynamic therapy compared to bilateral metal stenting alone. In one prospective trial endoprosthesis alone were compared with endoprosthesis plus photodynamic therapy [55] and another retrospective analysis demonstrated that photodynamic therapy can also be successfully applied percutaneously [56]. One year survival was 28 % with percutaneous drainage only (n = 20) and 52 % ($P < 0.05$) with additional photodynamic therapy (n = 27).

A large retrospective study [2] analyzed the outcome of 184 patients with hilar cholangiocarcinoma treated with either surgery, stenting alone or stenting with photodynamic therapy. Survival was longer after additional photodynamic therapy (Table 30.2). Photodynamic therapy and stenting resulted in lower serum bilirubin levels and better quality of life compared with stenting alone. Survival was similar after photodynamic therapy (360 days) and after incomplete resection (R1/R2) (366 days), although patients in whom photodynamic therapy was performed had more advanced tumor stages and higher Bismuth grades at inclusion. Best survival time was reported with R0 resection (684 days).

In a recent retrospective trial these results were confirmed [11]. It was shown that palliative photodynamic therapy resulted in survival similar to those with curatively intended R1/R2 resection, despite the fact that photodynamic therapy patients had more advanced tumor stages, higher Bismuth grades and were older. In patients undergoing attempted curative surgery the median survival time was 570 days compared with 360 days for photodynamic therapy, 240 days for radio/chemotherapy and 90 days for patients who received no additional treatment other than biliary drainage. One-year survival was 87 %, 69 %, 55 %, 51 %, 37 % and 20 % for R0 resection, attempted curative resection, R1/R2 resection, photodynamic therapy, chemo-and/or radiotherapy and biliary drainage only groups, respectively.

A prospective clinical cohort study [57] has demonstrated that radical surgery (mean survival 1,278 days) and palliative photodynamic therapy with Photofrin® (mean survival 512 days) are associated with an increased survival in patients with hilar cholangiocarcinoma compared to stent and chemotherapy (mean survival 173 days, $P < 0.0001$).

Two prospective randomised trials [38, 48], comparing PDT and endoprosthesis insertion with endoprosthesis insertion alone, confirmed the encouraging results of the pilot studies and comparative trials (Table 30.3).

In the first study 39 patients with large (<3 cm) advanced hilar tumors were included [48]. Exclusion criteria were porpyhria, previous chemo-or radiotherapy, recent use of photosensitizing or dermatotoxic drugs, prior insertion of metal stent, peritoneal carcinomatosis and diagnostic ERCP more than 1 month previously. Antioxidant products and bile stimulating herbal medicines interacting with the PDT effects were withheld from the 7th days before to the 7th days after photosensitizer administration.

Median survival times was 498 days with additional photodynamic therapy with Photofrin® (n = 20) and 98 days ($P < 0.0001$) with endoprosthesis insertion only (n = 19). Only patients with a bilirubin decrease of less than 50 % after successful stenting were included into the study. PDT relieved jaundice in these patients and improved quality of life. Enrollment was limited to patients with unsuccessful drainage, and this was criticized as a bias.

In a second randomised trial 32 unselected patients with less advanced non-resectable cholangiocarcinoma the survival advantage was confirmed [38]. The photosensitizer Photosan® was administered. Median survival was 630 days

Table 30.2 Retrospective trials comparing photodynamic therapy (PDT) plus drainage with drainage alone in nonresectable hilar cholangiocarcinoma

Author	Photosensitizer	Survival time PDT plus drainage versus drainage alone	P
Dumoulin et al. [49]	Photofrin®	Median 297 vs. 168 days	ns
Gerhardt et al. [39]	Photosan®	Median 495 vs. 369 days	<0.005
Kahaleh et al. [55]	Photofrin®	Mean 396 vs. 222 days	<0.004
Cheon et al. [56]	Photofrin®	Median 558 vs. 288 days	<0.05
Witzigmann et al. [2]	Photofrin®	Median 360 vs. 192 days	<0.01
Matull et al. [11]	Photofrin®	Median 360 vs. 90 days	<0.05

Table 30.3 Randomised trials comparing photodynamic therapy and endoprostheses versus endoprostheses alone as treatment for nonresectable hilar cholangiocarcinoma

Author	Photosensitizer	Median survival time Photodynamic therapy plus endoprostheses versus endoprostheses alone	P
Ortner et al. [48]	Photofrin®	498 vs. 98 days	<0.0001
Zopef et al. [38]	Photosan®	630 vs. 210 days	<0.05

with additional photodynamic therapy and 210 days with endoprosthesis alone ($P=0.019$).

In the first randomised trial patient's quality of life was poor at study entry and improved after PDT, whereas in the second trial patient's performance status was normal from the beginning and did not improve further. Only few specific side effects occurred in both trials (stenosis 0~10 %, photosensitivity 0~10 %). No difference in cholangitis rate was observed between the PDT and endoprosthesis only group. Hemobilia was observed in one patient.

The presence of a visible mass on imaging studies and increasing time between diagnosis and PDT predicted a poorer survival rate after PDT [58]. Photodynamic therapy should be performed within the first month after diagnosis [47, 48].

Repeat photodynamic therapy is safe [37] and effective. Local response defined as opening of more than 50 % of occluded segmental bile ducts, after the first, second, third and fourth PDT are 75 %, 70 %,58 %, and 50 %, respectively [2].

Multimodality strategies with chemotherapy and radiotherapy are feasible and well tolerated [36, 59]. However, at the moment it is unclear if combined treatment modalities prolong survival further.

30.3.4 Photodynamic Therapy for Recurrent Tumor After Resection or as Neoadjuvant Treatment

A small uncontrolled study showed marked destruction of the recurrent tumor with 75 % of patients disease free after 2-year [60].

Neoadjuvant PDT was evaluated in seven patients with advanced Bismuth type III and IV carcinoma which were thought to be unresectable after staging [61]. After PDT a curative resection could be performed in all patients; 83 % were recurrence free after 1- and 5-year survival was 71 %. No relevant side effects of PDT occurred except for a minor intraoperative phototoxicity in one patient.

Conclusion

PDT is the first palliative treatment option that has shown its efficacy in patients with nonresectable biliary cancer in two randomised prospective studies. PDT improves survival, jaundice and quality of life, is well tolerated and can be repeated without losing its efficacy. PDT can be combined with radiotherapy and chemotherapy. It has, however, to be shown if multimodality strategies improve survival further. PDT for recurrent tumors after surgery and neoadjuvant PDT is still experimental.

References

1. Jarnagin WR, Fong Y, DeMatteo RP, et al. Staging, resectability, and outcome in 225 patients with hilar cholangiocarcinoma. Ann Surg. 2001;234:507–19.
2. Witzigmann H, Berr F, Ringel U, et al. Surgical and palliative management and outcome in 184 patients with hilar cholangiocarcinoma: palliative photodynamic therapy plus stenting is comparable to R1/R2 resection. Ann Surg. 2006;244:230–9.
3. Neuhaus P, Jonas S, Settmacher U, et al. Surgical management of proximal bile duct cancer: extended right lobe resection increases resectability and radicality. Langenbecks Arch Surg. 2003;388: 194–200.
4. Otto G, Romaneehsen B, Hoppe-Lotichius M, et al. Hilar cholangiocarcinoma: resectability and radicality after routine diagnostic imaging. J Hepatobiliary Pancreat Surg. 2004;11:310–8.
5. Ristagno N, Knuth A, Pestalozzi BC. Is an aggressive surgical approach worthwhile in biliary cancer? Int Semin Surg Oncol. 2007;4:26–35.
6. Ballinger AB, McHugh M, Catnach SM, et al. Symptom relief and quality of life after stenting for malignant bile duct obstruction. Gut. 1994;35:467–70.
7. Robson PC, Heffernan N, Gonen M, et al. Prospective study of outcomes after percutaneous biliary drainage for malignant biliary obstruction. Ann Surg Oncol. 2010;17:2303–11.

8. Abraham NS, Barkun JS, Barkun AN. Palliation of malignant biliary obstruction: a prospective trial examining impact on quality of life. Gastrointest Endosc. 2002;56:835–41.
9. Sut M, Kennedy R, McNamee J, et al. Long-term results of percutaneous transhepatic cholangiographic drainage for palliation of malignant biliary obstruction. J Palliat Med. 2010;13:1311–3.
10. Mihalache F, Tantau M, Diaconu B, et al. Survival and quality of life of cholangiocarcinoma patients: a prospective study over a 4 year period. J Gastrointestin Liver Dis. 2010;19:285–90.
11. Matull WR, Dhar DK, Ayaru L, et al. R0 but not R1/R2 resection is associated with better survival than palliative photodynamic therapy in biliary tract cancer. Liver Int. 2011;31:99–107.
12. Farley DR, Weaver A, Nagorney DM. "Natural history" of unresected cholangiocarcinoma: patient outcome after noncurative intervention. Mayo Clin Proc. 1995;70:425–9.
13. Prat F, Chapat O, Ducot B, et al. Predictive factors for survival of patients with inoperable malignant distal biliary strictures: a practical management guideline. Gut. 1998;42:76–80.
14. Chang WH, Kortan P, Haber GB. Outcome in patients with bifurcation tumors who undergo unilateral versus bilateral hepatic duct drainage. Gastrointest Endosc. 1998;47:354–62.
15. Kassis M, Boyer J, Dumas R, et al. Plastic or metals stents for malignant stricture of the common bile duct? Results of a randomised prospective study. Gastrointest Endosc. 2002;57:178–82.
16. Glimelius B, Hoffman K, Sjoden PO, et al. Chemotherapy improves survival and quality of life in advanced pancreatic and biliary cancer. Ann Oncol. 1996;7:593–600.
17. Koeberle D, Saletti P, Borner M, et al. Patient-reported outcome of patients with advanced biliary tract cancers receiving gemcitabine plus capecitabine: a multicenter, phase II trial of the Swiss Group for Clinical Cancer Research. J Clin Oncol. 2008;26:3702–8.
18. Eckel F, Schmid RM. Chemotherapy in advanced biliary tract carcinoma: a pooled analysis of clinical trials. Br J Cancer. 2007;96: 896–902.
19. Valle J, Wasan H, Palmer DH, et al. Cisplatin plus gemcitabene versus gemcitabine for biliary tract cancer. N Engl J Med. 2010;362:1273–81.
20. Bowling TE, Galbraith SM, Hatfield ARW, et al. A retrospective comparison of endoscopic stenting alone with stenting and radiotherapy in non-resectable cholangiocarcinoma. Gut. 1996;39: 852–5.
21. Valek V, Kysela P, Kala Z, et al. Brachytherapy and percutaneous stenting in the treatment of cholangiocarcinoma: a prospective randomised study. Eur J Radiol. 2007;62:175–9.
22. Momm F, Schubert E, Henne K, et al. Stereotactic fractionated radiotherapy for Klatskin tumors. Radiother Oncol. 2010;95: 99–102.
23. Kopek N, Holt MI, Hansen AT, et al. Stereotactic body radiotherapy for unresectable cholangiocarcinoma. Radiother Oncol. 2010;94:47–52.
24. Lipson RL, Baldes EJ, Olsen AM. The use of a derivative of hematoporphyrin in tumor detection. J Natl Cancer Inst. 1961;26: 1–11.
25. Kato H, Katwaguchi M, Konako C. Evaluation of PDT in gastric cancer. Laser Med Sci. 1986;1:67–74.
26. Huang Z, Xu H, Meyers AD, et al. Photodynamic therapy for treatment of solid tumor potential and technical challenges. Technol Cancer Res Treat. 2008;7:309–20.
27. Foote CS. Definition of type I and type II photosensitized oxidation. Photochem Photobiol. 1991;54:659.
28. Buettner GR, Need MJ. Hydrogen peroxide and hydroxyl fee radical production by hematoporpyhrin derivate, ascorbate and light. Cancer Lett. 1985;25:297–304.
29. Athar MCA, Elmets CA, Bickers DR, et al. A novel mechanism for the generation of superperoxide anions in hematoporphyrin derivative-mediated cutaneous photosensitization: activation of the xanthine oxidase pathway. J Clin Invest. 1989;8:1137–43.
30. Abels C. Targeting the vascular system of solid tumors by photodynamic therapy (PDT). Photochem Photobiol Sci. 2004;3:765–71.
31. Nowis D, Stoklosa T, Legat M, et al. The influence of photodynamic therapy on the immune response. Photodiagn Photodyn Ther. 2005;2:283–98.
32. Castano AP, Mroz P, Hamblin MR. Photodynamic therapy and antitumor immunity. Nat Rev Cancer. 2006;6:535–45.
33. Cheon YK, Cho YD, Moon JH, et al. Diagnostic utility of interleukin-6 (IL-6) for primary bile duct cancer and changes in serum IL-6 levels following photodynamic therapy. Am J Gastroenterol. 2007;102:2164–70.
34. Kee W, Song LM, Wang KK, et al. Mono-l-aspartat chlorine e67 (Npe6) and haematoporphyrin derivate (HpD) in photodynamic therapy administered to a human cholangiocarcinoma model. Cancer. 1998;82:421–7.
35. Pahernik SA, Dellian M, Berr F, et al. Distribution and pharmacokinetics of Photofrin® in human bile duct cancer. J Photochem Photobiol B Biol. 1998;47:58–62.
36. Baisden JM, Kahaleh M, Weiss GR, et al. Multimodality treatment with helical tomotherapy intensity modulated radiotherapy and photodynamic therapy is feasible and well tolerated in patients with hilar cholangiocarcinoma. Gastrointestin Cancer Res. 2008;2:219–24.
37. Pereira SP, Ayaru L, Ackroyd R, et al. The pharmacokinetics and safety of porfimer after repeated administration 30–45 days apart to patients undergoing photodynamic therapy. Aliment Pharmacol Ther. 2010;32:821–7.
38. Zoepf T, Jakobs R, Arnold JC, et al. Palliation of nonresectable bile duct cancer: improved survival after photodynamic therapy. Am J Gastroenterol. 2005;100:2426–30.
39. Gerhardt T, Rings D, Hoeblinger J, et al. Combination of bilateral metal stenting and trans-stent photodynamic therapy for palliative treatment of hilar cholangiocarcinoma. Z Gastroenterol. 2010; 48:28–32.
40. Ofner JG, Schloegle H, Kostron H. Unusual adverse reaction in a patient sensitized with Photosan 3. J Photochem Photobiol B. 1996;36:183–4.
41. Kennedy JC, Pottier RH, Kennedy JC, et al. Endogenous protoporpyhrin IX: a clinical useful photosensitizer for photodynamic therapy. J Photochem Photobiol B. 1992;36:205–7.
42. Neumann J, Brandsch M. (Delta)-aminolaevulinic acid transport in cancer cells of the human extraheaptic biliary duct. J Pharmacol Exp Ther. 2003;305:219–24.
43. Zoepf T, Jakobs R, Rosenbaum A, et al. Photodynamic therapy with 5-aminolevulinic acid is not effective in bile duct cancer. Gastrointest Endosc. 2001;54:763–4.
44. Kiesslich T, Berland J, Plaetzer K, et al. Comparative characterization of the efficiency and cellular pharmacokinetics of Foscan- and Foslip-based photodynamic treatment in human biliary tract cancer cell lines. Photochem Photobiol Sci. 2007;6:619–27.
45. Kiesslich T, Neureiter D, Alinger B, et al. Uptake and phototoxicity of meso-tetrahydroxyphenyl chlorine are highly variable in human biliary tract cancer cell lines and correlate with markers of differentiation and proliferation. Photochem Photobiol Sci. 2010;9:734–43.
46. Peireira SP, Ayaru L, Rogowska A, et al. Photodynamic therapy of malignant biliary stricture using meso-tetrahydroxyphenylchlorin. Eur J Gastroenterol Hepatol. 2007;19:479–85.
47. Ortner MA, Liebetruth J, Schreiber S, et al. Photodynamic therapy of nonresectable cholangiocarcinoma. Gastroenterology. 1998;114: 536–42.
48. Ortner MA, Caca K, Berr F, et al. Successful photodynamic therapy for nonresectable cholangiocarcinoma: a randomised prospective study. Gastroenterology. 2003;125:1355–63.

49. Dumoulin FL, Horst E, Sauerbruch T, et al. Phase II study of photodynamic therapy and metal stent as palliative treatment for nonresectable hilar cholangiocarcinoma. Gastrointest Endosc. 2003;57:860–7.
50. Wang LW, Li LB, Li ZS, et al. Self-expandable metal stents and trans-stent light delivery: are metal stents and photodynamic therapy compatible? Lasers Surg Med. 2008;40:651–9.
51. Shim CS, Cheon YK, Cha SW, et al. Prospective study of the effectiveness of percutaneous transhepatic photodynamic therapy for advanced bile duct cancer and the role of intraductal ultrasonography in response assessment. Endoscopy. 2005;37:425–33.
52. Berr F, Wiedmann M, Tannapfel, et al. Photodynamic therapy for advanced bile duct cancer: evidence for improved palliation and extended survival. Hepatology. 2000;31:291–8.
53. Rumalla A, Baron TH, Wang KK, et al. Endoscopic application of photodynamic therapy for cholangiocarcinoma. Gastrointest Endosc. 2001;53:500–4.
54. Harewood GC, Baron TH, Rumalla A, et al. Pilot study to assess patient outcomes following endoscopic application of photodynamic therapy for advanced cholangiocarcinoma. J Gastroenterol Hepatol. 2005;20:415–20.
55. Kahaleh M, Mishra R, Shami VM, et al. Unresectable cholangiocarcinoma: comparison of survival in biliary stenting alone vs. stenting with photodynamic therapy. Clin Gastroenterol Hepatol. 2008;6:290–7.
56. Cheon YK, Cho YD, Baek SH, et al. Comparison of survival of advanced hilar cholangiocarcinoma after biliary drainage alone versus photodynamic therapy with external drainage. Korean J Gastroenterol. 2004;44:280–7.
57. Quyn AJ, Ziyaie D, Polignano FM, et al. Photodynamic therapy is associated with an improvement in survival in patients with irresectable hilar cholangiocraincoma. HPB (Oxford). 2009;11:570–7.
58. Prasad GA, Wang KK, Baron TH, et al. Factors associated with increased survival after photodynamic therapy for cholangiocarcinoma. Clin Gastroenterol Hepatol. 2007;5:743–8.
59. Fuks D, Bartoli E, Delceuserie R, et al. Biliary drainage, photodynamic therapy, chemotherapy for unresectable cholangiocarcinoma with jaundice. J Gastroenterol Hepatol. 2009;24:1745–52.
60. Nanashima A, Yamaguchi H, Shibasaki S, et al. Adjuvant photodynamic therapy for bile duct carcinoma after surgery: a preliminary study. J Gastroenterol. 2004;39:1095–101.
61. Wiedmann M, Caca K, Berr F, et al. Neoadjuvant photodynamic therapy as a new approach to treating hilar cholangiocarcinoma. Cancer. 2003;97:2783–90.

Radiation and Chemotherapy

31

H.A. Pitt and A. Nakeeb

31.1 Introduction

Cholangiocarcinoma is an uncommon tumor that may occur anywhere along the intrahepatic or extrahepatic biliary tree. In the United States approximately 5,000 cholangiocarcinomas are diagnosed per year while many more biliary malignancies occur in Asia. The hepatic duct bifurcation is the most frequently involved site, and approximately 50–70 % of cholangiocarcinomas are found in this perihilar region [1]. The role of radiation therapy, chemoradiation and chemotherapy as adjuvants to surgical resection in patients with perihilar cholangiocarcinoma remains controversial. Aggressive surgical resection obtaining a negative microscopic margin offers the only chance for long-term survival. However, many patients will only be candidates for nonoperative stenting or palliative surgery aimed to provide biliary drainage and prevent cholangitis and hepatic failure. Radiation therapy, chemoradiation and/or chemotherapy also can be used in these patients with nonresectable disease in an attempt to palliate symptoms and extend survival.

Five-year survivals of 30–40 % have been reported for perihilar cholangiocarcinomas in the subset of patients that can be resected with negative microscopic margins [1–12]. Despite recent advances in radiological imaging and improved staging of perihilar cholangiocarcinoma, in most series approximately half of the tumors are resectable at the time of exploration. In patients undergoing potentially curative resection for hilar cholangiocarcinomas local-regional recurrence is found approximately 60 % of the time while distant metastases are seen with or without local recurrence in almost 40 % [13]. Therefore, many authorities recommend the addition of adjuvant radiation, chemoradiation or chemotherapy for patients with resected perihilar cholangiocarcinoma.

31.2 Radiation Therapy

Initially, bile duct tumors were thought to be radioresistant, but several studies have shown that radiotherapy can palliate symptoms and may contribute to improvement in survival. Ionizing radiation likely acts by the production of free radicals that cause damage to deoxyribonucleic acid (DNA) resulting in double-stranded DNA breaks. These DNA lesions are unable to be repaired or are repaired inadequately in tumor tissue; and as a result, the malignant cells are unable to divide. Therapeutic gain is achieved by the difference in repair capacity and fidelity of repair of DNA lesions in tumor as opposed to normal tissue. Radiotherapy is delivered as a fractionated daily dose allowing normal tissue to repair DNA damage between treatments. Tumors repair this damage less well. Factors which limit the usefulness of radiotherapy in bile duct tumors include the inherent sensitivity of tumors to radiation, hypoxic radioresistant regions within tumor, the repopulation of surviving tumor cells, and the initial number of viable tumor cells in the resected field.

Radiation therapy has been evaluated in patients with cholangiocarcinoma using a variety of methods including external beam radiotherapy, intraoperative radiotherapy, internal radiotherapy, radioimmunotherapy, and charged particle radiation. External beam radiotherapy has been the most commonly used modality and is typically administered to a total dose of 45–60 Gy. Internal radiotherapy is normally delivered through either percutaneous or endoscopically placed biliary stents using iridium-192 as the radiation source. Total radiation doses may vary from 20 to 60 Gy up to 1 cm from the source. Radioimmunotherapy has also been performed with iodine-131 anti-CEA.

H.A. Pitt, MD (✉)
Temple University Health System,
Philadelphia, PA 19190
e-mail: hapitt@iupui.edu, henry.pitt@tuhs.temple.edu

A. Nakeeb, MD
Department of Surgery, Indiana University,
Indianapolis, IN, USA
e-mail: anakeeb@iupui.edu

W.Y. Lau (ed.), *Hilar Cholangiocarcinoma*,
DOI 10.1007/978-94-007-6473-6_31,

Several retrospective analyses have suggested that radiation therapy augments survival in patients with perihilar cholangiocarcinoma. In an analysis from Japan, Todoroki and colleagues [14] examined 63 patients who underwent resection of a perihilar cholangiocarcinoma. Twenty-one patients underwent resection alone, and 42 patients received adjuvant radiation therapy. Intraoperative radiation therapy (IORT) alone was given to 12 patients (mean dose 21.0±0.6 Gy), eight patients were treated with postoperative radiation therapy (PORT) (mean dose 43.6±1.4 Gy) and 22 patients received both IORT and PORT. The local-regional control rate was significantly better in the adjuvant therapy group compared to the resection alone group, 80 % vs. 31 % respectively. The actuarial 5-year survival also was significantly better in the resection+IORT+PORT group (39.2 %) compared to the resection alone group (13.5 %).

A 2003 report from the Academic Medical Center in Amsterdam [15] examined 91 patients with resected hilar cholangiocarcinoma. Twenty patients had no adjuvant radiation therapy, 30 patients had external beam radiotherapy (46.0±11.3 Gy), and 41 patients had combination external beam therapy (42.3±4.9 Gy) and intraluminal brachytherapy with Iridium seeds (10.4±1.7 Gy). Overall median survival was significantly longer in patients treated with adjuvant radiotherapy than in those who underwent resection without additional radiotherapy (24 vs. 8 months). The combination of external radiation and brachytherapy did not result in longer survival than external irradiation alone (21 and 30 months, respectively).

In many of these retrospective reports, patients receiving radiotherapy tended to have more favorable, often resectable tumors, and were relatively fit. These radiated patients, expected to have good outcomes, have been compared with patients with unresectable tumors, metastatic disease, or poor performance status who did not receive radiotherapy. Thus, the fact that patients receiving radiotherapy in these analyses have survived longer is not surprising. However, Sagawa and his Japanese colleagues [16] were unable to demonstrate any benefit for adjuvant radiation therapy after surgery in 69 patients with hilar cholangiocarcinoma.

To more objectively assess the benefit, if any, of adjuvant radiotherapy, we have previously reported the results of a prospective trial of adjuvant radiation therapy for patients with operable perihilar cholangiocarcinoma at the Johns Hopkins Hospital [17]. All patients were surgically staged and found to have cholangiocarcinoma localized to the perihilar biliary tree, with no evidence of intraperitoneal or distant metastases. All patients had histological confirmation of malignancy. Patients were included with either resected or unresected tumor, but were stratified on the basis of extent of resection. A Karnofsky Performance Status of at least 60 at the time of hospital discharge was required for inclusion. In addition, patients had to be fit to begin radiation therapy within 8 weeks after surgery.

During the 5-year study period, 50 patients were evaluated, whereas 34 were excluded. Radiation ranged from 45 to 63 Gy and consisted of external beam plus iridium-I92 seeds for resected patients and external beam plus cone down port for palliated patients. None of the patients received adjuvant chemotherapy. Patients undergoing curative resection survived significantly longer than patients undergoing operative palliation. Among 31 resected patients, radiation had no effect on mean (24 vs. 24 months), median, or actuarial survival. Similarly, among 19 palliated patients radiation had no effect on mean (10 vs. 13 months), median, or actuarial survival. Thus, for all 50 patients, adjuvant radiation therapy had no effect on overall survival (Fig. 31.1). Moreover, multivariate analysis identified resection as the only positive predictive factor for prolonged survival.

31.3 Chemoradiation

Combinations of chemotherapy with radiation have been attempted for many localized tumors. The benefit of combining chemotherapeutic agents with radiosensitizing properties such as 5-FU, mitomycin C, and cisplatin with radiation has been demonstrated with several gastrointestinal tumor types but not for biliary tract cancers. Nevertheless, chemoradiation has been applied to patients with cholangiocarcinoma at several centers. In general, these regimens are well tolerated; however, the number of patients has been small, both resected and unresected patients have been treated, and no control patients have been included. In a 2001 report from the University of South Florida, Serafini et al. [18] found no benefit for chemoradiation.

In another retrospective review Kim et al. [19] used adjuvant external beam radiotherapy (40 Gy) combined with concomitant bolus 5-FU (500 mg/m^2) chemotherapy for the first 3 days of each 2 weeks of radiation in 84 patients with extrahepatic cholangiocarcinoma. Monthly maintenance chemotherapy with 5-FU (500 mg/m^2, first 5 days of the month) was then administered for 1 year. The overall 5-year actuarial survival rate was 31 %. When patients were stratified by residual tumor, the 5-year survival rate was 36 % for patients with negative microscopic margins at the time of resection, 35 % for patients with positive microscopic margins, and zero for patients with gross residual disease. However, the 5-year actuarial survival was only 14 % overall for the subgroup with perihilar tumors. Thus, these results with adjuvant chemoradiation did not differ significantly from other reports of surgery alone.

In 2002 we reported 140 patients with biliary malignancies managed at the Medical College of Wisconsin over a

Fig. 31.1 Actuarial survival for 50 patients with perihilar cholangiocarcinoma with (n=23) and without (n=27) adjuvant radiation therapy (XRT) (From Pitt et al. [17])

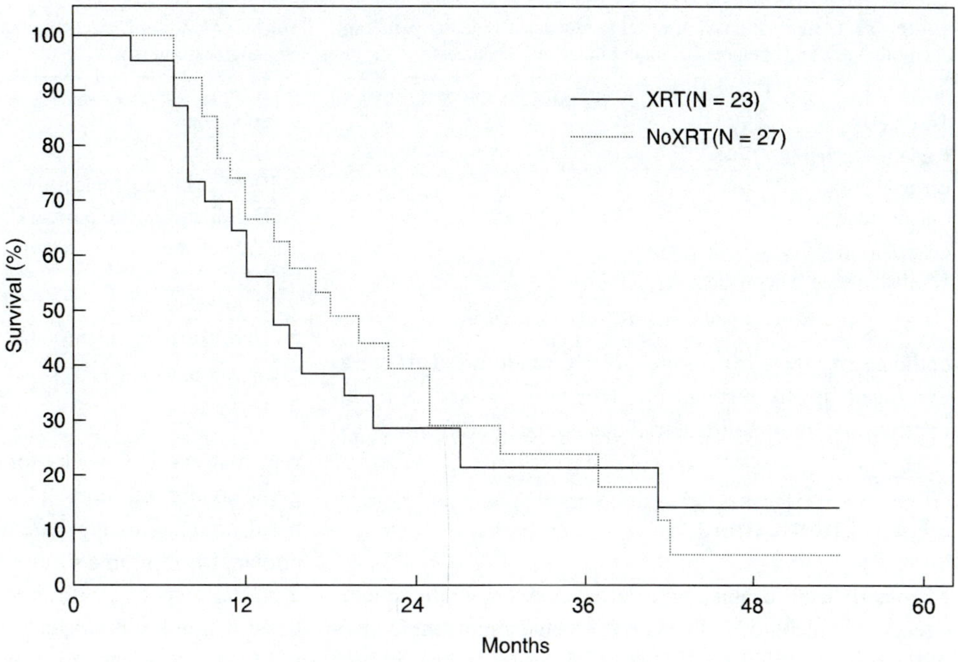

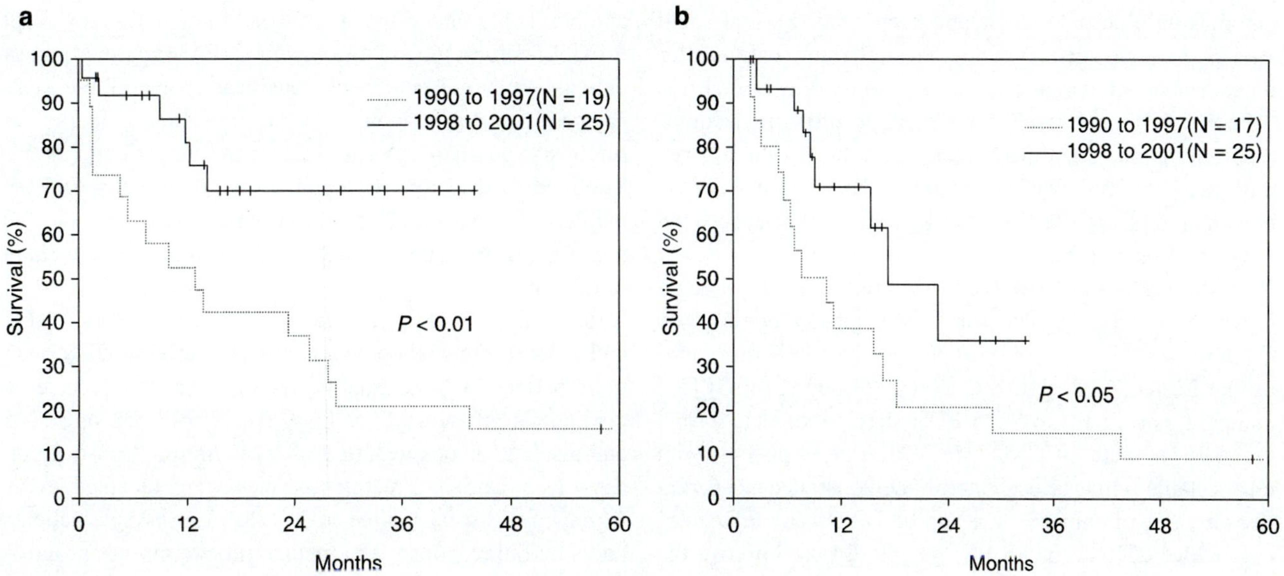

Fig. 31.2 (**a**) Actuarial survival for resected patients by time period (From Nakeeb et al. [2]). (**b**) Actuarial survival for patients treated with chemoradiation by time period (From Nakeeb et al. [2])

12-year period [2]. One hundred eleven (79 %) had cholangiocarcinomas, and 72 of these (65 %) were perihilar. Over the past 4 years of this analysis, improved staging, active biliary stenting and aggressive surgery led to improved survival ($P<0.01$, 70 % at 44 months) in resected patients (Fig. 31.2a). Chemoradiation with confocal radiation, 5-FU and gemcitabine was employed more frequently in the patients resected since 1998. In addition, this regimen of chemoradiation resulted in better survival ($P<0.05$) than a regimen with less sophisticated radiation and 5-FU alone which was used in the early 1990s (Fig. 31.2b).

In 2001–2002 a questionnaire was sent to members of the International Hepato-Pancreato-Biliary Association, the American Hepato-Pancreato-Biliary Association and the American College of Surgeons Oncology Group to assess current trends in adjuvant therapy for biliary malignancies [12]. Responses were received from 331 authorities at 262 centers in 39 countries worldwide. At that time, adjuvant chemoradiation is used at the majority of centers with this approach being employed most frequently in the Americas (71 %) followed by the Asia/Pacific region (55 %) and Europe (29 %) (Table 31.1). Interestingly, considerable

Table 31.1 International use of adjuvant radiation therapy, chemotherapy, and chemoradiation in biliary malignancies[a]

Treatment	Americas (%)	Asia/Pacific (%)	Europe (%)	Total (%)
Radiation therapy	70*	40	29	59
Chemotherapy	66	79	68	68
Chemoradiation	71*	55	29	63

[a]Adapted from Nakeeb et al. [20]
*$P<0.05$ versus other regions

Table 31.2 5-FU chemotherapy for unresectable perihilar cholangiocarcinoma[a]

Chemotherapy	N	Response rate (%)	Median survival
5-FU	12	9	6 months
5-FU, Cisplatin, Epirubicin	9	22	5 months
5-FU, Adriamycin, mitomycin C	14	29	11.5 months
5-FU, Methotrexate, Leukovorin, Cisplatin	10	30	4 months
5-FU, Interferon alpha	25	38	12 months
5-FU, Leukovorin, Mitomycin C	7	57	17 months

[a]Adapted from Todoroki [21]

enthusiasm (88 %) for a prospective randomised trial was expressed by the respondents. However, to date, a multi-institutional, multinational trial has not been performed.

31.4 Chemotherapy

Most early trials evaluating the efficacy of chemotherapeutic agents in cholangiocarcinoma represented small single institution phase II trials [20]. These trials often combined both gallbladder cancers and intrahepatic and distal cholangiocarcinomas with perihilar cholangiocarcinomas. Several small studies of single agent systemic chemotherapy regimens for unresectable cholangiocarcinoma using drugs such as 5-fluorouracil, methansulfon-m-anisidide, cisplatin, rifampicin, mitomycin C, and paclitaxel were reported. In general, these trials have shown little efficacy with partial response rates ranging from 0 % to 9 % and median survivals between 2 and 12 months [21].

In the 1980s and 1990s the most extensively investigated chemotherapeutic agent for cholangiocarcinoma was 5-fluorouracil (5-FU). An early prospective randomised trial by the Eastern Cooperative Oncology Group (ECOG) [22] comparing oral 5-FU to oral 5-FU + streptozotocin (Stz) and oral 5-FU + methyl-CCNU (MeCCNU) in 34 patients with unresectable cholangiocarcinoma demonstrated a partial response rate of only 9 %. The addition of either streptozotocin or MeCCNU to oral 5-FU therapy did not improve the response rate and was associated with a decrease in median survival from 26 weeks for 5-FU alone to 12 weeks for 5-FU+ Stz and 8 weeks for 5-FU+MeCCNU.

Because of the poor response rates with single agent 5-FU for cholangiocarcinoma, several authors have used combination chemotherapy in an attempt to achieve better response rates and longer survival (Table 31.2). Cholangiocarcinomas are believed to have a large percentage of hypoxic cells since they appear as hypovascular lesions on abdominal imaging and angiography. Therefore, Mitomycin C (MMC) had been proposed as a potential chemotherapeutic agent for cholangiocarcinoma because high levels of the drug can be achieved in bile and because it has a preferential toxicity in hypoxic cells.

In one study a regimen of intravenous bolus cisplatin (60 mg/m^2) and epirubicin (50 mg/m^2) on day one, and repeated every 3 weeks followed by 5-FU 200 mg/m^2/day given as a continuous 24 h infusion throughout the treatment course in nine patients with advanced extrahepatic cholangiocarcinoma (Table 31.2). Two patients (22 %) had a partial response with duration of response of 10 months, three patients (33 %) had stable disease, and four patients (44 %) had evidence of disease progression on therapy. The median survival was 5 months (range 3~13 months). In another study the efficacy of combination therapy with 5-FU, doxorubicin, and mitomycin C (FAM regimen) in 14 patients with unresectable cholangiocarcinoma (Table 31.2) showed a partial response (50 % or greater reduction in tumor size by imaging) was obtained in four patients (29 %). The median duration of response was 8.5 months, and the median survival was 11.5 months. An additional 6 (43 %) patients had evidence of disease stabilization for a median of 6.7 months.

Patt and colleagues [23] used systemic intravenous 5-FU and subcutaneous recombinant human interferon rIFN-α-2b in 25 patients with cholangiocarcinoma. Patients received a continuous infusion of 750 mg/m^2/d of 5-FU on days 1–5 and a subcutaneous injection of 5 MU/m^2 of rIFN-α-2b on days 1, 3, and 5. Treatment cycles were repeated every 14 days for 8 weeks. Nine of 24 (38 %) assessable patients had a partial response. The median time to disease progression was 9.5 months, and the median survival time 12 months. Unfortunately, none of the above regimens has been proven to enhance survival in patients with cholangiocarcinoma. The first phase III study of adjuvant chemotherapy compared 5-FU and mitomicin C to surgery alone in patients with biliary malignancies was published in 2002 [24]. In this multicenter Japanese trial, chemotherapy did not improve survival in patients with hilar or distal cholangiocarcinoma.

Over the past decade, however, several studies have demonstrated that gemcitabine [25–30], cisplatin [31, 32] and S-1 [11, 33, 34] all have activity against biliary malignancies. These observations have resulted in randomised phase II [35] and phase III [36] trials of gemcitabine alone versus gemcitabine plus cisplatin in patients with locally advanced or metastatic biliary cancer. In the phase II Advanced Biliary

Table 31.3 Gemcitabine plus cisplatin versus gemcitabine in advanced biliary cancers*

Variable	Gemcitabine plus cisplatin	Gemcitabine	P value
Patients	204	206	–
Metastatic	76 %	73 %	0.46
Resected	18 %	23 %	0.20
Palliative surgery	18 %	19 %	0.74
Biliary stenting	46 %	45 %	0.85
Overall survival	11.7 months	8.1 months	<0.001
Progression-free			
Survival	8.0 months	5.0 months	<0.001

*Adapted from Valle et al. [36]

Cancer (AISC-01) trial of 86 patients 6-month progression free survival increased from 48 % to 57 % when cisplatin was added to gemcitabine [35]. In the phase III ABC-02 trial, 410 patients were randomised [36]. The two groups were similar with respect to age, gender, extent of disease, performance status and extent of surgery as well as biliary stenting (Table 31.3). However, the patients who received gemcitabine plus cisplatin had increased overall and progression-free survival (Table 31.3). Adverse events were similar with the exception of neutropenia which was more common (25 vs. 17 %, $P<0.03$) in the gemcitabine plus cisplatin group. Thus, the combination of gemcitabine plus cisplatin is currently the chemotherapy regimen of choice for appropriate patients with hilar cholangiocarcinoma.

31.5 Summary

Despite significant advances in the surgical management of perihilar cholangiocarcinoma, the only chance for long-term survival remains complete resection with negative margins. Unfortunately, this goal is achievable in only a minority of patients. To date, radiation therapy alone has been disappointing in prolonging survival in these patients. While some studies suggest that adjuvant chemoradiation may be helpful, more studies are needed with gemcitabine as the primary chemotherapeutic agent. Both gemcitabine and cisplatin have been demonstrated in recent years to have activity against hilar cholangiocarcinomas. Moreover, a recent phase 3 trial suggests that the best results can be achieved with a combination of these two agents.

References

1. Nakeeb A, Pitt HA, Coleman J, et al. Cholangiocarcinoma: a spectrum of intrahepatic, perihilar, and distal tumors. Ann Surg. 1996; 224:463–75.
2. Nakeeb A, Tran KQ, Black MJ, et al. Improved survival in resected biliary malignancies. Surgery. 2002;132:555–64.
3. Tsao JI, Nimura Y, Kamija J, et al. Management of hilar cholangiocarcinoma: comparison of an American and Japanese experience. Ann Surg. 2000;232:166–74.
4. Jarnagin WR, Fong Y, DeMatteo RP, et al. Staging, resectability, and outcome in 225 patients with hilar cholangiocarcinoma. Ann Surg. 2001;234:507–17.
5. Sakamoto Y, Kosuge T, Shimada K, et al. Prognostic factors of surgical resection in middle and distal bile duct cancer: an analysis of 55 patients concerning the significance of ductal and radial margins. Surgery. 2005;37:396–402.
6. Woo SM, Ryu JK, Lee SH, et al. Recurrence and prognostic factors of ampullary carcinoma after radical resection: comparison with distal extrahepatic cholangiocarcinoma. Ann Surg Oncol. 2007;14: 3195–201.
7. DeOliveira ML, Cunningham SC, Cameron JL, et al. Cholangiocarcinoma: thirty-one year experience with 564 patients at a single institution. Ann Surg. 2007;245:755–62.
8. Igami T, Nishio H, Ebata T, et al. Surgical treatment of hilar cholangiocarcinoma in the "new era": the Nagoya University experience. J Hepatobiliary Pancreat Surg. 2010;17:449–54.
9. Hirano S, Kondo S, Tanaka E, et al. Outcome of surgical treatment of hilar cholangiocarcinoma: a special reference to postoperative morbidity and mortality. J Hepatobiliary Pancreat Surg. 2010;17: 455–62.
10. Lee SG, Song GW, Hwang S, et al. Surgical treatment of hilar cholangiocarcinoma in the new era: the Asian experience. J Hepatobiliary Pancreat Surg. 2010;17:476–89.
11. Unno M, Katayose Y, Rikiyama T, et al. Major hepatectomy for perihilar cholangiocarcinoma. J Hepatobiliary Pancreat Surg. 2010; 17:463–9.
12. Murakami Y, Uemura K, Sudo T, et al. Prognostic factors after surgical resection for intrahepatic, hilar and distal cholangiocarcinoma. Ann Surg Oncol. 2011;18:651–8.
13. Jarnagin WR, Ruo L, Little SA, et al. Patterns of initial disease recurrence after resection of gallbladder carcinoma and hilar cholangiocarcinoma: implications for adjuvant therapeutic strategies. Cancer. 2003;98:1689–700.
14. Todoroki T, Ohara K, Kawamoto T, et al. Benefits of adjuvant radiotherapy after radical resection of locally advanced main hepatic duct carcinoma. Int J Radiat Oncol Biol Phys. 2000;46:581–7.
15. Gerhards MF, van Gulik TM, Gonzalez Gonzalez D, et al. Results of postoperative radiotherapy for resectable hilar cholangiocarcinoma. World J Surg. 2003;27:173–9.
16. Sagawa N, Kondo S, Morikawa T, et al. Effectiveness of radiation therapy after surgery for hilar cholangiocarcinoma. Surg Today. 2005;35:548–52.
17. Pitt HA, Nakeeb A, Abrams RA, et al. Perihilar cholangiocarcinoma: postoperative radiotherapy does not improve survival. Ann Surg. 1995;221:788–97.
18. Serafini FM, Sachs D, Bloomston M, et al. Location, not staging, of cholangiocarcinoma determines the role for adjuvant chemoradiation therapy. Am Surg. 2001;67:839–44.
19. Kim S, Kim SW, Bang YJ, et al. Role of postoperative radiotherapy in the management of extrahepatic bile duct cancer. Int J Radiat Oncol Biol Phys. 2002;54:414–9.
20. Nakeeb A, Pitt HA. Radiation therapy, chemotherapy and chemoradiation in hilar cholangiocarcinoma. HPB. 2005;7:278–82.
21. Todoroki T. Chemotherapy for bile duct carcinoma in the light of adjuvant chemotherapy to surgery. Hepatogastroenterology. 2000; 47:644–9.
22. Falkson G, MacIntyre JM, Moertel CG. Eastern Cooperative Oncology Group experience with chemotherapy for inoperable gallbladder and bile duct cancer. Cancer. 1984;54:965–9.
23. Patt YZ, Jones Jr DV, Hoque A, et al. Phase II trial of intravenous flourouracil and subcutaneous interferon alfa-2b for biliary tract cancer. J Clin Oncol. 1996;14:2311–5.

24. Takada T, Amano H, Yasuda H, et al. Study group of surgical adjuvant therapy for carcinomas of the pancreas and biliary tract; is postoperative adjuvant chemotherapy useful for gallbladder carcinoma? A phase III multicenter prospective randomised controlled trial in patients with resected pancreaticobiliary carcinoma. Cancer. 2002;95:1685–95.
25. Patt YZ, Hassan MM, Aguayo A, et al. Oral capecitabine for the treatment of hepatocellular carcinoma, cholangiocarcinoma, and gallbladder carcinoma. Cancer. 2004;101:578–86.
26. Gebbia V, Giuliani F, Maiello E, et al. Treatment of inoperable and/or metastatic biliary tree carcinomas with single-agent gemcitabine or in combination with levofolinic acid and infusional fluorouracil: results of a multicenter phase II study. J Clin Oncol. 2001;19:4089–91.
27. André T, Tournigand C, Rosmorduc O, GERCOR Group, et al. Gemcitabine combined with oxaliplatin (GEMOX) in advanced biliary tract adenocarcinoma: a GERCOR study. Ann Oncol. 2004;15:1339–43.
28. Kornek GV, Schuell B, Laengle F, et al. Mitomycin C in combination with capecitabine or biweekly high-dose gemcitabine in patients with advanced biliary tract cancer: a randomised phase II trial. Ann Oncol. 2004;15:478–83.
29. Dingle BH, Rumble RB, Brouwers MC. The role of gemcitabine in the treatment of cholangiocarcinoma and gallbladder cancer: a systematic review. Can J Gastroenterol. 2005;19:711–6.
30. Murakami Y, Uemura K, Sudo T, et al. Gemcitabine-based adjuvant chemotherapy improves survival after aggressive surgery for hilar cholangiocarcinoma. J Gastrointest Surg. 2009;13:1470–9.
31. Rao S, Cunningham D, Hawkins RE, et al. Phase III study of 5FU, etoposide and leucovorin (FELV) compared to epirubicin, cisplatin and 5FU (ECF) in previously untreated patients with advanced biliary cancer. Br J Cancer. 2005;92:1650–4.
32. Ducreux M, Van Cutsem E, Van Laethem JL, et al. A randomised phase II trial of weekly high-dose 5-fluorouracil with and without folinic acid and cisplatin in patients with advanced biliary tract carcinoma: results of the 40955 EORTC trial. Eur J Cancer. 2005;41:398–403.
33. Ueno H, Okusaka T, Ikeda M, et al. Phase II study of S-1 in patients with advanced biliary tract cancer. Br J Cancer. 2004;91:1769–74.
34. Sasaki T, Isayama H, Nakai Y, et al. Multicenter, phase II study of gemcitabine and S-1 combination chemotherapy in patients with advanced biliary tract cancer. Cancer Chemother Pharmacol. 2010;65:1101–7.
35. Valle JW, Wasan H, Johnson P, et al. Gemcitabine alone or in combination with cisplatin in patients with advanced or metastatic cholangiocarcinomas or other biliary tract tumours: a multicentre randomised phase II study—the UK ABC-01 study. Br J Cancer. 2009;101:621–7.
36. Valle J, Wasan H, Palmer DH, et al. Cisplatin plus gemcitabine versus gemcitabine for biliary tract cancer. N Engl J Med. 2010;362(14):1273–81.

Index

A

Adjunctive measures, 171–173
Aminopyrine (dimethyl aminoantipyrine) test, 83
Anatomic basis/rationale, 213–214
Anatomic staging systems (Bismuth-Corlette), 43–45
Anesthesia, 155–164
Anomalies of the biliary system, 4
Anomalies of the portal venous system, 7
Arterial plexuses of the main bile duct wall, 13
Assessing resectability, 173–176

B

Benign lesions mimicking, 103–106
Biliary decompression, 162
Biliary drainage, effects of, 139–140
Biliary reconstruction after extended resections, 232
Biliary resection isolated *vs.* associated with hepatectomy, 255–260
Bioenergetic tests, 78–81
Bismuth–Corlette Type I, II and III tumors, central lobectomy, 219–220
Bismuth type I and II tumors
  local resection, 218–219
  major hepatectomy, 219
Bleeding: prevention and management, 160
Brush cytology and forceps biopsy, 95–96

C

Cahow's intrahepatic cholangiojejunostomy, 294
Central lobectomy, 211–220
Central lobectomy, outcomes of, 216–218
Chemoradiation, 319–320
Chemoradiation therapy (CRT), 282, 285–286
Chemotherapy (CT), 283–285, 320–321
Child-Pugh score, 76, 77
Cholangiocarcinoma
  risk factors, 18–22
  stage, 298–300
Chromosomal alteration, 121
Clearance tests, 81–82
Clinical course after PVE, 152
Clinical manifestations, 91–97
Clinical presentation, 26–37
Combined liver resection, 189–190
Complications, endoscopic approach, 300
Computed tomography (CT), 93–94
Conservative combined liver resection, 191–192
Curative surgery beyond liver resection, 190–191
Cytokeratin 19 (CK19), 120
Cytologic evaluation, 169–171

D

Developments in the advances in preoperative management, 190
Diagnosis, hilar cholangiocarcinoma, 91–97
Differences in drainage of distal and proximal bile duct tumors, 139–140
Differential diagnoses
  hilar cholangiocarcinoma, 99–106
  pathology, 39
Digitized image analysis (DIA), 96
Direct cholangiography, 55, 94–95
Distal cholangiocarcinoma, 303–304
Distal limit of bile duct resection line, 196–197
DNA hypermethylation, 96–97
Dynamic tests, 81–85

E

Early attempts of surgical treatment, 187–188
Embolization materials, 151–152
ENBD/ERCP/PTCD, efficacy of, 143–145
Endoscopic biliary drainage (ERCP), 140–141
Endoscopic nasobiliary drainage (ENBD), 143
Endoscopic ultrasonography-guided fine needle aspiration, 96
Endoscopy *vs.* percutaneous approach, 298–299
Epidemiology, 17–23
Epidermal growth factor receptor (EGFR) family ErbB-1 and ErbB-2, 116, 117
Ex situ ex vivo liver resection and autotransplantation, 191, 263–272
Ex situ ex vivo technique, variations, 267–268
Extended resections, 223–233

F

Feasibility and safety, 215–216
Fluorescence in situ hybridization (FISH), 96
Fluorodeoxyglucose-positron emission tomography (FDG-PET), 60
Fructose tolerance test, 83–84
Functional changes after PVE, 153
Fundamental principles of HCCa surgery, 195, 196
Future developments, 287

G

Galactose elimination capacity, 83
Glucose load: redox tolerance test, 83
Grading, 28
Gross appearance, cholangiocarcinoma, 26–27

H

Hepatectomy, local resection, 253–260
Hepatic arterial resection/reconstruction, 200–202

W.Y. Lau (ed.), *Hilar Cholangiocarcinoma*,
DOI 10.1007/978-94-007-6473-6, © Springer Science+Business Media Dordrecht and People's Medical Publishing House 2013

Hepatic artery
  reconstruction first approach, 247–250
  resection, 244–245
Hepatic hilar plate system, 15
Hepaticojejunostomy, 215, 216
Hepatobiliary uptake and excretion scintigraphy, 84
Hexose sugar metabolic capacity, 83–84
Hilar cholangiocarcinoma, 304–305
Histological changes after PVE, 153
History of photodynamic therapy, 309–310
History of surgery, 187–192
Homeostasis, 76–77

I

Image processing, 3D reconstructive, 66
Imaging
  findings, 60–61
  investigations, 92
  techniques, 54–60
  tools, advances, 65–66
Iminodiacetic acid, 84
Immunohistochemistry, 37–38
Impact of liver transplantation, 263–264
Indications for PVE, 148–149
Indications of laparoscopy, 128
Indocyanine green test, 81–82
Innervation of the biliary tract, 15
Intrabiliary therapies for palliation, 306
Intraluminal brachytherapy, 306
Intraoperative considerations, anesthesia, 157–160
Intraoperative techniques and decision-making, 176–177

L

Laparoscopic assisted surgery, 162–163
Laparoscopy and laparoscopic ultrasound, 127–131
Left hemihepatectomy
  with caudate lobectomy, 197, 199, 203–204
  extended, 229–231
Left hepatic duct, 292–293
  extrafascial, 292
Left trisectionectomy with caudate lobectomy, 201, 202, 206–207
Lidocaine and MEGX, 83
Ligamentum teres, segment III approach, 292–293
Limit of portal vein resection and reconstruction, 200–201
Liver and portal vein resection, 237–245
Liver function, assessment of, 75–88
Liver resection, 173–177, 212–213
  and liver transplantation, 167–182
  overall survival, 242–243
  volume, 198
Liver transplantation, 164, 177–181, 191, 213, 275–279
Liver tumors, 266–267
Local resection of hilar cholangiocarcinoma, 188
Local resection *versus* hepatic resection, 188–189
Longitudinal evaluation after hepatectomy, 85–87
Longmire procedure, 293–295
Long term results, extended resections, 233
Lymphadenectomy, 226–227
Lymphatic drainage of the extrahepatic biliary system, 14
Lymph node and nerve plexus dissection, 198–199

M

Magnetic resonance cholangiopancreatography (MRCP), 94
Magnetic resonance imaging (MRI), 55–60, 94
Magnetic resonance spectroscopy, 80–81
Major curative resection, 163–164
Malignant lesions mimicking, 101–103
Mayo protocol, 276–277
Microscopic appearances, 28–34
Microsomal capacity tests, 82–83
Model for end-stage liver disease (MELD), 77
Molecular carcinogenesis, 111–112
Molecular genetics, 38
Molecular markers, 111–123
  as target of therapy, 122
Multi-functional receptor Annexin A2 (ANXA2) in its ligand Tenascin, 118, 120, 121
Multi-row detector computed tomography (MDCT), 55

N

Navigation surgery, 72–73
Neoadjuvant/adjuvant therapy for liver resection and transplantation, 281–287
Neoadjuvant radiation therapy, complications, 277
Neoadjuvant treatment, 286–287
No touch resections, 243

O

Operative planning and simulation, 70
Orthotopic liver transplantation, 275–279
Outcomes ex situ ex vivo surgery, 268–271

P

Palliation by endoscopic approach, 297–300
Palliation, goals, 303
Palliative surgery, 191
Palliative surgical treatment, 291–295
Pathologic background, 254–260
Pathologic staging systems (AJCC, JSBS), 45–49
Pathology, cholangiocarcinoma, 25–39
P120 catenin and cadherin, 118, 119
Percutaneous palliation, 303–307
Percutaneous transhepatic biliary drainage (PTBD), 141–143, 305
Perioperative management, 207
Perioperative morbidity, 241–242
Perioperative mortality, 242
Peripheral blood redox state, 79
Peritoneal washings, 129–130
Photodynamic therapy (PDT), 282, 306, 309–314
  as palliative treatment, 312
  for recurrent tumor after resection or as neoadjuvant treatment, 314
Photosensitizers, 311–312
Plastic *versus* metal, 299–300
Populations at risk, 167
Portal pressure after PVE, 152
Portal vein
  embolization, 147–153
  reconstruction, 238
  resection, 244–245
Positron emission tomography (PET), 95
Postoperative complications and management, 232–233
Postoperative considerations, 160–161

Precursor lesions, 34
Preoperative biliary drainage, 133–134, 139–145
Preoperative clinical staging systems (Gazzaniga, Blumgart), 49–51
Preoperative considerations, 155–157, 223–227
Pre-operative evaluation, 238
  for anatomical variations, 66–68
  and staging, 61–62
Preoperative imaging, 53–62
Preoperative optimization of the liver for resection, 133–136
Preoperative portal vein embolization (PVE), 135
Preoperative staging, 197
  laparoscopy, 135–136
Prevailing pattern of the arterial blood supply, 7–15
Prevailing pattern of the portal venous system, 6–7
Prevailing patterns of the biliary system, 1–4
Principle of photodynamic therapy, 310–311
Prognostic and predictive factors, 39
Prognostic clinico-laboratory scoring, 77
Proto-oncogene K-ras mutation, 114, 118
Proximal limit of bile duct resection line, 195–196

Q
Quality of life benefits following endoscopic stenting, 300

R
Radiation and chemotherapy, 317–321
Radiation therapy (RT), 282, 283, 317–319
Radicality, 256
Radical resection and limits, 195–207
Radiological imaging and qualitative assessments, 77–78
Regenerative capacity: portal vein embolization, 84–85
Regional anesthesia and analgesia, 159–160
Remnant liver volume by 3D images, evaluation, 68–70
Resectability, assessment, 214
Resectional surgery, 202–203
Resection or transplantation, 181–182
Right hemihepatectomy
  with caudate lobectomy, 196, 199, 204–205
  extended, 227–229
Right hepatic duct, approach, 294–295
Right trisectionectomy with caudate lobectomy, 205–206
Right *vs.* left hepatectomy, 224–226
Right *vs.* left resections, 243–244

S
Screening and surveillance protocols, 177–179
Serological testing and imaging, 168–169
Serum tumor markers, 91–92, 121–123
Short-term outcomes, 255–256
Staging, 27–28
  laparoscopy, safety and complications, 129
  and selection of patients for transplant, 179–181
  systems, 43–51
Stents, technique, 297
Surgical anatomy of the hepatic hilum, 1–15
Surgical biliary bypass, 292–295
Surgical principle, central lobectomy, 214
Surgical technique
  biliary resection, 254
  hepatic artery reconstruction, 248–250
  liver resection, 238–241
Survival, local resection, 256–260

T
Technical aspects in ex situ ex vivo resection, 264–266
Technique of laparoscopy, 128–129
Technique of PVE, 149–151
3D reconstructive imaging, 65–73
Tissue adenine nucleotide and mitochondrial analysis, 79–80
Transhepatic approach, 151
Transileocolic venous approach, 149, 151
Tumor suppressor gene P53 mutation, 113–115
Tumor suppressor P16^{INK4A} alteration and methylation, 115–116
Types of PVE, 149

U
Ultrasonography, 54–55
Ultrasound, 92–93
Unilateral *versus* bilateral, 299
  drainage, 305–306
The University of California Los Angeles (UCLA) criteria and treatment protocol, 277–279

V
Variations in hepatic arterial blood supply, 8
Vascular endothelial growth factor (VEGF), 116
Venous drainage of the extrahepatic biliary system, 14
Volumetric Changes After PVE, 152

W
Widening the scope of endoscopy as a palliative tool, 300

Y
Yin-Yang negative-and positive-control hypothesis, 112–113